JOHNSON & EVERITT'S

Essential Reproduction

Martin H. Johnson

MA, PhD, FRCOG
Professor of Reproductive Sciences
Department of Physiology, Development and Neuroscience, University of Cambridge
Fellow of Christ's College, Cambridge
Honorary Academic Fellow of St Paul's College, Sydney, Australia

Sixth edition

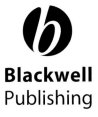

Blackwell
Publishing

First published 1980
Second edition 1984
Third edition 1988
Fourth edition 1995
Fifth edition 2000
Sixth edition 2007

1   2007

Library of Congress Cataloging-in-Publication Data

Johnson, M.H.
    Essential reproduction / Martin H. Johnson. – 6th ed.
    p. ; cm.
    includes bibliographical references and index.
    ISBN 978-1-4051-1866-8 (alk. paper)
    1. Mammals–Reproduction.   I. Title.
    [DNLM: 1. Reproduction–physiology.   2. Mammals—physiology.   WQ 205 J68e 2007]
    QL739.23.J64 2007
    573.6′19—dc22   2006036995

A catalogue record for this title is available from the British Library

Set in 9/12 pt Palatino by SNP Best-set Typesetter Ltd., Hong Kong
Printed and bound in Singapore by Markono Print Media Pte Ltd

Commissioning Editor: Vicki Noyes
Development Editor: Karen Moore
Production Controller: Debbie Wyer

For further information on Blackwell Publishing, visit our website:
http://www.blackwellpublishing.com

Contents

Preface to the Sixth Edition

There have been some spectacular advances in our understanding of the reproductive processes since the last edition. This progress has been due, in part, to the application to reproductive studies of the expanding range and sensitivity of the techniques of molecular biology, especially genomics, epigenetics and proteomics, as well as a much clearer understanding of the importance of systems biology in the integration of complex functions whether at cell, tissue, organism or social levels.

Four major heath issues place reproduction at the centre of scientific, clinical, political and ethical discourse. Continuing clinical developments in the field of assisted conception have expanded opportunities for the alleviation or circumvention of subfertility, genetic disability and, through stem cells, degenerative disease, but have also opened up new controversies. The threat posed by the human immunodeficiency virus continues to place reproduction and sexual behaviour high on the agenda of medical research, and is being accompanied by a rise in genitourinary infections in much of the world, with implications for future fecundity. The explosion of obesity and the realization that both child and adult health and well-being are affected enduringly by life *in utero* have focused work on pregnancy and the neonatal period of care. Finally, we are at last beginning to understand more fully how genetic expression interacts with environmental factors to influence complex behavioural phenotypes that include psychiatric disease and antisocial behaviour.

Two socio-legal changes have also been important influences on the science and medicine of reproduction. First, the changing roles of women and thus of men in developed societies has influenced thinking, research, social attitudes and legislation about sex and gender. A similar acknowledgement of the variety of sexual behaviour has also influenced attitudes to the types of research considered acceptable or important.

All chapters have been restructured, some of them substantially, to take these new developments into account. In places, more detailed information on deeper or applied aspects of some topics has been introduced in Boxes. In addition, requests for more specific references have hopefully been met better by longer reading lists divided into general and specific references. As before, many helpful comments, corrections and letters of advice have been received from readers, students and teachers all over the world. As always, in this sixth edition, I have tried to provide for students of reproduction a compact and comprehensive text that carves through the micro-detail of the subject to bring out its theoretical cores, but illustrates it with experiment, information and context.

It is sad that this sixth edition is also the first that has been prepared by myself alone. Barry Everitt, a long time friend and colleague, has been unable to co-author this volume due to changes of interest and the many work pressures in his life. I would like to thank him for the stimulation and friendship he has provided over the 27 years since the first edition of this book.

M.H.J.
Cambridge

How to Use this Book

This book represents an integrated approach to the study of reproduction. There can be few subjects that so obviously demand such an approach. During my teaching of reproduction at Cambridge University, the need for a book of this kind was clear to me and my colleagues. I know this volume goes some way towards filling this need because of the many appreciative comments I receive from colleagues at scientific meetings as well as from the Cambridge students.

I have written the book for medical, veterinary and science students of mammalian reproduction at all professional levels. Throughout, I have attempted to draw out the general, fundamental points common to reproductive events in all or most species. However, a great range of variation in the *details* of reproduction is observed amongst different species and, in some respects, very *fundamental* differences are also observed. Where the details differ, I have attempted to indicate this in the numerous tables and figures, rather than clutter the general emphasis and narrative of the text. Where the fundamentals differ, an explicit discussion is given in the text. These fundamental differences should not be ignored. For example, preclinical medical students may consider the control of luteal life in the pig, of parturition in the sheep or of ovarian cyclicity in the rat to be irrelevant to their future interests. However, as a result of extrapolation between species, in the past the human has been treated as a pig, a sheep and a rat (with much discomfort and detriment). If, on finishing this book, the student appreciates the dangers of uncritical extrapolations between species, I will have achieved a major aim.

Science is uncertain and provisional, and this provisionality has been illustrated in several places in this book. I have not tried to give a simple story where a simple story does not exist. Uncertainty can be hard to handle, especially in medicine, but it is a reality that is as important as those informational facts that we think we have certain knowledge of—indeed, knowing the boundary between the certain and the uncertain is perhaps the most important knowledge of all. For you students, this uncertainty also provides future research opportunities!

Confinements of space have unfortunately necessitated the omission of the subject of embryonic development from the text. To give only passing reference to this fascinating subject would be an injustice; to treat it fully would require a text of similar length to the present one. I recommend that the interested student seeks this information elsewhere.

I suggest that you first read through each chapter with only passing reference to tables, boxes and figures. In this way, I hope that you will grasp the essential fundamentals of the subject under discussion. Then re-read the chapter, referring extensively to the tables and figures and their legends, in which much detailed or comparative information is located. Finally, because my approach to reproduction is an integrated one, the book needs to be taken as a whole, as it is more than the sum of its constituent chapters.

Acknowledgements

I owe particular thanks to many people for help at many stages of the preparation of this edition: to present and former students for their interest, stimulation and responsiveness; to my colleagues at Blackwell Publishing for their help and advice; to John Bashford and his team in the Anatomy School at Cambridge for his advice and help with photographic illustrations; to the Histology section of the Department of Physiology, Development and Neuroscience, Cambridge for making available slides for photography; to Professor Peter Braude, Professor Graham Burton, Professor Tomas Hökfelt, J. Moeselaar, Dr Tony Plant, Dr J.M. Tanner and Dr Pauline Yahr for allowing me to use their original photographs and data; and to my many colleagues who read and criticized my drafts and encouraged me in the preparation of this edition, especially Jonathan Herring and Chi Wong.

CHAPTER 1

1 Sex

The reproduction of mammals involves sex. Sex is defined formally in biology as a process whereby a genetically novel individual is formed as a result of the mixing of genes from two or more individuals. So the essential feature of mammalian *sexual reproduction* is that the new individual receives its chromosomes in two equal portions: half carried in a *male gamete*, the *spermatozoon*, and half carried in a *female gamete*, the *oocyte*. These gametes come together at *fertilization* to form the genetically novel *zygote*. In order to reproduce itself subsequently, the individual must transmit only half its own chromosomes to the new zygotes of the next generation. In sexually reproducing species, therefore, a special population of *germ cells* is set aside. These cells undergo a *reduction division* known as *meiosis*, in which the chromosomal content of the germ cells is *reduced by half* and the genetic composition of each chromosome is modified as a result of the exchange of pieces of homologous chromosomes (Fig. 1.1). The increased genetic diversity that is generated within a sexually reproducing population may offer a richer and more varied source of material on which natural selection can operate. The population would therefore be expected to show greater resilience in the face of environmental challenge.

However, sex is not by any means an essential component of reproductive processes. Thus, *asexual* (or *vegetative*) reproduction occurs continuously within the tissues of our own bodies as individual cells grow, divide *mitotically* (Fig. 1.1) and generate two offspring that are genetically identical to each other and to their single parent. Many unicellular organisms reproduce themselves mitotically just like the individual cells of the body. Among multicellular organisms, including some complex vertebrates such as lizards, several reproduce themselves by setting aside a population of oocytes that can differentiate into embryos in the absence of a fertilizing spermatozoon to generate a complete new organism that is genetically identical or very similar to its parent. This asexual process of reproduction, often called *parthenogenetic* development, is simply not available to mammals. Although it is possible to stimulate a mammalian oocyte (including a human oocyte) in the complete absence of a spermatozoon, such that it undergoes the early processes of development and may even implant in the uterus, these parthenogenetic embryos always fail and die eventually. It seems that a complete set of chromosomes from a father and a complete set from a mother are an absolute requirement for normal and complete development to occur in mammals (see Chapter 9 for discussion as to why this is).

The consequences of obligatory sexual reproduction permeate all aspects of mammalian life. At the core of the process lies the creation and fusion of the two types of gamete. This occurs in mammals in two distinct types of

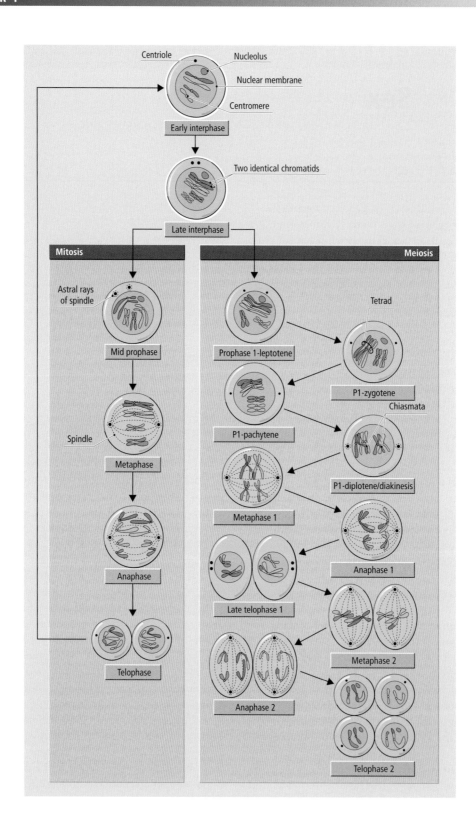

Fig. 1.1 Mitosis and meiosis in human cells. Each human cell contains 23 pairs of homologous chromosomes, making 46 chromosomes in total (see Fig. 1.2). Each set of 23 chromosomes is called a *haploid* set. When a cell has two complete sets, it is described as being *diploid*. In this figure, we show at the top a single schematized human cell with just 2 of the 23 homologous pairs of chromosomes illustrated, each being colour coded. Before division, the cell is in *interphase*, during which it grows and duplicates both its *centriole* and the DNA in each of its chromosomes. As a result, each chromosome consists of two identical *chromatids* joined at the *centromere*. Interphase chromosomes are not readily visible, being long, thin and decondensed (but are shown in this figure in a more condensed form for simplicity of representation).

In *mitotic prophase* (left-hand side), the two chromatids become distinctly visible under the light microscope as each shortens and thickens by a spiralling contraction; at the end of prophase the *nucleoli and nuclear membrane* break down. In *mitotic metaphase*, microtubules form a *mitotic spindle* between the two *centrioles* and the chromosomes lie on its *equator*. In *mitotic anaphase*, the centromere of each chromosome splits and the two chromatids in each chromosome each migrate to opposite poles of the spindle (*karyokinesis*). *Mitotic telophase* sees: the reformation of nuclear membranes and nucleoli; division of the cytoplasm into two daughters (known as *cytokinesis*); breakdown of the spindle; and decondensation of chromosomes so that they are no longer visible under the light microscope. Two genetically identical daughter cells now exist where one existed before. Mitosis is a non-sexual or vegetative form of reproduction.

Meiosis involves two sequential divisions (right-hand side). The *first meiotic prophase* (prophase 1) is lengthy and can be divided into several sequential steps: (1) *leptotene* chromosomes are long and thin; (2) during *zygotene*, homologous pairs of chromosomes from each haploid set come to lie side by side along parts of their length; (3) in *pachytene*, chromosomes start to thicken and shorten and become more closely associated in pairs along their entire length at which time *synapsis*, *crossing over* and *chromatid exchange* take place and nucleoli disappear; (4) in *diplotene* and *diakinesis*, chromosomes shorten further and show evidence of being closely linked to their homologue at the *chiasmata* where crossing over and the reciprocal exchange of DNA sequences has occurred, giving a looped or cross-shaped appearance. In *meiotic metaphase 1*, the nuclear membrane breaks down, and homologous pairs of chromosomes align on the equator of the spindle. In *meiotic anaphase 1*, homologous chromosomes move in opposite directions. In *meiotic telophase 1*, cytokinesis occurs; the nuclear membrane may re-form temporarily, although this does not always happen, yielding two daughter cells each with half the number of chromosomes (only one member of each homologous pair), but each chromosome consisting of two genetically unique chromatids (because of the crossing over at chiasmata). In the *second meiotic division*, these chromatids then separate much as in mitosis, to yield a total of four haploid offspring from the original cell, each one containing only one complete set of chromosomes. Due to chromatid exchange and the random segregation of homologous chromosomes, each haploid cell is genetically unique. At fertilization, two haploid cells will come together to yield a new diploid zygote.

individual, known as the two sexes: *male* and *female*. The gametes themselves take distinctive male or female forms (to prevent self-fertilization) and are made in distinctive male and female *gonads*: the *testis* and *ovary*, respectively. In addition, each gonad elaborates a distinctive group of hormones, notably the *sex steroid hormones*, which modify the tissues of the body to generate distinctive male and female somatic phenotypes suited to maturing and transporting their respective gametes. In most mammals, the sex steroids also affect the behaviour and physiology of the individuals of each sex to ensure that mating will only occur between different sexes at times of maximum fecundity. Finally, in mammals, not only do the steroids provide conditions to facilitate the creation of new individuals, they also prepare the female to carry the growing embryo for a prolonged period of *pregnancy* (*viviparity*), and to nurture it after birth through an extended period of *maternal lactation* and *parental care*.

Thus, the genetic mixing inherent in sexual reproduction has ramifying consequences for mammalian biology, shaping not just anatomy and physiology, but also aspects of behaviour and social structure. This ramification of sex throughout a whole range of biological and social aspects of mammalian life is mediated largely through the actions of the gonadal hormones. However, in humans and in other higher primates, social learning also plays an important role in generating sex differences. Children are taught how to behave as women or men, what is *feminine* and what is *masculine*. In this way they acquire a sense of their *gender*. Thus, although studies on mammals in general are relevant to humans, they are not in themselves sufficient. In order fully to understand human reproduction and sexuality, humans must be studied too. In this chapter, we examine how two sexes arise, differentiate and mature physically. In Chapter 2 we examine the related but distinct issues of gender development and sexuality.

The genesis of two sexes depends on genetic differences

The genetic determinant of sex is on the Y chromosome

In mammals, the genesis of two sexes has a genetic basis. Examination of human chromosomes reveals a consistent difference between the sexes in *karyotype* (or pattern of chromosomal morphologies). Thus, the human has 46 chromosomes, 22 pairs of *autosomes* and one pair of *sex chromosomes* (Fig. 1.2). Human females, and indeed all female mammals, are known as the *homogametic sex* because the sex chromosomes are both X chromosomes and all the gametes (oocytes) are similar to one another in that they each possess one X chromosome. Conversely, the male is termed the *heterogametic sex*, as his pair of sex chromosomes consists of one X and one Y, so producing two distinct populations of spermatozoa, one bearing an X and the other a Y chromosome (Fig. 1.2). Examination of a range of human patients with chromosomal abnormalities has shown that if a Y chromosome is present then the individual develops the male gonads (testes). If the Y chromosome is absent the female gonads develop (ovaries). The number of X chromosomes or autosomes present does not affect the primary determination of gonadal sex (Table 1.1). Similar

studies on a whole range of other mammals show that Y-chromosome activity alone is sufficient to determine gonadal sex. Thus the first step towards sexual dimorphism in mammals is the issuing of an instruction by the Y chromosome saying: 'make a testis'.

The Y chromosome itself is small. Moreover, most of its DNA is *heterochromatic* (that is, very condensed and incapable of synthesizing RNA). Therefore, the many structural genes required to make an organ as complex as the testis cannot be located on the Y chromosome alone. Indeed, these genes are known to lie on other autosomal chromosomes, and some even lie on the X chromosome. What the Y chromosome contains is a 'switching' or controller gene, which then somehow regulates the expression of all these other structural genes by determining whether and when they should become activated. The identity and location on

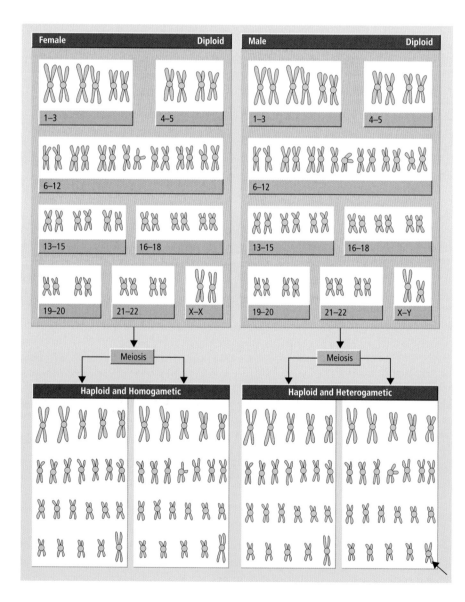

Fig. 1.2 Karyotypes of two mitotic human cells: one male and one female. Each cell was placed in colchicine, a drug that arrested them in mitotic metaphase when the chromosomes were condensed and clearly visible (see Fig. 1.1). The chromosomes were stained and then classified according to the so-called *'Denver' system*. The 44 *autosomes* (22 pairs of homologues) are grossly similar in size in each sex, but the pair of sex chromosomes are distinguishable by size, being XX (both large) in the female and XY (one large, one small) in the male. After meiotic division, all four female cells (only two shown) contain one X chromosome: the *homogametic sex*. In contrast, two of the male cells each contain an X chromosome and two contain a Y chromosome: the *heterogametic sex*. An arrow indicates the position of the *SRY* gene on the short arm of the human Y chromosome.

Table 1.1 Effect of human chromosome constitution on the development of the gonad.

Chromosomal number			
Autosomes	**Sex chromosomes**	**Gonad**	**Syndrome**
44	XO	Ovary	Turner's
44	XX	Ovary	Normal female
44	XXX	Ovary	Super female
44	XY	Testis	Normal male
44	XXY	Testis	Klinefelter's
44	XYY	Testis	Super male
66	XXX	Ovary	Triploids
66	XXY	Testis	(nonviable)
44	XX^{sxr}	Testis	Sex reversed*

*An X^{sxr} chromosome carries a small piece of Y chromosome translocated onto the X: see text.

the Y chromosome of this 'make a testis' gene was discovered initially by the study of some rare and atypical individuals.

Clinicians identified a few men with an XX sex chromosomal constitution and women with an XY chromosomal constitution—a situation called *sex reversal* At first sight, these sex-reversed people appear to contradict all that has been said above (see Table 1.1). However, careful examination of the DNA sequences on the short arm of the Y chromosome of many XY females has revealed either that short pieces of DNA are missing (*chromosomal deletions*) or that there are *mutations* of one or more nucleic acid bases. By comparing the DNA sequences in a large number of such patients, it is possible to find one region of the Y chromosome common to all of them that is affected by deletion or mutation. This region is a likely locus for a testis-determining gene. Supportive evidence comes from many of the XX males, who are found to have translocations of small pieces of the Y chromosome to one of their autosomes or X chromosomes. Again, the critical piece of Y chromosome that must be translocated to yield an XX male seems to come from the same region as is damaged in the XY females. This region contains a gene called *SRY* (in humans), which stands for 'sex-determining region of the Y gene'. The gene is located close to the end of the short arm of the human Y chromosome (see arrow in Fig. 1.2). Genes that code for a common sequence of 88 amino acids (the *Sry* box) have been found in other mammals, and are also associated with the development of a testis. In the mouse the gene is called *Sry* and also lies on the short arm but nearer to the centromere.

The identification of the mouse homologue was important, because it enabled a critical experimental test of the function of this region of the Y chromosome to be performed. Thus, a region of DNA containing only the *Sry* gene was excised from the Y chromosome and injected into the nuclei of one-cell XX mouse embryos. The excised material can integrate into the chromosomal material of the XX recipient mouse, which now has an extra piece of DNA. If this piece of DNA is functional in issuing the instruction 'make a testis', the XX mouse should develop as a male. This is what happened, strongly supporting the idea that the region containing the controller gene had been identified. This gene encodes a protein that binds DNA and localizes to the nucleus (Box 1.1). These features might be expected in a controller gene that influences other downstream genes. But when and where does *SRY* act to cause a testis to be generated?

The two gonads develop from a bipotential precursor plus three waves of ingressing cells

The early development of the gonad is indistinguishable in males and females. In both sexes the gonads are derived from common *somatic mesenchymal tissue* precursors called the *genital ridge primordia*. These primordia develop at about 3.5–4.5 weeks in human embryos, on either side of the central dorsal aorta, on the posterior wall of the lower thoracic and upper lumbar region (Fig. 1.3b,c). These two knots of mesenchyme form the basic matrices of the two gonads. Three waves of ingressing cells expand this matrix and do so in sex-specific ways to give the final forms of the ovary and testis.

One wave of migration consists of the gamete precursors called the *primordial germ cells* (PGCs). These are first identifiable in the human embryo at about 3 weeks in the epithelium of the yolk sac near the base of the developing allantois (Fig. 1.3a). By the 13–20-somite stage, the PGC population, expanded by mitosis, can be observed migrating to the connective tissue of the hind gut and from there into the gut mesentery (Fig. 1.3b). From about the 25-somite stage onwards, 30 days or so after fertilization, the majority of cells have passed into the region of the developing kidneys, and thence into the adjacent genital ridge primordia. This migration of PGCs is completed by 6 weeks and occurs primarily by amoeboid movement. The genital ridges may produce a chemotactic substance to attract the PGCs, as PGCs co-cultured in a dish with a genital ridge move towards it. Moreover, gonad primordial tissue grafted into abnormal sites within the embryo attracts germ cells to colonize it.

At about the same time as the PGCs are entering the genital ridges, a second group of cells also migrates in. These cells are derived from the columnar *coelomic* (or *germinal*) *epithelium* that overlies the genital ridge mesenchyme. They migrate in as columns called the *primitive sex cords* (Fig.

BOX 1.1 The molecular biology of SRY* action

There is uncertainty as to how SRY protein acts

In some mammals it binds DNA and localizes in the nucleus, which may suggest an action as a *conventional transcription factor* by binding to target gene promoter sites. However, few genes have been identified that it activates or represses directly in this way. It also has the property of opening up or remodelling chromatin (so-called *DNA bending*), thereby making genes accessible to conventional transcription factors, which has suggested a possible action as an *'architectural' transcription factor*. There is also some evidence that it can affect RNA stability and/or pre-RNA splicing.

Sry may not be quite the master gene that we first thought

Studies of naturally occurring or induced mutations in humans and mice have implicated a number of other genes in the 'make a testis' instruction. These include genes called *Sox9*, *Dax1* and *Wnt4*. Deletions or mutations of *Sox9* lead to XY human and mouse females, while deletions or mutations of *Dax1* and *Wnt4* lead to XX males. These findings have led to the suggestion that *Sox9* enhances and *Dax1* and *Wnt4* oppose Sry activity. In support of this idea, *Sox9* expression rises in males shortly after *Sry*, while *Dax1* and *Wnt4* expression decline in males over the same period of embryogenesis.

Interestingly, over-expression of *Sox9* in XX embryos leads to XX males and over-expression of *Dax1* and *Wnt4* in XY embryos to XY females. These dosage effects suggest that it may not be the absolute amount of Sry protein that is important for the instruction 'make a testis' so much as the ratio of Sry and/or Sox9 to Dax1 and/or Wnt4. In normal development, perhaps *Sry* expression promotes *Sox9* and depresses *Dax1* and *Wnt4* expression, but disturbances in the expression levels of these down-stream genes can override the original *Sry* push to 'make a testis'.

Finally, downstream of all these 'make a testis' genes there seem to be at least two 'confirm a testis' genes. One of these, encoding fibroblast growth factor 9 (*Fgf9*) is discussed in the main text; in embryos genetically lacking *Fgf9* genes, mesonephric cell invasion fails, myoid cells do not develop, the emergent seminiferous cords collapse and the gonad reorganizes as an XY ovary. The second gene is *prostaglandin D synthase* (*Ptgds*), which is produced by both pre-Sertoli and primordial germ cells and catalyses synthesis of prostaglandin D (PGD). Exogenous PGD can convert female gonads at least partially to XX male gonads, and endogenous PGD is thought to have a testicular reinforcement role in the developing testis.

Overall, the developing testis seems to use multiple genes in a 'belt and braces' approach triggered by *Sry* expression (the belt). However, this approach leaves testis development vulnerable to rare genetic mutations in the downstream 'braces' genes, which, helpfully, are also facilitating elucidation of the molecular web of male testis formation.

Advanced reading

Adams IR, McLaren A (2002) Sexually dimorphic development of mouse primordial germ cells: switching from oogenesis to spermatogenesis. *Development* **129**, 1155–1164 (prostaglandin D synthase).

Chaboissier M-C *et al.* (2004) Functional analysis of *Sox8* and *Sox9* during sex determination in the mouse. *Development* **131**, 1891–1901 (Sox 9).

Colvin JS *et al.* (2001).Male-to-female sex reversal in mice lacking fibroblast growth factor 9. *Cell* **104**, 875–889 (*Fgf9* mutants).

Grosschedl R *et al.* (1994) HMG domain proteins: architectural elements in the assembly of nucleoprotein structures. *Trends in Genetics* **10**, 94–100. (DNA bending properties of the Sry box).

Ohe K *et al.* (2002) A direct role of SRY and SOX proteins in pre-mRNA splicing. *Proceedings of the National Academy of Sciences of the USA* **99**, 1146–1151 (evidence about the molecular mechanism of action of Sry).

Swain A *et al.* (1998) *Dax1* antagonizes *Sry* action in mammalian sex determination. *Nature* **391**, 761–767.

Vainio S *et al.* (1999). Female development in mammals is regulated by *Wnt-4* signalling. *Nature* **397**, 405–409.

Vidal VPI *et al.* (2001) *Sox9* induces testis development in XX transgenic mice. *Nature Genetics* **28**, 216–217 (*Sox9* dosage effect).

*Gene/Protein notations

Throughout the book uses the following gene/protein notation (Sry as example):

Human genes/mRNAs – *SRY*; Human protein SRY.

Mouse genes/mRNAs – *Sry*; mouse protein Sry.

Where a generic statement about mammals is made, the mouse notation is used.

1.3d). The further development of these cells depends on whether the *Sry* gene is expressed or not. In the developing males, *Sry* expression is *restricted to the cells of the sex cords*. These cells proliferate vigorously and penetrate deep into the medullary mesenchyme, surrounding most of the PGCs to form *testis cords* (Fig. 1.4a). They will eventually become *Sertoli cells*, the main supporting cell for spermatogenesis. Because *Sry* expression is limited to the precursor Sertoli cells (*pre-Sertolic cells*), it has been suggested that the *Sry* gene actually issues the instruction: *'make a Sertoli cell'*. Now enclosed within the cords, the PGCs are known as *prospermatogonia* and will later give rise to spermatozoa.

In contrast, females lack *Sry* expression, and their sex cords are ill-defined and do not penetrate deeply into the ridge. Instead, the cells condense cortically as small clusters around the PGCs, now called *oogonia*. This clustering initiates formation of the *primordial ovarian follicles* (Fig. 1.4c,d). In these follicles the condensing cord cells will give rise to the *granulosa cells* of the primordial follicle, while the oogonia will give rise to *oocytes* (see Chapter 5).

The third wave of migratory cells comes from the mesonephric primordia, which lie just lateral to the genital ridges (Fig. 1.3c), and, like the sex cords, they show major sex differences. In the male, mesonephric cells are thought

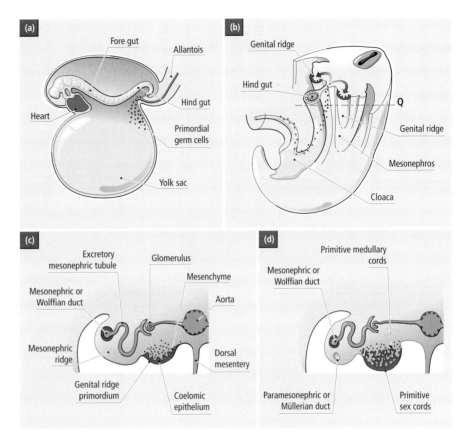

Fig. 1.3 A 3-week human embryo showing: (a) the origin of the primordial germ cells; and (b) the route of their migration. Section Q is the plane of transverse section through the lumbar region shown at 4 weeks in (c). In (d) the same plane of section is shown at 5 weeks of development: the 'indifferent gonad' stage.

to contribute at least three major cell types to the testis. Some cells contribute the vasculature tissue of the testis. Other cells synthesize steroid hormones and cluster between the cords to form *Leydig cells*—the main source of androgens. The third group of mesonephric cells condenses on the developing testis cords and stimulates formation of a basement membrane on which they then sit as *myoid cells*, thereby forming the *seminiferous cords*, the forerunners of the adult *seminiferous tubules* (Fig. 1.4b). The inward migration of this latter group of mesonephric cells giving rise to myoblasts is attributable to the chemotactic action of a growth factor called *fibroblast growth factor 9 (Fgf9)*, which is produced by the developing Sertoli cells. Should this migration fail (for example, in mice lacking *Fgf9* genes), the testis cords regress, emphasizing the important role of myoid cells in testis formation. The mesonephric tissue also forms the *rete blastema* or *rete testis cords*, later becoming the *rete testis*, which forms part of the male sperm-exporting duct system (Fig. 1.4a,b). In the female, no myoid cells migrate and the rete blastema is vestigial and transient, leaving only a vestigial *rete ovarii* in the adult (Fig. 1.4c,d). However, the mesonephric vascular and Leydig cell precursors in males may be paralleled in females by equivalent cells that will eventually form respectively blood vessels and condensations around the developing follicles called *thecal cells*.

With these three waves of inward migration completed, the basic patterns of testis and ovary are established. However, although the initial decision as to whether to make an ovary or a testis depends on the presence or absence of the *SRY* activity in developing Sertoli cells, subsequent development of the gonad, particularly of the ovary and its follicles, is dependent on the presence of a population of normal germ cells. For example, women suffering from *Turner's syndrome* (see Table 1.1), who have a normal autosomal complement but only one X chromosome, develop an ovary. Subsequently, however, normal oocyte growth requires the activity of both X chromosomes, and the activity of only one X in individuals with Turner's syndrome leads to death of the oocyte. Secondary loss of the follicle cells follows, leading to *ovarian dysgenesis* (abnormal development), and a highly regressed or *streak* ovary. Conversely, men with *Klinefelter's syndrome* (see Table 1.1) have a normal autosomal complement of chromosomes but three sex chromosomes, two X and one Y. Testes form normally in these individuals as a result of the expression of *SRY*. However, most of the germ cells die much later in life when they enter meiosis and their death is the result of the activity of two X chromosomes rather than one. These syndromes provide us with two important pieces of clinical evidence. First, *initiation* of gonad formation can occur when sex *cord cells* have only *one* Y (testis) or *one* X (ovary)

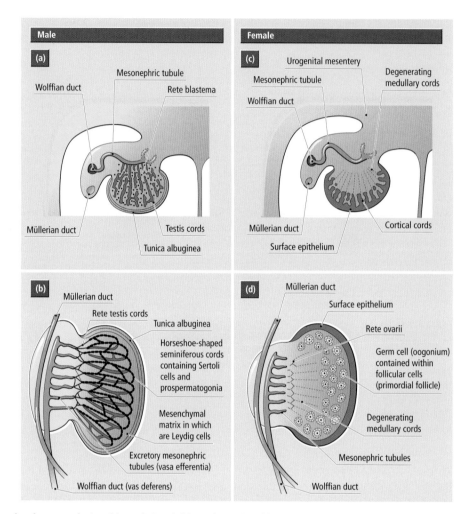

Fig. 1.4 Testicular development during (a) week 8 and (b) weeks 16–20 of human embryo-fetal life. (a) The *primitive sex cords* proliferate into the medulla, establish contact with the *mesonephric medullary cords* of the rete testis blastema and become separated from the coelomic epithelium by the *tunica albuginea* (fibrous connective tissue), which eventually forms the *testicular capsule*. (b) Note the horseshoe shape of the *seminiferous cords* and their continuity with the *rete testis cords*. The *vasa efferentia*, derived from the mesonephric tubules, connect the seminiferous cords with the *Wolffian duct*.

    Comparable diagrams of ovarian development around (c) week 7 and (d) the weeks 20–24 of development. (c) The primitive sex cords are less well organized and cortical, while medullary mesonephric cords are absent or degenerate. The cortical coelomic epithelial cells condense around the arriving primordial germ cells to yield *primordial follicles* shown in (d). In the absence of medullary cords and a true persistent *rete ovarii*, no communication is established with the mesonephric tubules. Hence, in the adult, oocytes are shed from the surface of the ovary, and are not transported by tubules to the oviduct (compare with the male, see Chapters 4 & 5).

chromosome. Second, *completion* of normal gonad development requires that the *germ* cells have *two X* chromosomes in an *ovary* but *do not have more than one X* chromosome in a *testis*.

Primary hermaphrodites have both ovarian and testicular tissues

We have established that *Sry* activity on the Y chromosome converts an indifferent gonad into a testis, whereas the absence of its activity results in an ovary. *Genetic maleness* leads to *gonadal maleness*. This primary step in sexual differentiation is remarkably efficient, and only rarely are individuals found to have both testicular *and* ovarian tissue. Such individuals are called *primary* (or *true*) *hermaphrodites* and arise in many cases because of the presence of a mixture of XY and XX (or XO) cells.

    The main role of the *Sry* gene in sexual determination is completed with the establishment of the fetal gonad, and the gene is no longer expressed in the fetus. From this point onwards, the gonads themselves assume the pivotal role in directing sexual differentiation both pre- and postnatally.

Again, it is the male gonad, like the Y chromosome before it, which plays the most active role, taking over the 'baton of masculinity' in this sexual relay.

The differentiation of two sexes depends on the endocrine activity of the fetal testis

Endocrine activity in the ovaries is *not* essential for sexual differentiation during fetal life. In contrast, the testes actively secrete two *essential* hormones. The interstitial cells of Leydig secrete steroid hormones, the *androgens*, and the Sertoli cells within the seminiferous cords secrete a dimeric glycoprotein hormone called *Müllerian inhibiting hormone* (MIH; also called MIS for Müllerian inhibiting substance and AMH for anti-Müllerian hormone). These hormones, which are discussed in more detail in Chapter 3, are the messengers of male sexual differentiation sent out by the testis. In their absence, female sexual differentiation occurs. Thus, sexual differentiation must be actively diverted along the male line, whereas differentiation along the female line again seems to reflect an inherent trend requiring no active intervention.

The male and female internal genitalia develop from different unipotential precursors through the actions of androgens and MIH

Examination of the primordia of the male and female *internal genitalia* (see Figs 1.4 & 1.5) shows that instead of one indifferent but bipotential primordium, as was the case for the gonad, there are two separate sets of primordia, each of which is *unipotential*. These are both located in the mesonephros adjacent to the developing gonad, and are called the *Wolffian* or *mesonephric* (male) and *Müllerian* or *paramesonephric* (female) ducts. In the female, the Wolffian ducts regress spontaneously and the Müllerian ducts persist and develop to give rise to the *oviducts, uterus* and *cervix* and *upper vagina* (Fig. 1.5). If a female fetus is *castrated* (its gonads removed), internal genitalia develop in a typical female pattern. This observation demonstrates that ovarian activity is not required for development of the female tract.

In the male, the two testicular hormones prevent this spontaneous development of female genitalia. Thus androgens, secreted in considerable amounts by the testis, actively maintain the Wolffian ducts, which develop into the *epididymis, vas deferens* and *seminal vesicles*. If androgen secretion by the testes should fail, or be blocked experimentally, then the Wolffian duct system regresses and these organs fail to develop. Conversely, exposure of female fetuses to androgens causes the development of male internal genitalia.

Testicular androgens have no influence on the Müllerian duct system, however, and its regression in males is under the control of the second testicular hormone, MIH. Thus, *in vitro* incubation of the primitive internal genitalia of female embryos with MIH provokes abnormal regression of the Müllerian ducts.

The male and female external genitalia develop from a single bipotential precursor through the actions of androgens

The primordia of the external genitalia, unlike those of the internal genitalia, are bipotential (Fig. 1.6). In the female, the *urethral folds* and *genital swellings* remain separate, thus forming the *labia minora* and *majora*, while the *genital tubercle* forms the *clitoris* (Fig. 1.6). If the ovary is removed, these changes still occur, indicating their independence of ovarian endocrine activity. In contrast, androgens secreted from the testes in the male cause the urethral folds to fuse (so enclosing the *urethral tube* and contributing, together with cells from the genital swelling, to the *shaft of the penis*); the genital swellings to fuse in the midline (so forming the *scrotum*); and the genital tubercle to expand (so forming the *glans penis*) (Fig. 1.6). Exposure of female fetuses to androgens will 'masculinize' their external genitalia, while castration, or suppression of endogenous androgens, in the male results in 'feminized' external genitalia.

Secondary hermaphrodites have genitalia that are not of the sex expected from their gonads

Failure of proper endocrine communication between the gonads and the internal and external genital primordia can lead to a dissociation of gonadal and genital sex. Such individuals are called *secondary* (or *pseudo*) *hermaphrodites*. For example, in the genetic syndrome of *androgen insensitivity syndrome* (*AIS*; also called *testicular feminization* or *Tfm*) the genotype is XY (male), and testes develop normally and secrete androgens and MIH. However, the fetal genitalia are genetically insensitive to the action of androgens (see detailed discussion in Chapter 3), which results in complete regression of the androgen-dependent Wolffian ducts and in the development of female external genitalia. Meanwhile, the MIH secreted from the testes exerts its action fully on the Müllerian ducts, which regress. Thus, this genetically male individual, bearing testes and having androgens circulating, nonetheless appears female with labia, a clitoris and a vagina, but totally lacks other components of the internal genitalia (Fig. 1.7a).

A naturally occurring counterpart to testicular feminization is the genetically based *adrenogenital syndrome* (*AGS*; also called *congenital adrenal hyperplasia* or *CAH*) in female fetuses, in which the XX female develops ovaries as usual. However, as a result of genetic defects in the corticosteroid synthesizing enzymes, the fetal adrenal glands become

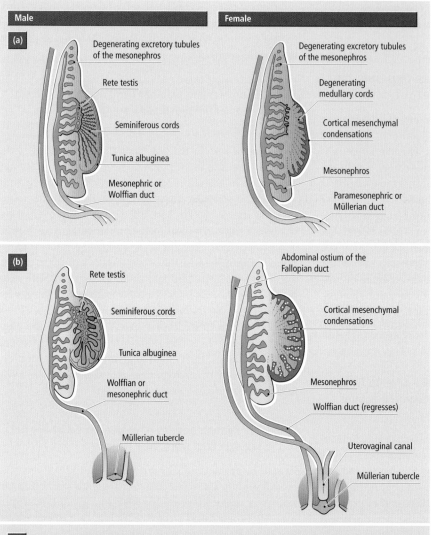

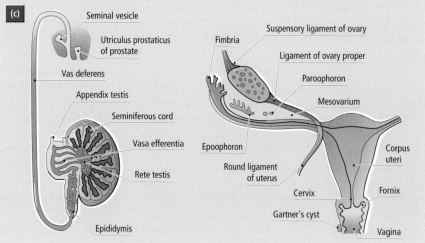

Fig. 1.5 Differentiation of the internal genitalia in the human male (left) and female (right) at: (a) week 6; (b) the fourth month; and (c) the time of descent of the testis and ovary. Note the *paramesonephric Müllerian* and *mesonephric Wolffian* ducts are present in both sexes early on, the former eventually regressing in the male and persisting in the female, and vice versa. The *appendix testis* and *utriculus prostaticus* in the male, and *epoophoron, paroophoron* and *Gartner's cyst* in the female are thought to be remnants of the degenerated Müllerian and Wolffian ducts, respectively.

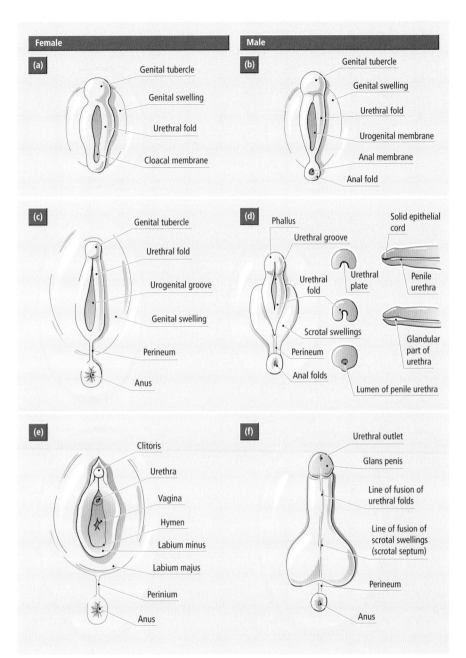

Fig. 1.6 Differentiation of the external genitalia in the human female (left) and male (right) from common primordia shown at: (a) 4 weeks; and (b) 6 weeks. (c) In the female, the *labia minora* form from the *urethral folds* and the *genital tubercle* elongates to form the *clitoris*. (d) Subsequent changes by the fifth month are more pronounced in the male, with enlargement of the genital tubercle to form the *glans penis* and fusion of the urethral folds to enclose the *urethral tube* and form the *shaft of the penis* (the genital swellings probably also contribute cells to the shaft). (e) The definitive external genitalia of the female at birth. (f) The definitive external genitalia of the male at birth.

hyperactive in an attempt to overcome the lack of corticosteroids, and secrete large quantities of precursor steroids, some with strong androgenic activity (see Chapter 3 for details of steroid biosynthetic pathways). These androgens stimulate development of the Wolffian ducts, and also cause the external genitalia to develop along the male pattern. The Müllerian system remains, as no MIH has been secreted. Thus, the individual appears partially or even wholly masculinized with a penis and scrotum, but is genetically and gonadally *female* and possesses the internal genitalia of *both* sexes (Fig. 1.7b).

Individuals with *persistent Müllerian duct syndrome* present as genetic males in whom either MIH production, or responsiveness to it, is inadequate. They therefore have testicular androgens that stimulate external genitalia and Wolffian ducts, but *retain* Müllerian duct structures. These men are thus genetically and gonadally *male* but possess the internal genitalia of *both* sexes.

Apart from the problems of immediate clinical management raised by diagnosis of these syndromes, abnormalities of development of the external genitalia may have important long-term consequences. The single, most

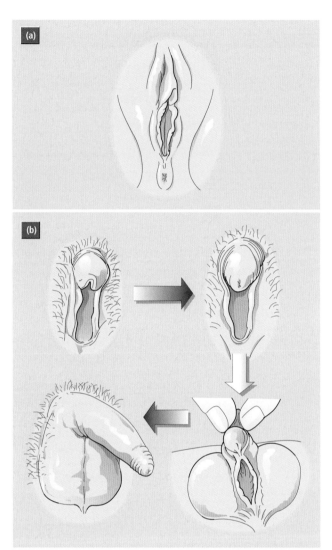

Fig. 1.7 (a) External genitalia of an XY adult with complete *androgen insensitivity syndrome (testicular feminization)*. Although an androgen-secreting testis is present internally, the external genitalia are indistinguishable from those of a female, and at birth the child would be classified as a girl (see Chapters 2 & 3 for more details). (b) The external genitalia from XX girls with *adrenogenital syndrome* show varying degrees of masculinization, from an enlarged clitoris to development of a small penis and (empty) scrotum. Ovaries are present internally. The adrenal cortex has inappropriately secreted androgens at the expense of glucocorticoids during fetal life and directed development of the genitalia along the male line. Clearly, the more severe cases could lead to sex assignment as a boy, or to indecision (see Chapter 2).

important event in the identification of sex of the newborn human is examination of the external genitalia. These may be unambiguously male or female, regardless of whether the genetic and gonadal constitutions correspond. They may also be ambiguous as a result of partial masculinization during fetal life. Sex assignment at birth is one important step that contributes to the development of an individual's *gender identity*, so uncertainty or error at this early stage can have major consequences for an individual's self-perception later in life as a man or a woman. This issue is discussed in more detail in Chapter 2.

Pre- and postnatal growth of the gonads is slow until puberty

We have seen how phenotypic features of the male and female develop. The female path of development is taken

unless there is intervention via genetic (*SRY*) and then endocrine (androgens and MIH) activities, when a male develops. During the remainder of prenatal life and during postnatal life up to puberty, further sexual divergence of physical phenotypes occurs only at a very slow pace and both internal and external genitalia remain immature, growing slowly in line with general body growth. In the male (but not the female) this process is dependent on low and variable levels of gonadal hormones. Despite the relative quiescence, some important reproductive changes do occur over this period.

The testes migrate to a scrotal position

The gonad develops in the upper lumbar region of the embryo, yet by adulthood in most mammalian species, including humans, the testes have *descended* through the abdominal cavity, and over the pelvic brim through an inguinal canal to arrive in the scrotum (Fig. 1.8). Evidence of this extraordinary migration is found in the nerve and blood supplies to the testis, which retain their lumbar origins and pass on an extended course through the abdomen to reach their target organ. The transabdominal descent of the testis towards the inguinal canal involves two ligamentous structures: at the superior pole of the testis is the *suspensory ligament* while inferiorly is the *gubernaculum*, which attaches the testis to the posterior abdominal wall (Fig. 1.8). As the fetal male body grows, the suspensory ligament elongates but the gubernaculum does not, and thus in the male the relative position of the testis becomes increasingly caudal or pelvic. Two hormones, both secreted by the developing Leydig cells, are responsible for these male-specific effects. Androgens act on the suspensory ligament, allowing its elongation, while *insulin-like growth factor 3* (Insl3) acts on the gubernaculum to mature and stabilize it.

Testicular migration in humans may be arrested developmentally at some point on the migratory route resulting

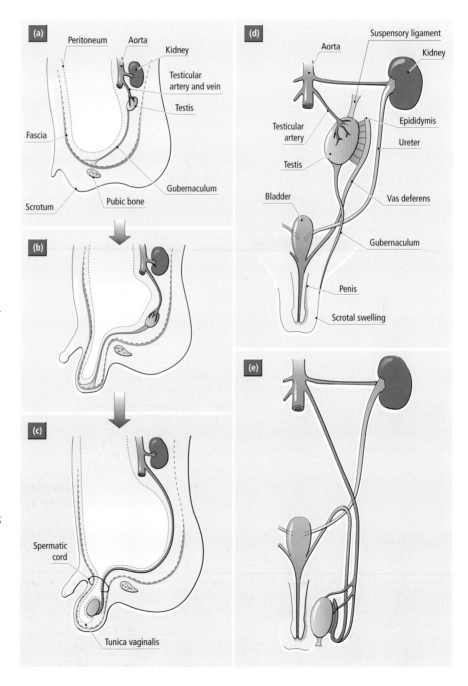

Fig. 1.8 (a–c) Parasagittal sections through a developing male abdomen. The initial retroperitoneal, abdominal position of the testis shifts pelvically between 10 and 15 weeks, extending the blood supply (and Wolffian duct derivatives, not shown) as the *gubernaculum* shortens and the *suspensory ligament* (d) (connecting the testis to the posterior abdominal wall) lengthens and regresses. A musculofascial layer evaginates into the scrotal swelling accompanied by peritoneal membrane, which forms the *processus vaginalis*. Between weeks 25 and 28 of pregnancy in the human, the testis migrates over the pubic bone behind the processus vaginalis (which wraps around it forming a double-layered sac), reaching the scrotum by weeks 35–40. The fascia and peritoneum become closely apposed above the testis, obliterating the peritoneal cavity leaving only a *tunica vaginalis* around the testis below. The fascial layers, obliterated stem of the processus vaginalis, vas deferens and testicular vessels and nerves form the *spermatic cord*. (d, e) Front view of the migration, showing the extended course ultimately taken by the testicular vessels and vas deferens.

in one or both testes being non-scrotal, a condition known as *cryptorchidism* (hidden gonad). The consequences of cryptorchidism in men demonstrate that a scrotal position is essential for normal testicular function. Although adult endocrine activity is not affected in any major way, spermatogenesis is arrested, testicular metabolism is abnormal and the risk of testicular tumours increases. These effects can be simulated by prolonged warming of the scrotal testis experimentally or by wearing thick tight underwear. The normal scrotal testis functions best at temperatures 4–7°C lower than abdominal 'core' temperature. Cooling of the testis is improved by *copious sweat glands in the scrotal skin* and by the blood circulatory arrangements in the scrotum. The *internal spermatic arterial* supply is coiled (or even forms a rete in marsupials) and passes through the *spermatic cord* in close association with the draining venous *pampiniform plexus*, which carries peripherally cooled venous blood (Fig. 1.9). Therefore, a heat exchange is possible, cooling the arterial and warming the venous blood (see also Box 1.2).

Testicular growth and activity are important for male development

By weeks 16–20 of human fetal life, the testis consists of an outer *fibrous tunica albuginea* enclosing vascularized stromal tissue, which contains condensed Leydig cells and solid seminiferous cords comprised of a basement membrane, Sertoli cells and prospermatogonial germ cells. These germ cells are quiescent and mitotic divisions are rarely observed.

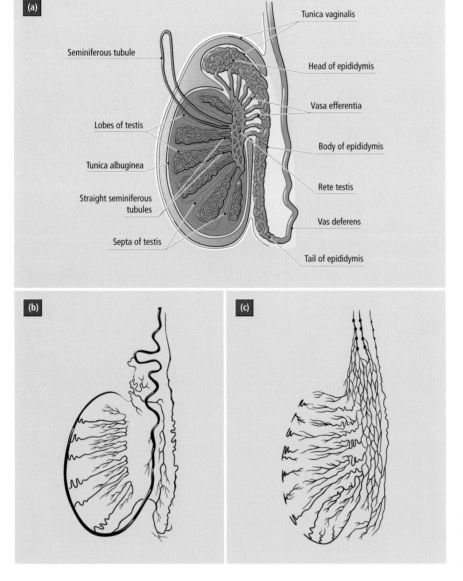

Fig. 1.9 Section through an adult human testis to show: (a) general structure; (b) arterial supply; and (c) venous drainage.

BOX 1.2 Evolutionary evidence of testis migration

Comparative biological study of the male testis provides evidence of 'evolutionary cryptorchidism'. Thus:
- in elephants, hyraxes and the monotremes (platypus and echidna), the testes normally do not descend at all from the lumbar site
- in armadillos, whales and dolphins, the testes migrate only part of the route to the rear of the lower abdomen
- in hedgehogs, moles and some seals, they lodge in the inguinal canal
- in most rodents and wild ungulates, they retain mobility in the adult, migrating in and out of the scrotum to and from inguinal or abdominal retreats.

In animals, such as humans, that have scrotal testes, a null mutation of the *Insl3* gene results in no Insl3 expression and failure of gubernacular maturation and testicular descent. It would be interesting to look at *Insl3* gene expression in the above non-scrotal species!

The human scrotal testis clearly *requires* a lower ambient temperature for normal function, but this requirement may be a secondary *consequence* of its scrotal position rather than the original evolutionary *cause* of its migration. Thus, those species in which testes remain in the abdomen survive, flourish and reproduce despite the high testicular temperature. It remains unclear as to why testes are scrotal in so many species, given their greater physical vulnerability!

Advanced reading

Nef S, Prada LF (1999) Cryptorchidism in mice mutant for *Insl3*. *Nature Genetics* **22**, 295–299.

Zimmermann S *et al.* (1999) Targeted disruption of the *Insl3* gene causes bilateral cryptorchidism. *Molecular Endocrinology* **13**, 681–691.

The seminiferous cords connect to the cords of the *rete testis*, the *vasa efferentia* and thereby to the *epididymis*.

The Leydig cells in the human testis actively secrete testosterone from at least weeks 8–10 of fetal life onwards, with blood levels peaking at 2 ng/ml at around weeks 13–15. Thereafter, blood levels decline and plateau by 5–6 months at a level of 0.8 ng/ml. This transient *prenatal peak* of blood testosterone is a feature of many species, although in some, for example the rat and sheep, the peak may approach, or span, the period of parturition, and only begin its decline postnatally. The males of some primate species, including humans, show a *postnatal peak* in plasma testosterone, concentrations reaching 2–3 ng/ml by 3 months postpartum, but declining to around 0.5 ng/ml by 3–4 months. A second modest infantile rise in androgens occurs at 1 year and extends to puberty, when a prepubertal peak in androgen output occurs, reaching levels of about 9 ng/ml. The capacity to secrete testosterone is, as we have seen, essential for establishment of the male phenotype. It is also important for the continuing development of the male phenotype and, in many if not all species, can also influence the development of masculine behaviour patterns (see Chapter 2). The Sertoli cells continue to produce MIH throughout fetal life up until puberty, when levels drop sharply.

Throughout fetal and early postnatal life, testis size increases slowly but steadily. The prospermatogonial germ cells undergo only limited mitotic proliferation and contribute little to this growth. At puberty there is a sudden increase in testicular size to which all parts of the testis contribute: the solid seminiferous cords canalize to give rise to tubules; the intratubular Sertoli cells increase in size and activity; the germ cells resume mitotic activity and begin the process of spermatozoal formation; and endocrine secretion by the intertubular Leydig cells increases sharply. These changes herald the onset of sexual maturity and the development of fertility. The causes and consequences of this sudden growth at puberty will be discussed in detail in Chapter 7. The details of how the mature testis functions are described in Chapter 4.

Most ovarian germ cells die before puberty and all of them enter meiosis

The ovary, unlike the testis, retains its position within the abdominal cavity, shifting slightly in some species, such as the human, to assume a pelvic location. It is attached to the posterior abdominal wall by the *ovarian mesentery* or *mesovarium*. The ovary, like the testis, grows slowly but steadily in size during early life. As in the testis, little of this growth is due to the germ cells themselves. However, quite unlike the situation in the testis, the ovarian germ cells undergo three major changes.

- First, whereas in the male the prospermatogonial germ cells remain in a mitotic cell cycle, albeit rarely dividing, in the female *all the oogonial germ cells cease dividing mitotically* either before birth (human, cow, sheep, goat, mouse), or shortly thereafter (rat, pig, cat, rabbit, hamster), to *enter into their first meiotic division*, thereby becoming *primary oocytes*. The termination of mitosis and entry into meiosis seems to be programmed into all PGCs, since even XY-bearing PGCs enter meiosis spontaneously when cultured in female genital ridges or within the extragonadal parts of the male embryo itself should they have gone astray and not reached the male genital ridge. It seems that the Sry-driven enclosure of the XY germ cells within the seminiferous cords *suppresses meiotic onset* and maintains the PGCs as mitotic cells. There is a major consequence for women of this early termination of mitosis in that by the time of birth *a woman has all the oocytes within her ovaries that she will ever have*. If these oocytes are lost, for example by exposure to X-irradiation, they cannot be replaced from stem cells and the woman will be infertile. This situation is distinctly different from that in the male in which the mitotic proliferation of spermatogonial stem cells continues throughout adult reproductive life (see Chapter 4).

• Second, having entered meiosis so prematurely, the germ cells, as described earlier, form primordial follicles as a result of the condensation of surrounding granulosa cells derived from invading sex cords (Fig. 1.4c). The formation of the primordial follicles precipitates the second major change. The oocytes abruptly arrest their progress through first meiotic prophase at *diplotene*, their chromosomes still enclosed within a nuclear membrane called the *germinal vesicle* (Fig. 1.10b; see also Fig. 1.1 for details of meiosis). The oocyte halted at this point in meiosis is said to be at

the *dictyate stage* (also called *dictyotene*). The primordial follicle may stay in this arrested meiotic state for up to 50 years in women, with the oocyte metabolically ticking over and waiting for a signal to resume development. The reason for storing oocytes in this extraordinary protracted meiotic prophase is unknown. Although a few follicles may resume development sporadically and incompletely during fetal and neonatal life, regular recruitment of primordial follicles into a pool of growing follicles occurs first at puberty.

• The third remarkable feature occurring over this prepubertal period is the death of most of the meiotically arrested oocytes at or around the time of birth, depending on the species (Fig. 1.11). The cause of death is unknown and the reasons for it are unclear. The consequence of it is that

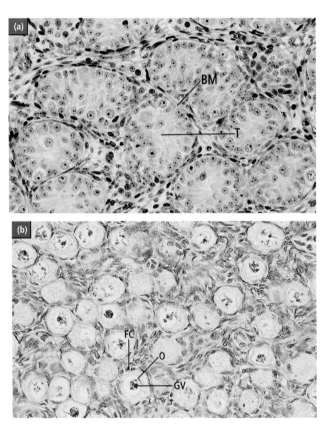

Fig. 1.10 Sections through immature (a) testis and (b) ovary, both at the same magnification. Note in (a) that each tubule is surrounded by a basement membrane (BM) and within the tubule there is no lumen (T) and a relatively homogeneous-looking set of cells comprising a very few spermatogonial stem cells and mostly Sertoli cells as seen here. Note in (b) that each oocyte (O) is relatively large and contains within it a distinctive nucleus (the germinal vesicle, GV). The ooctye is surrounded by a thin layer of follicle granulosa cells (FC) to form the primordial follicle.

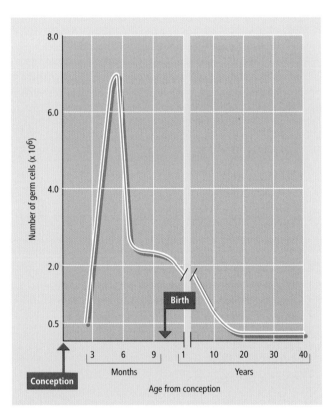

Fig. 1.11 Numbers of ovarian germ cells during the life of a human female. After an initial period of migration, mitotic proliferation commences at around days 25–30. The first meiotic prophases can be detected at around days 50–60, and the first diplotene-stage chromosomes at around day 100. All germ cells are at the *dictyate stage* by birth. *Atresia* of oocytes in the meiotic prophase is first obvious by about days 100, and continues throughout fetal and neonatal life. The period from entry of first germ cells into meiosis to full attainment of the dictyate stage by all germ cells varies between species, being in days after conception (date of birth in brackets): sow 40–150 (114); ewe 52–110 (150); cow 80–170 (280); rat 17.5–27 (22).

the stock of female germ cells available for use in adult life is reduced even further.

The ovary is not essential for prepubertal development

Over the prepubertal period the output of steroids by the ovary is minimal and, indeed, removal of the ovary does not affect prepubertal development. In some species, including humans, there may be a transitory stimulation of ovarian endocrine activity spanning the period of birth, but this does not appear to be important for female development. However, at puberty marked changes in both the structure and endocrine activity of the ovary occur, and for the first time the ovary becomes an essential and positive feminizing influence on the developing individual. How it does so is discussed further in Chapters 5, 7 and 8.

Summary

In this chapter we have seen that sexual differentiation is an enduring process of divergence, which begins with the expression of a genetic message that establishes the structure and nature of the fetal gonad, and then extends from the gonad via its hormonal secretions to many tissues of the body. Thus, sex may be defined at several levels and by several parameters. Concordance at all levels may be incomplete, and the medical, social and legal consequences of this 'blurring' of a clear, discrete sexual boundary may pose problems. However, in this chapter we have been able to define, by a broad set of criteria, how the two sexes are established. In the next chapter, we examine the issues of gender and sexuality and how they are related to the establishment of the two sexes.

KEY LEARNING POINTS

- Sexual reproduction in mammals involves the creation of a genetically novel individual by the contribution of equal numbers of chromosomes from two parents of different sexes.

- Sexual reproduction requires the production of male and female gametes (spermatozoa and oocytes) by the process of meiosis during which the chromosome number of somatic cells is halved and genetic recombination occurs.

- The male and female gametes are made in male and female gonads (testis and ovary) in male and female individuals (men and women).

- Males and females are distinguished simply by the presence or absence of a Y chromosome.

- A single gene called *Sry* on the Y chromosome acts by issuing the instruction 'make a testis'.

- The developing gonad arises from a unipotential genital primordium of mesenchymal tissue and three invading cell populations: the primordial germ cells, the germinal epithelial cells, and mesonephric cells.

- Sertoli cell precursors in the testis derive from the male germinal epithelial cells and are the sole site of *Sry* expression: so 'make a testis' may be expressed as 'make a Sertoli cell'.

- The granulosa cells of the follicle derive from the female germinal epithelial cells.

- Mesonephric-derived myoid cells migrate into the male genital ridge under the influence of fibroblastic growth factor 9 and are essential for stabilizing testis tubule development.

- Leydig cells in the male and thecal cells in the female are also derived from ingressing mesonephric cells, as are the vascular cells of the gonads.

- The embryonic testis makes two main hormones (androgens in Leydig cells and Müllerian inhibiting hormone, MIH, in Sertoli cells).

- The androgens stimulate the Wolffian ducts to make the epididymis, vas deferens and prostate.

- MIH causes the Müllerian ducts to regress.

- In the absence of MIH, the Müllerian duct becomes the oviduct, uterus, cervix and upper vagina.

- Common bipotential precursors of the external genitalia are stimulated to become the scrotum and penis by the testicular androgens, but become the labia and clitoris in the absence of androgens.

- The ovary is not required for the development of the prepubertal female, but the testis is required for the development of the prepubertal male.

- A sex reversed individual has an XX testis or an XY ovary.

- A primary hermaphrodite has both ovarian and testicular tissue.

- A secondary hermaphrodite has internal and/or external genitalia at variance with the sex of their gonads.

- In the fetal/neonatal ovary, the germ cells enter meiosis and then arrest in prophase of first meiosis at the germinal vesicle stage.

- Most female germ cells die around the time of birth.

- The testes migrate caudally under the combined influence of androgens and insulin-like growth factor 3 (Insl3), and, in most male mammals, assume a scrotal position.

FURTHER READING

General reading

Brennan J, Capel B (2004) One tissue, two fates: molecular genetic events that underlie testis versus ovary development. *Nature Reviews in Genetics* **5**, 509–521.

Capel B (2000) The battle of the sexes. *Mechanisms in Development* **92**, 89–103.

Carrillo AA, Berkovitz GD (2004) Genetic mechanisms that regulate testis determination. *Reviews in Endocrine and Metabolic Disorders* 5, 77–82.

Crow JF (1994) Advantages of sexual reproduction. *Developmental Genetics* **15**, 205–213.

Josso N (1994) Anti-Müllerian hormone: a masculinizing relative of TGF-β. *Oxford Reviews of Reproductive Biology* **16**, 139–164.

Ostrer H (2001) Identifying genes for male sex determination in humans. *Journal of Experimental Zoology* **290**, 567–573 (a general review of strategies for identifying genes of interest).

Ostrer H (2001) Sex determination: lessons from families and embryos. *Clinical Genetics* **59**, 207–215 (a human-focused review on genetics of sex determination).

Ramkisson Y, Goodfellow PN (1996) Early steps in mammalian sex determination. *Current Opinions in Genetics & Development* **6**, 316–321.

Schafer AJ, Goodfellow PN (1996) Sex determination in humans. *BioEssays* **18**, 955–963.

Sutton KA (2000) Molecular mechanisms involved in the differentiation of spermatogenic stem cells. *Reviews of Reproduction* **5**, 93–98.

More advanced reading (see also Boxes)

Albrecht KH, Eicher EM (2001) Evidence that *Sry* is expressed in pre-Sertoli cells, and Sertoli cells and granulosa cells have a common precursor. *Developmental Biology* **240**, 92–107.

Berta P *et al.* (1990) Genetic evidence equating *Sry* and the testis-determining factor. *Nature* **348**, 448–450 (an early mutation study confirming role of *Sry* in testis formation).

Jeans A *et al.* (2005) Evaluation of candidate markers for the peritubular myoid cell lineage in the developing mouse testis. *Reproduction* **130**, 509–516.

Koopman P *et al.* (1990) Expression of a candidate sex-determining gene during mouse testis differentiation. *Nature* **348**, 450–452 (the original mouse evidence supporting *Sry* identification as testis-determining gene).

Koopman P *et al.* (1991) Male development of chromosomally female mice transgenic for *Sry*. *Nature* **351**, 117–121 (the transgenic experiment).

Lovell-Badge R, Robertson E (1990) XY female mice resulting from a heritable mutation in the murine primary testis determining gene, *Tdy*. *Development* **109**, 635–646 (an early mutation study confirming role of *Sry* in testis formation).

McLaren A (2000) Germ and somatic cell lineages in the developing gonad. *Molecular and Cellular Endocrinology* **163**, 3–9.

Sinclair AH *et al.* (1990) A gene from the human sex-determining region encodes a protein with homology to a conserved DNA-binding motif. *Nature* **346**, 240–244 (the original paper describing *SRY* as the testis-determining gene).

2 Gender and Sexuality

In Chapter 1, sex was defined in biological terms as the creation of a genetically unique individual as a result of the equal contribution of chromosomes from two parents: hence, two types of gamete (oocytes and spermatozoa) are produced from two types of gonad (ovary and testis) in two types of individual (female and male). What then is gender, how does it relate to sex, and where does sexuality fit in to all of this? This chapter examines these questions. At the outset, it must be emphasized that there exists considerable variation in the ways that these terms are used. The discussion that follows attempts to clarify the issues, explain common usage and provide a consistent framework through which to consider gender and sexuality.

Gender is a system of classification based on sex

The features by which the two sexes were described and differentiated in Chapter 1 included their chromosomes, genes, gonads, gametes, hormones and anatomical structures (upper part of Table 2.1), and we explored the developmental relationships between them. There is an assumption, broadly universal across cultures and history, that the identification of one of these features as male or female could reasonably be expected to predict that all the other features would also be concordantly male or female. Thus, the presence or absence of a penis at birth is taken generally as diagnostic of males or females, respectively. Of course, as described in Chapter 1, discordances can and do exist, and we now understand more of the nature and origin of many of them. Estimates of the incidence of ambiguous external genitalia are understandably problematic, but figures of 0.1–0.2% of babies with major ambiguity and 1–2% with less severe ambiguity have been suggested (Box 2.1). Although small in percentage terms, this amounts to a large number of intersex individuals. The traditional approach to genital ambiguity in Americo-European cultures has been to intervene as early in childhood as possible to remove or reduce ambiguity and assign a clear anatomical and thus social sex to the baby. An intersex state was not considered acceptable. However, other cultures have taken a different approach, and accepted intersex individuals for who they are, often according them a special social status as a distinctive 'third sex', for example, the hijra in India or the berdache among some North American indigenous peoples. A move towards a more flexible approach to the clinical management of genital ambiguity has recently occurred in Americo-European society, in part through pressure from people who were assigned a 'sex' medically, and in their view inappropriately, as babies (see later).

The bipolar biological classification of individuals as either men or women is paralleled by a bipolar allocation of many other traits, some of which are summarized in the lower part of Table 2.1 as *gender attributes*. Unlike the features characterizing sex, these attributes are based more on attitudes, expectations, behaviour and roles; some of them may appear contentious or less absolute; many are complex; and many vary in detail or substance with different cultures or, within a culture, over historical time. In the table, these attributes have been grouped under the broad heading of gender because they are associated with sex, but not obviously, invariably or simply so. Moreover, any causal relationships between those features listed under sex and those attributes listed under gender are not always immediately obvious. It is for this reason that gender is defined

here as a system of classification *based on* sex. In order to distinguish sex from gender, we reserve the terms *male* and *female* to describe sexual features and the words *masculine* and *feminine* to describe gender attributes. The nature of the relationship between sex features and gender attributes forms the substance of this chapter. First, we will examine in a little more detail some of the gender differences summarized in Table 2.1. Then we will explore the basis of gender differences in behaviour since, collectively, these will influence social interactions and thereby the socially based gender attributes. Lastly we will examine the reproductive and sexual attributes of gender and explore their interrelationship with sexuality.

Gender stereotypes and gender identities

Two quite complex concepts need to be grasped for a sound understanding of gender.

A gender stereotype is the set of beliefs about what it means to be a man or a woman in a particular society

The gender attributes listed in Table 2.1 constitute the elements of *gender stereotypes*. Gender stereotypes provide a

Table 2.1 Sex and gender: oppositional descriptions.

Sexual features	Male	Female
Chromosome	Y present	Y absent
Gene	*SRY* active in Sertoli cell	*SRY* inactive
Gonad	Testis	Ovary
Gamete	Spermatozoon	Oocyte
Hormone	Androgens, MIH	No androgens or MIH
External phenotype	Penis, scrotum	Clitoris, labia
Internal phenotype	Vas deferens, prostate, etc.	Oviduct, uterus, vagina

Gender attributes	Masculine	Feminine
Inter-/intra-gender interaction patterns	Pre- and proscribed contact and relational patterns	Distinctive patterns
Social role	Public, extrovert, in the workplace, powerful, independent, forceful, outspoken	Private, domestic, powerless, quiet, care provider
Reproductive role	Disposable and transitory	Essential and enduring
Sexual role	Active, insertive, dominant	Passive, receptive, submissive
Work role	Rule setting and enforcing, leadership, military, ritualistic and priesthood, artistic	Constructive, agricultural, food preparation, domestic, creative, nurturant
Appearance	Characteristic and uniform hairstyle, body decoration, clothes, ornamentation	Characteristic and varying hairstyle, body decoration, clothes, ornamentation
Temperament and emotion	Competitive, combative, aggressive, ambitious, not expressive of vulnerable emotions	Cooperative, consensual, expressive, empathic, affectionate, emotionally free
Intellect and skills	Better mathematical and spatial skills, systematizing	Better linguistic skills, people oriented
Language used	Words reserved for use by men	Words reserved for use by women

BOX 2.1 How frequently is concordance for chromosomal, gonadal and genital sex absent?

Cause	Estimated frequency/ 1000 live births
Non-XX females or non-XY males	1.93
Complete or partial androgen insensitivity	0.08
Congenital adrenal hyperplasia	15.08
True hermaphrodites	0.01
Vaginal agenesis	0.17

In the UK, the birth certificate has to record the baby's sex as male or female; intersex is not a legal option (Births and Deaths Registration Act of 1953). Interestingly, the Adoption and Children Act of 2002 does allow parents to be registered by the 'sex neutral' term 'parent'. This neutrality accommodates adoption by same-sex couples (both male or both female), thereby avoiding two mothers or two fathers. It will be interesting to see whether this precedent leads to pressure for sex-neutral birth and/or death registrations, or even for the recording of 'intersex'. Such pressure may come from the increasingly prevalent clinical practice of conservative surgical and endocrinological intervention in cases of sex ambiguity until the child grows and expresses a gender identity as masculine, feminine or intermediate.

Data adapted from Blackless M *et al.* (2000) How sexually dimorphic are we? Review and synthesis. *American Journal of Human Biology* **12**, 151–166.

description which is broadly recognizable as defining what it means to be *masculine* or *feminine* in a society. The precise attributes appropriate to each gender will vary from one society to another, or in the same society over time. However, social, historical and anthropological studies reveal a remarkable consistency in the extent to which each of those attributes listed recurs with greater or lesser emphasis in the gender stereotypes of a range of different societies. For example, the exclusion of women from public life or from particular social or work roles is more evident in strict Islamic societies or traditional Judaeo-Christian societies than in modern secular societies. However, in the latter societies such gender stereotyping still persists in that certain roles remain associated strongly with men (e.g. consultant surgeons, priests) or women (e.g. nurses, midwives) even if many of these associations are much weaker than they once were. The behaviour expected of men and women also differs. Rowdy, aggressive behaviour from men is resignedly expected and often excused ('boys will be boys'), whereas the same behaviour from women is considered 'unladylike'. On a more trivial level, the wearing of earrings by men or of trousers by women was until recently in British society very gender astereotypic: there were social rules about what constituted appropriately gendered body decoration and clothing, many of which still linger in today's attitudes and values, albeit much attenuated.

Although it may appear difficult in a society in flux to define the current gender stereotypes in terms acceptable to all, nonetheless there tends to be a normative social view about those elements constituting masculine and feminine behaviour. The cohesiveness of that view can be particularly strong for the members of each generation: a person's peers. In framing a gender stereotype, no claim is being made that this stereotype is true for all or indeed for any female or male. It is rather a shared cultural belief about what men and women are like. This social consensus about what it means to be a man or a woman is important for individuals' perceptions of themselves and of those around them. It provides a yardstick against which to measure their own masculinity or femininity and that of those whom they meet.

This measuring process is important because those who appear to stray too far from the stereotype are generally regarded negatively or as a focus for rebellion. In societies in which gender plays a strong social role, it is less acceptable for men to appear feminine than for women to appear masculine, although there are boundaries in both directions. This asymmetry may result from the fact that men tend to be more powerful than women, and so their attributes are more valued socially. So in societies in which gender stereotypes are being eroded, there tends to be more acceptance of the perceived masculinization of women's stereotypes and more resistance to the feminization of men's stereotypes. However, as economies shift increasingly towards a service function, in which traditionally feminine attributes are more valued, the employment opportunities for traditionally masculine men are reduced and these men become marginalized as their masculine attributes are less valued. A key message from this brief discussion is the strong cultural contingency of gender attributes.

Gender stereotyping provides a social shorthand for classifying people by sex

We are presented with a bewildering array of social information. Part of the process of our development as children is to learn how to interpret the world around us. Sex differences are an important part of that world. By learning a gender stereotype, or indeed any other stereotype (ethnicity, race, class, age, employment), one is provided with a social shorthand or sketch that enables some rapid preliminary assessments to be made of each individual encountered. Recognizing someone as male or female allows us to associate the various attributes of gender stereotypes and thereby conditions our immediate behaviour patterns in ways that are socially appropriate for our and their gender. Of course, this process will tend to reinforce the gender stereotype of the society. It does not, however, preclude later reactions to the individual as an individual. If you doubt the importance of social sketching of this sort, consider your reaction on being introduced to someone whose sex and gender are not immediately obvious. How comfortable are you, and how does it affect your behaviour? Or consider how you react when, in a different culture, you find that the accepted gender stereotypes conflict with those of your own culture: for example, men holding hands or kissing in public or women being excluded from public life? Humans are social beings and the rules by which societies function are therefore very important.

Gender identity describes the personal concept of 'me as a man or a woman'

We have a social view that there are two genders defined broadly by the gender stereotypes of our society. Each of us is part of that society. It therefore follows that each of us has a view of ourselves as being masculine or feminine and of conforming to a greater or lesser degree to the stereotype. The extent to which each individual feels confident of his or her position within this bipolar gender spectrum is a measure of the strength and security of their *gender identity*. Most individuals have gender identities that are fully congruent with their sex. Thus, most women and men who are physically female and male, respectively, have *strong gender identities*. Some individuals may feel less certain about their gender identities, although they nonetheless identify congruently with their physical sex: they may be said to have *weak gender identities*. A few individuals may feel that their gender identities are totally at variance with their otherwise congruent genetic, gonadal, hormonal and genital sex. Such people are described as being *transsexual* or *transgendered*. Transgendering may occur in either direction, the *male-to-female transgendered* consider themselves to be females with a female gender identity and brain but with otherwise male bodies, whereas the *female-to-male transgendered* feel themselves to be men in an otherwise woman's body. Traditionally, more male-to-female transgendered individuals have been identified than female-to-male, although this may represent differential reporting more than real prevalence. The transgendered may adopt the gender roles of the physically different sex, and some may undergo surgical and hormonal treatments so as to bring their bodies and their bodily functions (their sex) as closely congruent to their gender identity as is possible (females becoming *trans men* and males becoming *trans women*) (Box 2.2). Transgendered men and women provide us with perhaps the strongest justification for making the distinction between sex and gender. A better

> **BOX 2.2 The law and trans men and women**
>
> Recent legislative changes across Europe permit recognition of trans men and women in their 'new' identities. In the UK, the relevant law is the Gender Recognition Act 2004, which provides for a 'gender recognition certificate' meaning that their legal sex does not match that on their birth certificate. In order to qualify for a certificate, 'expert evidence' must be produced to establish the person's gender identity, effectively a gatekeeper role for clinicians. Then, only after 2 years living in one's 'acquired gender' (the terminology the Act uses) can the person get a certificate. Third, the person's birth certificate remains unamended. Although legally this is not a problem, some trans people argue that this is a failure to accept that the surgery or treatment is to match them to their true sex and that the sex on the birth certificate was an error.

understanding of the basis of trans people may also help us to refine more clearly the boundary between sex and gender.

Gender differences may not be as great as they first appear to be

Intuitively, when looking at the gender attributes in Table 2.1, it is possible simultaneously to recognize the gender stereotypes as familiar while rejecting them as an oversimplification. For example, whereas men in general might not readily express vulnerable emotions through crying and admissions of helplessness, many individual men do express such emotions and show such behaviour. Individual women can be just as competitive and aggressive as men, although overall these attributes are associated much less with women than with men. Many studies have attempted to make objective and quantitative measurements of gender differences, through the use of behavioural and cognitive function tests and the use of questionnaires to address attitudes. For most attributes, the degrees of variation *within* populations of men and of women are so great that the *overlap between* men and women is too large to produce significant differences between the sexes (see Box 2.3). Moreover, rarely if ever do any differences observed have predictive validity: it is not possible from the measurement of a gender attribute in an individual to predict whether that individual is a man or a woman.

There is thus a paradox. Society has a clear and polarized concept of what it means to be masculine and feminine within society. Moreover, most individuals profess a very clear concept of themselves as masculine or feminine and an understanding of what that means for their place in society. Yet both objectively and subjectively it is not

BOX 2.3 Summary of findings from a meta-analysis of studies on sex differences in humans

124 traits were analysed in a range of published studies to see whether there were significant differences between populations of men and women.

- For 78% of these traits, there was effectively no difference.
- For 15% of them, there was a moderate population difference. Traits observed more frequently in the male population included spatial perception, mental rotation, physical and verbal aggression, assertiveness, body esteem, sprinting, activity level, self-efficacy of computer use. Traits more frequently observed in women included spelling and language skills, and smiling when aware of being observed.
- For only 6% of traits were large differences observed. Observed more frequently for men were mechanical reasoning, masturbation, permissive attitudes to casual sex, and for women agreeableness.
- Only 2% of traits showed very large sex differences, throw velocity/distance and grip strength being significantly more frequent in males.

Conclusions and qualifications

It is important to note that for all traits there was overlap. Some are clearly related to the anabolic actions of androgens on muscles, and others may be culturally conditioned—expectations from gender stereotypes perhaps influencing attribute acquisition.

Where statistically significant sex differences are found, it is important to note that scores for some traits may vary with factors such as age and experience, mood, motivation, practice and ambient hormone levels, and that these may differ for the two sexes.

Overall, what impresses is how similar the two sexes are. Humans do not seem very dimorphic!

Gender differences nonetheless are often highlighted

There are two types of reaction to the evidence that men and women show big overlaps in attributes. One reaction

is to focus on those statistically significant average differences that are observed and to seek to understand their origins—the 'women are from Venus, men are from Mars' approach. This reaction may also be used to justify the perceived different needs/treatments of men/boys and women/girls in education, health, employment, etc.

The alternative approach, while accepting that some average differences do exist between the sexes, is to focus on people first and foremost, given the overlap between sexes and complex biological and social origins of sex differences. This approach accepts the notion of a less gendered society than hitherto in which people of either sex are freer to flourish without constraint of stereotype. A recent debate about biological sex differences among scientists illustrates these distinctive reactions (see Further reading). These two differing approaches take us into political and social theory, and we simply alert readers to read and interpret the evidence base as objectively as possible despite the strong academic and social reactions that discussion of sex differences evokes.

Further reading

Baron-Cohen S (2003) *The Essential Difference: Male and Female Brains and the Truth about Autism.* Basic Books, New York (takes quite a strong position about innate biological differences between male and female brains, and relates the analysis to the higher incidence of autism among males; acknowledges considerable overlap and sex-atypical patterns).

Barres BA (2006) Does gender matter? *Nature* **442**, 133–136 (questions biological origins of sex differences in scientific success).

Shibley Hyde J (2005) The gender similarities hypothesis. *American Psychologist* **60**, 581–592 (the meta-analysis that emphasizes the similarities rather than the differences between the sexes).

Lawrence PA (2006) Men, women and ghosts in science. *PLoS Biol.* **4**, e19, 13–15 (takes the approach that biological sex differences are inevitably a part of our makeup as humans and scientists and cannot be ignored).

possible to sustain a strongly bipolar description of a gendered society. Men and women overlap greatly in the attitudes that they express, in their patterns of behaviour, in their skills and, increasingly, in the roles they adopt. There is more a continuum of attributes than a bipolar segregation. Some societies reflect this reality and are relatively non-gendered, but most societies have a bipolar gendered organization despite the lack of evidence for its inevitability. Why? Presumably such social organization is seen to have advantages, for example for the production and raising of children, controlling patterns of inheritance, the division of labour, or the ability to resist external threats.

In order to take this discussion further, we will turn to a consideration of how a gendered society might arise.

The origins of gender

It will be clear from the foregoing discussion that gender is a concept applicable to humans. Does this therefore mean that studies on the origin of sex differences in the behaviour of animals are of no use to us in trying to understand gender differences in humans? We examine this question first for non-primates, and then for non-human primates, before finally considering whether and how this evidence applies to humans.

Hormones, the brain and behavioural dimorphism

In animals hormones condition sex differences in behaviour and brain structure

Exposure of animals to sex hormones during a critical period of early life is associated with *sexually dimorphic behaviour* displayed later in adulthood, for example, the distinctive urination patterns shown by the dog (cocked leg) and bitch (squatting). This critical period may be in late fetal life (e.g. guinea-pig, sheep) or neonatally (e.g. rat, mouse, hamster). The most intensively studied behaviour patterns are those associated with copulation. Thus, during sexual interaction with females, adult male rats show *courtship behaviour* (e.g. *pursuing females* and *anogenitally investigating* them), *mounting*, *intromission* and *ejaculation* (Fig. 2.1). Conversely, adult females display *soliciting* and *receptive postures*, such as *lordosis* (Fig. 2.1). These behaviours are *predominantly, but not exclusively*, typical for each sex. Thus, normal males will occasionally solicit and even accept mounts by other males, while females in heat will often mount one another. *The differences in behaviour are not absolute but quantitative.*

Treatment of female rats with testosterone during the first 5 days of life increases their display of masculine patterns of sexual behaviour in adulthood and reduces their display of feminine patterns. Castration of male rats to remove the influence of androgens during this same critical period has the reverse effects. Thus, 'masculinization' in the rat (and other non-primates) is accompanied by 'defeminization'. How do androgens influence the development of these behavioural differences?

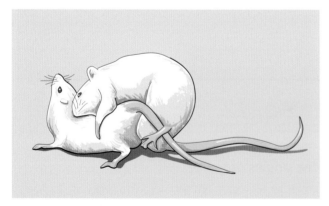

Fig. 2.1 Sex-dependent behaviour patterns in male and female rats. Note the immobile *lordosis* posture shown by the *receptive* female, which enables the male to *mount* and achieve *intromissions* which will result in *ejaculation*. Receptivity and lordosis are shown predominantly by females; mounting, intromission and ejaculation patterns of behaviour are shown predominantly by males.

Exposure to steroids over the critical period affects the *structure of the developing brain*, generating many neuroanatomical sex differences, some of which seem to explain the sex differences in behaviour. Most attention has focused on structural sex differences in a region of the brain called the *anterior hypothalamus* and adjacent *medial preoptic area* (the anatomy of these regions is discussed in more detail in Chapter 6). Both of these areas are known to be intimately involved with the control of sexual behaviour in adult animals (see Chapter 8). Indeed, neonatal implantation of androgens directly into the anterior hypothalamus of female rodents not only masculinizes the local brain structure but also results in increased reproductive male behaviour in adulthood (Fig. 2.2).

In animals, then, there is clear evidence that hormones lead to neuroanatomical and behavioural changes, in much the same way that they also lead to the development of sexually dimorphic genitalia. However, it is important to remember that it is *quantitative* sex differences in behaviour that are observed, not *absolute* differences of a qualitative nature. It is therefore oversimplistic to believe that particular sexually dimorphic areas of the brain are *reliably* associated with specific behavioural functions. Some behavioural flexibility persists. However, our broad understanding of these animal studies enables us to fit sex differences in brain structure and in behaviour into the same conceptual framework of sex, as we did for the gonads, hormones and genitalia in Chapter 1. There is then no need for a 'gender category' in these species.

Non-human primates show sex differences in behaviour which appear to be influenced by hormonal exposure early in life

To what extent do androgens exert the same effects on the development of sexually dimorphic behaviour in non-human primates? Results from experiments on rhesus monkeys suggest some similarities. Young females, exposed to high levels of androgens during fetal life, display levels of sexually dimorphic behaviour in their patterns of childhood play that are intermediate between normal males and females (Fig. 2.3). Moreover, although both male *and* female infant monkeys will mount other infants (Fig. 2.4a), only males progressively display mounts of a mature pattern (Fig. 2.4b). Androgenized females, however, do develop this mature mounting pattern. Moreover, as adults they attempt to mount other females at a higher frequency than do non-androgenized females. Thus, neonatal androgenization produces persistent 'masculinization' of behaviour. However, the androgenized female monkeys as adults show normal menstrual cycles and can become pregnant. They must therefore display patterns of adult feminine sexual behaviour at least adequate for them to interact

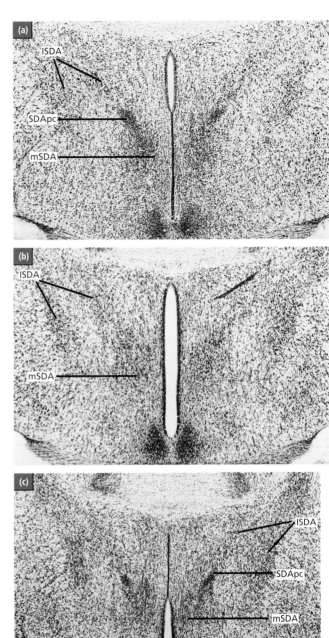

Fig. 2.2 Photomicrographs of coronal sections through the preoptic area of three 21-day-old gerbils (*Meriones unguiculatus*). Section (a) is taken from a male, (b) from a female and (c) from a female treated neonatally with androgens (testosterone propionate: 50 mg on the day of birth and 50 mg the next day). The sexually dimorphic area (SDA) can be divided into several regions: medial (mSDA); lateral (lSDA); and pars compacta (SDApc). The SDA differs between males and females in a number of aspects: prominence (not necessarily size); acetylcholinesterase histochemistry; steroid binding; and various other neurochemical characteristics, but most obviously in the presence or absence of the SDApc. Thus, the SDApc is virtually never found in females (compare a with b). Note that in females treated neonatally with testosterone, there is a clear SDApc (compare c with b). These pictures provide clear evidence of the impact of hormones during a critical period of early life on the differentiation of this part of the brain. The medial preoptic area in general is closely involved with the regulation of sexual behaviour (see Chapter 8), and some progress has been made in relating specific aspects of sexual behaviour to subdivisions of the SDA. It is also important to note that such sex differences in the structure of the preoptic area are found in many species, from rats to humans, but the precise details of the dimorphism vary considerably.

successfully with males, suggesting that they are not totally or permanently 'defeminized'.

These results suggest a less complete or persistent effect of androgens on the development of sexually dimorphic behaviour in primates than in non-primates. Why might this be? One explanation lies in the timing of the critical androgen-sensitive effect on brain structure. In rats, this occurs neonatally, after genital phenotype is established, so making it easily accessible to selective manipulation. If a critical period exists in primates, it occurs during fetal life, and may be prolonged. Attempts to androgenize primate fetuses *in utero* often lead to abortion if doses of administered androgens are too high. The genitalia also tend to be masculinized, which might affect the subsequent social interactions and learning of the infant. Thus, a specific selective effect of androgen on the brain may not yet have been achieved. Alternatively, it is possible that in non-human primates, the rather rigid hormonal determination

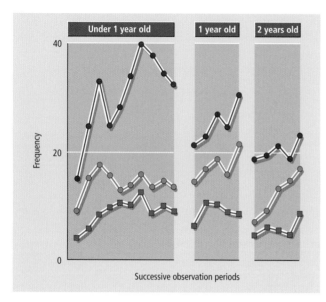

Fig. 2.3 Frequency of 'rough-and-tumble play' during the first, second and third years of life of a rhesus monkey male (red circles), female (blue squares) and female that had been treated with androgens prenatally (green circles). Note that males display this behaviour at a higher frequency than females and that androgenized females are intermediate.

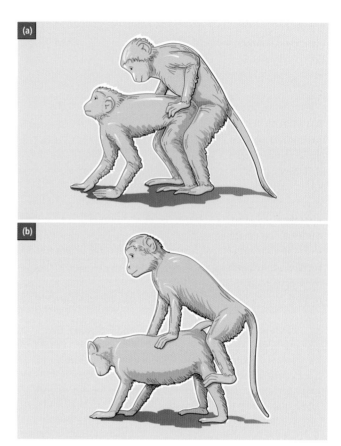

Fig. 2.4 Sexually dimorphic patterns of mounting behaviour in young rhesus monkeys. (a) Early in life, both males and females show immature mounts by standing on the cage floor.
(b) During development, males show progressively more mature mounts in which they clasp the female's calves so that she supports his weight entirely. Androgenized females display more of the latter type of mature mounts than do untreated females.

of sexually dimorphic behaviour seen in non-primates simply does not occur. Androgens may predispose to masculine patterns of behaviour, but other factors may also influence the degree to which they are expressed.

What about sex differences in brain structure in non-human primates? As for non-primates, a few such differences exist, including some in the hypothalamic region particularly concerned with reproductive and sexual behaviours. However, although it seems probable that most of these neuroanatomical differences result from endocrine exposure in early life, this has not been demonstrated formally. Neither has a strict association between sexually dimorphic brain structures and behaviour been shown.

In humans there may be both sex and gender differences in brain structure and the expression of gender attributes, but the underlying causes are uncertain

Not surprisingly, the difficulty in studying non-human primates is exacerbated further when the human is considered. The requirement to use post-mortem brains for neuroanatomical analysis restricts both the amount and quality of the material, and observations are complicated by variations in age, pathology, experience and structural

artefacts. Although studies are limited and often conflicting, a few consistent sex differences in the structural organization of the brain have been reported, for example in a small region of the anterior hypothalamus called the *3rd interstitial nucleus (INAH3)*. However, the significance of these sex differences for gender identity and attributes is less clear. A claim has been made that the size and organization of the *central bed nucleus of the stria terminalis (cBST)* is associated specifically with *gender identity* as opposed to sex. Thus, it is reported as being smaller in women than in men, and also smaller in trans women (male-to-female transgendered; Fig. 2.5). However, the number of individual brains studied is small, as are the measured gender differences, and there is overlap between genders such that nuclear size is not predictive for gender. It is also not clear when these size differences first appear or what causes them. Until we know more about the time at which brain differences emerge and we are able to study more brains from a larger range of individuals with gender or endocrine anomalies, it will be difficult to draw firm conclusions.

More recently, neuroanatomical imaging techniques have been used to search for male/female differences in the functional organization of the living brain. A number of these studies has now shown that there are population sex differences in brain lateralization of some functions, females showing more left-lateralized language and emotion processing, whereas males tend to show right-lateralized visuospatial activity. There is also evidence for sexual dimorphism in the *amygdala*, a region of the brain involved in emotional processing. Overall, more study is needed for secure identification of sex and/or gender based brain organizational differences. Certainly, claims as to the hormonal cause(s) of any differences must be viewed cautiously. For example, genetic differences (one versus two X chromosomes) have been claimed as responsible for amygdala dimorphism.

What about the relationship between hormones and gendered *behaviour* in humans? This question has been studied in both adults and children using various of the gendered attributes summarized in Table 2.1. It is important to re-emphasize that in humans the two sexes differ quantitatively in gender attributes, with much overlap. The influence of prenatal hormones on subsequent behaviour

has been fruitfully investigated in genetic females with adrenogenital syndrome (AGS; see Chapter 1)—nature's counterpart to experimental animals treated exogenously with androgens during the critical period of neural differentiation. However, it is important to note that we are not dealing with 'pure' androgen effects in these girls/women, as under- or (therapeutic) overexposure to corticosteroids is known to affect brain structure and behaviour directly. Studies of girls with AGS has revealed *increased* levels of energy expenditure and athletic interests more characteristic of boys, and a *decreased* incidence of 'rehearsals' of maternal behaviour and doll-play activities, together with diminished interest in dresses, jewellery and hairstyles. This spectrum of behaviour, termed *tomboyism*, is well recognized and accepted in Western culture, and provides few if any problems for children so affected. Tomboyism might be thought to be a consequence of the effects of androgens on the fetal brain, rather like the changes in rough-and-tumble play in infant monkeys exposed prenatally to androgens. However, as a group, AGS girls had *stronger* feminine gender identities than a group of non-AGS tomboys, and only slightly weaker gender identities than control girls. Moreover, among AGS girls there was no clear relationship between weak feminine gender identity and the degree of genital virilization. Further study of AGS females as adults has revealed only slender evidence of enduring behavioural consequences. Thus, they show only slight evidence of a higher incidence of dissatisfaction with their female gender identity and of lesbianism than did controls, but again not related to the degree of presumptive androgenization. A small group of AGS women do identify as trans men, but again not necessarily the most androgenized. Thus, overall the studies on AGS girls/women provide little support for either androgens or masculinized genitalia being an exclusive or necessary determinant of defeminization in humans. However, it is important to note that the AGS girls and women studied will, by definition, span the low to moderate part of the androgenization scale, where genital virilization is incomplete.

How to summarize? It seems clear that there *are* some sex differences and even perhaps a gender difference in brain structure in humans, but these differences are small. It is unclear when they arise and what causes them. There is no direct evidence relating them *causally* to particular behavioural differences between genders. Evidence from animals suggests that hormones *can* influence brain organization and thereby behaviour, but even in animals there is a not a rigid and absolute causal relationship between the two. In humans, where there is even greater flexibility and overlap of sex-related behaviour patterns and of gendered attributes, a role for hormones prenatally or neonatally is plausible but more research is needed to find out the full extent and nature of any influence (see also p. 119).

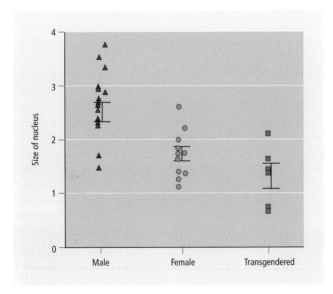

Fig. 2.5 The scatter of sizes of the central bed nucleus of the stria terminalis (cBST) in human adult males, females and trans males (male-to-female transgendered). Error bars ±SEM. Note the sex difference and that the trans male nuclear volume is closer to the female pattern. Data redrawn from Zhou *et al.* (1995).

Gender development may form part of social learning in humans

In the discussion above, we referred again to the significance of the assignment of sex to a baby as a boy or a girl depending on the presence or absence of a penis. It was pointed out that this assignment might then affect both how the individual saw him- or herself and how the parents and peers viewed and treated the developing child. We now explore this area further in our analysis of gender development.

Patterns of interaction between babies and those around them emphasize gender differences

Starting from birth, mothers attribute different characteristics to male infants than to female infants. Thus, when individual adults are handed the same baby, having been told variously that it is a girl or a boy, *their play, handling of and communication with it differ according to their perception of its sex*. This sort of study shows that babies of different sexes are likely to be treated differently simply because they are of different sexes. A second example makes an additional point. When adults are shown the same video sequence of a child playing, and some are told that it is a boy and others a girl, *their interpretations of its behaviours depend on the sex that they believe it to be*. For example, when the child was startled and believed to be a boy, it was perceived more often as being angry, whereas the same startled behaviour, when believed to be that of a girl, was perceived as fearful distress. This sort of study tells us that expectations about how a male or female baby *should* behave can lead adults to interpret the same behaviour very differently. It raises the possibility that some behaviours may be reinforced or responded to in different gender-specific ways as a result of the expectations of others. Several studies have shown very clearly that the expectations that adults have of a boy differ from those expected of a girl; and men tend to be much more prone to gender stereotyping in this regard than women. Thus, girls are expected to be softer and more vulnerable and are played with more gently. They are also expected to be more vocal and socially interactive, and parents spend more time in these sorts of behaviours with girls. Boys in contrast are encouraged to do things, are less directly communicated with and are disciplined or roughly handled more often.

These sorts of observations emphasize how important and subtle gender stereotypes are and how they are applied to children from the moment of birth. Indeed, parents seem quite anxious to encourage differences between boys and girls by the types of toys they offer them, the clothes they provide for them, and the activities they encourage and discourage. Rewards and approval are offered when children conform to parental gender stereotypes. These parental gendering activities are particularly marked for the first 2–3 years of a child's life. It is precisely over this period that a child develops its own sense of gender identity. By 2 years children label themselves consistently as male or female, and soon thereafter reliably associate certain sorts of behaviour and activities with males and females. They appear to have both a gender identity and a gender stereotype. They also by 5 years of age seem to realize that gender is fixed and cannot be changed across time or situation: they have a sense of *gender constancy*. Indeed, if 3–6-year-old children are shown a video of another child, their descriptions of its behaviour are very different if told that it is a boy than if told it is a girl. They actually seem to be even more rigidly gender stereotyping than their parents when performing the same task! Since children spend a lot of time with one another, they are likely to reinforce gender stereotypes in each other: peer pressure in action.

Children are, of course, cognitive beings. They do not simply absorb subconsciously impressions of the world around them, although that does occur. They see and hear what goes on around them in the household, in the media, at school. They see men and women and what they do and don't do. Models of male and female behaviour are provided all round them. So there may also be a copying element in the development and elaboration of their growing gender identity and the ways in which they express it. However, copying a model implies identification with that model in the first place and so it is likely that copying is a secondary process that may relate more to the expression of a gender identity than its initial establishment.

Thus, a lot of evidence supports the view that gender stereotypes are applied to babies and children very early in life, and that children also use them and apply them to their world from an early age. The child's environment is thus immersed in gender stereotyping. Does this mean that the way in which babies are treated and gender stereotyped *causes* their own gender to develop? It is entirely plausible to suggest that at least some gendered patterns of behaviour that develop in boys and girls may be induced differentially by the way in which they are treated by others and as a result of the expectations of others. In effect, the gender stereotype of a society may be 'taught' to its children by the way they are treated. If this were so, it might be suggested that ambiguity on the part of parents about the sex of their child could affect the development of gender identity. Cases of transgendering might be associated with a sexually ambiguous childhood: for example, parents treating their son more as a girl, clothing him in dresses and not reinforcing 'boyish' activities in play and sport. The evidence on this suggestion is far from clear. Just because a suggestion is plausible, it does not mean that it is true. What is the evidence?

Gendered behaviour by babies may affect the way that they are treated

In an earlier section, the evidence that exposure to androgens during fetal or neonatal life might influence gendered behaviour was reviewed. The evidence was consistent with there being a possible influence on childhood play patterns. There are indeed claims of intrinsic behavioural differences between newborn male and female babies, although these are not yet strong enough to convince. However, it is at least plausible to suggest that just as babies may respond differently to adults who show gender-specific behaviour towards them, so sex differences in baby behaviour might induce different responses in adults. Clearly, the experiments described above, in which adults were (correctly or incorrectly) 'told' the sex of a child and responded in ways typical for the believed gender, cannot be explained in this way. However, in these experiments when a male baby was handled by adults, half of whom thought it was male and the other half of whom thought it was female, and they were then asked about their experiences, there were differences. Thus where reality and belief were congruent the adults had felt more 'comfortable' than when there was conflict. This may mean that they were picking up on inconsistencies in the baby's behaviour that conflicted with expectations. What this may be telling us is that adults are sensitive to the baby's behaviour as being boy-like or girl-like. It does not, of course, tell us whether these sensed differences in behaviour were due to hormonal influences on the baby or to previous social learning by it. Here is the core of our dilemma. From the moment of birth, boys and girls are likely to be treated differently, so how can we separate cleanly the effects of hormones from those of learning?

One way to achieve this might be to look at babies who were born boys but 'became' girls postnatally (or rarely vice versa). A single highly influential case was provided in the 1960s by monozygotic male twins—the so-called Money twins, named after the clinician who described the case. One twin (John) was genitally damaged at circumcision. This boy was reassigned as a girl (Joan), given genital plastic surgery, provided with hormone therapy and brought up as a girl. Joan was described as having a female gender identity and was taken by John Money as decisive evidence that sex of rearing 'trumped' genetic, endocrine and gonadal sex in the establishment of gender identity. However, it was later found that in adulthood, Joan rejected her female identity, reverted to John, married and had an adopted child. Amazingly, this one case determined pae-

---

---

diatric policy on genital ambiguity until the late 1990s (see Box 2.4).

Recently, more systematic prospective studies on the development of gender identity in a range of patients with different combinations of genetic, gonadal, genital and rearing sex have begun to appear. These are based on thorough descriptions of each sex-variable in relation to the measured outcome of gender identity. At best, conclusions are highly provisional, but suggest that many XY individuals exposed to normal prenatal androgens but reared as females are likely to declare male sexual identities later in life. XX individuals exposed to high prenatal androgens and reared as males are more likely to develop male identities. Such evidence is important if assignment of sex at birth or soon thereafter is to be attempted. Of course, the alternative, as described earlier, is to accept the intersex state as a valid interim and/or long-term option—a situation that would require both social and legal sanction for it to be acceptable to many parents.

These studies indicate that the establishment of gender identity is clearly complex and roles for both the gender of rearing and fetal androgens are likely, perhaps interacting in ways we do not yet understand. In this context, the male transgendered are of particular interest. We need to understand whether their exposure to androgens was normal and whether they were reared unambiguously as boys according to their genital sex. They develop a feminine gender identity, but why? Understanding how the transgendered develop may throw interesting and important light on the relative roles of hormones and environment in gender development.

Summary

Four potential elements that might contribute towards the establishment of gender have been considered: sex chromosome constitution, hormones, social learning and brain structure. The brain is central since the expression of attitudes and behaviour, which form the basis of social interactions, is the result of neural processes. Both the organization and function of the brain can be influenced by genes, hormones and learning. Hormones affect brain structure and behaviour in non-primates and modulate behaviour sex-dependently in primates, although their impact is less rigid. The patterns of usage of neuronal circuits that come from interactions with the environment, including social learning, can affect brain organization and function, so that learning and rehearsal are associated with changes to the 'hard wiring' of the brain. When we consider the development of gender, a clear separation of endocrine and social factors has not been achieved. It might be suggested that such a rigid separation is also impossible, since each may interact with and reinforce the other. Small gender differences in the behaviour of newborn babies may be induced by androgens. These subtle differences may be detected by parents and peers who also have clear expectations and beliefs derived from gender stereotypes that condition their behaviour towards the baby's actions and anatomy. These interactions tend to amplify small differences into larger ones. Soon the baby/child engages in the process actively. The process is a dynamic one, susceptible and responsive to cultural difference and change, based on the undoubted cognitive flexibility of humans, and well suited to the development of a social mammal.

Gender and reproduction

Gender has been defined and discussed as a system of classifying individuals based on their sex. Sex in mammals, as we saw in Chapter 1, is fundamentally about reproduction and genetics. The process of reproduction involves the bringing together of a male and a female (*courtship*) so that their haploid gametes can unite at fertilization. In mammals, one of each type of gamete is obligatory for the successful production of a new individual. As we will discuss further in Chapter 9, in mammals fertilization is *internal*: it involves the process of *coition* in which the spermatozoa are deposited in the vagina. Courtship and coition can involve elaborate rituals and behaviours in which males and females express sex- or gender-dependent patterns of behaviour. Even a brief look at the gender attributes listed in Table 2.1 reveals that many can be related plausibly to the different reproductive roles of males and females. The generally nurturant, emotional, consensual, creative and private attributes of females and the more aggressive, competitive, powerful attributes of males seem well suited to the explicitly reproductive gender roles. Thus, males are essentially disposable. Their only *necessary* role in reproduction is briefly discharged, whereas females have an *extended essential* role. Because of this, females are a *precious resource* who, in times of danger, must be given protection if the social group is to survive. A single male could, in principle, provide all the sperm needed for many females. Moreover, all those unnecessary males will be a drain on resources if food is limited: males are costly biologically. They are therefore *disposable* in war or in risky competition with one another. It is thus tempting to *explain* gender differences in human societies entirely in terms of their value to the reproductive process. It is also tempting to conclude that the broad similarities between the reproductive roles of animals and humans must mean that gender differences in humans, like sex differences in animals, are the product of an evolutionary process which is, at its heart, genetically programmed and so ultimately genetically determined. These temptations should be resisted.

Undoubtedly the genetic inheritance of humankind exerts powerful effects on us and our behaviour. However, what distinguishes humans from most other animals is the powerful additional legacy left to us by our culture. Humans are distinguished by our capacity to use information around us, to learn as we grow, to conceptualize and to establish and transmit cultures, including complex language, in ways not open to most animals. This mental flexibility may operate within limits imposed by our genetic inheritance, but it also operates on opportunities presented by that same inheritance. Even a superficial view of the widely different cultural roles that men and women have in different societies, how they are treated, are valued and behave, shows the power of cultural inheritance. This is not surprising, given what we saw of how children learn about gender stereotypes from the society around them.

So reproduction and sex are tightly, inevitably and invariably linked through our biological and genetic inheritance, whereas reproduction and gender are linked more loosely and elastically through our cultural inheritance. This point is made more clearly when we examine the varied functions associated with courtship and coition in humans. Reproduction is obviously one such function. However, erotic pleasure quite distinct and separable from reproduction is another: humans can and do mate regardless of their fertility. The process of mating is an object in itself. Courtship and coition can also serve a wider emotional purpose, involving feelings such as dependence, power, self-worth, and security. Courtship and coition also have social and economic functions: when formalized in kinships they establish patterns of inheritance and power in a society. We should also remember that coition has a consequence not always welcomed by humans, but essential for some microorganisms, of transmitting them and the diseases they may cause through a society. These varied and wide-ranging functions of and consequences for courtship and coition mean that society tries to control the processes with customs and laws (see Chapter 15). These then of course form part of the cultural inheritance that we learn as part of the gender stereotype of our society.

The relationship between sex, gender and reproduction raised in this section will be revisited in many chapters later in this book. Now, however, we will complete our preliminary consideration of sex, reproduction and gender by looking at the relationship of all three to sexuality.

Sexuality involves the erotic

As mentioned in the previous section, courtship and coition can involve intense and pleasurable sexual fantasies and feelings. This state of sexual excitement in humans is described as the *erotic*. In this book, we reserve the use of the term *sexuality* for this erotic experience and its expression in human lives. This definition is not uniformly agreed and would be considered by some to be controversial and too narrow. Sometimes, sexuality is used to describe all that it means to be a man or a woman, a sort of all-pervasive state that is difficult to distinguish clearly from gender itself. We find this definition too diffuse to be useful. Of course, the erotic and its associations can be very pervasive and, as we will see, not limited simply to the events surrounding courtship and coition. However, at heart, our sexuality is about inner erotic excitement and fantasy and its outward expression in sexual erotic behaviour. A *sexual individual* is one who is erotically functional mentally and/or behaviourally, an *asexual individual* lacks erotic experience and fantasy.

The biology of erotic arousal seems to be similar for men and women, and descriptions of what it is like to be in an erotically aroused state are not gender specific (see Chapter 9 for further discussion). What then distinguishes erotic experiences in different individuals and genders?

Sexuality can be classified by the stimulus of erotic arousal

A commonly used system for classifying sexuality uses the object of sexual arousal as its starting point. Examples of such a classification are shown in Table 2.2. Four things are striking about the contents of this table.

• First, there is a wide range of erotically arousing stimuli. It is important to note that they are not necessarily *mutually exclusive*. For example, a person may be aroused by both men and women (*bisexual*), or by the opposite sex *and*

Table 2.2 A classification system for sexualities.

Object causing arousal	Classification of person aroused	Comments
Person of opposite sex	Heterosexual	Social norm in most cultures
Person of same sex	Homosexual	Acceptable in some forms in many societies; illegal or disapproved in others
Immature person	Paedophiliac	Generally unacceptable
Inanimate objects	Paraphiliac	Acceptable if not causing harm to others or distress to paraphiliac him- or herself
Excrement	Coprophiliac	Generally disapproved of
Wearing clothing of other gender	Fetishistic transvestite	Often confused with transgendered but is not a gender issue; may be accepted or ridiculed
Watching others naked and/or engaged in sex	Voyeur	Broadly disapproved of unless 'formalized' or paid for
Self displaying naked or engaged in sex	Exhibitionist	Broadly disapproved of unless 'formalized' or paid for
Receiving or inflicting pain during sex	Sadomasochist	Recently held to be illegal in Europe

by objects or cross-dressing, or be sadomasochistic with the same and/or opposite sex partner(s). The sexuality of humans is complex. Moreover, the stimuli of erotic arousal may change for an individual with age, experience or social expectation. So this labelling system is imperfectly rigid, and the use of labelling as a shorthand can be misleading.

• Second, the stimuli are a mixture of objects, people and activities and in some cases are described in terms of how they are used erotically but in others are not. When we deal with the sexual, there are two levels of description. There is the inner world of conscious arousal, imagination and fantasy: this is usually given the name *sexual identity*, akin to the conceptual inner state of gender identity we described earlier. It is an acknowledgement by a person of their own state of being as a sexual individual. Their own state may or may not fit with the categories used in Table 2.2, although most people will tend to use the labels that society provides for them. Thus, someone might say 'I am a heterosexual/homosexual/bisexual being': that would be the verbal expression of their sexual identity. This inner world may or may not be expressed through behaviour and sexual attitudes. Society usually has a clear expectation of how people with different sexualities will behave and what their attributes will be, a sexual stereotype, and this will be absorbed as a part of the sexual identity of people.

• Third, most of the stimuli clearly have nothing to do with procreative sex, since procreation is impossible or unlikely in the context of arousal by them. This emphasizes the clear separation of reproductive and erotic activities that can be observed in humans compared with other mammals in which reproduction and sexual arousal (especially in females) are very closely co-regulated (see Chapter 8). In this regard humans resemble their closest evolutionary relatives among the higher primates and especially chimpanzees and bonobos. Thus, these species show quite clearly that sexual interactions, both within and between sexes and across age groups, can have a social role in addition to a sexual role. Genital showing and looking, touching and rubbing, erection and mounting are commonly observed between individuals of the same sex, and are seen as pleasurable and reassuring. Such same sex interactions are often called *socio-sexual* to distinguish them from the *eroto-sexual* interactions between males and females, although it is unclear how real this distinction is. The main point to understand is that sexual stimulation can form part of the social cement for social species.

• Fourth, the social acceptability of different sexual stimuli varies with the stimuli, the type of person involved and the society in which they are experienced. Thus, homosexual acts between men have been viewed variously as essential, desirable, acceptable, immoral, illegal and pathological in different cultures and at different times, whereas those between women have been ignored, ridiculed, politicized,

accepted, encouraged and celebrated. Similarly, paedophilia has been, and still is, variously defined according to a wide range in the age of sexual consent in different societies—both historical and contemporaneous. Heterosexuality, although a social norm in most societies, is circumscribed heavily by restrictions on its expression in many, for example within marriage, caste or ethnic group or by the relative age differentials of the partners. The social regulation of sexual expression is usually strict, whether by law or social sanction. In many cases, it is so strict that individuals will hide or deny any sexual feelings that do not conform to approved sexual stereotypes, or may only express those feelings covertly. This strong social and self-censorship makes research in the area of sexuality very difficult. People may lie, distort or remember selectively in retrospective studies using questionnaires or interviews. Even in prospective studies, the behaviour and attitudes observed and recorded may reflect a strong impact of social expectations, as we will see in the next two sections, which consider how we acquire sexual identities.

Genetics, brain anatomy, androgens and social learning have all been implicated in the formation of sexualities

Given the wide range of erotic stimuli, it would seem very unlikely that there is a direct genetic basis for our sexualities. It is difficult to see why evolution should have selected genes for fetishistic transvestism. It would be more reasonable to expect that evolution might have selected genes that encouraged sexual arousal in general and by the opposite sex in particular, since that would presumably promote the most effective transmission of those same genes to future generations. So might there be something qualitatively different about the basis of sexual arousal by people as stimuli as opposed to by objects or situations? There is little clear evidence on this point. However, just as in humans there appears to be considerable emancipation of our gender from our genes, such that social learning plays a larger role, so the same may have happened with our sexuality. There may be evolutionary advantages to flexible and adaptive social and sexual structures that came with this emancipation. Thus, whether or not there are genetic or anatomical correlates and even causes of human sexualities, there seems likely to be an element of social learning too. As with gender identity, it is difficult to disentangle the threads.

Twin and familial studies have suggested that there may be a genetic element in the establishment of our sexuality—a finding much trumpeted in the popular press. However, the results are far from decisive. The studies have focused almost exclusively on the question of how male homosexuality is determined. Monozygotic twins are reported to show a higher concordance of homosexuality than same-sex dizygotic twins. However, this finding does not demonstrate a 'gene for sexuality'. Indeed, although some familial studies have suggested that some homosexual men are more likely to carry a particular set of genetic markers on the X chromosome, none of these results has been confirmed in other studies. Caution is required in interpreting these sorts of genetic study of complex behavioural traits. Thus, genetically more similar individuals are likely to share common experiences because they have similar characteristics. This might predispose them to responses more likely to lead to development of a particular sexuality. Imagine that our sexuality is learnt in early childhood. The way in which it is learnt may depend on the maturation of the nervous system as well as the social surroundings. Imagine a gene or genes that advanced slightly the maturation of one part of the nervous system over another part. That might change the learning pattern and so influence the probability of a particular sexuality developing. This hypothetical scenario is presented to illustrate that, although there must be a *genetic influence* on sexuality, this does not mean that there is a *genetic cause*. The origins of sexuality are likely to be more complex and multifactorial.

A second line of evidence comes from studies on the structure of the brain. Earlier, examples were given of suggested sexual dimorphism in brain structure and organization in humans. There are reports that the 3rd interstitial nucleus of the anterior hypothalamus (INAH3), which is larger in men than in women, is of intermediate size in the brains of self-declaring homosexual men. However, the number of men in the studies is small and the overlap in the size values between gay men and non-gay men is too great to be significant in some studies. The validity of these much publicized claims needs to be established more carefully. If they do prove to be true, then the origins and time of development of the size differences must be established. At present, the evidence certainly does not warrant any suggestion that size differences in hypothalamic nuclei either cause or are caused by homosexuality. There are no experimental data from animals to suggest a direct relationship between this area of the brain and something as complex as homosexual orientation and behaviour. Indeed, studies in animals (see Chapter 8) suggest this to be very unlikely, as this hypothalamic area appears to be much more concerned with the organization of copulatory reflexes than with the expression of partner preference.

Since, in animals, some hypothalamic nuclei differ in size as a result of perinatal androgen exposure, is there any evidence linking exposure to androgens to sexual attraction towards women? We have the same problems here that we encountered when considering androgens and gender development. However, although women who have adrenogenital syndrome do show a higher incidence of attrac-

tion towards other women, *most* such women have a heterosexual attraction to men. Numerous other women with *no* evidence of androgen exposure are attracted to women. Conversely, gay men show no evidence of reduced androgens in comparison with heterosexual men. So androgens seem unlikely to cause lesbianism, although they might predispose to it indirectly, and lack of androgens is unlikely to cause male homosexuality.

So where does social learning fit? There is some evidence from work on paraphilias and fetishisms relating sexual arousal experiences in early childhood to the stimuli likely to arouse in the adult: associative learning. Children do show evidence of arousal, such as phallic erection, from an early age, and seem to derive pleasure from phallic stimulation. It is possible that the coincidence of arousal with an emotionally charged event or object in childhood might lead to the association of eroticism with that event or object in later life. However, the evidence on this point is far from clear, and we simply do not know how we become eroticized to particular stimuli. The question of social learning in the development of sexuality is considered further in the next section.

The relationship between sexuality and gender

Highly gendered societies, in which heterosexuality is the social norm and homosexuality is disapproved of, place a strong emphasis on the link between gender and heterosexuality. Thus, an integral part of being feminine is to be attracted to men and of being masculine is to be attracted to women. A heterosexual identity thus becomes subsumed into a gender identity such that the two are conflated conceptually. This conflation is evident in the sexual stereotypes of traditional Judaeo-Christian-Islamic societies. Thus, *masculine men* are seen as sexually dominant, active, insertive and initiating whereas *feminine women* are sexually passive, receptive and submissive. Deviations from these stereotypes are stigmatized, witness the stereotypes of the sexually passive, effeminate and 'unmanned' gay and the sexually aggressive, masculine and defeminized lesbian. However, in practice heterosexual individuals show a much wider range of astereotypical sexual behaviours and, as we have already seen, heterosexuality need not be 'pure' but can coexist within an individual with wider sexual interests such as sadomasochism, paraphilias and bisexuality. Moreover, although some gay men and lesbians may have insecure gender identities as men and women and may indeed conform to effeminate and butch stereotypes, respectively, many others, especially those who are confident of their homosexuality (are 'out'), do not. There are many gay men who are both homosexual and masculine, and lesbians who are both homosexual and feminine. Insecurity of gender identity for homosexuals is, of course, a likely outcome in a society in which sexual and gender stereotypes are conflated and variation from accepted gender and sexual stereotypes is stigmatized. In other societies, in which this conflation of gender and sexuality does not occur, there appears little problem in masculine men and feminine women expressing homosexual emotions and behaviour. In this regard, the transgendered are again instructive. Both male-to-female and female-to-male transgendered individuals may find men, women or both sexually arousing. Thus, a transgendered individual of the male sex with a feminine gender identity may find men sexually attractive, in which case he is homosexual before surgery and hormone treatment and she is heterosexual afterwards. Trans people emphasize the importance of uncoupling sexuality from gender conceptually, even if in Judaeo-Christian and Islamic cultures they have been conflated socially.

The conflation of sexuality and gender further complicates study of the possible social learning of sexuality. A number of retrospective studies suggest that gays and lesbians recall having more ambiguous gender experiences in childhood than do self-defining heterosexual men and women. For example, gay men recalled playing with girls and girls' toys and games, and lesbians recalled being tomboyish. However, retrospective studies suffer from the dangers of selective recall and denial, which, as we saw earlier, is a dangerous possibility in an area as sensitive as this. Prospective studies of children referred to clinicians precisely because they were displaying gender-atypical play patterns have shown that as adults these individuals manifest a higher incidence of homosexuality than control children. It is difficult to know how to interpret these findings, especially as they are based on children so seriously different (or perceived to be so) as to be referred to a gender clinic. Precisely because society, parents and children themselves associate gender and sexual stereotypes, they are more likely to develop in tandem: there is after all the basis of a socially learned element to each. The results do not mean that they *must* develop in tandem or that having one identity *causes* a person to have the other (in either direction).

Summary

We do not understand how people acquire a sexual identity. Indeed, our understanding of the complex nature of sexual identity is incomplete. Our systems for classifying sexuality are at best approximate and still based largely on a historical view of all sexual deviation from a narrowly defined heterosexuality as being pathological and socially undesirable. This is not a helpful starting point for looking at the natural expression of sexuality. There undoubtedly are influences of genes, hormones, brain structure and social learning on how our sexualities develop, but there is

little evidence that any one of these actually causes each of us to have a particular sexual identity. The fact that different societies construct different systems of sexual stereotypes and that these become absorbed (internalized) through social learning into each individual's sexual identity implies that social learning must play a large part in the construction of sexuality, perhaps building on or interacting with the various influences of genes and hormones to affect brain function and structure.

It is perhaps not surprising that the relatively simple rules governing the development of sex differences in the behaviour of rodents cannot easily be applied to primates and humans. The finding in animals that exposure to androgens during a critical period of early life both alters the structure of the brain and affects patterns of sex-dependent and sexual behaviour in adulthood, does not find a simple counterpart in monkeys or humans. In both the latter species, behavioural evidence of the effects of exposure of the fetal female brain to androgens is present in the form of sexually dimorphic childhood behaviour, but affected individuals can display apparently typical patterns of feminine gender identity and heterosexual behaviour as adults. Sex assignment at birth and the subsequent gender-specific patterns of social behaviours and interactions that flow from gender and sexual stereotypes seem to play a major role in shaping behavioural dimorphism, gender identity and sexual identity.

In these first two chapters, we have examined both the foundations of sexual reproduction in mammals and the many and wide-ranging aspects of the social life of mammals that flow from them. In subsequent chapters, we will look at the physiological processes regulating fertility and sexual behaviour that result in conception, pregnancy, parturition, lactation and maternal care.

FURTHER READING

General reading

Golombok S, Fivush R (1994) *Gender Development*. Cambridge University Press, Cambridge (an excellent account of gender development, despite its age).

Hinde R (1996) Gender differences in close relationships. In: *Social Interaction and Personal Relationships* (ed. D. Miell & R. Dallos), pp. 324–335. Sage, London (an account of gender relationship patterns by an eminent behavioural scientist).

Hines M (2004) *Brain Gender*. Oxford University Press, Oxford (a measured account of the behavioural and neuroanatomical studies on sex and gender).

More advanced reading (see also Boxes)

Bancroft J (1989) *Human Sexuality and its Problems*. Churchill Livingstone, London (despite its age, a rich repository in which to dip).

KEY LEARNING POINTS

- Gender is a system of classification based on sex.

- A gender stereotype is a set of social beliefs about what it means to be a man or a woman. It may include appearance, behaviour, role (social, sexual and employment) and emotional and attitudinal attributes. It provides a shorthand for classifying people socially by sex.

- A gender identity is an inner state of awareness of one's own identity as a man or a woman in society. It is usually congruent with one's sex. Trans people have a gender identity that is not congruent with their sex.

- Although gender is a bipolar system based on two distinct sexes, when gender differences are measured in populations of men and women they are not found to be bipolar. Indeed, most attributes show large overlap between genders and none are reliably predictive of gender.

- In non-primate animals, hormones condition sex differences in both brain structure and behaviour. However, the behavioural differences are not absolute but quantitative.

- In higher primates and humans, there is evidence of differences in brain structure between both the sexes and the genders but these differences are not large and their cause is unknown. Likewise it is not clear whether the differences have any direct effect on behaviour.

- The hormonal environment of higher primate and human fetuses and neonates has some effects on behaviour in infancy, some of which may persist into adult life. It is not known how these endocrine effects are exerted. It is not clear whether they are exerted directly on the brain, indirectly via effects on, for example, genital anatomy, or by a combination of both routes. The effects are not absolute but quantitative.

- In humans, the newborn baby is treated differently from the moment of its birth according to its perceived gender.

- In humans, the behaviour of a baby is interpreted to mean different things depending on its perceived gender.

- Babies of different sexes seem to show different behaviours quite early in neonatal life, but it is not clear whether the origin of these differences is endocrine, genetic, socially learnt or a mixture of all three.

- Human infants establish a gender identity by 3 years of age and start to develop a gender stereotype shortly thereafter. They develop a sense of gender constancy by 5 years of age. They then develop the expression of their gender identity by copying the sex-stereotyped behaviour that they observe around them.

- Gender stereotypes in most societies include reproductive roles and share attributes relevant to these reproductive roles. However, gender stereotypes are not limited to reproduction and reflect the fact that in humans sexual activity is not exclusively or even primarily a reproductive activity. There appears to be a large element of social learning in the construction of gender stereotypes and identities, and this forms part of the cultural inheritance that is transmitted transgenerationally.

- Sexuality involves the erotic and may be classified by the stimulus of erotic arousal. This system of classification is unsatisfactorily rigid. Many people find a range of stimuli arousing and the range may change with time. Asexual people are not aroused erotically.

- A sexual stereotype is the constellation of attributes and behaviours associated with people whose erotic arousal is classified according to a particular type of stimulus.

- The sexual identity of a person describes their inner state of feeling as a sexual being.

- Genes, brain structure, hormones and social learning have all been implicated in the development of sexuality, but there is no clear evidence directly linking any one element causally to a particular sexual identity.

- In some societies, attributes of sexuality and gender have been conflated implying that heterosexual arousal and a strong sense of gender identity are linked.

- Anthropological and social studies, as well as studies on trans people, show that it is possible to separate out sexuality from gender identity.

Berenbaum SA, Bailey JM (2003) Effects on gender identity of prenatal androgens and genital appearance: evidence from girls with Congenital Adrenal Hyperplasia. *Journal of Clinical Endocrinology & Metabolism* **88**, 1102–1106 (studies on AGS girls/women that suggest no simple link between either androgen exposure or genital masculinization and the defeminization of identity).

Byne W *et al.* (2001) The interstitial nuclei of the human anterior hypothalamus: an investigation of variation with sex, sexual orientation, and HIV status. *Hormones and Behavior* **40**, 86–92 (a study that confirms a correlation between brain structure and sex, but not with sexuality).

Chau P-L, Herring J (2004) Men, women, people: the definition of sex. In: *Sexuality Repositioned: Diversity and the Law* (ed. B. Brooks-Gordon *et al.*), pp. 187–214. Hart Publishing, Oxford (reviews legal and historical approaches to intersex people).

Deaux K (1985) Sex and gender. *Annual Review of Psychology* **36**, 49–81 (a classic text on gender).

Good CD *et al.* (2003) Dosage-sensitive X-linked locus influences the development of amygdala and orbitofrontal cortex, and fear recognition in humans. *Brain* **126**, 2431–2446 (brain sex and chromosomal constitution).

Dixson AF (1998) *Primate Sexuality: Comparative Studies of the Prosimians, Monkeys, Apes and Human Beings.* Oxford University Press, Oxford (a classic text comparing sexual behaviours of different primates; dip into it highly selectively).

Greenberg JA (2002) Deconstructing binary race and sex categories: a comparison of the multiracial and transgendered experience. *San Diego Law Review* **39**, 917–942 (an interesting legal analysis of sex and gender in relation to biology, using race as a comparator).

Johnson MH (2004) A biological perspective on sexuality. In: *Sexuality Repositioned: Diversity and the Law* (ed. B. Brooks-Gordon *et al.*), pp. 155–186. Hart Publishing, Oxford (reviews studies on the origins and nature of sexuality, focusing on homo- and heterosexuality).

Kruijver FPM *et al.* (2000) Male-to-female transsexuals have female neuron numbers in a limbic nucleus. *Journal of Clinical Endo-crinology & Metabolism* **85**, 2034–2041 (a study claiming a correlation between brain structure and gender).

McDowell L (2004) Sexuality, desire and embodied performances in the workplace. In: *Sexuality Repositioned: Diversity and the Law* (ed. B. Brooks-Gordon *et al.*), pp. 85–108. Hart Publishing, Oxford (provides an example of how gender stereotypes mutate in a changing society, by examining the roles of men and women in the workplace).

Mustanski BS *et al.* (2005) A genomewide scan of male sexual orientation. *Human Genetics* **116**, 272–278 (a recent example of a study looking for a genetic basis for homosexuality).

Pasterski VL *et al.* (2005) Prenatal hormones and postnatal socialization by parents as determinants of male-typical toy play in girls with congenital adrenal hyperplasia. *Child Development* **76**, 264–278 (a paper that attempts to distinguish social and endocrine influences on gender attributes).

Zhou JN *et al.* (1995) A sex difference in the human brain and its relation to transexuality. *Nature* **378**, 68–70.

3 Reproductive Messengers

In Chapter 1 we saw that the gonads are the pivotal organs in the reproductive process, translating genetic sex into phenotypic sex. This translation is mediated by the chemical messengers: androgens, Müllerian inhibiting hormone (MIH) and insulin-like growth factor 3 (Insl3). These messengers provide three examples from a large and diverse family of *hormones*, which mediate a complex network of communication within the reproductive system, some of the main routes of which are shown in Fig. 3.1. Each of these routes will be considered in more detail in later chapters. In this chapter, the main hormones themselves will be introduced and some general principles underlying their activities explained.

Hormones act at variable distances from the cells that produce them

Coordination of function within the body requires effective communication over a range of distances. A variety of hormonal secretion and transport patterns has developed to meet these needs. For example, in Chapter 2 we saw that androgens produced by the testis influence the structure and function of the rat brain. To achieve these pervasive effects, the steroids are secreted into the bloodstream, in which they are distributed rapidly throughout the tissues of the body. This secretory process is called *endocrine*, meaning literally 'secreted inwards'. However, not all steroid actions are achieved in this way. For example, androgens and oestrogens within the adult testis also pass into the fluids within its duct system (the seminiferous tubules), in which they are carried to the epididymis and vas deferens (see Chapters 4 & 9). In this cases, these hormones exert more localized actions within the duct systems themselves. This sort of secretion is termed *exocrine*, meaning 'secreted outwards'.

Hormones can also act very close to their site of secretion on adjacent cells and tissues. For example, MIH, Insl3 and androgens influence the differentiation of the internal genital primordia by local diffusion from the fetal testis (Chapter 1). In this case, the secretion is said to be *paracrine*, or acting 'close by'. Indeed, hormones secreted by a cell may act back on the same cell to influence its own function. This autostimulation is described as *autocrine* activity. Finally, some hormones, which in certain circumstances can be released from a cell to act on other cells at a distance, can sometimes appear anchored to the surface of the secreting cell, in which case they can act on adjacent cells only. This latter very localized action has been termed *juxtacrine*. This versatility of hormones is well captured in members of the *epidermal growth factor* (EGF) family. These are

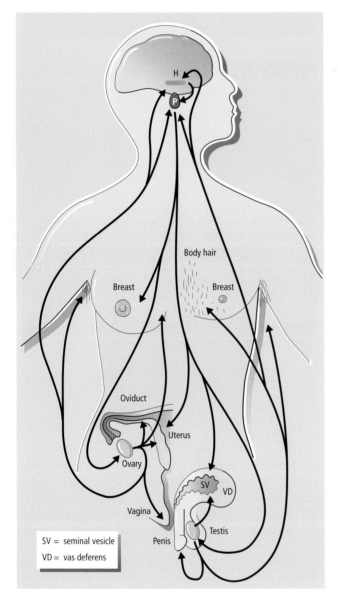

Fig. 3.1 A schematic view of the main routes of communication by chemical messengers within the reproductive system. The hypothalamic region (H) of the brain influences the pituitary gland (P), which in turn influences the breasts (Chapter 14), the uterus, cervix and seminal vesicle (Chapters 8 & 13) and the gonads: testis and ovary (Chapters 4 & 5). The gonads themselves exert feedback influences on the pituitary and brain (see Chapters 6 & 7 for details). The gonads also influence multiple sites in the internal and external genitalia (Chapters 8–14), and at least some of these sites send feedback messages to the gonads directly or indirectly. Finally, in a number of tissues or organs messages are passed around internally between different cell types or even fed back on the very cells that produced them (see e.g. Chapter 5).

membrane-anchored molecules, the outer portion of which can be cleaved by metalloproteinases, to be released locally or systemically. EGFs thereby act auto-, juxta-, para- *and* endocrinologically!

Clearly, from what we have seen already, the same hormone can use a variety of routes 'to spread the message'. Whether it acts locally or pervasively will depend not only on the *nature* and *direction* of its secretion, but also on the *blood supply* of its secreting tissue and the *solubility* of the hormone itself in the fluids bathing this tissue. These latter points will be considered after the main hormones themselves have been introduced.

Hormones can be classified into three main chemical classes

The hormones involved in reproductive activity can be subdivided broadly into lipids, proteins and monoamines. In this section, the main family members of each of these classes of hormone are introduced and their general properties described. Detailed discussion of their actions and the control of their production follows in later chapters, as indicated in the text and tables.

Lipids

There are two classes of lipid-based reproductive hormones, the *steroids* and the *eicosanoids*. Lipids are in general less soluble in the aqueous fluids of the body than are proteins and monoamines. They therefore tend to partition preferentially to hydrophobic environments such as cells and are often either modified for transport through the body fluid or carried on transporters (see later).

Steroids

The steroid hormones comprise a large group of molecules all derived from a common sterol precursor: *cholesterol* (Fig. 3.2). Cholesterol is synthesized from acetate in many tissues of the body, and is an important structural component of cell membranes. Indeed, if the cholesterol content of mammalian cells is manipulated to abnormal levels experimentally or varies pathologically, then the cell membranes malfunction, destabilize and rupture more easily. In steroidogenic tissues, most of the steroid output is derived from acetate with cholesterol as an intermediate product (Fig. 3.2). Cholesterol itself can also be used as a starting substrate, being acquired either from intracellular stores of esterified cholesterol or from cholesterol circulating in the blood.

The pathway for steroid biosynthesis from cholesterol is illustrated in Fig. 3.3, which also provides a visual framework of the molecular relationships of the different steroid family members. The conversion of cholesterol to *pregne-*

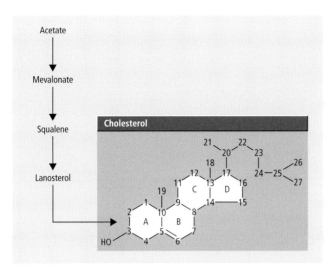

Acetate

↓

Mevalonate

↓

Squalene

↓

Lanosterol

Cholesterol

Fig. 3.2 The basic structure of the cholesterol molecule. Each of the 27 carbon atoms is assigned a number, and each ring a letter. The individual carbon atoms are simply carrying hydrogen atoms unless otherwise indicated (e.g. C-1 and C-19 are –CH_2– and –CH_3 residues, whereas C-3 is –CHOH–). Cholesterol is converted to pregnenolone by cleavage of the terminal 6 carbons, leaving a steroid nucleus of 21 carbons. This conversion occurs within the mitochondria, and requires NADPH and oxygen.

nolone marks the first and common step in the formation of all the major steroid hormones. This conversion is rate-limiting and therefore an important point of regulation. The conversion occurs on the inner mitochondrial membrane and requires NADPH, oxygen and cytochrome P-450. Pregnenolone is then converted to the sex steroids in the adjacent smooth endoplasmic reticulum. There are four main families of steroid: the *progestagens, androgens, oestrogens* (American spelling estrogens) and *corticosteroids* (Fig. 3.3), of which only the first three are regarded as the sex steroids. Although there are three distinctive classes of sex steroids, they are related structurally to each other. Indeed, they can be seen as different generations of a biosynthetic family, the progestagens being 'grandparental' and the androgens being 'parental' to the oestrogens (Fig. 3.3). Interconversion from one class of steroid to another is undertaken by a series of enzymes arranged together as a *biosynthetic unit*, taking in substrate and passing the molecule along a production line with little 'leakage' of any intermediates. For example, the enzymes 17α-hydroxylase, 17,20-desmolase, 17-ketosteroid reductase and 3β-hydroxy steroid dehydrogenase would form an enzyme package for the synthesis of testosterone from pregnenolone.

The close relationship of the different classes of steroids means that an enzymatic defect at one point in the synthetic pathway may have far-reaching effects. For example, not uncommon genetic deficiencies in the fetal adrenal gland are reduced activity of 21α-hydroxylase (which converts 17α-hydroxyprogesterone to 11-desoxycortisol; Fig. 3.3) or of 11β-hydroxylase (which converts 11-desoxycortisol to cortisol). In either case, there is a resulting deficiency of corticosteroids which leads to further compensatory stimulation of the corticosteroid biosynthetic path (*congenital adrenal hyperplasia*), which in turn leads to the accumulation of high levels of 17α-hydroxyprogesterone. This steroid is then converted by 17,20-desmolase to androgen, which masculinizes female fetuses (see Chapters 1 and 2, adrenogenital syndrome). Conversely, genetic deficiency of 17,20-desmolase itself results in depressed androgen output, and the failure of male fetuses to masculinize.

Within each class of sex steroids there are several natural members. There are two criteria for membership of each class: similarity of chemical structure and sharing of common functional properties. Structurally, natural progestagens are characterized by 21 carbons (C_{21} steroids), a double bond between C4 and C5, a β-acetyl at C17 and a β-methyl at C13. Natural androgens are characterized by 19 carbons (C_{19} steroids); strong androgenic activity is associated with a β-hydroxylated C17 and a ketone structure (–C=O) at C3. Natural oestrogens have 18 carbons (C_{18} steroids), an aromatized A ring hydroxylated at C3, and a β-hydroxyl group at C17.

The structural features shared by members of each steroid class are reflected in common functional properties. Tables 3.1–3.3 summarize the principal natural progestagens, androgens and oestrogens, together with some of the functional characteristics of each class. It is commonly said that progestagens are associated with the preparations for pregnancy and its maintenance, androgens with the development and maintenance of male characteristics and fertility, and oestrogens with the development and maintenance of female characteristics and fertility. Although broadly correct, this statement is a simplification, and we will encounter a number of exceptions, for example, androgens stimulate secondary sex patterns and behaviour in females (Chapters 7 & 8) and oestrogens stimulate epididymal function in males (Chapter 9).

Eicosanoids

The eicosanoids comprise two major classes of messenger: the *prostaglandins* (PGs), which are of principal interest for reproductive processes, and the *leukotrienes*, which play a lesser role. The pathway of their biosynthesis is shown in Fig. 3.4. The essential polyunsaturated fatty acid, *arachidonic acid*, is the common precursor. It is derived from glycerophospholipids in the cell membranes by the actions of two enzymes: *phospholipase A2* (PLA_2, acting primarily on phosphatidyl-choline and phosphatidyl-ethanolamine); and *phospholipase C* (PLC, acting on phosphatidyl-inositol). Arachidonic acid is converted to the leukotrienes by the

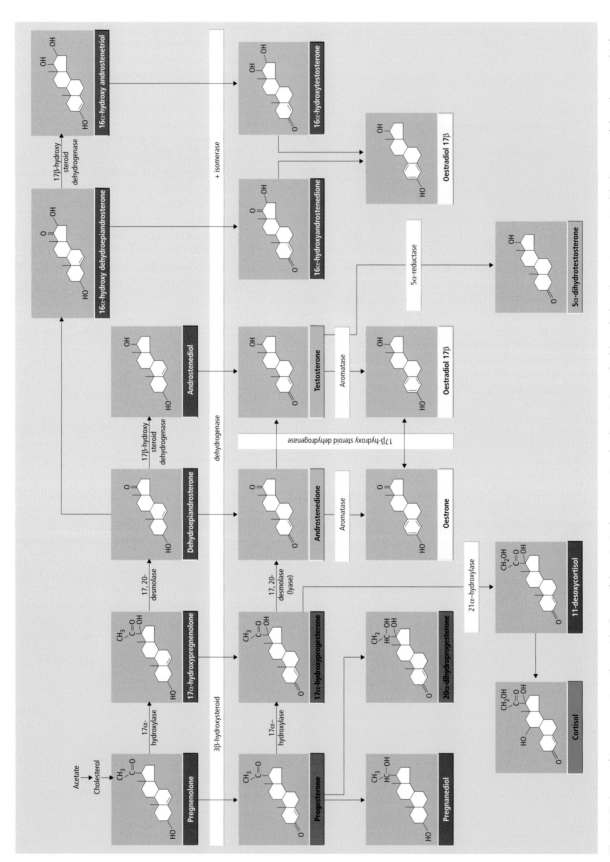

Fig. 3.3 Pathway of interconversion of steroids. Some of the principal enzymes involved are indicated, although the scheme is very simplified, many of them have multiple isoforms. Note that extensive interconversions are possible; however, in any given tissue, absence of certain enzymes will mean that only parts of the matrix will be completed. Clearly, the enzymes present will therefore determine which steroids can and cannot be made from which available substrates. The members of the four major classes of sex steroids are shown with distinct colour bars: progestagens, red; androgens, green; oestrogens, yellow; and corticosteroids, blue. Note that in steroid terminology the suffixes denote the following: -ol = hydroxyl group; -diol = two hydroxyl groups; -one = ketone group; -dione = two ketone groups. An unsaturated —C-C-link is indicated by -ene; two such links are indicated by -diene. Note also that aromatase denotes 19-hydroxysteroid dehydrogenase + C-10,19 lyase.

Table 3.1 Principal properties of natural progestagens and their receptors.*

Progestagens	Relative potency (%)	Some key properties	Receptors
Progesterone (P4)	100	1 Prepare uterus to receive conceptus	Two isoforms PR-A and –B, sharing 780 identical amino acids, but with PR-B having an additional 164 amino acids. Each receptor, on binding P4, transcriptionally activates different genes by binding to sequences in their promoters.
17α-Hydroxyprogesterone (17α-OHP)	40–70	2 Maintain uterus during pregnancy	
20α-Hydroxyprogesterone (20α-dihydroprogesterone or 20α-OHP)	5	3 Stimulate growth of mammary glands, but suppress secretion of milk	
		4 Mild effect on sodium loss via distal convoluted tubule of kidney	
		5 General mild catabolic effect	
		6 Regulate secretion of gonadotrophins	

*In Tables 3.1–3.3 the relative potencies are only approximate since they vary with species and with the assay used. This variation is due partly to differences in the relative affinity of receptors in different tissues, partly to differences in local enzymic conversions of steroids within tissues and partly to differences in systemic metabolism: see text for discussion of these factors. Common abbreviations or alternative names encountered in the literature are also recorded in Tables 3.1–3.3.

Table 3.2 Principal properties of natural androgens.*

Androgens	Relative potency (%)	Some key properties	Receptor
5α-dihydrotestosterone (DHT)	100	1 Induce and maintain differentiation of male somatic tissues	A single androgen receptor isoform, AR, of 918 amino acids
Testosterone (T)	50	2 Induce secondary sex characters of males (deep voice, body hair, penile growth) and body hair of females	
Androstenedione (A 4)	8	3 Induce and maintain some secondary sex characters of males (accessory sex organs)	
Dehydroepiandrosterone (DHEA)	4	4 Support spermatogenesis	
		5 Influence sexual and aggressive behaviour in males and females	
		6 Promote protein anabolism, somatic growth and ossification	
		7 Regulate secretion of gonadotrophins(testosterone)	
		8 Anticorticosteroid effects (DHEA)	

*As for Table 3.1.

action of cytosolic *5-lipoxygenase*, and to the prostaglandins by the microsomal *cyclooxygenases 1 and 2* (*cox 1 and cox2*; Fig. 3.4). The rate-limiting step appears to be the availability of arachidonic acid, which thus forms the principal control point, exerted mainly by varying the activity of PLA_2. This enzyme is present in an inactive membrane-bound form in lysosomes, and its release and activation depend primarily on reduction of the stability of the lysosomal membranes. The type of prostaglandin synthesized varies in different tissues at different times, as a result of variation in the relative activities of the downstream enzymes.

Table 3.3 Principal properties of natural oestrogens.*

Oestrogens	Relative potency (%)	Some key properties	Receptors
Oestradiol 17β (estradiol or E_2)	100	1 Stimulate secondary sex characters of female 2 Prepare uterus for spermatozoal transport 3 Increase vascular permeability and tissue oedema	Two receptors exist, ERα (c.595 amino acids) and ERβ, which has several isoforms arising from slice variants giving a size range of c.480–530 amino acids.
Oestriol (estriol or E_3)	10	4 Stimulate growth and activity of mammary gland and endometrium	
Oestrone (estrone or E_1)	1	5 Prepare endometrium for progestagen action 6 Mildly anabolic; stimulate calcification 7 Active during pregnancy 8 Regulate secretion of gonadotrophins 9 Associated with sexual behaviour in some species	

*As for Table 3.1.

PGs are synthesized in most tissues of the body, including the ovary and the uterine myometrium, cervix, ovary, placenta and fetal membranes (see Chapters 5, 10, 11 & 13). They have half-lives of the order of 3–10 min, and so act mainly as local hormones, either paracrinologically or after a short passage through the local bloodstream. They are inactivated totally by a single passage through the systemic circulation, and particularly through the lungs.

Proteins

The protein hormones can be subgrouped into gonadotrophic glycoproteins, somatomammotrophic polypeptides, cytokines and small peptides.

Gonadotrophic glycoproteins

There are three gonadotrophins, so called because they stimulate the gonads, namely *follicle-stimulating hormone* (FSH), *luteinizing hormone* (LH) and *chorionic gonadotrophin* (CG) (Table 3.4). They are closely related to a fourth hormone, only indirectly involved in reproductive processes, called *thyroid-stimulating hormone* (TSH or *thryotrophin*). FSH, LH and TSH are produced in the pituitary gland, while CG is produced in the placenta. Each of these hormones is a heterodimeric globular protein consisting of two glycosylated polypeptides (α- and β-chains) linked non-covalently. The same α-chain is used in all four hormones, but the β-chain is unique to each, conferring most of the specific functional properties of each hormone. Each polypeptide has complex *O*- or *N*-linked carbohydrate side chains that are unique for each hormone (Table 3.4). The removal or modification of the carbohydrate side chains

does not appear to reduce appreciably binding to target receptors and indeed may even increase it. However, carbohydrate changes can influence hormone biosynthetic and secretion rates (*N*-linked), stability and half-life in the circulation (especially *O*-linked on tail of HCG), as well as the ability of the hormone to activate receptors after binding (*N*-linked). This latter property means that hormones lacking some carbohydrate chains can occupy receptors non-functionally and thereby act as *antagonists*. This property may be useful therapeutically and also important physiologically, because analysis of plasma and urinary gonadotrophins reveals a wide range of molecular sizes for each hormone that reflects modifications to the glycosylation pattern. Moreover, the balance of modifications varies under different conditions. Understanding the full functional importance of the variation and how it is controlled naturally is a current challenge for clinical research.

Somatomammotrophic polypeptides

This family is named for the pervasive effects its members have on tissue growth and function, including effects on the mammary gland. The family has three main members all evolved from an ancestoral gene through duplication and modification and so structurally and functionally related: *prolactin* (PRL), *placental lactogen* (PL; also called *placental somatomammotrophin*) and *growth hormone* (GH; also called *somatotrophin*). Each consists of a single polypeptide chain. PRL and PL are particularly concerned with lactation, GH plays a role in puberty, and a placental variant called GH-V is active in pregnancy (Table 3.5). However, in addition to these very specific reproductive functions, these polypeptides have a widespread, generally

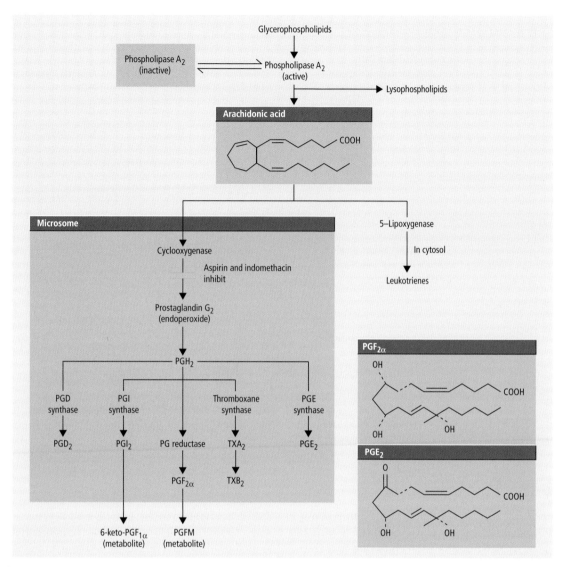

Fig. 3.4 Biosynthesis of prostaglandins (PGD_2, $PGF_{2\alpha}$ and PGE_2) and leukotrienes. The rate-limiting step is arachidonic acid availability. Factors such as steroids, which affect the activity of phospholipase A_2, are therefore critical determinants of the rate of PG synthesis. Cycloxoygenase has two isoforms: cox1 is constitutive and cox2 is inducible. Leukotrienes stimulate myometrial contractility; PGE_2 stimulates myometrial activity, cervical ripening and autocrine output of PGE_2 from the amnion; $PGF_{2\alpha}$ stimulates myometrial activity and cervical ripening; PGI_2 may inhibit myometrial activity and is essential for decidualization. Each PG can act either through intracellular nuclear peroxisome proliferator-activated receptors (PPARs) or through G-protein-coupled cell surface receptors specific for each PG (called PGE1–4 for PGE_2, FP for $PGF_{2\alpha}$, DP for PGD_2, IP for PGI_2 and TP for thromboxanes) Abbreviations: PGI_2 = prostacyclin; TXA_2 and TXB_2= thromboxane A_2 and B_2. Box lower right shows PG structure.

supportive role, helping other hormones to achieve their effects more fully and influence growth, angiogenesis, immune regulation, and metabolism. In this way, they resemble cytokines, with which they also share a similar mode of interaction with their target cells.

Cytokines

Cytokines are also polypeptides, having one or two chains, and molecular weights usually less than 100 kDa. Conven-

tionally, they are distinguished from the 'classical' protein hormones (gonadotrophic glycoproteins and somatomammotrophic polypeptides, described above) by several criteria: (1) they are made in a variety of cell types, not a defined gland; (2) they act on a multiplicity of target cell types; (3) different cytokines interact to modulate each other's effects; (4) several cytokines may have identical or overlapping effects, that is, they show considerable *functional redundancy*; (5) they tend to act mainly in an autocrine, paracrine

Table 3.4 Properties of human gonadotrophins.

	Luteinizing hormone (LH) (also called Lutropin; interstitial cell-stimulating hormone (ICSH))	Follicle-stimulating hormone (FSH) (also called Follitropin)	Chorionic gonadotrophin (CG)
Secreted from	Anterior pituitary gonadotrophs	Anterior pituitary gonadotrophs	Placental trophoblast
Acts upon	Leydig cells (Ch. 4)	Sertoli cells (Ch. 4)	Luteal cells (Ch. 11 & 12)
	Thecal cells—antral follicles (Ch. 5)	Granulosa cells—follicles (Ch. 5)	
	Granulosa cells—preovulatory follicles (Ch. 5)		
	Luteal cells—corpus luteum (Ch. 5)		
	Interstitial glands of ovary (Ch. 5)		
Molecular mass (kDa)	c.28	c.28	c.37
Composition	α-chain* (92 aminoacids and 2 N-linked[1] carbohydrate chains; β-chain† 121 amino acids and one N-linked carbohydrate chain	α-chain* as LH; β-chain† 111 amino acids and 2 N-linked[1] carbohydrate chains	α-chain* as LH; β-chain† of 150 amino acids (a 29 carboxy addition to LHβ) with 2 N-linked[1] + O-linked[1] carbohydrate chains
Receptor	85–92 kDa glycoprotein; G-protein coupled; adenyl cyclase linked	75 kDa (675aa) receptor that dimerizes on FSH binding; G-protein coupled; adenyl cyclase linked	As for LH

*The common or backbone subunit chain—encoded in a single gene with four exons on chromosome 6.
†The subunit chain conferring specificity. For LH and FSH, single genes on chromosome 19. For CG, three genes expressed and three with low activity, all on chromosome 19; three exons in each. There is 80% homology between the common parts of CG and LH β-chains, but only 36% homology between LH and FSH β-chains.
[1]O-linked carbohydrate chains are attached to a serine or threonine residue via N-acetylgalactosamine; N-linked chains to asparagines via N-acetylglucosamine.

and/or juxtacrine way, and less often in an endocrine way; and (6) they often seem to function to modulate or mediate the actions of more conventionally endocrine hormones, such as LH and FSH. However, as more is being learnt about both cytokines and classical hormones, these distinctions become increasingly blurred. For example, *inhibin* is a cytokine that functions in both endocrine and paracrine roles in reproduction (see below), and we have already mentioned the resemblance that the somatomammo-trophins have to cytokines.

Like the steroids, cytokines can be grouped into families on the basis of both their molecular structure and their overlapping activities. The main cytokine families and their members relevant for reproductive processes are recorded in Table 3.6. Note that many of the cytokines have names that appear unconnected with reproduction. This apparent anomaly reflects the wide range of effects that cytokines have in many tissues, and often they were named after the first tissue or function by which they were discovered (e.g. bone morphogenetic protein and leukaemia inhibitory factor). Note also that we have already encountered two of these cytokines (MIH and

Insl3) in Chapter 1. The *inhibins* and *activins* are in the same family as MIH, and form a series of heterodimers from three basic subunits made on three genes, one encoding an α-subunit and two encoding β-subunits as shown in Fig. 3.5.

Small peptides
There are four small peptides that have important roles in reproduction. Each of them is made in the form of a larger polypeptide precursor, the active hormone (or hormones) being cleaved out just before they are secreted.

Gonadotrophin-releasing hormone (GnRH) is a member of a large family of peptides, produced in neurosecretory cells in a part of the brain called the *hypothalamus* (see Fig. 3.1 & Chapter 6). The family also includes releasing hormones for thryotrophin, corticotrophin and somatotrophin and, as their names imply, they are concerned with release of these hormones from cells in the *anterior pituitary*. GnRH is a decapeptide derived by cleavage from a larger precursor called *prepro-GnRH* (Fig. 3.6).

Oxytocin is a nonapeptide, which is also mainly produced by neurons in the hypothalamus. Like *arginine vaso-*

Table 3.5 Properties of human somatomammotrophic polypeptides.

	Prolactin (PRL)	Placental lactogen (PL) (also called Chorionic somatomammotrophin (CSA1/2))	Growth hormone (GH-N) (also called Somatotrophin; also GH-V, a second GH placental gene)
Secreted	Anterior pituitary lactotrophs and placental deciduas + other tissues	Cytotrophoblast to week 6, then syncytiotrophoblast + invasive mononuclear trophoblast. (In farm animals, binucleate cells)	Ant. pituitary somatotrophs (GH-N) Syncytial trophoblast placental variant (GH-V) + 3 chorionic somatomammotrophin-like CSA, B and L; Act via IGF system (Table 3.6)
Acts upon	Leydig cells (Ch. 4) Seminal vesicle and prostate (Ch. 8) Ovarian follicles (Ch. 5) Corpus luteum (Ch. 5) Mammary gland (Ch. 14) Amnion (Ch. 12)	Maternal intermediary metabolism (Ch. 11 & 12) Mammary gland (Ch. 14) Fetal growth (Ch. 12) (In farm animals, glands in pregnancy Ch. 11)	General follicle support (Ch. 5) Puberty (Ch. 7) Breast development (Ch. 14) (In farm animals, glands in pregnancy Ch. 11) CS genes of uncertain function
Molecular mass (kDa)	23 (isoforms of 25, 16, 50–60, 100 kDa by splicing, post-translational modification and aggregation)	22 kDa (Several prolactin-like proteins or PLPs also made in placenta, as are proliferin and proliferin-related protein, PRP)	GH-N 22 kDa, 121 aa; GH-V 22 kDa, 121 aa (93% homology with GH-N but with an N-linked glycosylated form of 25 kDa)
Composition	Single polypeptide chain of 199 aas. Post-translationally modified → multiple isoforms	Single polypeptide chain of 191 amino acids non-glycosylated (25% homology to PRL, 85% to GH)	191 amino acids (single glycosylation site in GH-V)
Genes	A single 10 kb gene on chr. 6 with 5 exons. Exon 1 only expressed in deciduas + other tissues	Two genes on chr. 17 (each with 5 exons) encoding same polypeptide	Two genes (5 exons each) on chr. 17 in PL cluster
Receptor	Binds PRL receptor: long and short forms (591 and 291 amino acids in the rat) by alternative splicing	Binds PRL-R (same affinity) and GH-R (affinity 1/2000 < GH)	Binds GH-R and PRL-R (GH-V binds PRL-R > GH-N and GH-R < GH-N)

pressin (AVP; also called *antidiuretic hormone*, ADH), a similar hormone with a less direct involvement in reproductive processes, oxytocin is transported along long neuronal processes from the hypothalamus into the *posterior pituitary* (Fig. 3.7c), where it is released into the blood to act on the uterus (see Chapter 13) and the mammary gland (see Chapter 14). Like GnRH, oxytocin and AVP are each derived from a larger precursor consisting of an N-terminal signal peptide (which is removed before packaging occurs), followed by the hormone itself and then a *neurophysin* sequence (shown for oxytocin in Fig. 3.7a). The neurophysin is able to bind oxytocin, and in this way the hormone is packaged for transport along the axon to the terminals of the neurons in the posterior pituitary. Neurophysin is

released, along with oxytocin, into the bloodstream, but it has no clear function in the body.

Recently, production of both GnRH and oxytocin has been identified at several other sites; for example, GnRH has been found in the placenta, ovary and other regions of the brain, and oxytocin has been found in the ovary, testis and uterus and widespread sites in the forebrain and brainstem. These findings have suggested a more diverse role for these hormones, or neurotransmitters, and this will be discussed later in the book.

The other important peptides that we will encounter are β-*endorphin* and *vasoactive intestinal peptide* (VIP), which is a member of the large *glucagon–secretin* peptide family and may be important in controlling the release of prolactin

Table 3.6 Cytokine families and family members (alternative names shown in brackets).

Families and members	Abbreviation	General structure (amino acids/kDa)	Receptor (R) type	Reproductive involvement
Epidermal growth factor family				
Epidermal GF	EGF	Single-chain glycoprotein Juxtacrine: 1207 aa Paracrine: 53 aa (6 kDa)	EGF-R (tyrosine kinase)	Follicular, pre- and postimplantation development (Ch. 5, 10 & 11); breast development (Ch. 14)
Transforming growth factor (44% homology with EGF)	TGF-α	Single-chain glycoprotein Juxtacrine: 160 aa Paracrine: 50 aa	EGF-R (tyrosine kinase)	Pre- and postimplantation development (Ch. 10); breast development (Ch. 14)
Heparin-binding EGF-like growth factor (41% homology with EGF)	HB-EGF	Single-chain glycoprotein Juxtacrine: 204 aa Paracrine: 22 kDa	EGF-R + heparan sulfate	Implantation (Ch. 10) (also amphiregulin, epiregulin, neuroregulin-1)
Insulin family				
Insulin		Disulfide-linked A and B chains, A 24 aa, B 29 aa	Insulin R	Preimplantation development (Ch. 10); fetal growth and development (Ch. 12); breast development (Ch. 14)
Insulin-like growth factors or somatomedins	IGF-1, IGF-2	Single chains; IGF-1 70 aa, IGF-2 67 aa	IGF1R-I for IGF-1; IGF2R for IGF-2	Follicular development (Ch. 5); growth and development (Ch. 12)
Relaxin H2		Disulfide-linked A and B chains	RXFP1 and 2 (LGR7 and 8; relaxin family peptide receptors 1 and 2)	Parturition in animals, and implicated in early pregnancy (Chs 11 & 13) (Relaxin H1/3 non-functional?)
Insulin-like protein 3, (relaxin-like factor)	Insl3 (RLF)	A/B heterodimer A 26 aa, B 37 aa (14 kDa)	RXFP2 (LGR8)	Constitutively produced by Leydig cells under influence of LH. Essential fetally for testis descent (Ch. 1) and spermatogenesis (Ch. 4)
Transforming growth factor β (all produced from the C-terminal region of a precursor protein)				
Transforming growth factors	TGFs β1, β2, β3	Homodimers, disulfide-linked (25 kDa)	TGFβ R types I, II and III	Testis (Ch. 4); Ovary (Ch. 5); implantation (Ch. 10); preimplantation development (β1), extraembryonic membranes (β2), fetal tissues especially heart (β1, β2, β3) (Ch. 10)
Activins (5 subunits, B-A to –E, of which only A and B important)		Two disulfide-linked β-chains (Fig. 3.5) forming homo- or heterodimers	Binds activin-RI and then recruits activin-RII	Intraovarian activity (Ch. 5); intratesticular activity (Ch. 4); gonad–pituitary interactions (Ch. 6); postimplantation development (Ch. 11)
Inhibin		Heterodimer of 1α chain + 1activin A or Bβ chain (Fig. 3.5)	Inhibin-Rs (two low-affinity described) + betaglycan; a high-affinity TGFβ type III receptor	Endocrine regulation of spermatogenesis and with activin A folliculogenesis (Chs. 4, 5, 6); whilst activins are produced in many tissues, inhibin is limited to gonads

Factor	Abbreviation	Structure	Receptor	Function
Müllerian inhibitory hormone	MIH (MIS, AMH)	Homodimer +13.5% carbohydrate (140 kDa)	MIS-R (also called AMHR2)	Development of internal genitalia; descent of testis (Ch. 1); follicular restraint (Ch. 5)
Bone morphogenetic proteins (at least 15 family members)	BMPs	Dimers, 110–140 aa	Serine-threonine kinases types I (Alk2, 3, 6) and II (BMPRII and BMPRIIb)	Germ cell specification (Ch. 1); spermatogensis (BMP4, 7, 8; Ch. 4); follicle growth (Ch. 5)
Glial-derived neurotropic growth factor	GDNF	Homodimer, 2×134 aa, 30 kDa (non-glycosylated)	GRFRα1 (GPI-linked)	Spermatogonial stem cell maintenance (Ch. 4)
Growth differentiation factor	GDF-9	Dimer, 139 aa	ALK5 and BMPRII	Oocyte growth factor (Ch. 5)
Fibroblastic growth factor family FGF (7 members) aFGF, bFGF, kFGF, int-2	FGF	Single-chain glycoprotein (17 kDa)	Flg/bek R (four classes)	Follicles and corpus luteum of ovary (Ch. 5); preimplantation development (kFGF); organogenesis (Ch. 10)
Leukaemia inhibiting factor	LIF	Single-chain glycopeptide (32–67 kDa)	LIF-Rβ	Implantation (Ch. 10)
Leptin	Leptin	Single chain peptide (16 kDa, 167 aa)	LEPR$_{L\&S}$ (also called Ob-R (obese-receptor)) (short, long and secreted forms)	Puberty (Ch. 7); pregnancy? (Chs 11 & 12); lactation? (Ch. 14)
Tumour necrosis factor α (cachectin)	TFNα	Membrane monomer (26 kDa, 233aa) Secreted as homotrimer ($3 \times$ 17 kDa)	TNF-R (3 receptors)	Spermatogenesis (Ch. 4); follicular atresia (Ch. 5)
Various				
Platelet-derived growth factor	PDGF	Homo/heterodimeric glycoproteins AA, AB, BB. Disulfide bonded (25 kDa)	PDGF-α and β class	Preimplantation development; fetal and placental development (Ch. 10)
Placental growth factor	PlGF	Glycosylated dimeric peptide (two splice sites) (46–50 kDa) 149 or 170aa	Vascular endothelial GF-R	Implantation (Ch. 10)
Endothelins 1–4		Peptides, 21 aa	Two subtypes, ET$_A$ and ET$_B$ cleaved from BigET precursor	Luteal regression (Ch. 5); pregnancy? (Ch. 11)
Stem cell factor	SCF	2 forms by alt splicing; juxtacrine/paracrine	c-Kit receptor	Spermatogonial proliferation in testis and folliculogenic initiator in ovary (Chs 4 & 5)
Type 1 interferons (Trophoblastin or trophoblast protein 1)	IFN-τ	172aa	Type I IFN-AR1 & 2	Antiluteolytic and pregnancy promoting (Ch. 11)
Grhelin	Grhelin	28 aas (from 117 pre-proprotein)	GH-secretogogue receptor (GHS-R1a)	Puberty? (Ch. 7); pregnancy? (Ch. 11)

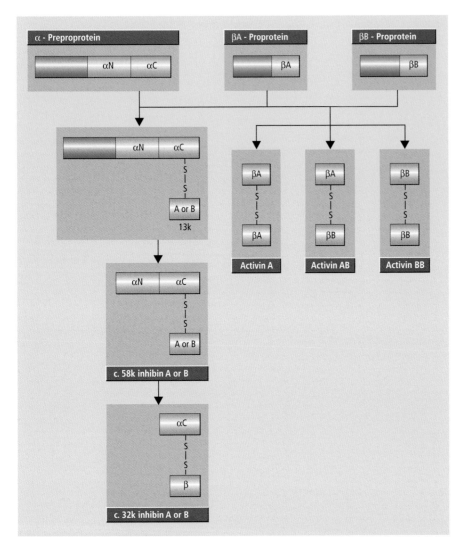

Fig. 3.5 The biosynthesis of inhibins and activins occurs from three genes producing one α-preproprotein (specific for inhibin) and two β-proproteins (which can form part of either activin or inhibin). In each case, the N-terminus (dark blue) is cleaved off and the subunit peptides are then linked in different combinations. Activins take three forms depending on the β chain composition: activin A (AA β homodimer), activin B (BB β homodimer) and activin AB (AB β heterodimer). Two forms of inhibin (A and B) exist, depending on whether pairing is with an activin A or B β-subunit. The presence of glycosylation sites on the peptides means that the molecular weights of the hormones can vary considerably. Activin activity can be modulated by the inhibin chain sequestration of β chains, and the two hormones seem to exist in a functional equilibrium. Additionally, *follistatin*, a binding protein for activin, can sequestering the cytokine in high-affinity complexes.

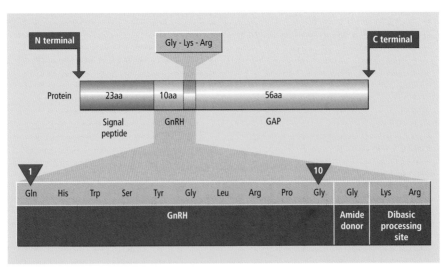

Fig. 3.6 Structure (upper blue bar) of human cDNA for prepro-GnRH (molecular weight 10000), which comprises the decapeptide GnRH preceded by a signal sequence of 23 amino acids and followed by a Gly-Lys-Arg sequence necessary for enzymatic processing and C-terminal amidation of GnRH. The C-terminal region of the precursor is occupied by a further 56 amino acids that constitute the so-called GnRH-associated peptide or *GAP*, the function of which, if any, is unknown. The amino acid sequence of the GnRH is shown in the lower part of the figure. Recently, a second GnRH gene has been identified (GnRH-II) differing at three amino acids from GnRH-I (pGlu-His-Trp-Ser-**His**-Gly-**Trp-Tyr**-Pro-Gly). There is a suggestion that it may preferentially release FSH, but the evidence is unclear.

Fig. 3.7 (a) Oxytocin is synthesized as a precursor molecule (central yellow bar) with: a leader sequence (S); the oxytocin nonapeptide sequence (OT); a Gly-Lys-Arg linker sequence, serving the same function as described for GnRH in the legend to Fig. 3.6; and a neurophysin sequence. (b) The nine amino acids comprising oxytocin contain a hexapeptide 'ring' and a tripeptide 'tail'. (c) A schematized structure of a hypothalamic neurosecretory neuron indicating the cellular location of the various synthetic and processing stages that result in the release of oxytocin (OT) and neurophysin (NP) from neurohypophyseal terminals.

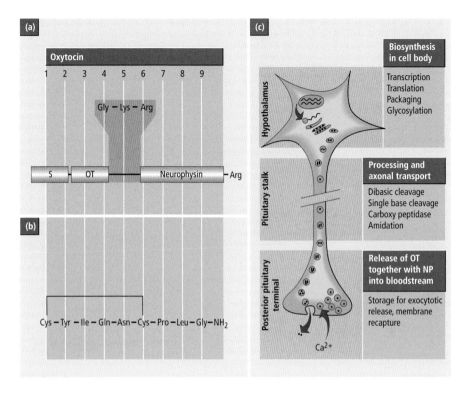

from the pituitary (see Chapter 6). As with GnRH and oxytocin, both are also derived from large precursor molecules within neurons in the hypothalamus and elsewhere. The synthesis of β-endorphin is especially interesting. Its precursor molecule, *prepro-opiomelanocortin*, undergoes extensive intracellular post-translational processing to yield β-endorphin (which is an opioid peptide), as well as several other biologically active hormones, especially *adrenocorticotrophic hormone* (ACTH; also called *corticotrophin*). Figure 3.8 illustrates the processing of prepro-opiomelanocortin and emphasizes the complex nature of post-translational processing that occurs during peptide secretion, and which sometimes results in neurons producing and releasing several biologically important messengers. The effects of β-endorphin on reproduction are mediated entirely via intrahypothalamic interactions (see Chapter 6).

Monoamines

The catecholamines, *dopamine, noradrenaline* and *adrenaline*, as well as the indolamine, *N*-acetyl-5-methoxytryptamine or *melatonin*, have all been implicated in reproductive neuroendocrine control mechanisms. Dopamine is synthesized from tyrosine and is also the precursor of noradrenaline, which in turn is the precursor of adrenaline (Fig. 3.9a). These catecholamines are found in many neurons in the brainstem and, in the case of dopamine, in the hypothalamus, and they have a well-established role as neurotrans-

mitters. Dopamine is also an important hormone; it is released from terminals in the hypothalamus and reaches the anterior pituitary where it is an important modulator of prolactin secretion (see Chapter 6). Melatonin (Fig. 3.9b) is synthesized from serotonin (5-hydroxytryptamine) in the *pineal gland* and is under environmental control. It is released into the bloodstream and exerts important actions within the hypothalamus in order to regulate reproductive activity in seasonally breeding mammals (see Chapter 6).

Having introduced most of the main messengers used to relay information in the reproductive system, we will now consider some of the general properties of messengers that influence how we interpret and understand their activities.

Hormonal actions involve receptors

In the last section, we introduced a bewilderingly wide variety of molecules that act as reproductive messengers. Despite this diversity, some useful and important *general* conclusions can be drawn about how these chemical messengers act. The hormones were grouped according to their general chemical structure and their functional activities. These two systems of classification are directly interrelated, as each of these messengers exerts its influence by combining with a specific *receptor*. This receptor has a molecular conformation that matches some three-dimensional physical feature(s) on the messenger molecule (which is often described as the *ligand*, in the context of its receptor). The

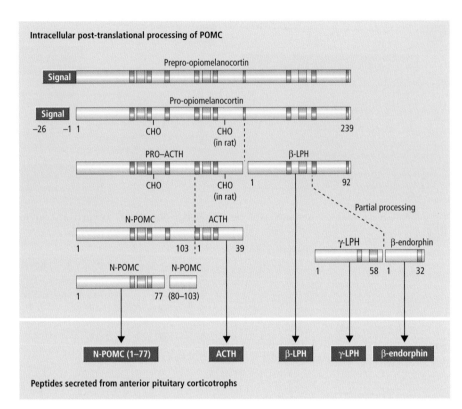

Fig. 3.8 The post-translational processing of prepro-opiomelanocortin and pro-opiomelanocortin (POMC). Note that there are several processing products including the opioid peptide β-endorphin, the non-opioid peptide ACTH (corticotrophin) and lipoproteins (LPH). CHO = carbohydrate side chains; yellow areas = melanocyte-stimulating hormone core sequences; blue areas = sites for proteolytic cleavage.

interaction between the two, like a key in a lock, then leads to secondary changes in the receptor (or in a molecule adjacent to it) that alert the cell to the arrival of the ligand. This information can then be incorporated by the cell into its pattern of behaviour. Thus, the cell responds to the hormone via the mediation of its receptor. Since ligand–receptor interaction depends on a good stereochemical fit between the two molecules, it is not surprising that the general molecular *structure* of messengers correlates with their general *biological activities*.

We have already grouped and subgrouped hormones according to their structural relatedness. The more closely related molecules are, the more likely they are to bind to each other's receptors, albeit perhaps not as well as to their own. For example, human GH and prolactin each have specific receptors (GH-R and PRL-R) to which they bind. Placental lactogen binds to *both* these receptors; additionally, placentally derived GH (GH-V) binds much better to PRL-R than does pituitary GH. These binding patterns reflect structural variations at the level of their amino acid sequences.

Sometimes these effects can appear paradoxical; thus, progesterone will also bind to the glucocorticoid receptor and so function as a glucocorticoid agonist! Similarly, several closely related members of a family may all work through the same receptor, but they may not be equally effective. For example, the 'strong' oestrogen, oestradiol

17β, is much more effective at binding and activating the oestrogen receptors than are oestriol and oestrone, which are therefore said to be 'weak' oestrogens. In Tables 3.1–3.3, the natural members of each steroid class are ranked in order of decreasing potency, and details of the receptors with which they interact are also given. This concept of *strong and weak hormone activity* is often encountered, and can be understood in terms of patterns of interaction with and activations of receptors.

Finally, some molecules may have the required structure to bind to a given receptor, but may not be able to activate it. This can happen if one part of the natural ligand is involved in receptor binding, but a second structurally and spatially distinct domain of the ligand is required for receptor activation. If a molecule is generated that retains only the first domain, it can occupy the receptor without activating it. In so doing, it may prevent the natural ligand(s) from binding and thus act as an *antagonist*. For example, we saw earlier that gonadotrophins from which sugar residues had been removed were inactive biologically. They can, however, bind to receptors. Thus, deglycosylation has affected selectively the domain(s) concerned with activation. Similarly, progesterone will compete with dihydrotestosterone to bind the androgen receptor, and so function as an antiandrogen.

Pharmacologists have taken advantage of both the blocking and mimicking effects that can operate through recep-

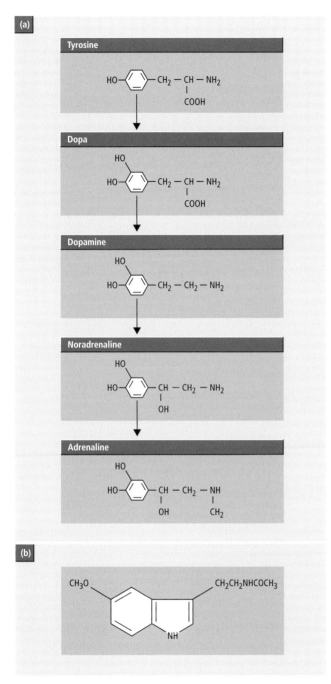

Fig. 3.9 (a) The biosynthetic pathway (from top downwards) and molecular structures of the catecholamines: dopamine, noradrenaline and adrenaline. (b) The structure of the indolamine = melatonin.

tors to develop drugs for therapeutic use, such as controlling fertility or hormone-dependent tumour growth. Chemical synthesis of 'analogues' of natural hormones can be achieved most easily for steroids and small peptides, and these provide the best examples, some of which, in clinical or experimental use, are listed in Table 3.7.

A side effect of some synthetic chemicals (food additives, plastics, pesticides) released into the general environment and/or food chain is the ability to bind to hormone receptors and thereby to block them or to activate them inappropriately. Most attention has focused on possible developmental reproductive abnormalities in male fetuses, but acute exposure in adulthood is also claimed to affect male fertility. For example, dieldrin and endosulfan have oestrogen receptor-binding properties and have been associated with lowered sperm counts and increases in testicular cancer, cryptorchidism and *hypospadias* (urethral opening not at penis tip), although a causal relationship remains to be proven. Naturally occurring phyto-oestrogens, such as genistein found in soya beans, may also have mildly stimulatory effects, although with disputed adverse or even beneficial consequences in, for example, postmenopausal women, where claims for bone strengthening and protection against cardiovascular accidents have been made.

Hormone activity can be regulated by controlling receptor expression

As the tissue specificity of hormonal action depends on both the hormone and its receptor being present, hormonal activity can be regulated *either* by controlling the availability of the hormone *or* by controlling the expression of the receptor. The latter control is extremely important in reproduction and can be achieved either by varying the *amount* of receptor available for binding to the ligand or the *structure* of the receptor as a result of different types of post-translational modification that affect its stability and how it interacts with the ligand and/or the intracellular second messenger signalling system. Thus, the maturation of the ovarian follicle (see Chapter 5), the changing uterine function during the menstrual cycle (see Chapters 6 & 8) and the changes in the female tract at birth (see Chapter 13) are all critically dependent on the acquisition, loss or modification of particular receptors on relevant tissues at appropriate times. Details of these patterns of receptor regulation will be discussed later. For the moment, it is important to note that the *measurement of variation in hormone levels alone will not provide an adequate basis for understanding reproductive function*. The receptor profile must also be known.

The importance of this conclusion is underlined by reference to the genetic deficiency condition of androgen-insensitivity syndrome described in Chapters 1 and 2. You will recall that affected individuals are phenotypic females with normal external genitalia, breasts and a female gender identity. On examination, these women are found to have an XY chromosome constitution, abdominal testes and blood levels of androgens in the male range. Examination of the usual androgen target tissues of these women reveals

Table 3.7 Some synthetic agonists/antagonists in clinical or experimental use.

Progestagens	1	Derivatives of 19-nortestosterone (testosterone lacking the C19-methyl group attached to C10 and with an ethynyl group –C–CH at C17) active as progestagens: norethisterone (also called norethindrone), norethisterone acetate norethynodrel/ethynodiol diacetate: converted to norethisterone before active as progestagens norgestrel (also called levonorgestrel)
	2	Derivatives of 17α-hydroxyprogesterone by esterification of the 17-hydroxyl group (have progestagenic activity): medroxyprogesterone acetate chlormadinone acetate magestrol acetate provera
	3	Desogestrel, gestodene, norgestimate, levonorgestrel (so-called third-generation progestins which have little androgen activity and can be used at much lower doses)
	4	RU486 (mifepristone), onapristone (ZK 98299): antiprogestins
Oestrogens	1	Derivatives of oestradiol 17β having oestrogenic activity: ethinyloestradiol with an ethinyl group at C17α, and mestranol with an ethinyl group at C17α and an –OCH3 group at C3
	2	Clomiphene citrate (clomid): initial stimulation, then antioestrogenic
	3	Diethylstilboestrol: agonist
	4	Nafoxidine, tamoxifen, 4-hydroxytamoxifen, MER 25: all antioestrogens (nafoxidine binds to the receptor but the complex fails to bind to chromatin; in contrast, the tamoxifen–receptor complex binds to the chromatin but is ineffective in stimulating the acceptor site)
	5	Letrozole, anastrozole, exemestane: aromatase inhibitors
Androgens	1	17β-ester derivatives (fat soluble/injectable agonists): stanozolol, methenolone, boldenone, trenbolone, dromostanolone, various testosterone and nandrolone esters
	2	17α-alky derivatives (oral agonists): oxymetholone, oxandrolone, fluoxymesterone, ethylestrenol, danazol, stanozolol, methyltestosterone, methandrostenolone, antiandrogens; cyproterone and cyproterone acetate
Peptides		GnRH analogues (buserelin, nafarelin, histrelin, goserelin, lupon) used to suppress gonadotrophin output during infertility treatment (see Chapter 15) or, in conjunction with selective sex steroid replacement, in the control of a range of steroid-dependent pathologies
LH/FSH/HCG		Genes for α and β chains cloned and co-expressed in cell lines to produce bioactive recombinant hormones. Fusing unique terminal 29aas from HCG β-chain to extend β-chains of LH or FSH dramatically increases their stability in blood and thus their bioactivity. Removal of N-linked carbohydrate chains can lead to receptor occupancy without activation and thus function as antagonists.

an absence or deficiency of androgen receptors. Thus, although the androgens are produced and present, the body is blind to them and masculinizing activity is lost.

Finally, as we learn more about small inter-individual variations in receptor gene structure through, for example, single nucleotide polymorphisms, we are finding that the different resultant haplotypes may have slightly different ligand binding properties. For example, at least four FSH receptor haplotypes are now known which affect the sensitivity of women to FSH. It has long been known from experience with the clinical induction of ovulation with FSH (see Chapters 5 and 15) that women vary greatly in their sensitivity, and now we are beginning to understand why. This understanding opens the possibility of haplotyping women in advance and then tailoring the stimulation

regime to their haplotype—a real advance in avoiding ovarian hyper- or hypostimulation (see Chapter 15).

Receptor stimulation activates target cell transducer systems

The coupling of a hormone and its receptor leads to activation of the complex. This activation can take different forms depending on the chemical structure of the hormone (Fig. 3.10).

Thus, steroids and prostaglandins, being lipid soluble, can pass *into* a target cell to combine with the C-terminal region of its free specific *intranucleoplasmic receptor*, thereby activating it. Activation involves phosphorylation of the receptor and a conformational change so that the steroid/

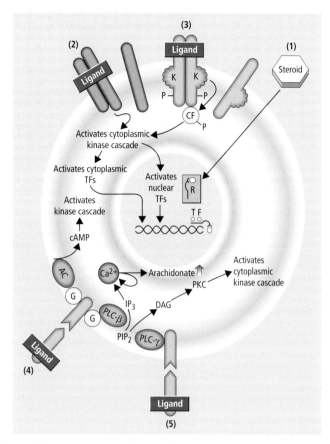

Fig. 3.10 Receptor activation and second messengers. Ligands can influence cell function, and ultimately nuclear gene expression, in a variety of ways. Here we summarize in a very simplified form a very complex and rapidly evolving field of study. (1) Steroid hormones, being lipid soluble, pass freely into cell nuclei where they bind receptors (R), displacing associated stabilizing proteins, such as HSP90, leading to receptor activation by phosphorylation; the activated complex can then bind to steroid-specific response elements (SREs) in the DNA and to transcription factors (TF) to activate steroid-specific genes. (2) Some ligands (prolactin, growth hormone, placental lactogen, LIF, leptin, TNF-α) cross-link two receptor chains (as hetero- or homodimers). The cross-linked complex then activates the Jak-Stat cytosolic kinase cascade, resulting in either the phosphorylation of TFs in the cytoplasm and their translocation to the nucleus, or the translocation of the kinases themselves to the nucleus where they phosphorylate and activate TFs. Hormonal ligands that act in this way can cross-link overlapping spectra of receptor monomers to induce overlapping spectra of downstream cascades, so accounting for some of the redundancy seen amongst cytokines (see text). (3) Other ligands (cytokines of the EGF and TGFβ families) bind to, and multimerize, receptors that *are themselves kinases* (K). Multimerization leads to kinase activation and both autophosphorylation of the receptor (–P) and phosphorylation of cytoplasmic factors (CF–P), and thereby to a cascade of kinase activity culminating in TF activation. Again, there is some overlap of downstream kinases and their targets both within this class of ligand–receptor interaction and between this class and class 2 above. The EGF family receptors are tyrosine kinases and are dimerized on ligand binding. Their activation then triggers numerous down stream second messenger pathways including phospholipase Cγ, ras/MAP kinases, and multiple STAT isoforms. The TGFβ family members form a complex with two type II receptors and then recruit two type I receptors, all four receptors having serine/threonine kinase activity. The activated kinases phosphorylate the receptors themselves and the intracellular signalling Smad proteins. The activated Smads translocate to the nucleus to bind with co-factors to response elements in cytokine target gene promoters. (4) Some ligands (LH, FSH, CG, GnRH, oxytocin, arginine vasopressin) bind to receptors which then associate with G proteins (G). G proteins can then act in at least two ways: (i) to stimulate phospholipase Cβ (PLC-β) to hydrolyse phosphatidylinositol phosphate (PIP_2) to 1,4,5-triphosphate (IP_3) and diacylglycerol (DAG), which release Ca^{2+} and activate protein kinase C (PKC) respectively; or (ii) to modulate activity of adenyl cyclase (AC) and so the output of cAMP. (5) Some ligands (EGF) may activate phospholipase Cγ (PLC-γ) directly, without G-protein mediation.

receptors form homodimers. This complex, but not the steroid or receptor alone, can then bind to specific DNA sequences in the chromatin: the so-called acceptor sites or *steroid response elements* (SREs) specific for each steroid (e.g. ARE, PRE and ERE for androgens, progestagens and oestrogens respectively). Binding of adjacent transcription factors also occurs, leading to a rapid rise in the activity of RNA polymerase II, production of mRNA species specific for the steroid, and, in the continuing presence of the complex, a more general stimulation of nucleolar and transfer RNA synthesis. Protein synthesis increases within 30 min of steroid stimulation, and includes proteins specifically and selectively induced by the stimulating steroid.

Protein hormones and growth factors cannot enter cells, and so use a different sort of receptor mechanism. Their receptors are located at the surface of the cell. After binding of the hormone to its receptor, different sorts of transmembrane activation events can occur (summarized in Fig. 3.10). In each of these cases, the receptor is acting as a *transducer*, passing the information on the arrival of the hormonal ligand *outside* the cell to effect metabolic responses *inside* the cell. The intracellular molecular systems mediating these responses are called *second messenger systems*. Figure 3.10 does not do justice to the complex interactions of different second messenger systems or to the variety of systems that each ligand–receptor complex activates. Unravelling this complexity is important for an understanding of just how the cells of the body integrate the large variety of extracellular messages that they receive.

Apparent target tissues may be affected only secondarily

A final word of caution! When studying the effects of hormones on reproduction, it is important to show not just that the hormone exerts a biological effect on tissue function or structure, but also to determine whether it does so *directly*. For example, progesterone exerts powerful effects on the surface luminal epithelium of the uterus in early pregnancy to inhibit oestrogen-induced proliferation. However, this effect *requires progesterone receptors on the cells of the underlying uterine stromal tissue*. Thus, if mice are studied which lack luminal epithelial progesterone receptors, they are nonetheless inhibited from proliferating by progesterone. Only a lack of P4 receptors restricted to stromal cells prevents this inhibition. Similarly, in humans the integrin expression in the epithelium at the time of implantation depends on the influence of progesterone on the stroma that stimulates production of a member of the epidermal growth factor family, which then acts on the overlying epithelium. Thus, steroids (and other hormones) may act indirectly by stimulating paracrine mediators in adjacent tissues.

There may be more receptor systems than we think!

An increasing variety and complexity of receptors has been discovered with the sequencing of the human and mouse genome, increasing our understanding of how genes are used and, most importantly, enabling us to knock out genetically known receptors and yet find that the hormone still has biological effects. Some of this receptor variety is due to differential splicing of gene transcripts and/or processing of proteins, and some is due to the presence of homologous receptor genes. However, quite a different level of variety has come from studying the cell biology of ligand–receptor–second messenger systems. These studies not only reveal that multiple second messenger systems may be activated by the same ligand–receptor interactions, they also have led to discovery of qualitatively quite different receptor families and thus mechanisms of hormone action. As yet, these studies are at early stages, examples of which we briefly give here. The actions of progesterone through its classical receptors (Table 3.1) cannot explain all its biological activities, some of which persist in receptor knockout mice and others of which show kinetics and inhibitor sensitivities that are incompatible with traditional receptor function. A cell-surface membrane receptor has been postulated to be involved. A similar novel cell-surface receptor for oestradiol, sensitive to both oestradiol-17β *and* its natural enantiomer oestradiol-17α, and functioning via a MAP kinase second messenger system, has been described in cells lacking conventional nuclear receptors ERα and β. We mention these examples to illustrate an important cautionary point: if a hormone has a direct effect on a tissue, you should not assume it is operating through known receptors until you demonstrate their exclusive involvement directly!

We have considered some of the ways in which the presence or activity of receptors can influence the biological activity of hormones. We end this chapter by looking at the factors influencing the levels of hormone available to interact with these receptors.

The levels of a hormone in its target tissues depend on its turnover

The levels of a hormone in the fluids bathing potential target cells depend on the balance between its arrival and its removal. These in turn depend on the local blood circulation, the nature and proximity of its secreting cells (local and paracrine or distant and endocrine), its circulating blood levels and its stability. A high local blood flow will tend to dissipate autocrine and paracrine secretions but facilitate the local distribution of endocrine secretions. We will examine in more detail the factors influencing blood levels of endocrine secretions and the stability of hormones in tissues.

Blood levels of hormones may fluctuate because their secretion may fluctuate

To a clinician, the hormones most directly visible are those measured in a sample of systemic blood. Measurements may be made by *bioassays*, which provide a direct test of the hormone's functional activity (example in Fig. 3.11), or by use of a *protein-binding radioassay* (example in Fig. 3.12). What interpretation can be placed on such measurements?

Observations on one sample of blood represent a single static measurement taken from a highly dynamic system. Figure 3.13 shows a series of values of blood testosterone taken from a man over a 24-h period. Two important points emerge from inspection of these values. First, mean blood levels of testosterone, and indeed of other hormones such as prolactin, vary over a 24-h period, showing *circadian rhythmicity*. Thus, samples should generally be taken for comparison at similar times. Second, testosterone (like many other hormones such as gonadotrophins, GnRH and prolactin) is secreted not continuously but in a pulsatile

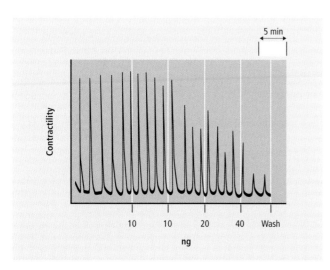

Fig. 3.11 Bioassay of hormones: various doses of a biological sample are compared with known hormonal standards for their effects in a biological system. In this example, increasing amounts (10, 20 and 40 ng) of a preparation of the cytokine relaxin are investigated for their inhibitory effects on the spontaneous contractility of a segment of oestrous mouse uterus. From this experiment a plot of inhibition vs. concentration can be made. Unknown samples can then be used in the same system, and the concentration estimated from the standard plot. The disadvantage of bioassays is that the endpoints can be variable and susceptible to influence by extraneous factors, including the inherent variability of the biological material in the assay itself and contaminating agents that interfere with the assay. The advantage of bioassays is that they actually measure biological activity (see legend to Fig. 3.12).

manner at intervals of between 1 and 3 h. The amplitude of these pulses is often large. A single blood sample taken at one point in time does not take this pulsing into account and may be misleading. This pulsatile secretion pattern can be crucial to hormonal function. As we will see in Chapter 6, a change from pulsatile to continuous expression of GnRH results in suppression of the output of LH from the pituitary. It seems that when receptors are occupied constantly by ligand, they become 'exhausted' and are uncoupled from the internal second messenger systems that would normally operate. This uncoupling is called *receptor downregulation*. Several other examples of receptor down-regulation in the face of continuous stimulation (both physiological and pharmacological) will be encountered later.

Thus, care must be taken in interpreting values for hormone levels in the blood. Moreover, even when a reliable measurement has been made, its interpretation depends on understanding that the value depends not simply on hormone production rates but on the balance between the rate of hormone secretion and its rate of clearance by various routes.

Hormones can be metabolized as they pass round the body

Most, but not all, hormones detectable in the blood are produced from a single major source, and so hormone levels will usually reflect the activity of that source. However, some hormones may come from multiple sources, either naturally (e.g. during pregnancy when fetal, placental and/or maternal sources of many hormones are present; see Chapters 11 & 12) or pathologically (e.g. tumours commonly secrete chorionic gonadotrophin and placental lactogen). Additionally, other hormones may be produced by a mixture of direct secretion and interconversion from other hormonal substrates (e.g. oestrone, 10–30% from ovaries directly, the remainder derived from metabolic conversion of ovarian oestradiol 17β and of adrenal androstenedione by peripheral tissues, notably the liver). This distinction between primary secretion and metabolic conversion can be important in interpreting changes in the mean blood levels of a steroid, particularly in pathological conditions.

The rate at which a hormone is removed from the blood is reflected in its half-life. An awareness of hormonal half-lives is important in interpreting changes in hormone levels (Table 3.8). Thus, short half-lives mean that hormonal levels are more responsive to secretory changes. Changes in half-life may also inform about the state of the hormone itself (e.g. whether it has been modified to increase its rate of clearance) or about the functional competence of the organs effecting clearance. Removal of hormones from the blood is affected only marginally by utilization in receptor

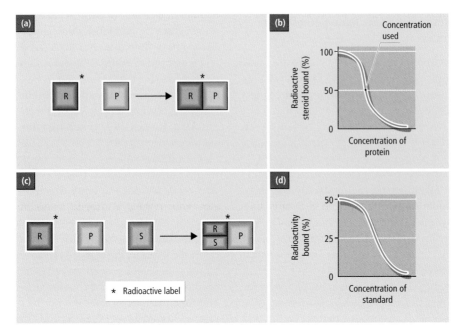

Fig. 3.12 Radioassay of hormones. (a) A sample of pure, radioactive hormone (R*) is mixed with different amounts of a binding protein (P), which may be a specific antibody (radioimmunoassay) or an isolated plasma-binding protein or cell receptor (radio receptor assay). The bound and free hormones are then separated. This may be accomplished in several ways: the protein can be used fixed to the side of the sample tube (solid phase assay), in which case the free hormone is easily washed away; alternatively, proteins in solutions may be precipitated by adding salts or a second antibody directed against the protein. The proportion of the hormone binding to the protein can then be plotted (b). Usually, a binding protein amount that binds about half the radioactive hormone is selected for assay use as shown in (c), in which the selected amount of binding protein (P) is incubated with radioactive hormone (R*) in the presence of various dilutions of a sample of plasma containing a known level of non-labelled standard hormone (S). The unlabelled standard hormone competes with the labelled hormone for the binding protein, and so the percentage of bound radioactivity declines as the amount of S increases. In this way a calibration curve can be constructed as shown in (d). Dilutions of samples of plasma containing *unknown* levels of hormone can now be used instead of the standard hormone, and the concentration of hormone thereby determined from the standard curve. Protein-binding assays are more reliably quantitative than bioassays, but may only measure one feature of the hormone, which is not necessarily equivalent to its activity. Thus, immunoassays are measuring the antigenic activity of the hormone not its biological activity, but, for example, quite large amounts of free gonadotrophin α-chain are present in the circulation, as well as non-functional polymorphic gonadotrophins. Receptor assays measure binding to the receptor, but as we saw, deglycosylated LH binds but does not activate. Thus, the results of radioassays must be interpreted carefully.

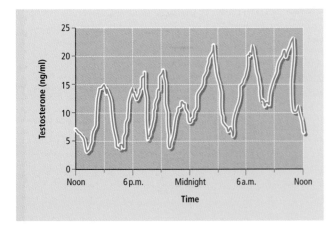

Fig. 3.13 Testosterone levels in blood samples taken from a male patient at 45-min intervals over a 24-h period. Note that there are pronounced oscillations and the mean level is higher between midnight and noon.

complexes, and mainly by metabolic conversion (e.g. steroids in the liver or prostaglandins in the lung) to a range of biologically inactive or less active derivatives.

Levels of hormones can be affected by the presence of binding proteins

The mean blood level of some hormones is also influenced by the presence of binding proteins. Thus, the lipid hormones and their precursors are relatively insoluble in water. In order for them to reach their target cells, they must either bind to *carrier proteins* or be *chemically modified* to increase their solubility in plasma. Thus, most of the cholesterol and sex steroids in the blood are bound with carrier protein molecules in equilibrium, with much lower levels of free steroid in aqueous solution, rather in the way that haemoglobin carries reservoirs of bound oxygen (Table 3.9). Steroids are also rendered more soluble in plasma by conjugation to give steroid glucosiduronates and sulfates. In such a state, they show reduced biological activity and must be deconjugated again in target tissues in order to become fully active.

In contrast, protein hormones are more freely soluble in the aqueous fluids of the body, but do not readily enter cells, tending to act at their surfaces. Nonetheless, some protein hormones do complex with binding proteins in the blood and/or tissues, and this binding can affect their availability for binding to receptors. Thus, the cytokines insulin and insulin-like growth factor 1 (IGF-1) bind to a number of different *insulin growth factor-binding proteins* (IGFBPs), and the levels of these proteins modulate both the plasma/tissue concentration and the activity of the cytokines, complicating the interpretation of their actions.

Table 3.8 Half-lives of some hormones in the blood.

Hormone	Half-life
Steroids	2–3 min
Prostaglandins	3–10 min
Gonadotrophins	
LH, FSH	1–3 h and 36 h (biphasic)
CG	6 h and 36 h (biphasic) – stabilized by the O-linked carbohydrate chains on tail of β-chain
Prolactin and placental lactogen	10–20 min and 24 h (biphasic)

Similarly, *follistatin* (a single-chain glycopolypeptide with size variants 32–39 kDa produced in the ovary) binds to activin and modulates its capacity to influence follicular development in the ovary (see Chapter 5) and to release FSH from the pituitary (see Chapter 6). Thus, the activity of a hormone can be regulated by varying the level of its binding hormone.

The presence of variable levels of binding proteins also complicates the interpretation of hormone measurements. Thus, when the levels of the binding proteins themselves vary, the bound hormone levels will vary accordingly. For example, cases of androgenization in women can be associated with normal androgen levels but *reduced* levels of sex-steroid-binding globulin. In these cases, the proportion of androgen readily available to receptors has risen and androgenization occurs. Conversely, during pregnancy, the levels of steroid-binding proteins rise six-fold (see Chapter 11 for details), leading to a corresponding increase in total, measurable steroid levels, although not of free steroid. It is difficult to determine accurately the ratio of free to bound steroid in blood samples. However, samples of body secretions, such as saliva, contain levels of steroids that reflect primarily the levels of unbound blood steroid available for equilibration. Analysis of saliva for steroid levels is also useful because frequent sampling on an outpatient basis is possible.

Hormones may be metabolized in their target tissues

Tissue levels of a hormone may be affected not only by its rate of delivery to the tissue, but also by its metabolism once it arrives there. Some tissues can take a circulating hormone, transform it enzymically and then utilize it locally, and three examples are provided here.

Table 3.9 Steroid-binding proteins in human plasma.

Binding protein	Percentage of non-conjugated steroids bound*			
	Progestagens	Androgens	Oestrogens†	Cortisol
Albumin	48	32	63	20
Cortisol-binding globulin§	50	1	—	70
Sex steroid-binding globulin	—	66	36	—
Free steroid	2	1	1	10

*Steroids conjugated as sulfates or glucosiduronates bind weakly to albumin only.
†Oestrone and oestriol bind mainly to albumin.
§Also called transcortin.
Note: Albumin is a low-affinity/high-capacity binding protein whilst the globulins are high-affinity/low-capacity binding proteins. There are sex differences, females in general binding proportionately more androgens/oestrogens to sex steroid-binding globulin than to albumin.

The enzyme 5α-reductase is present in many of the androgen target tissues, for example the male accessory sex glands and the skin and tissues of the external genitalia. This enzyme converts testosterone, the main circulating androgen, to 5α-dihydrotestosterone (Fig. 3.3), which has a much higher affinity for the androgen receptor in these target cells, and thus is a much 'stronger' androgen than testosterone. In the prenatal and immature male, in whom both the testicular and blood levels of testosterone are relatively low, testosterone is secreted and converted to 5α-dihydrotestosterone in the tissues possessing 5α-reductase. The low levels of this highly active androgen then exert local effects on the external genitalia, increasing phallic and scrotal size and rendering them clearly distinguishable from the clitoris and labia in females. The importance of this 5α-reductase activity is revealed in people who are genetically deficient in it. Affected male infants have poorly developed male external genitalia, and at birth may be classed as females. At puberty, the external genitalia are suddenly exposed to much higher levels of circulating testosterone, and respond with a sudden growth to normal size. This so-called 'penis-at-twelve' syndrome illustrates vividly the role of local 5α-reductase activity in mediating many of the actions of testosterone (see also Chapter 8).

A second example of local steroid interconversion appears even more dramatic. The hypothalamus of male and female rodents, and indeed primates, is able to take circulating testosterone and convert it to oestradiol 17β by local aromatizing activity (Fig. 3.3). The high local levels of oestradiol 17β then interact with a local oestrogen receptor to stimulate activity. Thus, paradoxically, the actions of testosterone to masculinize the neonatal rat brain (see Chapters 2 & 6) and to maintain masculine sexual behaviour in adulthood (see Chapter 8) are accomplished only after aromatization to oestradiol. This phenomenon emphasizes that the terms 'male' and 'female' hormones should be used with care.

A final example is provided by local tissue enzymic action that synthesizes oestradiol from either androstenedione (aromatase) or oestrone (oestradiol-17β-dehydrogenase) (Fig. 3.3). The presence of different isotypic variants of these enzymes in different tissue allows the tissue-specific accumulation of high levels of the more potent oestrogen from circulating substrate. For example, breast tumours commonly have high oestradiol content derived by local conversion and providing a potent stimulus to tumour growth. Targeting such local tissue enzyme isotypes may provide a route to cancer control.

Hormones may self-regulate by feedback

The pervasive importance of hormones for the reproductive process will already be clear, and so understanding how hormone production is controlled is important for understanding reproduction. Many of the major endocrine hormones are regulated by feedback mechanisms (see Fig. 3.1), and so before leaving this general introduction to reproductive messengers, some key features of feedback control are discussed.

A feedback system requires that some functional consequence of an output signal is detected and that the information so detected then influences the output signal itself. During *negative feedback*, the influence will be to depress the output signal while during *positive feedback* the output signal will be enhanced.

Negative feedback is characteristically used to maintain an even physiological state—*homeostasis*. For example, it is easy to see how detection of low blood glucose might advantageously stimulate its restoration by its synthesis and/or release so as to maintain metabolic activity. Reproductive events, as we will see, also use negative feedback mechanisms. For example, ovarian function requires both FSH and LH activity. Secretion of each of these hormones is sensitive to negative feedback from the ovary in the form of signals indicating *the rate of growth of follicles*. This ensures that follicle growth is regulated properly (see Chapter 5 for details). However, a key characteristic of negative feedback systems is that the *set- or balance-point* of the feedback system can be changed. A useful analogy is the thermostat in a house: if it is set high the heating system feedback system responds to keep the house hot; if set low, then a cooler house prevails. The body can also reset the balance-point of its feedback systems by changing the sensitivity of hormone-regulating tissues to the negative feedback signal—for example during different phases of the menstrual cycle the feedback sensitivity to ovarian signals is varied, thereby varying the output of LH and FSH during the cycle (details in Chapter 5).

Positive feedback contrasts with negative feedback in that, rather than stabilizing the system, the greater the impact of the output signal the more that signal is stimulated and so an *explosive runaway* situation develops. Such a situation will inevitably be self-limiting when it runs out of steam or destroys itself. We will see several examples of positive feedback in reproduction, for example during the build up to ovulation (an explosive event)—so again ovarian activity providing us with a clear example (Chapter 5).

Summary

Although the hormones involved in reproduction are diverse, an understanding of the activities of each of them is helped if two fundamentally important general points are grasped. First, hormonal activity in the body (tissue, fluids or blood) may reflect changing primary secretion, secondary interconversions, metabolic clearance or the

KEY LEARNING POINTS

- Hormones act as reproductive messengers throughout the body via endocrine, exocrine, paracrine, autocrine and juxtacrine activities.

- There are different kinds of hormones: lipids such as steroids and eicosanoids; proteins, glycoproteins and peptides including cytokines; and monoamines.

- Different kinds of hormones differ in both their chemical structures and their biological properties.

- These two distinguishing properties are interrelated because hormones work through receptors.

- The chemical structure of the hormone determines both the goodness of its fit as a receptor ligand and the effectiveness with which it activates the receptor, although different parts of the hormone molecule may be responsible for each of these properties.

- Receptors are activated when the hormone binds and its activation initiates a downstream cascade of intracellular responses: a second messenger system.

- Most receptors are on the cell surface, but some, for steroids and eicosanoids, are intracellular.

- Some receptors will bind more than one hormone.

- The functional effectiveness with which a hormone binds and activates a receptor determines whether it is a strong- or weak-acting hormone.

- Where more than one hormone can bind and activate a receptor they are called agonists.

- Some molecules bind but do not activate receptors: these function as antihormones or antagonists.

- Naturally occurring and manufactured analogues of and antagonists to hormones exist, and may exert toxic or therapeutic effects via their interactions with receptors.

- The type and level of receptors present in a cell or tissue determine the sensitivity of that tissue to different hormones.

- Some tissues may appear to be regulated by a hormone, when in fact an adjacent tissue may be the hormone target which then locally stimulates the adjacent tissue by paracrine activity.

- Tissues can regulate their receptors and so control their responsiveness to hormones.

- If a hormone is present constantly, many receptors down-regulate and the cell becomes refractory to the presence of the hormone.

- Blood levels of hormones can fluctuate with time of day and from hour to hour.

- Hormones are metabolized as they pass through the body; this may make them more or less active or soluble, or may clear them completely from the blood giving them a short half-life.

- Hormones may be bound to carrier molecules that stabilize them, neutralize them or increase their total amount in the blood.

- Variation in the levels of carrier molecules can lead to variations in the blood levels of hormones measured.

- Local target tissues can metabolize hormones before they interact with receptors to increase or decrease their potency locally.

- Secretion of many hormones is regulated by feedback mechanisms. Negative feedback stabilizes a feedback system, but the level of its activity can also be regulated through balance- or set-point control. Positive feedback systems are explosive and self-limiting.

---

levels of binding proteins. Second, hormone activity may also be regulated at the level of the target tissues by altering the level or activity of endogenous receptors or by changing patterns of paracrine stimulation between adjacent tissues. These important conclusions will be revisited in following chapters as we explore reproductive function in more detail.

FURTHER READING

General reading

Beato M *et al.* (1995) Steroid hormone receptors: many actors in search of a plot. *Cell* **83**, 851–857.

Hull KL, Harvey S (2001) Growth hormone: roles in female reproduction. *Journal of Endocrinology* **168**, 1–23.

Ivell R (1997) Biology of the relaxin-like factor (RLF). *Reviews of Reproduction* **2**, 133–138.

Fares F (2006) The role of O-linked and N-linked oligosaccharides on the structure-function of glycoprotein hormones: development of agonists and antagonists. *Biochimica Biophysica Acta* **1760**, 560–567.

Feng X-H, Derynck R (2005) Specificity and versatility in TGF-β signaling through Smads. *Annual Reviews in Cell and Developmental Biology* **21**, 659–693.

Freeman ME *et al.* (2000) Prolactin: structure, function and regulation of secretion. *Physiological Reviews* **80**, 1523–1631.

Fruhbeck GFR (2006) Intracellular signalling pathways activated by leptin. *Biochemical Journal* **393**, 7–20.

Harrison CA *et al.* (2005) Antagonists of activin signaling: mechanisms and potential biological applications *Trends in Endocrinology and Metabolism* **16**, 73–78.

Hsueh AJ *et al.* (2005) Hormonology: a genomic perspective on hormonal research. *Journal of Endocrinology* **187**, 333–338.

Lessey BA (2003) Two pathways of progesterone action in the human endometrium: implications for implantation and contraception. *Steroids* **68**, 809–815.

Linzer DIH, Fisher SJ (1999) The placenta and the prolactin family of hormones: regulation of the physiology of pregnancy. *Molecular Endocrinology* **13**, 837–840.

Lu C (2005) New members of the insulin family: regulators of metabolism, growth and now . . . reproduction. *Pediatric Research* **57**, 70R–73R.

Nilsson S *et al.* (2001) Mechanisms of estrogen action. *Physiological Reviews* **81**, 1535–1565.

Picard D. (1998) Steroids tickle cells inside and out. *Nature* **392**, 437–438.

Pike AC (2006) Lessons learnt from structural studies of the oestrogen receptor. *Best Practice Research in Clinical Endocrinology & Metabolism* **20**, 1–14.

Robinson ICAF (1986) The magnocellular and parvocellular oxytocin and vasopressin systems. In: *Neuroendocrinology* (ed. S.L. Lightman & B.J. Everitt), pp. 154–176. Blackwell Scientific Publications, Oxford.

Sharpe RM (2001) Hormones and testis development and the possible adverse effects of environmental chemicals. *Toxicology Letters* **120**, 221–232.

Singh AB, Harris RC (2005) Autocrine, paracrine and juxtacrine signaling by EGFR ligands. *Cellular Signalling* **17**, 1183–1193.

Wehling M. (1997) Specific nongenomic actions of steroid hormones. *Annual Reviews in Physiology* **59**, 365–393.

Woodruff TK, Rather JP. (1995) Activins, inhibins and reproduction. *Annual Reviews in Physiology* **57**, 219–244.

More advanced reading

Bathgate RA *et al.* (2006) International Union of Pharmacology LVII: Recommendations for the nomenclature of receptors for relaxin family peptides. *Pharmacological Reviews* **58**, 7–31.

Cassidy A *et al.* (2006) Critical review of health effects of soyabean phyto-oestrogens in post-menopausal women. *Proceedings of the Nutrition Society* **65**, 76–92.

Costagliola S *et al.* (2005) Specificity and promiscuity of gonadotropin receptors. *Reproduction* **130**, 275–281.

Farooqui AA, Horrocks LA (2006) Phospholipase A2-generated lipid mediators in the brain: the good, the bad, and the ugly. *Neuroscientist* **12**, 245–260.

Fraser LR *et al.* (2006) Effects of estrogenic xenobiotics on human and mouse spermatozoa. *Human Reproduction* **21**, 1184–1193.

Gromoll J, Simoni M (2005) Genetic complexity of FSH receptor function. *Trends in Endocrinology and Metabolism* **16**, 368–373.

Imamov O *et al.* (2005) Estrogen receptor beta in health and disease. *Biology of Reproduction* **73**, 866–871.

Kahn SM *et al.* (2002) Sex hormone-binding globulin is synthesized in target cells. *Journal of Endocrinology* **175**, 113–120.

Kumar TR (2005) What have we learned about gonadotropin function from gonadotropin subunit and receptor knockout mice? *Reproduction* **130**, 293–302.

Linzer DIH, Fisher SJ (2000) The placenta and the prolactin family of hormones: regulation of the physiology of pregnancy. *Molecular Endocrinology* **13**, 837–840.

Mangelsdorf DJ *et al.* (1995) The nuclear receptor superfamily: the second decade, *Cell* **83**, 835–839.

Mazerbourg S, Hsueh AJ (2006) Genomic analyses facilitate identification of receptors and signalling pathways for growth differentiation factor 9 and related orphan bone morphogenetic protein/growth differentiation factor ligands. *Human Reproduction Update* **12**, 373–383.

Mulac-Jericevic B, Conneely OM (2004) Reproductive tissue selective actions of progesterone receptors. *Reproduction* **128**, 139–146.

Peluso JJ (2006) Multiplicity of progesterone's actions and receptors in the mammalian ovary. *Biology of Reproduction* **75**, 2–8.

Penning TM (2003) Hydroxysteroid dehydrogenases and pre-receptor regulation of steroid hormone action. *Human Reproduction Update* **9**, 193–205.

Reed MJ (2004) Role of enzymes and tissue-specific actions of steroids. *Maturitas* **48** (Suppl. 1), S18–S23.

Rispoli LA, Nett TM (2005) Pituitary gonadotropin-releasing hormone (GnRH) receptor: Structure, distribution and regulation of expression. *Animal Reproduction Science* **88**, 57–74.

Themmen APN (2005) An update of the pathophysiology of human gonadotrophin subunit and receptor gene mutations and polymorphisms. *Reproduction* **130**, 263–274.

Toran-Allerand CA (2005) Estrogen and the brain: beyond ERα, ERβ, and 17β-estradiol. *Annals of the New York Academy of Sciences* **1052**, 136–144.

Tung L *et al.* (2006) Progesterone receptors (PR)-B and PR-A regulate transcription by different mechanisms: AF-3 exerts regulatory control over coactivator binding to PR-B. *Molecular Endocrinology* **20**, 2657–2670.

Yong EL *et al.* (2003) Androgen receptor gene and male infertility. *Human Reproduction Update* **9**, 1–7.

CHAPTER 4

Testicular Function in the Adult

In Chapter 1, we described how the fetal testis formed from an indifferent genital ridge and how endocrine function in the fetal testis was critical for the establishment of male phenotype. We saw that postnatal growth of the testis was slow and the output of androgens low, albeit higher than in females. At puberty, however, a rapid growth and maturation of the testis occurs as it assumes its adult form, accompanied by increases in the output of both androgens and spermatozoa. The way in which this pubertal transition is controlled will be considered later, in Chapter 7. First, however, we consider how the adult testis functions.

The testis is divided into compartments

The testis has two major products (1) spermatozoa, which transmit the male's genes to the embryo, and (2) hormones, required for the maintenance of male reproductive functions in adulthood. Androgens are the most important of these hormones, although oestrogens, inhibin, activin and Insl3 are also produced. The production of androgens and spermatozoa occurs in two discrete compartments within the testis. Spermatozoa develop *within* the tubules in close association with *Sertoli cells*, while androgens are synthesized *between* the tubules in the *Leydig cells*. These two com-

partments are not only structurally distinct but are also separated physiologically by cellular barriers, which develop during puberty and limit the free exchange of water-soluble materials. The precise cellular location of these barriers has been analysed by injection of dyes or electron-opaque materials into the blood, thus allowing the visualization of their distribution within the testis. Fairly free equilibration occurs between blood and the *interstitial* and lymphatic tissues (marked I in Fig. 4.1), but penetration through the peritubular wall into the *basal compartment* of the tubule (marked B in Fig. 4.1) is slower. Surprisingly, however, the major barrier to diffusion lies not at the peritubular boundary itself but between the basal compartment of the tubule and an *adluminal compartment* (marked A in Fig. 4.1). The physical basis for this barrier comprises multiple layers of adherens (inter-Sertoli cell anchoring), gap (inter-Sertoli cell communicating) and tight (para-Sertoli cell occluding) junctional complexes completely encircling each Sertoli cell, and linking it firmly to its neighbours (Fig. 4.1, upper insert). Marker molecules are rarely seen penetrating through these junctional barriers between the adjacent Sertoli cells. The barrier constitutes the main element of the so-called *blood–testis barrier*. It is absent prepubertally, but develops before the initiation of spermatogenesis.

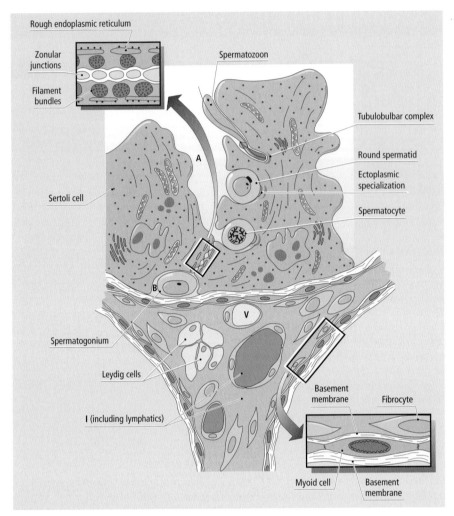

Fig. 4.1 Cross-section through part of an adult testis to show the four compartments, which are: vascular (V); interstitial (I), including the lymphatic vessels and containing the Leydig cells; basal (B); and adluminal (A). The latter two compartments lie within the seminiferous tubules. The interstitial and basal compartments are separated by an acellular basement membrane surrounded externally by myoid cells and invested with a loose coat of interstitial fibrocytes (see lower insert box). Myoid cells are linked to each other by punctate junctions. No blood vessels, lymphatic vessels or nerves traverse this boundary into the seminiferous tubule. Within the tubule, the basal and adluminal compartments are separated by rows of zonular tight, adherens and gap junctional complexes (see upper insert box), linking together adjacent Sertoli cells round their complete circumference and forming the *blood–testis barrier*. Intracellular to these junctional complexes are bundles of actin filaments running parallel to the surface around the 'waist' of the Sertoli cells, and internal to the filaments are cisternae of rough endoplasmic reticulum. Within the basal compartment are the spermatogonia, whilst spermatocytes, round and elongating spermatids and spermatozoa are in the adluminal compartment, in intimate contact with the Sertoli cells with which they form special junctions.

The presence of this barrier has two major functional consequences. First, it prevents intratubular spermatozoa from leaking out into the systemic and lymphatic circulations. This function is important because the body's immune system is not tolerant of spermatozoal antigens, which are capable of eliciting an immune response. Such a response can lead to *antispermatozoal antibodies* and even to an autoimmune inflammation of the testis (*autoallergic orchitis*), both of which are associated with subfertility. Second, the composition of *intratubular fluid* differs markedly from that of the *intertubular fluids*: blood, interstitial fluid and lymph (Fig. 4.2). If radioactive 'marker molecules' are injected into the blood and their equilibration between blood, lymph and interstitial fluid is measured over time, it is found that ions, proteins and charged sugars enter the interstitial fluid and lymph rapidly, confirming the absence of a significant barrier at the capillary level. In contrast, these molecules do not gain free diffusional access to the tubular lumen.

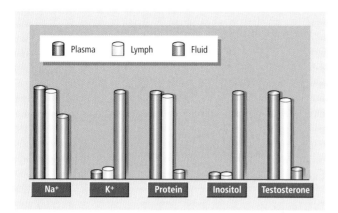

Fig. 4.2 Relative concentrations of substances in the venous plasma (vascular compartment), lymph (interstitial compartment) and testicular fluid leaving the seminiferous tubules (adluminal compartment). Note that seminiferous tubule fluid differs markedly from plasma and lymph.

The intratubular fluid has a quite distinct composition that results from a mix of actively transported and secreted molecules and in both cases the key player is the Sertoli cell. Secreted molecules include androgen-binding protein (ABP), testicular transferrin and sulfated glycoproteins 1 and 2 (SGP1 and 2). The barrier means that the later stages of spermatogenesis occur in a quite distinct and controlled chemical microenvironment.

The testicular fluid secretion can occur against considerable hydrostatic and diffusional gradients. Thus, if the outflow of fluid from the tubules towards the epididymis is blocked pathologically or by ligation of the vasa efferentia, secretion continues nonetheless, and the seminiferous tubules dilate with fluid and spermatozoa, generating a hydrostatic pressure that, if unrelieved, will lead eventually to pressure necrosis and atrophy of intratubular cells.

In summary, the testis may be divided into two major compartments, each of which is further subdivided. The *extratubular* compartment consists of an *intravascular* component, in free communication with an *interstitial* component, including the lymphatics, and in which androgen synthesis occurs in Leydig cells. The *intratubular* compartment consists of a *basal* component, in restricted communication with the interstitium. A unique feature of the seminiferous tubule is that it also has a distinct *adluminal* intratubular compartment, which is effectively isolated from the other three compartments, and in which most of the spermatogenic events occur.

Spermatogenesis has three main phases

The mature spermatozoon is an elaborate, highly specialized cell. *Spermatogenesis*, the process by which spermatozoa are formed, has three elements which occur sequentially.

• First, *mitotic proliferation* produces large numbers of cells.
• Second, *meiotic division* generates genetic diversity and halves the chromosome number.
• Third, *cytodifferentiation* packages the chromosomes for effective delivery to the oocyte.

Large numbers of these complex cells are produced, between 300 and 600 sperm per gram of testis per second! How is this achieved?

Mitotic proliferation increases cell number

The quiescent interphase prospermatogonial germ cells of the immature testis (see Fig. 1.10) are reactivated at puberty to enter rounds of mitosis in the basal compartment of the tubule. Henceforth they are known as *spermatogonial stem cells* (*As spermatogonia*). From within this reservoir of self-regenerating As spermatogonia emerge, at intervals, groups of cells with a distinct morphology called *A1 spermatogonia*. Their emergence marks the beginning of spermatogenesis. Each of these A1 spermatogonia undergoes a limited number of mitotic divisions at about 42-h intervals, thus producing a *clone* of cells. The number of divisions is characteristic for the species, and clearly will determine the total number of cells in the clone. Thus, in the rat there are six divisions leading to a maximum clone size of 64 cells, although cell death during mitosis can reduce this number considerably. The morphology of the cells produced at each mitotic division can be distinguished from that of its parent, enabling us to subclassify spermatogonia (e.g. in the rat) as *type A1–4* during the first three mitoses, *type intermediate* after the fourth mitosis, and *type B* after the subsequent fifth division (Fig. 4.3). All the spermatogonia type B of the clone then divide to form *resting primary spermatocytes* (see Box 4.1 for discussion of pluripotent spermatogonial stem cells).

A remarkable feature of this mitotic phase of spermatogenesis is that although nuclear division (*karyokinesis*) is completed successfully, cytoplasmic division (*cytokinesis*) is incomplete. Thus, all the primary spermatocytes derived from one type A1 spermatogonium are linked together by thin cytoplasmic bridges, constituting effectively a large syncytium. Even more remarkable is the fact that this syncytial organization persists throughout the further meiotic divisions, and individual cells are only released during the last stages of spermatogenesis as mature spermatozoa.

Meiosis halves the chromosome number and generates genetic diversity

The proliferative phase of spermatogenesis takes place in the basal intratubular compartment of the testis. Each

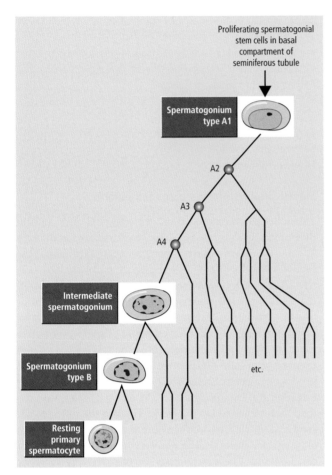

Proliferating spermatogonial
stem cells in basal
compartment of
seminiferous tubule

Spermatogonium
type A1

A2

A3

A4

Intermediate
spermatogonium

Spermatogonium
type B

etc.

Resting
primary
spermatocyte

Fig. 4.3 Cells in the mitotic proliferative phase of spermatogenesis in the rat (present in the basal intratubular compartment). From the population of proliferating spermatogonial type As stem cells arise type A spermatogonia, which have large, ovoid, pale nuclei with a dusty, homogeneous chromatin. The intermediate spermatogonia have a crusty or scalloped chromatin pattern on their nuclear membranes, and this feature is heavily emphasized in type B spermatogonia, in which the nuclei are also smaller and rounded.

resting preleptotene primary spermatocyte so formed duplicates its DNA content and then pushes its way into the adluminal intratubular compartment by transiently disrupting the zonular tight junctions between adjacent Sertoli cells. This brief breach of the blood–testis barrier, which may be regulated by the germ cells themselves, seems to involve the action of the cytokines TNFα and TGFβ3 (see Table 3.6). The spermatocytes then enter the first meiotic pro-phase which is very prolonged (Fig. 4.4; for details of meiosis see Fig. 1.1). During prophase, the sister chromatid strands on the paired homologous chromosomes come together to form synaptonemal contacts at pachytene, during which the chromatids break, exchange segments of genetic material and then rejoin, thereby shuffling their

genetic information, before pulling apart (Figs 1.1 & 4.4). Primary spermatocytes at different steps in this sequence can be identified by the characteristic morphologies of their nuclei, reflecting the state of their chromatin (Fig. 4.4). During this prolonged meiotic prophase, and particularly during pachytene, the spermatocytes are especially sensitive to damage, and widespread degeneration can occur at this stage.

The first meiotic division ends with the separation of homologous chromosomes to opposite ends of the cell on the meiotic spindle, after which cytokinesis yields, from each primary spermatocyte, two *secondary spermatocytes* containing a single set of chromosomes. Each chromosome consists of two chromatids joined at the centromere. The chromatids then separate, move to opposite ends of the second meiotic spindle, and the short-lived secondary spermatocytes divide to yield haploid *early round spermatids* (Fig. 4.4). Thus, from the maximum of 64 primary spermatocytes that entered meiosis (in the rat), 256 early spermatids could result. Again, the actual number is much less than this, as, in addition to any losses at earlier mitotic stages, the complexities of the meiotic process result in the further loss of cells. Yet again, the whole cluster of spermatids is linked syncytially via thin cytoplasmic bridges. With the formation of the early round spermatids, the important chromosomal reduction events of spermatogenesis are completed.

Cytodifferentiation packages the chromosomes for delivery

The most visible and major changes during spermatogenesis occur during a remarkable cytoplasmic remodelling of the spermatid that is called *spermiogenesis* (Fig. 4.5). During this process, spermatids change shape from round to *elongating* spermatids. A *tail* is generated for forward propulsion; the *midpiece* forms, containing the mitochondria (energy generators for the cell); the *equatorial and postacrosomal cap* region forms, and is important for sperm–oocyte fusion; the *acrosome* (a modified lysosomal structure) develops and functions like an 'enzymatic knife' when penetrating towards the oocyte; the nucleus contains the compact packaged haploid chromosomes; and the *residual body* acts as a dustbin for the residue of superfluous cytoplasm, and is phagocytosed by the Sertoli cell after the spermatozoon departs. The spermatid centrioles are of particular interest. They reduce to a central core structure linking the midpiece to the sperm head. All or most of their pericentriolar material, that normally nucleates microtubules, is lost. The opposite happens in the oocyte (Chapter 5), in which pericentriolar material is retained but centrioles are lost. This reciprocal pattern of reduction means that at fertilization there is centriolar complementarity of gametes (Chapter 9).

BOX 4.1 Potency and spermatogonial stem cells

- *Spermatogonial (As) stem cells form a small self-renewing population* from which some cells periodically divert to form the spermatogenic lineage. The stem cells can now be isolated from the testis and studied *in vitro* or transplanted to other sites. When placed into a seminiferous tubule, the stem cells can populate it and produce fertile spermatozoa—definitive proof of their stem cell potential.

- *How do the stem cells 'decide' to proliferate or differentiate?* Members of the TGFβ family are implicated in this decision (Table 3.6). Stem cell pluripotency is promoted by glial derived neurotrophic growth factor (GDNF) secreted from the Sertoli cells. In contrast, activin A suppresses the pluripotency of stem cells, and their differentiation as spermatogonia A and B is promoted by BMP4, also from Sertoli cells. BMP4 probably acts by stimulating the appearance of c-Kit receptors on the spermatogonia, and these receptors then bind stem cell factor (SCF), which is itself produced by the Sertoli cell. This interaction helps to maintain the mitotic divisions of the differentiating spermatogonia. Once spermatogonial proliferation is completed, BMP7, 8a and 8b seem to be required for successful meiosis, as their genetic deletion leads to the loss of meiotic germ cells.

- *Microenvironmental niches within the testis?* It will immediately be apparent that the Sertoli cell plays a key role and produces several growth factors, each with different consequences. It is not clear how it achieves this. Some of these growth factors act juxtacrinologically and so their spatial organization on the cell surface may be important in determining which GFs are expressed locally. The Sertoli cell also oscillates its activities with the spermatogenic cycle, so there may be temporal regulation of GF expression patterns too. These findings have given rise to the idea of the 'micro-environmental niche' experienced by stem cells and their descendants, determining the decision whether to remain a stem cell or to differentiate into spermatozoa.

- *How pluripotent is the spermatogonial stem cell?* If, instead of being placed into seminiferous tubules, the stem cells are held *in vitro* or transplanted to other sites in the body, they are found to have a broader stem cell potential than simply the spermatogenic lineage, being able to give rise to multiple cell types. In this regard, they resemble embryonic stem (ES) cells derived *in vitro* from the epiblast of the blastocyst (see Chapter 10). Conversely, pluripotential embryonic stem cells themselves have now been shown capable under the influence of cytokine BMP4 of giving rise to primordial germ cells, which in conjunction with seminiferous tubule cells then can form spermatogonial stem cells and spermatozoa. BMP4 is also important *in vivo* for the formation of primordial germ cells (see Chapter 1 for details of the development of the testis *in vivo*). Thus spermatogonial and embryonic stem cells seem to be closely related, and so the potential use of spermatogonial stem cells therapeutically to treat degenerative disorders is being explored as an alternative to the use of ES cells, which is more controversial ethically (see Chapter 15).

Advanced reading

de Sousa Lopes SM *et al.* (2004) BMP signaling mediated by ALK2 in the visceral endoderm is necessary for the generation of primordial germ cells in the mouse embryo. *Genes and Development* **18**, 1838–1849.

Guan K *et al.* (2006) Pluripotency of spermatogonial stem cells from adult mouse testis. *Nature* **440**, 1199–1203.

Loveland KL, Hime G (2005) TGFβ superfamily members in spermatogenesis: setting the stage for fertility in mouse and *Drosophila*. *Cell and Tissue Research* **322**, 141–146.

Ohta H *et al.* (2000) Regulation of proliferation and differentiation in spermatogonial stem cells: the role of c-kit and its ligand SCF. *Development* **127**, 2125–2131.

Toyooka Y *et al.* (2003) Embryonic stem cells can form germ cell in vitro. *Proceedings of the National Academy of Sciences of the USA* **100**, 11457–11462.

Zhao G-Q (2002) Consequences of knocking out BMP signaling in the mouse. *Genesis* **35**, 43–56.

Zhao G-Q, Garbers DL (2002) Male germ cell specification and differentiation throughout the phylogeny from invertebrates to mammals. *Developmental Cell* **2**, 537–547.

Spermiogenesis is completed with the formation of a fully mature spermatozoon (Fig. 4.6). With the appearance of the spermatozoa, the thin cytoplasmic bridges that make up the syncytium rupture, and the cells are released into the lumen of the tubule in a process called *spermiation*. They are washed along the seminiferous tubules in the testicular fluid secreted by Sertoli cells.

Genetic activity during spermatogenesis is special

Spermatogenesis is a complex and specialized process and, not surprisingly, requires a large number of genes for its successful completion. The processes of mRNA production and translation continue throughout spermatogonial mitosis and meiosis (except on the sex chromosomes, which cease transcription from meiosis onwards); indeed, after the completion of meiosis there is a large transcriptional surge. Autosomal transcription ceases during the transition from round to elongated spermatids. The burst of transcription immediately *after meiotic completion* is characterized by two features not observed in somatic cells: the use of specialized transcriptional machinery and the expression of large numbers of spermatogenic-specific genes (Box 4.2). Because this postmeiotic burst occurs from the *haploid genomes*, it raises the possibility that the spermatozoa might differ from each other phenotypically in ways that reflect

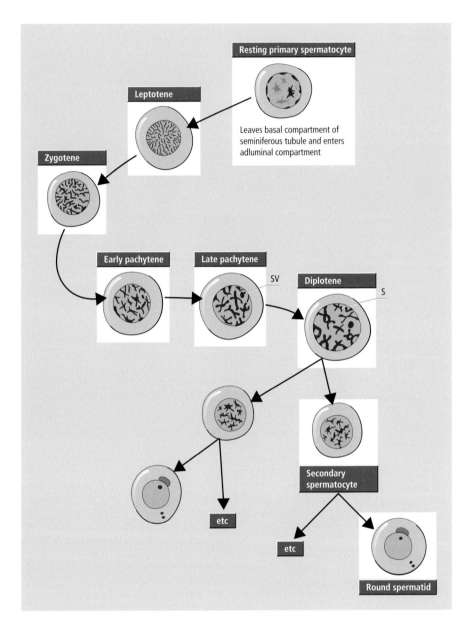

Resting primary spermatocyte

Leptotene

Leaves basal compartment of seminiferous tubule and enters adluminal compartment

Zygotene

Early pachytene

Late pachytene

SV

Diplotene

S

etc

Secondary spermatocyte

etc

Round spermatid

Fig. 4.4 Progress of a rat primary spermatocyte through meiosis in the adluminal intratubular compartment. DNA synthesis is completed in the resting primary spermatocyte, although limited 'repair DNA' associated with crossing over occurs in late zygotene and early pachytene. In leptotene, the chromatin becomes filamentous as it condenses. In zygotene, homologous chromosomes thicken and come together in pairs (synapsis) attached to the nuclear membrane at their extremities, thus forming loops or 'bouquets'. In pachytene, the pairs of chromosomes (bivalents) shorten and condense, and nuclear and cytoplasmic volume increases. It is at this stage that autosomal crossing over takes place (the two sex chromosomes are paired in the *sex vesicle*, SV). The synapses (S) can be seen at light-microscopic level as chiasmata during diplotene and diakinesis, as the chromosomes start to pull apart and condense further. The nuclear membrane then breaks down, followed by spindle formation, and the first meiotic division is completed to yield two secondary spermatocytes each containing a single set of chromosomes. These are very short lived and rapidly enter the second meiotic division, the chromatids separating at the centromere to yield four haploid round spermatids.

their unique haploid genetic composition. Were this so, it might then be possible to separate later spermatids and spermatozoa into subpopulations based on their carriage of distinctive genetic alleles. Such a separation might occur in the female genital tract, thereby exerting 'natural selection' on a population of spermatozoa that was genetically and, via haploid expression, phenotypically heterogeneous. Selection might also be made in the laboratory, were spermatozoal enrichment for particular characteristics wanted. For example, the separation of X- and Y-bearing spermatozoa might allow prefertilization sex 'selection'. However, successful evidence of haploid spermatozoal selection has been hard to come by. This is not entirely

surprising as spermatids exist in a syncytial mass of cytoplasm, giving opportunity for mRNAs and proteins to diffuse into all spermatids regardless of their genotype. Additionally, the premeiotic inactivation of the X and Y chromosomes (see above) makes selection for sex by this approach very unlikely. Recently, the separation of X- and Y-bearing spermatozoa has been claimed not on the basis of the *differential expression* of the sex chromosomes, but as a result of their *different total DNA contents*. Thus, the percentage difference in DNA content of X- and Y-bearing human spermatozoa is 2.9% (boar 3%; bull 3.8%; stallion 4.1%; ram 4.2%). The separation of fertile spermatozoa by flow cytometry can achieve enrichment rates of over 75%

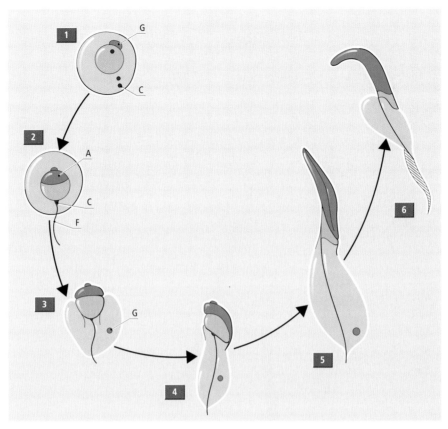

Fig. 4.5 Progress of a rat round spermatid through the packaging phase of the spermatogenic lineage. The Golgi apparatus (G) of the newly formed round spermatid (1) gives rise to glycoprotein-rich lysosomal-like granules, which coalesce to a single acrosomal vesicle (A) that grows over the nuclear surface to form a cap-like structure (2). Between the acrosome and the nucleus, a subacrosomal cytoskeletal element, the perforatorium, forms in many species. The nuclear membrane at this site loses its nuclear pores. The two centrioles (C) lie against the opposite pole of the nuclear membrane, and a typical flagellum (F) (9 + 2 microtubules) grows outwards from the more distal centriole (2), while from the proximal centriole the neck or connecting piece forms, linking the tail to the nucleus. The nucleus moves with its attached acrosomal cap towards the cytoplasmic membrane and elongation begins (3 and 4). Chromatin condensation commences (Box 4.3) beneath the acrosomal cap, generating a nuclear shape, which is characteristic for the species (3–6), and superfluous nuclear membrane and nucleoplasm is lost. The Golgi apparatus detaches from the now completed acrosomal cap and moves posteriorly as the acrosome starts to change its shape. Nine coarse fibres form along the axis of the developing tail, each aligned with an outer microtubule doublet of the flagellum (see Fig. 4.6 for details). In the final phase, the mitochondria migrate to the anterior part of the flagellum, and condense around it as a series of rods forming a spiral (see Fig. 4.6). The superfluous cytoplasm appears 'squeezed' down the spermatid and is shed as the spermatozoa are released (hatched) (6). The mature spermatozoon has remarkably little cytoplasm left.

in large farm animals. However, the prospects for a 100% successful separation of human spermatozoa for therapeutic use by this approach seem poor.

Spermatozoal chromatin is modified during spermatogenesis

The cessation of transcriptional activity during spermiogenesis is due to a massive repackaging of the spermatogenic DNA, such that the chromatin becomes highly condensed (to about 5% of the volume of a somatic cell nucleus). This form of DNA is described as being *hetero-chromatic*. Condensation is achieved by the replacement of the histones that characterize somatic cell chromatin by *protamines* (Box 4.3). In this way, spermatozoa develop tightly compressed chromatin in which genetic expression is completely absent. As pointed out above, the sex chromosomes go through this process earlier than the autosomes and end up in a special nuclear compartment, the *sex vesicle*, which lacks RNA polymerase II. This repackaging and silencing of chromatin is preparing the male genome for life in the zygote (see Chapter 10).

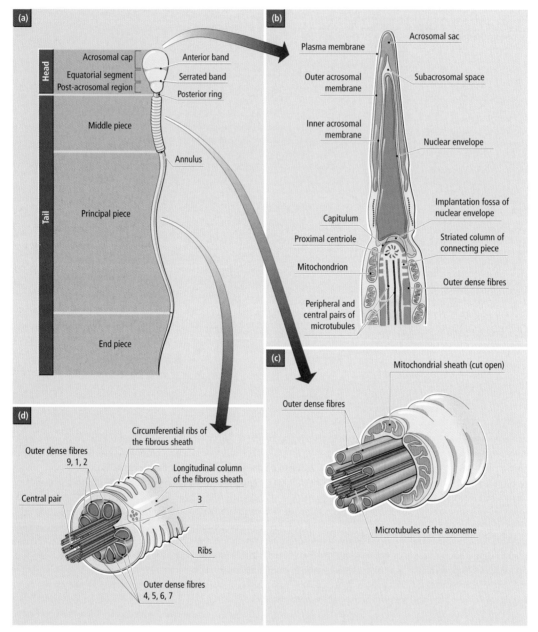

Fig. 4.6 (a) Diagram of a primate spermatozoon (50 μm long) showing on the left, the main structural regions; and on the right, the boundaries between them. The surface membrane structure within each region is highly characteristic, having a unique lipid, sugar, surface charge and protein composition that differs from those in adjacent regions. These differences are probably maintained both by the inter-regional boundary structures and by underlying molecular attachments to cytoskeletal elements. The differences are important functionally (Chapter 9). (b) Sagittal section of the head, neck and top of the midpiece. Note the elongated (green) nucleus with highly compact chromatin and the acrosomal sac. The posterior end of the nuclear membrane is the only part to retain nuclear pores and forms the implantation fossa, which is connected to the capitulum by fine filaments. The capitulum, in turn, is connected to the outer dense fibres by two major and five minor segmented columns and is also the site of termination of the two central microtubules of the flagellum. The more distal of the two centrioles degenerates late in spermiogenesis. In a few species both centrioles are lost; they are not essential for sperm motility, only for the initial formation of the axoneme during spermiogenesis. (c) Sketch of the midpiece (surface membrane removed). Note the sheath of spiral mitochondria, and the axoneme of the tail comprising nine circumferential doublets of microtubules and two central microtubules; peripheral to each outer doublet is a dense fibre. (d) Section and sketch of the principal piece (surface membrane removed). The mitochondria are replaced by a fibrous sheath, comprising two longitudinal columns interconnected by ribs. The two fibrous sheath columns connect to underlying outer dense fibres 3 and 8. The outer dense fibres terminate towards the end of the principal piece, and the fibrous sheath then attaches directly to outer microtubules 3 and 8 before itself fading away in the end piece.

BOX 4.2 Gene expression during spermatogenesis

- *Highly distinctive processes occur during spermatogenesis* such as pluripotency retention; meiosis; genetic recombination; haploid gene expression; chromatin remodelling and condensation; and acrosome and flagellum formation. These processes involve unique gene products, many of which have been identified recently through expression profiling of different spermatogenic cells isolated and purified by centrifugation and gravity sedimentation, combined with tests of function/expression using transgenic and knockout mouse models. Here we focus on haploid expression.

- *The transcription machinery of the haploid spermatogenic lineage* shows several unique features. For example, TATA-binding protein (TBP), transcription factor IIB (TFIIB), and RNA polymerase II all accumulate in much higher amounts (approximately 100×) in post-meiotic cells than in somatic cells. In addition, testis-specific isoforms exist of many transcriptional complex proteins including TBP, TAFII (TBF associated factors, such as TFIIAτ and, TAFIIQ) and TBP-related protein (TRF2). This highly characteristic complex of molecular machinery then facilitates expression of an equally characteristic set of spermatogenic genes.

- *Many genes expressed in somatic cells are also expressed in male germ cells*, but use alternative promoters and/or splice isoforms, or are usurped by expression of homologous genes specific for the spermatogenic lineage. Other genes are uniquely expressed in that lineage. Many of the wave of genes activated after meioisis have promoters containing cAMP-responsive elements (CREs), DNA sequences which recruit members of the CRE-binding (CREB) family of transcription factors. In somatic cells, CREBs bind to CREs, are phosphorylated, and recruit a co-activator (CREB-binding protein or CBP). The CBP has a dual function, as it acetylates histones, thereby contributing to the chromatin decondensation that precedes transcription, and it also provides a link to the transcription machinery complex. However, there is little CREB expression in the testis (and most of it is in Sertoli cells). Instead, a protein called cAMP response element modulator (CREM; mostly present as its CREMτ isoform) is highly expressed and interacts specifically with testis-specific TFIIAτ and TRF2 in the spermatogenic transcription complex.

- *Mice null for CREM and TRF2* (but not CREB) block in early spermiogenesis, indicating their critical role in post-meiotic transcriptional control. Moreover, both proteins are located in the nuclei of round spermatids (genes expressing) but become cytoplasmic in elongating spermatids (genes shut down). CREMτ levels increase under the influence of FSH, but interestingly the hormone acts by stabilizing the mRNA encoding the protein. CREM-controlled genes include many essential for mature sperm function, such as those encoding protamines 1 and 2 (essential for sperm DNA packing: see Box 4.3) and proacrosin (a sperm-specific protease precursor important in zona penetration: see Chapter 9).

Further reading

Daniel PB *et al.* (2000) Novel cyclic adenosine 3',5'-monophosphate (cAMP) response element modulator theta isoforms expressed by two newly identified cAMP-responsive promoters active in the testis. *Endocrinology* **141**, 3923–3930.

Eddy EM (2002) Male germ cell gene expression. *Recent Progress in Hormone Research* **57**, 103–128.

Grimes SR (2004) Testis-specific transcriptional control. *Gene* **343**, 11–22.

Monaco L *et al.* (2004) Specialized rules of gene transcription in male germ cells: the CREM paradigm. *International Journal of Andrology* **27**, 322–327.

Sassone-Corsi P (2002) Unique chromatin remodeling and transcriptional regulation in spermatogenesis. *Science* **296**, 2176–2178.

Schlecht U *et al.* (2004) Expression profiling of mammalian male meiosis and gametogenesis identifies novel candidate genes for roles in the regulation of fertility. *Molecular Biology of the Cell* **15**, 1031–1043.

Venables JP (2002) Alternative splicing in the testes. *Current Opinion in Genetics and Development* **12**, 615–619.

Spermatogenesis is highly organized both temporally and spatially

Each mature spermatozoon is one sibling in a large family, derived from one parental spermatogonium type A. The family is large because of the number of premeiotic mitoses, and the spermatozoa are only siblings and not 'identical twins' because meiotic chiasmata formation ensures that each is genetically unique despite having a common ancestral parent. Within each testis tubule, hundreds of such families develop side by side, and there are 30 or so tubules within each rat testis. How is the development of these families organized temporally and spatially?

Spermatogenesis proceeds at a constant and characteristic rate for each species

One way to measure the length of time it takes to complete parts of the spermatogenic process is to 'mark' cells at different points during the process, and then to measure the rate of progress of the labelled cells through its completion. For example, if radioactive thymidine is supplied to the resting primary spermatocytes as they engage in the final round of DNA synthesis before they enter into meiosis, the cell nuclei will be labelled and their progress through meiosis, spermiogenesis and spermiation can be followed. In this way, the amount of time required for each

BOX 4.3 Spermatogenic chromatin remodelling

- *In somatic cells, the nucleosome is the basic unit of chromatin* and consists of 146 base pairs of DNA wrapped round an octamer of core histones: two molecules of H2A, H2B, H3 and H4. A fifth histone, H1, protects the DNA fragments linking adjacent nucleosomes. The chromatin structure undergoes structural alterations fit for different local or global functions (gene expression/suppression, DNA repair/reproduction, chromosomal nuclear localization). These alterations include use of different non-allelic histone variants and various post-translational histone modifications (acetylation, methylation, phosphorylation, etc.), some of which may even be retained heritably across cell division cycles as *chromatin imprints* (see Chapters 9, 12 & 14). The rich combinatorial possibility of multiple histone variants, each susceptible to multiple post-translational modifications, provides highly complex nucleosomal microenvironments—an informational treasure chest of 'epigenetic' information to rival the genetic code itself.
- *Histone changes occur during spermatogenesis.* First, there is an incorporation, mainly during meiosis, of histone variants, including testis-specific variants of H1 (H1t and HILS1), H2A (TH2A) and H3 (H3t). Their incorporation is also accompanied by a range of histone modifications. These changes seem to be associated with the events of meiosis (especially the H2A and H3 variants), the segregation of the sex chromosome to the sex vesicle (especially H2A variants), and the preparation for the next phase of chromatin remodelling during condensation (especially H1 variants).
- *The condensation of chromatin* that occurs during the transition from round to elongating spermatid is accompanied by hyperacetylation and ubiquitination of histones, which is linked strongly to their removal and replacement with *transition nuclear proteins* (TNPs 1 and 2), small basic proteins unique to the testis. These appear to facilitate the subsequent change, during which they in turn are replaced during spermatid elongation with *protamines 1 and 2* (small basic proteins comprising 50% arginine). The protamine molecules on adjacent regions of DNA are cross-linked to each other via disulfide bonds on their constituent cysteines. The end result is inactive condensed hetero-chromatin.

Further reading

Govin J et al. (2004) The role of histones in chromatin remodelling during mammalian spermiogenesis. *European Journal of Biochemistry* **271**, 3459–3469.

Khochbin S (2001) Histone H1 diversity: bridging regulatory signals to linker histone function. *Gene* **271**, 1–12.

Tanaka H, Baba T (2005) Gene expression in spermiogenesis. *Cellular and Molecular Life Sciences* **62**, 344–354.

spermatogenic step can be measured. In Fig. 4.7 the times required for each step in the rat are represented visually in blocks, the length of each being a measure of relative time. The absolute time for the whole process, from entry into first mitosis to release of spermatozoa, is recorded for several species in Table 4.1 (column 1). It is a lengthy process, taking several weeks.

There are differences between species in the total time required to complete spermatogenesis. However, it is striking that within a species the rate of progression of cells through spermatogenesis is remarkably constant. Thus, the spermatogonia type A within any testis of a given species seem to advance through spermatogenesis at the same rate, and take the same total time for completion of the process. Hormones, or other externally applied agents, do not seem to speed up or slow down the spermatogenic process. They may affect whether or not the process occurs at all, but not the rate at which it occurs. This remarkable constancy suggests a high level of intrinsic organization.

Rounds of spermatogenesis are initiated at time intervals that are constant and characteristic for each species

So far we have considered the process of spermatogenesis from the viewpoint of a single spermatogonium type A, generating a family of descendant spermatozoa at a constant and characteristic rate. Once this process has been commenced at a particular point in any tubule, new spermatogonial stem cells at the same point do not commence the generation of their own clones until several days have elapsed. Remarkably, it has been found that this interval between successive entries into spermatogenesis is also constant and is also characteristic for each species (Table 4.1, column 2). Somehow, the stem cell population measures, or is told, the length of this time interval. This cyclic initiation of spermatogenesis is called the *spermatogenic cycle*.

In the case of the rat, the spermatogenic cycle is about 12 days long. This period is one-quarter of the 48–49 days required for completion of mature spermatozoal production, so it follows that four successive spermatogenic processes must be occurring at the same time (Fig. 4.7). The advanced cells, in those spermatogenic families that were initiated earliest, are displaced progressively by subsequent rounds of developing spermatogenic cells from the periphery towards the lumen of the tubule. Thus, a transverse section through the tubule will reveal spermatogenic cells at four distinctive stages in the progression towards spermatozoa, each cell type representing a stage in separate, successive cycles (Fig. 4.7).

As both the spermatogenic cycle and the spermatogenic process are of constant length, it follows that the cells in successive cycles will always develop in parallel.

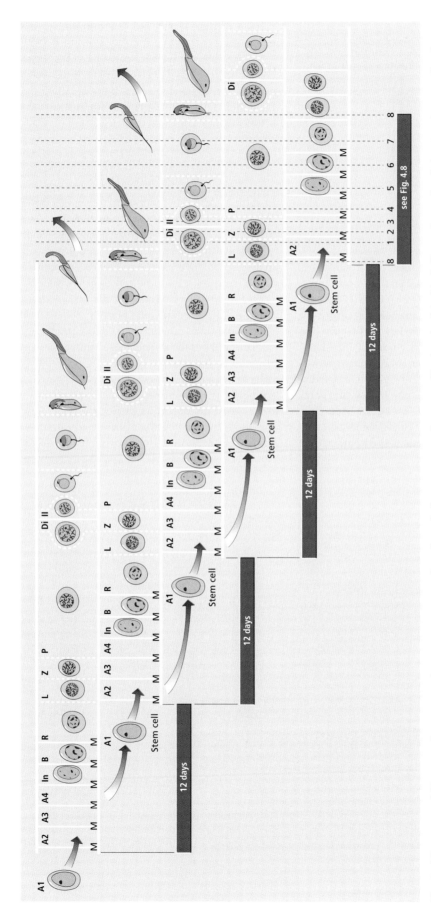

Fig. 4.7 The top panel illustrates the passage of one rat spermatogonium through the spermatogenic process. The length of the block illustrating each cellular stage is proportional to the amount of time spent in that stage. When a new cell type arises by division, vertical white bars separate adjacent blocks (M, mitosis). During meiotic prophase and spermiogenesis, however, cells change morphology by progressive differentiation, not quantal jumps. This continuum of change is indicated by the use of vertical broken white lines to delineate blocks. A, In and B, spermatogonia; R, L, Z, P and Di, resting, leptotene, zygotene, pachytene and diplotene primary spermatocytes; II, secondary spermatocytes. Each of the lower panels shows the history of other spermatozoa, which commenced development by cyclic generation of new type A spermatogonia from the stem cell population at progressively later time intervals. The interval between each of these events is about 12 days. Note that four such events occur before the upper spermatozoon (and its siblings in the family) has completed development and been released. As cells progress through spermatogenesis, they move progressively from the basal tubule to the luminal centre. Thus, several different cell types will be present in one cross-section of a tubule at the same time, although at different points on the radial axis through the tubule. This feature is illustrated more compactly in Fig. 4.8, in which the sections indicated by the dashed lines numbered 1–8 are summarized.

Table 4.1 Kinetics of spermatogenesis.

Species	Time for completion of spermatogenesis (days)	Duration of cycle of the seminiferous epithelium (days)
Man	64	16
Bull	54	13.5
Ram	49	12.25
Boar	34	8.5
Rat	48	12

Therefore, the sets of cell associations in any radial cross-section through a segment of tubule taken at different times will always be characteristic (Figs 4.7 & 4.8). For example, as the cycle interval is 12 days and it also takes 12 days for the six mitotic divisions, entry into meiosis will always be occurring just as a new cycle is initiated by the first division of a spermatogonium type A (Fig. 4.8, column 8). Similarly, it takes 24 days (i.e. two cycles) for the premeiotic spermatocyte to complete meiosis and the early phase of spermatid modelling. So not only will entry into mitosis and entry into meiosis coincide, but so will the beginning of spermatid elongation (Fig. 4.8, column 8). These events will also coincide with release of spermatozoa at spermiation, as it

takes a further 12 days for the completion of spermatid elongation.

Up to this point, we have considered the organization of the spermatogonial stem cells and their descendants at one point in the tubule. However, there are thousands of spermatogonia type A throughout the tubules in any one testis at any one time: how are they organized in relation to each other?

The seminiferous epithelium cycles

Imagine all of the spermatogonial stem cells throughout the testis entering mitotic activity at exactly the same time. As the time to complete spermatogenesis is constant, there would be a simultaneous release of all the resulting spermatozoa. Moreover, as the spermatogenic cycle is constant for all stem cells, periodic pulses of spermatozoal release would occur (every 12 days in the rat, for example). This could result in an episodic pattern of male fertility. This problem could be circumvented if the spermatogonial stem cells throughout the testis initiated mitotic activity not synchronously but randomly. Then, their relative times of entry into spermatogenesis would be staggered, thus eliminating the pulsatile release of spermatozoa and smoothing it into a continuous flow. In fact, the testis functions in a manner somewhat between these two extremes, although the end result is continuous spermatozoal production.

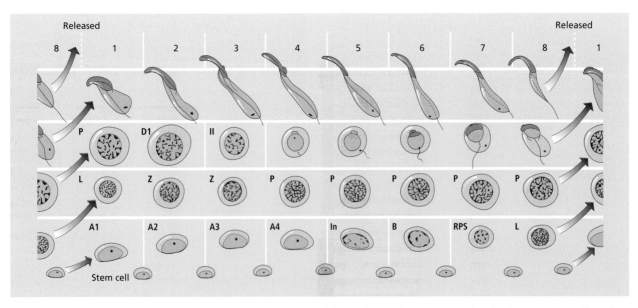

Fig. 4.8 The sections indicated in Fig. 4.7 are summarized here. Read from left to right. A vertical white bar between two cells in the sequence indicates a cell division; otherwise the changes are not quantal but occur by progressive differentiation. Abbreviations as for Fig. 4.7. RPS, resting primary spermatocyte. (Note: because the spermatogenic process is continuous, it can be subdivided more or less finely. The subdivision pattern used here is a basic one. A commonly used, more finely divided and thus more complex pattern uses 16 rather than 8 subdivisions numbered I to XVI. A rough equivalence is stage 1: IX–XI, stage 2: XII–XIII, stage 3: XIV, stage 4: I, stage 5: II–IV, stage 6: V–VI, stage 7: VII, and stage 8; VIII).

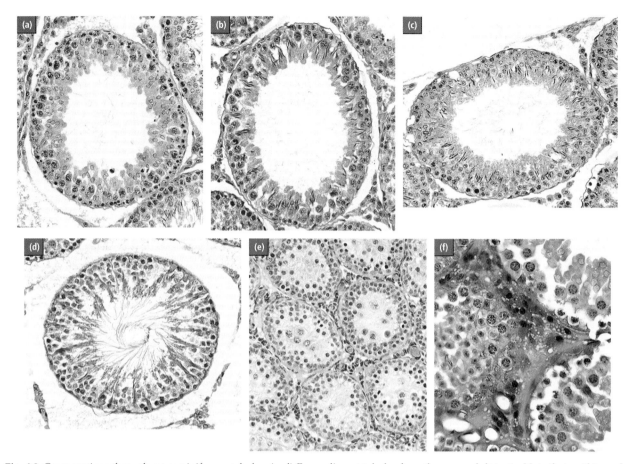

Fig. 4.9 Cross-sections through rat seminiferous tubules. (a–d) Four adjacent tubules from the same adult testis. Note that, within each tubule, the sets of cell associations along all radial axes are the same. However, each tubule has a different set of cell associations from its neighbour. Thus, tubule (a) is at stage 8/1 in Figs 4.7 and 4.8, tubule (b) is at stage 2, tubule (c) is at stage 5, and tubule (d) is at stage 7. Tubule (e) is from an adult rat testis 4 weeks after hypophysectomy. Note that spermatogenesis fails during the early meiotic stage with no cells more mature than a primary spermatocyte present. Note also the lack of a tubular lumen, indicating cessation of fluid secretion. Panel (f) shows staining of the intertubular region of an adult intact testis for the Leydig cells. Note their reddish foamy cytoplasm indicative of steroidogenesis.

Examination of cross-sections through the testes of most mammals shows that within a tubule the same set of cell associations is observed, regardless of the point on the circumference studied (Fig. 4.9a–d). This means that all the stem cells in that section of tubule must be synchronized in absolute time. It is almost as though a message passes circumferentially around the segment of tubule activating the stem cell population in that segment to initiate spermatogonial type A production together. This spatial coordination of adjacent spermatogenic cycles gives rise to the *cycle of the seminiferous epithelium*, as the whole epithelial cross-section goes through cyclic changes in patterns of cell association (see Fig. 4.8).

The human testis (together with the testes of New World monkeys and great apes) is somewhat atypical, as a cross-section through an individual tubule reveals a degree of spatial organization that is more limited to 'wedges'. It is as if

the putative activator message does not get all the way round a cross-section of tubule, and so the coordinated development of different spermatogonial stem cells is initiated over a smaller area. This does not mean, of course, that the control of either the spermatogenic cycle or the rate of spermatogenesis in man differs fundamentally from control mechanisms in other species. It means merely that the spatial coordination between adjacent individual stem cells is not so great.

Spermatogenesis in adjacent regions along a seminiferous tubule appears to be phase advanced or retarded

If an individual seminiferous tubule is dissected and laid out longitudinally, and cross-sections are taken at intervals along it and classified according to the set of cell associations in it, a pattern, similar to that in Fig. 4.10, will then

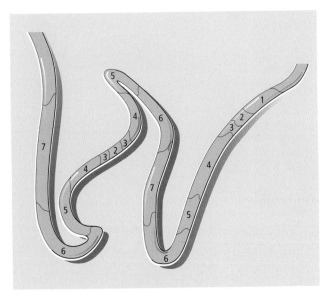

Fig. 4.10 Dissected seminiferous tubule from a rat testis. Note that whole segments of the tubule are at the same stage (numbered) of the cycle of the seminiferous epithelium, and that adjacent segments tend to be either just advanced or just retarded.

often result. Adjacent tubule segments, each containing synchronized populations of spermatogenic stem cells, seem to have entered the spermatogenic process slightly out of phase with each other. For example, in Fig. 4.10, the most advanced segment (7) is at the centre; moving along the tubule in either direction leads to sets of cell associations characteristic of progressively earlier stages of the cycle of the seminiferous epithelium. It is as though the central segment has been activated first, and then another hypothetical 'activator message' has spread along the tubule in both directions, progressively initiating mitosis and, thereby, spermatogenic cycles. The resulting appearance in the adult testis, as shown in Fig. 4.10, is sometimes called the *spermatogenic wave*.

It is important not to confuse the wave with the cycle of the seminiferous epithelium, although both phenomena appear very similar. Imagine that, whereas the sequence of cell associations forming the *wave* could be recorded by travelling along the tubule with a movie camera running, the same sequence of cell associations would only be captured in the *cycle* by setting up the movie camera on time-lapse at a fixed point in the tubule. Thus, *the wave occurs in space, while the cycle occurs in time.*

The Sertoli cell may control the temporal and spatial organization of spermatogenesis

These observations on spermatogenesis imply a remarkable degree of temporal and spatial organization among

the spermatogenic cells. The Sertoli cell is the probable organizer. Thus, the cytoplasms of adjacent Sertoli cells are in continuity with one another via extensive gap junctional contacts. These effectively provide a continuous cytoplasmic network along and around the tubule through which communication and synchronization might occur (see Fig. 4.1). In addition, each Sertoli cell spans the tubule from peritubular basement membrane to lumen, thereby providing a potential radial conduit for communication, through which all its associated spermatogenic cells could be locked into the same rate of developmental progression. This latter possibility is made more attractive by the observation that the Sertoli cell engages in intimate associations with all the cells of the spermatogenic lineage. These associations are of three types: (1) Pachytene spermatocytes communicate with, and receive material from, the Sertoli cell via gap junctional complexes. (2) Most spermatocytes and spermatids form unique *ectoplasmic specializations* with Sertoli cells (ECs; adherens-like junctions which replace desmosomal junctional complexes present at spermatogonial stages; Fig. 4.1), and these are largely thought to be concerned with anchoring and then releasing the spermatogenic cells and perhaps remodelling them during spermiogenesis. They are lost at spermiation. (3) Elongating spermatids and Sertoli cells also form heavily indented *tubulobulbar complexes* (also adherens-like junctions) through which the Sertoli cell is thought to remove material during cytoplasmic condensation (Fig. 4.1). Finally, the Sertoli cell itself shows characteristic changes in morphology and biochemistry in concert with the cycle of the seminiferous epithelium. For example, the volume, lipid content, nuclear morphology, and number and distribution of secondary lysosomes vary cyclically, as do the synthesis and output of a number of testicular proteins, such as ABP, SGP1 and 2, transferrin and plasminogen activator. Interestingly, the output of the latter protein is high at around the time of spermiation and the passage of preleptotene spermatocytes into the adluminal compartment, suggesting a potential function for its proteolytic activities. Moreover, Sertoli cell cycling is initiated at puberty ahead of spermatogenesis, suggesting that it leads and the spermatogenic process follows. Failure of Sertoli cell maturation or inadequate Sertoli cell proliferation results in aspermatogenesis. However, although the evidence implicating Sertoli cell activity in the organization of the spermatogenic cycle is highly persuasive, such a role remains to be proven decisively.

Summary

The production of spermatozoa is a complex and highly organized process, which is now well described, even if its coordinating control remains imperfectly understood.

Whether or not the Sertoli cell plays a role in the control of spermatogenic rates, cycles and waves remains to be established. In contrast, it *is* established that the Sertoli cell plays a critical role in mediating the actions of hormones and other agents on spermatogenesis. We will now consider endocrine activity within the testis and its relationship to the process of spermatogenesis.

Testicular endocrine activity and the control of spermatogenesis

The testis produces hormones

The most important hormones produced by the testis are the androgens, which, as discussed in Chapter 1, play a major and essential role both during development and in reproductive and sexual function in the mature male (see Chapter 8). In addition, the testis produces oestrogens—in some species, such as the horse, in large amounts. The cytokines inhibin, activin, MIH and Insl3 are also testicular products, as is the peptide hormone, oxytocin. Where does each of these come from and what does each do locally and systemically?

Steroids of the testis

As discussed in Chapter 3, the androgens comprise a class of steroid with distinct structural and functional features (see Table 3.2). The principal testicular androgen is testosterone. It is synthesized from acetate and cholesterol (Fig. 4.11) by the Leydig cells of the interstitial tissue (Fig. 4.9f). Thus, Leydig cells isolated in culture produce testosterone. The enzyme 3β-hydroxysteroid dehydrogenase, involved in Δ5 to Δ4 conversions (Fig. 4.11), is localized to Leydig cells, and in pathological conditions and seasonal breeders, changes in testosterone output correlate with changes in the morphology of the smooth endoplasmic reticulum in Leydig cells.

In man, 4–10 mg of testosterone are secreted daily, and leave the testis by three routes. The hormone rapidly enters both the blood (in the ram, 80 ng/mL of testicular venous blood) and lymph (50 ng/mL). Although the concentrations in each are similar, the major quantitative output is

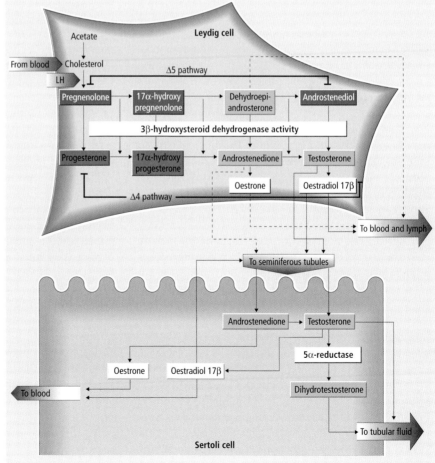

Fig. 4.11 Summary of the steroidogenic pathways in the human testis. The principal (Δ5) path for testosterone synthesis in the Leydig cells of the human is indicated by heavy lines, but the Δ4 pathway is also used and may be more important in other species. In addition to testosterone, some of the intermediates in the pathway are released into the blood: androstenedione at 10% and dehydroepiandrosterone at about 6% of testosterone levels in man. Some testosterone and androstenedione enter Sertoli cells. Here they may bind to androgen receptors directly or after conversion to the more potent dihydrotestosterone. Androgens may also be converted to oestrogens. In humans prepubertally, this occurs predominantly in the Sertoli cells, but postpubertally in the Leydig cells. Oestrogen also enters the seminiferous tubule fluid (see Chapter 9).

to the blood, with its greater flow (17 mL blood/min and 0.2 mL lymph/min in the ram). However, the lymphatic flow is important as the lymph drainage pathways carry testosterone adjacent to the testicular excurrent ducts and the male accessory sex glands, which are stimulated by it. The third route is exocrine. Testosterone, being relatively lipid soluble (see Chapter 3), passes freely through the tissues of the testis and enters the tubule lumen where it binds to the androgen-binding protein (ABP) secreted by the Sertoli cells. The ABP carries it in the testicular fluid flowing into the excurrent ducts, which are stimulated by it (see Chapter 8).

However, androgens also act *within* the testis, where three cell types are targets, each possessing androgen receptors (ARs). First, androgens act autocrinologically on the Leydig cells themselves in a short negative feedback loop. Androgens also act on myoid cells to sustain tubular functional integrity. Finally, androgen within the seminiferous tubules enters Sertoli cells, where much of it is converted by 5α-reductase activity to the more active dihydrotestosterone. Both DHT and testosterone then bind to ARs within the Sertoli cell itself. Interestingly, whereas both Leydig and myoid cells show constitutive levels of AR, Sertoli cells show oscillations in AR levels in phase with the cycle of the seminiferous epithelium, peaking as stage 8 and sperm release is approached. These spermatogenic stages are also the ones most sensitive to androgenic deficit and it is during these stages that the production of most androgen-dependent proteins occurs. It is known that the promoter of the AR gene is sensitive to the androgen:AR complex, and so androgens themselves appear able to regulate AR expression and cyclical Sertoli cell activity. The cells of the spermatogenic lineage do not seem to need to express AR for sperm fertility.

Testosterone can also be converted to oestrogen in the Sertoli cells, although recent evidence suggests that this pathway operates mainly in fetal life in humans. As the testis matures, most testicular oestrogen is derived directly from Leydig cell activity. In adult humans the output is relatively small, but in the boar and stallion it matches the androgen output. Oestrogen's main function is not in the testis, but in the epididymus (see Chapter 9 for details).

Cytokines and peptides of the testis

The growth factors inhibin B and activin A (see Table 3.6 & Fig. 3.5) are both produced by the Sertoli cells. About 25% leaves the testis via lymphatic flow, with most of the remainder passing into the fluid of the seminiferous tubule, from which they are absorbed during passage through the epididymis. In the systemic circulation, these peptides bind to target cells in the pituitary (see Chapter 6), and thereby function as endocrine hormones. However, they also have

paracrine and autocrine roles within the testis, receptors binding inhibin being located on Leydig cells, and those binding activin on both Sertoli and spermatogenic cells. Output of MIH from the adult testis is low, its primary role being in embryonic, fetal and neonatal life (see Chapter 1). Insl3 is one of the most abundant peptide products of the Leydig cells, but its precise role in adulthood is unclear.

Oxytocin (see Chapter 3, 'Small peptides') is also produced in the Leydig cells and has been shown to stimulate seminiferous tubule motility, via an action on the peritubular myoid cells. Its passage from the testis in the lymph may give it a further paracrine function: the stimulation of epididymidal motility.

Spermatogenesis is dependent on endocrine support

The production of androgens and spermatozoa is interrelated functionally. Thus, at puberty, androgen levels rise and spermatogenesis commences. In some adult mammals, androgen and sperm production do not occur throughout the year (e.g. the roe deer, ram, vole, marine mammals and possibly some primates). Rather, the behaviour and morphology of the males show seasonal variations, which reflect the changing levels of androgen output. In these *seasonal breeders*, the spermatogenic output also varies in parallel with the changing endocrine pattern. If androgens are neutralized, spermatogenesis proceeds only as far as the very early preleptotene stages of meiosis. The male becomes *aspermatogenic*. Restoration of androgens restores spermatozoal output. The Sertoli cells are the likely target for androgen action, given their capacity to bind androgens, to generate more potent ones via 5α-reductase activity, and their central role in spermatogenesis.

The causal association between the presence of androgens and the process of spermatogenesis ensures that mature spermatozoa are always delivered into an extragonadal environment suitably androgenized for their efficient transfer to the female genital tract. Given the importance of androgens for spermatogenesis and male function, how is their output regulated?

Luteinizing hormone acts on Leydig cells

It has been known for many years that removal of the pituitary gland (hypophysectomy) causes the testes to shrink, sperm output to decline and spermatogenesis to arrest at the primary spermatocyte stage (Fig. 4.9e). The Leydig cells become involuted, testosterone output falls and the testosterone-dependent male genitalia hypotrophy. If testosterone is given at the time of hypophysectomy, spermatogenesis continues, albeit at a slightly reduced level, and the secondary sex characteristics show little sign of regression, although the Leydig cells do still involute.

These experiments established that the secretion of testosterone by the Leydig cells was under the control of the pituitary.

In experiments on the rat, it was shown that if, after hypophysectomy, luteinizing hormone (LH; see Table 3.4 for details) is administered instead of testosterone, then not only are secondary sex characteristics and spermatogenesis maintained, but the Leydig cells do not involute and testosterone output is maintained. Further confirmation of the role of LH comes from the effect of administration to an intact adult male of an antiserum to bind free LH. The level of plasma testosterone falls and regression of the androgen-dependent secondary sex characteristics follows. The results of these two experiments suggest strongly that pituitary-derived LH stimulates the Leydig cells to produce testosterone. Subsequently, LH has been shown to bind specifically to high-affinity LH receptors on the surface of the Leydig cells, the only testicular cells to express them. As a result, intracellular cAMP levels rise within 60 s, and testosterone output rises within 20–30 min. LH does not act alone on the Leydig cells; two other hormones also influence its activity. Both prolactin, a second anterior pituitary hormone (see Table 3.5), and inhibin bind to receptors and facilitate the stimulatory action of LH. Neither hormone alone, however, stimulates testosterone production.

It seems clear, then, that LH stimulates Leydig cells to produce testosterone, which passes into the tubules, binds to androgen receptors within the Sertoli cells and thereby supports spermatogenesis. However, it is important to stress that, although testosterone or LH administered immediately after hypophysectomy can prevent aspermatogenesis in rats, some reduction in testis size and a 20% reduction in sperm output occur. In many other species, including primates, the decline in sperm output after hypophysectomy is even more severe, despite administration of high doses of testosterone or LH. Moreover, if aspermatogenesis is allowed to develop after hypophysectomy of any species, sperm production cannot be restored with LH or testosterone alone. For complete restoration and maintenance of spermatogenesis, LH stimulation of Leydig cells is not sufficient. The same requirement applies to the restoration of spermatogenesis in seasonally fertile animals. Taken together, this evidence suggests another pituitary hormone is required for full testicular function and recovery. This is follicle-stimulating hormone (FSH; Table 3.4).

Follicle-stimulating hormone acts on Sertoli cells

FSH binds to receptors (FSH-Rs) on the basolateral surface of Sertoli cells, and is thus freely accessible to the large blood-borne glycoprotein hormone. The FSH-R levels vary with the cycle of the seminiferous tubule, but do so in opposite phase to the ARs (see above), being lowest on the days when ARs are highest (stages 6–8). The main second messenger system stimulated by binding is adenyl cyclase, and so cAMP generation also cycles antiphase to ARs. This reciprocal temporal relationship may be explained in part because FSH stimulates the production of intracellular ARs, as well as inhibiting its own FSH-R production. Androgens in turn stimulate the appearance of FSH-Rs. Thus, FSH and testosterone oscillate to act synergistically on the Sertoli cell to allow spermatogenesis to go to completion, explaining why, once androgen levels have fallen after hypophysectomy, neither androgen nor LH alone can fully restore testicular activity. Both hormones also stimulate calcium signalling in Sertoli cells. Thus, they are intimately entwined functionally.

These observations provide further evidence for a central coordinating role for the Sertoli cell in the events of spermatogenesis. There is a final piece of evidence that supports this conclusion. Vitamin A has long been recognized as essential for spermatogenesis; its deficiency is associated with subfertility, and in its complete absence spermatogenesis arrests at preleptotene stages. Receptors for vitamin A are present in Sertoli cells.

Paracrine actions by cytokines work locally with FSH and androgens

FSH and androgens interact to stimulate and regulate Sertoli cell function and thereby the proteins and cytokines that it produces. The cytokines then influence spermatogenesis (see Boxes). Over 300 FSH-inducible proteins have been described including ABP (carries androgen in testicular fluid), transferrin (transports iron into germ cells), GDNF (regulates proliferation of spermatogonial stem cells: Box 4.1), SCF (potentiates survival of spermatogonia A and B: Box 4.1), aromatase (converts androgens to oestrogens) and CREMτ (critically regulates postmeiotic gene expression: Box 4.2). However, given the complex interplay between FSH and androgen, and the cytokines they also influence, it is not clear whether these genes are induced directly or indirectly by FSH and to what extent other hormones are also involved.

Summary

In this chapter we have considered the two major products of the testis and their relationship. The main endocrine secretion of testosterone by the Leydig cells is dependent primarily on pituitary LH. Some of the testosterone enters the seminiferous tubules, where it acts on the Sertoli cells, together with FSH, in order to help maintain the cellular product of the testis: the spermatozoa. Without testosterone, spermatogenesis ceases. Although both FSH and testosterone are essential for full spermatogenesis, their

KEY LEARNING POINTS

- The adult testis has two main products: spermatozoa and hormones.

- The testis has two main physiological compartments (inside and outside seminiferous tubules) each of which is subdivided: the extratubular compartment into intravascular and interstitial; and the intratubular compartment into basal and adluminal.

- A major physiological barrier (blood–testis barrier) separates the basal and adluminal intratubular compartments.

- Leydig cells make androgens, oxytocin and Insl3 and are in the interstitial compartment.

- Sertoli cells make inhibin, activin and MIH and are in the intratubular compartment.

- Spermatozoa are made within the tubules.

- Spermatogonial stem cells provide a pluripotent self-replenishing pool of spermatogenic precursor cells, and can also give rise to embryonic stem cells.

- Spermatogenesis has three main phases: proliferative, meiotic and cytodifferentiative.

- The proliferative mitotic phase occurs in the basal compartment and comprises spermatogonia A, intermediate and B.

- The meiotic phase occurs in the adluminal compartment and comprises primary and secondary spermatocytes.

- The cytodifferentiative phase occurs in the adluminal compartment and comprises round and elongating spermatids. It is called spermiogenesis.

- As the spermatozoa from a single spermatogonium develop, they remain in contact with each other through cytoplasmic bridges.

- As spermatids elongate, they form an acrosome, condensed heterochromatin, a midpiece containing mitochondria and centrioles, and a mainpiece tail.

- The chromosomal condensation involves replacement of histones first with basic transition nuclear proteins (TNPs) and then with protamines.

- Heterochromatization results in transcriptional inactivity in elongated spermatids and spermatozoa.

- Distinctive species of mRNA are made after meiosis (haploid expression) and survive in mature spermatozoa.

- It does not appear to be possible to separate haploid spermatozoa according to their genetic expression patterns.

- Surplus cytoplasm is discarded in the residual body.

- Not all the developing spermatozoa survive.

- When spermatogenesis is completed, the cytoplasmic bridges are broken and the spermatozoa are released into the tubular lumen in a process of spermiation.

- They are washed along the seminiferous tubules in testicular fluid secreted by the Sertoli cells.

- The process of spermatogenesis takes a time characteristic for the species and is remarkably constant.

- A new round of spermatogenesis is initiated at a time interval characteristic for the species and is remarkably constant. It is usually about 25% of the time taken to undergo spermatogenesis.

- This regular periodicity of spermatogenic initiation is called the spermatogenic cycle.

- Spermatogenesis is initiated at different times in different regions of the testis thereby giving a smooth, non-pulsatile flow of spermatozoa.

- Spermatogenesis is initiated at the same time in closely adjacent regions of the same seminiferous tubule. Thus, cross-sections of tubule seem to 'cycle' together: the cycle of the seminiferous epithelium.

- Nearby sections of seminiferous tubule initiate spermatogenesis with a slight phase advance or retardation, giving the appearance of a spermatogenic wave.

- The Sertoli cells also cycle with their adjacent spermatogenic cells.

- Sertoli cells cycle in the absence of spermatogenic cells in both adults and pubertally, suggesting that they may coordinate the temporal and spatial organization of spermatogenesis.

- Spermatogenesis fails in the absence of the gonadotrophins: luteinizing hormone (LH) and follicle-stimulating hormone (FSH).

- In the absence of LH, androgens fall and spermatogenesis ceases.

- Prepubertal or quiescent testes cannot initiate spermatozoal production without both LH and FSH.

- Once spermatogenesis is under way, removal of FSH results in a significant fall in spermatozoal production and a reduction in testis size.

- LH binds to receptors on the Leydig cells and is required for synthesis of androgens.

- Prolactin and inhibin enhance the stimulation of Leydig cells by LH.

- Androgens enter Sertoli cells where they are converted to dihydrotestosterone, bind to androgen receptors and are essential for Sertoli cell function.

- Spermatogenesis fails during meiosis in the absence of androgens.

- FSH binds to receptors on the Sertoli cells and is required for synthesis of inhibin and activin.

- FSH also stimulates androgen receptors in the Sertoli cell.

- Androgens also stimulate receptors for FSH on Sertoli cells.

- FSH and androgens act synergistically on Sertoli cells to promote Sertoli cell function and the support of spermatogenesis.

- Androgens pass out of the testis in blood, lymph and testicular fluid (bound to ABP) and act systemically and locally in the male genetic tract.

actions appear to be purely permissive. They determine whether or not spermatogenesis will take place, but do not regulate the rate at which cells develop along the spermatogenic lineage, the frequency with which the stem cells provide spermatogonia type A, or the spatial coordination between adjacent clones of spermatogenic cells. These processes appear to be regulated internally by the Sertoli cells.

FURTHER READING

General reading

Cupps PT (ed.) (1991) *Reproduction in Domestic Animals,* 4th edn. Academic Press, London.

De Kretser DM *et al.* (2004) The role of activin, follistatin and inhibin in testicular physiology. *Molecular and Cellular Endocrinology* **225**, 57–64.

Fawcett DW, Bedford JM (1979) *The Spermatozoon.* Urban & Schwarzenberg, Munich.

Holdcraft RW, Braun RE (2004) Hormonal regulation of spermatogenesis. *International Journal of Andrology* **27**, 335–342.

Loveland KL *et al.* (2005) Drivers of germ cell maturation. *Annals of the New York Academy of Sciences* **1061**, 173–182.

Siu MKY, Cheng CY (2004) Dynamic cross-talk between cells and the extracellular matrix in the testis. *BioEssays* **26**, 978–992.

Walker WH, Cheng J (2005) FSH and testosterone signaling in Sertoli cells. *Reproduction* **130**, 15–28.

More advanced reading (see also Boxes)

Bedall MA, Zama AM (2004) Genetic analysis of Kit ligand functions during mouse spermatogenesis. *Journal of Andrology* **25**, 188–199.

Bremner WJ *et al.* (1994) Immunohistochemical localization of androgen receptors in the rat testis: evidence for stage-dependent expression and regulation by androgens. *Endocrinology* **135**, 1227–1234.

Gorczynska-Fjälling E (2004) The role of calcium in signal transduction processes in Sertoli cells. *Reproductive Biology* **4**, 219–241.

Luetjens CM *et al.* (2005) Primate spermatogenesis: new insights into comparative testicular organisation, spermatogenic efficiency and endocrine control. *Biological Reviews of the Cambridge Philosophical Society* **80**, 475–488.

Mruk DD, Cheng CY (2004) Cell–cell interactions at the ectoplasmic specialization in the testis. *Trends in Endocrinology and Metabolism* **15**, 439–447.

Parvenin M *et al.* (1986) Cell interactions during the seminiferous epithelial cycle. *International Reviews in Cytology* **1**, 115–151.

Roosen-Runge EC (1962) The process of spermatogenesis in mammals. *Biological Review* **37**, 343–377.

Sharpe RM *et al.* (2003) Proliferation and functional maturation of Sertoli cells, and their relevance to disorders of testis function in adulthood. *Reproduction* **125**, 769–784.

Xia W *et al.* (2005) Cytokines and junction restructuring during spermatogenesis—a lesson to learn from the testis. *Cytokine & Growth Factor Reviews* **16**, 469–493.

Fertility in the adult female is episodic

In Chapter 1, we described how the fetal ovary formed from an indifferent genital ridge. It differentiates later than the testis and its endocrine activity is not required during fetal and neonatal life for development of the female phenotype. Significant ovarian endocrine activity occurs first during full sexual maturation at puberty with two main steroid secretions: *oestrogens* and *progestagens*. From puberty onwards, the ovary also produces haploid oocytes for fertilization by spermatozoa. As in the adult testis, the endocrine activity of the ovary is coordinated with the production of its gametes. However, adult ovarian function differs fundamentally from testicular function in two ways. First, relatively few oocytes are released, and second their release is not in a continuous stream but occurs *episodically* at *ovulation*. Moreover, the pattern of release of the *oestrogens* and *progestagens* reflects this episodic release of oocytes. Thus, the period before ovulation is characterized by *oestrogen dominance*, and the period after ovulation is characterized by *progestagen dominance*. Once this sequence of oestrogen–ovulation–progestagen has been completed, it is repeated. Therefore we speak of a *cycle of ovarian activity*.

The cyclic release of steroids imposes a corresponding cyclicity on the whole body and, in most species, on the behaviour of the adult female. These cycles are called the *oestrous cycle* in most animals and the *menstrual cycle* in higher primates. Why is female reproductive activity cyclic? The genital tract of the female mammal, unlike that of the male, must serve two quite distinct reproductive functions, each with distinctive physiological requirements. It must act to transport gametes to the site of fertilization, and it also provides the site of implantation of the conceptus and its subsequent development. The distinct phases of the female cycle reflect these two roles. During the first, oestrogenic part of the cycle, the ovary prepares the female for receipt of the spermatozoa and fertilization of the oocyte. During the second, progestagenic part of the cycle, the ovary prepares the female to receive and nurture the conceptus should successful fertilization have occurred. Sandwiched between these two endocrine activities of the ovary, the oocyte is released at ovulation.

In this chapter, we will consider the sequence of changes *within the ovary itself* by which a coordinated and cyclic pattern of production of the oocyte and ovarian steroids is achieved. In later chapters, we will consider how this ovarian cyclicity leads to the oestrous and menstrual cycles.

The adult ovary consists of follicles and interstitial tissue

The adult ovary is organized on a pattern comparable to the testis (Fig. 5.1b) with an interstitial tissue made up of glandular tissue, the so-called *interstitial glands* (homologous to Leydig cells), set in *stroma*. The interstitial tissue

surrounds *follicles* (homologous to tubules). In contrast to the testis, in which the contents of the tubules show cyclic changes as the spermatozoa form (the cycle of the seminiferous epithelium), the whole ovary cycles. However, each ovarian cycle is made up of an interconnecting series of events in a subset of follicles as they mature. In the first part of this chapter, we will follow the maturation of a single follicle in some detail. In the second part of the chapter, we will relate the activity in a single follicle to the activity of the ovary as a whole in order to describe and explain the ovarian cycle itself.

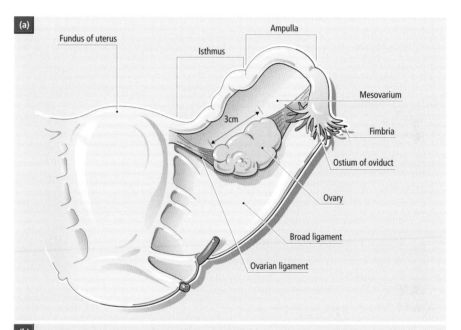

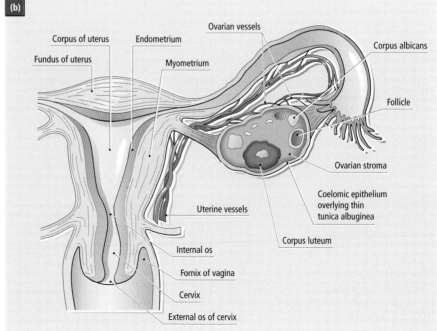

Fig. 5.1 Posterior views of the human uterus and one oviduct and ovary: (a) intact; (b) sectioned. The ovaries have been pulled upwards and laterally, and would normally have their long axes almost vertical. Note that all structures are covered in peritoneum *except* the surface of the ovary and oviducal ostium. The ovary has a stromal matrix of cells, smooth-muscle fibres and connective tissue containing follicles, corpora lutea and corpora albicans, and interstitial glands. Anteriorly at the hilus the ovarian vessels and nerves enter the medullary stroma via the mesovarium.

The pattern of gamete production in the female, like that in the male, shows processes of proliferation by *mitosis*, genetic reshuffling and reduction by *meiosis*, and cytodifferentiation during *oocyte maturation*. In the female, however, the need for mitotic proliferation is not as great because only one or a few oocytes are shed during each cycle, unlike the massive and continuous sperm output of the testis. Thus, as we saw in Chapter 1, the female completes the proliferative phase during fetal and/or neonatal life, when the primordial germ cells or *oogonia* (equivalent to spermatogonia in the male) all cease dividing and enter meiosis where they arrest in the dictyate germinal vesicle stage (first meiotic prophase) to become *primary oocytes* (equivalent to primary spermatocytes) (but see Box 5.1). They do this within the *primordial follicle*, which consists of

flattened mesenchymal cells (granulosa cells) condensed around what is first the oogonium and then the primary oocyte (Figs 5.2a & 5.3a), all enclosed within a basement membrane, the *membrana propria*. The primordial follicle constitutes the fundamental functional unit of the ovary.

The follicle is the fundamental reproductive element of the ovary

The primordial follicles can stay in this arrested state for up to 50 years in women, with the oocyte metabolically ticking over and waiting for a signal to resume development. The reason for storing oocytes in this extraordinary protracted meiotic prophase is unknown. Although a few follicles may resume development sporadically and incom-

---

BOX 5.1 Postnatal oogenesis—a contemporary controversy?

- *Science operates by hypothesis, challenge and reformulation.* An enduring problem for modern science is that the public wants certainty, whereas scientists work with probability. In Chapter 1, we summarized the conventional wisdom of many decades: that *all* the PGCs in the human fetal ovary enter meiosis and then arrest in leptotene on being surrounded by granulosa cells, so that by birth a woman has all the eggs/follicles she will ever have. No interphase PGC stem cells capable of mitotic proliferation remain to replenish depleted stocks—contrast the testis with its spermatogonial type A stem cells (see Chapter 4). However, this long-established dogma has recently been challenged.

- *Do the numbers add up?* The above dogma predicts that one oocyte = one follicle, so counts of follicles throughout the reproductive life of a female should steadily decline as the follicles are used up during ovulation or death (atresia). The most rigorous and recent life course follicle count (in the mouse; Kerr *et al.*) confirms that once follicle numbers are stabilized postnatally, they actually stay constant for at least 100–120 days! Only then do they decline as female mouse fertility begins to fall (the murine equivalent of 35 for women). How are they stabilized over this period of maximum fecundity?

- *One possibility is stem cell replenishment.* In primates, which are more difficult to study rigorously, it has long been suggested that some ovarian oogonia (free of follicle cells) exist and are potentially or actually mitotic. Johnson *et al.* have now suggested that in mice something similar may happen. They experimentally depleted primordial follicles more rapidly than would occur naturally and suggest that numbers were capable of rapid recovery (of the order of 12 h, which is

implausibly rapid). If the observations are indeed correct, could the replacement oocytes come from entry of adult oogonia into meiosis and granulosa condensation? The problem is that far too few free oogonia are available to replenish the follicular losses so rapidly. It was therefore suggested that in the mouse haemopoietic stem cells are recruited from the circulation and converted to oogonia—but again, so rapidly?

- *So could there be some limited capacity for oocyte/follicle replenishment*—the stem cell used differing with species? It remains to be proved one way or the other. But if there is such a capacity, what are the intraovarian signals that regulate whether, when and how it occurs? A long-established dogma is under the microscope. Uncertainty is one of the joys and excitements of science, if also infuriating for non-scientists!

Further reading
For?
Bukovsky A *et al.* (2005) Oogenesis in cultures derived from adult human ovaries. *Reproductive Biology and Endocrinology* **3**, 17 doi:10.1186/1477–7827-3-17.

Johnson J *et al.* (2004) Germline stem cells and follicular renewal in the postnatal mammalian ovary. *Nature* **428**, 145–150.

Johnson J *et al.* (2005) Oocyte generation in adult mammalian ovaries by putative germ cells in bone marrow and peripheral blood. *Cell* **122**, 303–315.

Johnson J *et al.* (2005) Setting the record straight on data supporting postnatal oogenesis in female mammals. *Cell Cycle* **4**, 1469–1475.

Kerr JB *et al.* (2006) Quantification of healthy follicles in the neonatal and adult mouse ovary: evidence for maintenance of primordial follicle supply. *Reproduction* **132**, 95–109.

Spradling AC (2004) More like a man. *Nature* **428**, 133–134.

Unconvinced?
Greenfeld C, Flaws JA (2004) Renewed debate over postnatal oogenesis in the mammalian ovary. *BioEssays* **26**, 829–832.

Telfer EE *et al.* (2005) On regenerating the ovary and generating controversy. *Cell* **122**, 821–822.

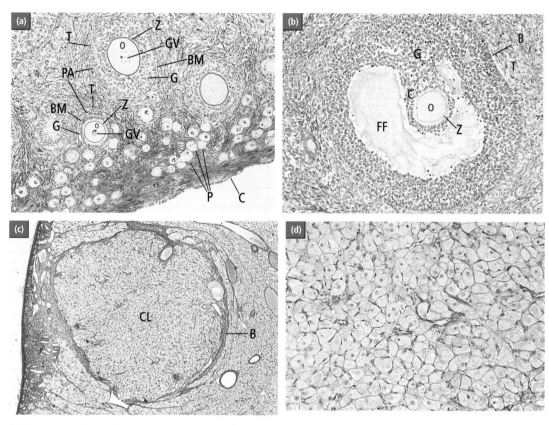

Fig. 5.2 (a) Primordial follicles (P) in the cortical stroma of the ovary, lying adjacent to the coelomic epithelium (C), grow in size to give preantral follicles (PA) which contain an enlarged oocyte (O) containing a 'nucleus' or germinal vesicle (GV) surrounded by a zona pellucida (staining blue; Z) and proliferated granulosa cells (G) which in one follicle are only one layer thick but in the other are several layers thick. Outside the granulosa cells is a basement membrane (BM) on which the theca (T) forms. (b) Further follicular growth leads to antral follicles in which the granulosa cells (G) have proliferated further and the fully grown oocyte (O) is surrounded by a zona (Z) and cumulus cells (C), set in the follicular antrum containing follicular fluid (FF). The thecal tissues (T) differentiate and remain separated from the granulosa cells by the basement membrane (B), which is not penetrated by blood vessels leaving the granulosa cells avascular. (c) After a preovulatory growth spurt by the follicle and the process of ovulation, the remaining granulosa cells increase in size and fill the emptied follicular antrum as they luteinize within a fibrous thecal capsule (B) to form a corpus luteum (CL). (d) A higher power view of the luteal cells. Note the relatively large size of the luteal cells and the vascularization of the previously avascular granulosa area, now luteinized. (a, b, d, same magnification; c, magnification 25% that of others.)

pletely during fetal and neonatal life, regular recruitment of primordial follicles into a pool of growing follicles occurs first at puberty. Thereafter, a few follicles recommence growth every day, so that a continuous trickle of developing follicles is formed. When a primordial follicle commences growth it passes through three stages of development *en route* to ovulation: first it becomes a *primary* or *preantral* follicle; then a *secondary* or *antral* follicle (also called a *vesicular* or *Graafian* follicle); and finally a *preovulatory* follicle in the run-up to ovulation itself. The times taken to traverse each of these stages differ (Table 5.1), the preantral phase being the longest and the preovulatory phase the shortest. We will now trace the development of one such primordial follicle.

Follicles grow and mature

Primordial to preantral transition

The earliest *preantral* phase of follicular growth is characterized by an increase in the diameter of the primordial follicle from 20 μm to between 200 and 400 μm, depending on the species (Fig. 5.3a,b). A major part of this growth occurs in the primary oocyte, which increases its diameter to its *final size* of 60–120 μm. This oocyte growth is *not* accompanied by the reactivation of meiosis. Rather, the dictyate chromosomes are actively synthesizing large amounts of ribosomal and mRNA, the latter being used to build organelles and to generate stores of proteins, all of which are essential for later stages of oocyte maturation and for the first few days

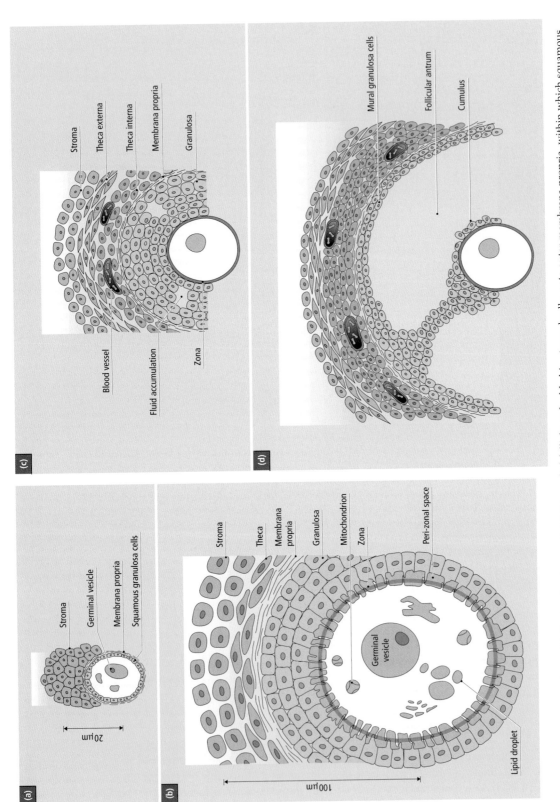

Fig. 5.3 Stylized morphology of follicular development. (a) Primordial follicle embedded in stromal cells: note outer membrana propria, within which squamous granulosa cells enclose a primary oocyte at the dictyate stage with a germinal vesicle (equivalent to the nucleus). (b) Preantral follicle: stromal cells condense on the membrana propria to form a thecal layer; the granulosa cells divide and become cuboidal; the oocyte grows and secretes the zona pellucida. Contact between granulosa cells and the primary oocyte is maintained by cytoplasmic processes through the zona. Within the oocyte: mitochondria increase in number and are small and spherical with columnar cristae; the smooth endoplasmic reticulum breaks up into numerous small vesicles; the Golgi complex breaks into small vesicular units often associated with lipid droplets. The genes are transcriptionally active. (c) Early antral follicle in which the granulosa and thecal cells have proliferated. The thecal cells now comprise two layers, an outer fibrous theca externa and an inner theca interna, rich in blood vessels and large, foamy cells with abundant smooth endoplasmic reticulum. Within the avascular granulosa layer, coalescing fluid drops are evident. (d) Expanded antral follicle, with a fully developed follicular antrum, leaving the oocyte surrounded by a distinct and denser layer of granulosa cells, the cumulus oophorus, and the walls lined by mural granulosa cells. The oocyte itself shows only a small further increase in size.

Table 5.1 Cytokines and follicular development (see Table 3.6 for details of cytokines and their receptors).

Cytokine	Source	Actions
Faciliate follicle growth		
SCF	GCs	Initiates oocyte growth in primordial follicle and stimulates TC mitosis; maintains growth of preantral and antral GCs; boosts A output from TCs
FGF2	Primordial and growing oocytes; GCs	Promotes primordial follicle recruitment; suppresses GC apoptosis; stimulates T/ICs
IGF 1 (pig, rat), IGF 2 (human, cow, sheep)	Mitotic GCs at antral stage (rat, pig, human) or TCs (cow, sheep) (ICs in primates?)	Promotes FSH-induced mitosis, differentiation and E2 output of GCs and LH-induced A synthesis by TCs
Inhibin B	GCs in early/mid antral follicle and declines thereafter	Enhances FSH stimulation of GCs
GDF9	Preantral and antral oocytes	Co-stimulates with FSH GC mitosis, stimulates E2 and depresses P4 output to prevent premature luteinization; may interact with BMP15
Inhibin A	GCs in large antral and preovulatory follicles; also LCs	Enhances LH-induced A rise in TCs and P4 rise in LCs
TGF-β	TCs in antral follicles	Inhibits G/TC proliferation but stimulates GC differentiation and production of inhibin and E2
Antagonize follicle growth and/or promote atresia		
MIH	GCs up to early antral stage	Depresses recruitment of primordial and preantral follicles
Activins	GCs in preantral phase, declining as follicle matures (can block further growth if stay high)	Promote FSH receptor expression on early GCs and stimulate GC proliferation; attenuate LH-induced rise in A output from TCs; depress P4 output from LCs
IGFBPs	GCs (sheep, pigs); TCs (cow). Depressed by FSH; higher in atretic follicles	Bind and attenuate IGFs (which can be released through action of IGFBP protease-pregnancy-associated protein A (PAPP-A) made by GCs under FSH control
TNFα and leptin		Promote atresia and antagonize FSH effects to depress follicle growth and steroidogenesis
Involved in dominant follicle selection?		
BMP15	Preantral and antral oocytes	Depresses PAPP-A output and may be involved in selection of dominant follicle

A, androgens; E2, oestrogen; GCs, granulosa cells; ICs, interstitial cells; LTs, luteal cells; P4, progesterone; TCs, thecal cells.

of development after fertilization (see Chapter 10). This period thus represents part of the cytodifferentiative phase, occurring *in tandem with* the arrested meiosis, not *after* meiotic completion as in the male.

Early during growth of the oocyte, it secretes glycoproteins, which condense around it to form a translucent acellular layer called the *zona pellucida*. The zona separates the oocyte from the surrounding granulosa cells, which divide to become several layers thick (Fig. 5.3b). However, contact between granulosa cells and oocyte is maintained via granulosa cytoplasmic processes, which penetrate the zona and form gap junctions at the oocyte surface. Gap junctions also form in increasing numbers between adjacent granulosa cells, thus providing the basis for an extensive network of

intercellular communication. Through this network, biosynthetic substrates of low molecular weight, such as amino acids and nucleotides, are passed to the growing oocyte for incorporation into macromolecules. This nutritional network is important, because the granulosa layer is completely *avascular*, with no blood vessels penetrating the membrana propria. The granulosa:oocyte complex thereby resembles the Sertoli cell–spermatogenic complex, in which a similar avascular close relationship occurs (Chapter 4), perhaps reflecting their shared developmental origins (Chapter 1).

In addition to oocyte growth and granulosa cell proliferation, the preantral follicle also increases in size and complexity through the condensation of ovarian stromal cells on the outer membrana propria. This loose matrix of spindle-shaped cells is called the *theca* of the follicle (Fig. 5.3b). With further development and proliferation, the thecal cells can be distinguished as two distinct layers (Fig. 5.3c): an inner glandular, highly vascular *theca interna*, surrounded by a fibrous capsule, the *theca externa*.

Preantral to antral transition

During this phase, the granulosa cells continue to proliferate, resulting in a further increase in follicular size. As they do so, a viscous fluid starts to appear between them (Fig. 5.3c). This *follicular fluid* is composed partly of granulosa cell secretions, including mucopolysaccharides, and partly of serum transudate. The drops of fluid coalesce to form a single *follicular antrum* (Figs 5.3d & 5.2b). The appearance of the follicular antrum marks the beginning of the *antral phase* of development. Increase in follicular size from now on depends mainly on an increase in the size of the follicular antrum and the volume of follicular fluid, although granulosa cells do continue to proliferate.

Although the oocyte does not increase in size over the antral period, it continues to actively synthesize RNA and turnover protein. As the follicular antrum grows, the oocyte is left suspended in fluid surrounded by a dense mass of granulosa cells called the *cumulus oophorus*. It is connected to the rim of peripheral, or *mural*, granulosa cells only by a thin 'stalk' of cells (Fig. 5.3d).

This maturing antral follicle is now ready to enter its preovulatory phase and to approach ovulation. However, before this remarkable process is described, the underlying control of growth from primordial to expanded antral follicle will be examined.

Early follicular growth can occur independent of external regulation

We do not understand fully how each day a few primordial follicles start to develop as preantral follicles, or how those that do are selected. It is clear that preantral follicular development can occur independently of any direct *extraovarian* controls, although growth hormone (GH) is generally facilitatory for early follicle growth and survival, probably mediated by IGF1 production from granulosa cells. *Intraovarian cytokines* are certainly involved in the earliest stages of growth (Table 5.1). Stem cell factor, which in the testis is produced by the Sertoli cells and potentiates survival of spermatogonia A and B, is also produced by granulosa cells and binds to its Kit receptor on the oocyte to initiate oocyte growth in primordial follicles. SCF production may be enhanced by the action of FGF2 produced by the oocyte itself. MIH, in contrast, appears inhibitory to primordial follicle recruitment. However, there comes a point when further follicular development *does* require external support, and, as was found for spermatogenesis

in the male, this external support is provided by the pituitary.

Removal of the pituitary (hypophysectomy) prevents the completion of antral follicle development. The precise stage at which follicles arrest in the absence of a pituitary depends on the species: in the rat, arrest occurs at late preantral to early antral stages, but in the human, it occurs when antral follicles are slightly more advanced, with a diameter of 2 mm. The granulosa cells in arrested follicles show reduced protein synthetic activity, accumulation of lipid droplets and pyknotic nuclei. Apoptotic death of the oocyte and granulosa cells follows. Leukocytes and macrophages invade and fibrous scar tissue forms. This process is called *atresia*.

A similar follicular phenotype is also observed in mice genetically lacking gonadotrophins, indicating their obligatory involvement. Accordingly, atresia is prevented by follicle-stimulating hormone (FSH) and luteinizing hormone (LH). These hormones bind to follicular *FSH and LH receptors* that first appear on cells in the late preantral and early antral follicles. FSH alone is sufficient for initial follicular growth, but LH assists further antral expansion. Thus, FSH-knockout mice arrest follicular development preantrally, whereas LH knockout mice block at the antral stage. *So, the gonadotrophins pick-up preantral follicles and stimulate antral growth.* What do the gonadotrophins do and where in the follicle do they do it?

FSH and LH stimulate steroid synthesis during the antral stage

When the distribution of receptors in early antral follicles is analysed, it is found that *only the cells of the theca interna bind LH* whereas *only the granulosa cells bind FSH*. Moreover, the effects of hormone binding at each of these sites produce very different consequences.

The antral follicles produce and release increasing amounts of steroids as they grow under the influence of the gonadotrophins. The main oestrogens produced are oestradiol 17β and oestrone. Antral follicles also account for 30–70% of the circulating androgens found in women, mainly androstenedione and testosterone (the remainder coming from the adrenal). These various sex steroids are produced in different parts of the follicle. The antral follicle can be dissected surgically, so that its granulosa cells become separated from the cells of the theca interna. When grown separately *in vitro*, the *thecal cells are found to synthesize androgens* from acetate and cholesterol. This conversion is greatly stimulated by LH (Fig. 5.4). Only very limited oestrogen synthesis by these cells is possible, particularly in the early stages of antral growth. The granulosa cells, in contrast, are incapable of forming androgens. If, however, the granulosa cells are supplied with exogenous androgens, they possess enzymes that will readily aromatize them to oestrogens. *This aromatization is stimulated by FSH* (Fig. 5.4).

Thus, the androgens produced by developing follicles are derived exclusively from thecal cells, whereas the oestrogens can arise via two routes. One involves *cell cooperation* in which *thecal androgens are aromatized by the granulosa cells*. The other route is by *de novo* synthesis from acetate in thecal cells. The balance between these two potential sources of oestrogen varies with different species, but it seems probable that *all* of the oestrogen within the follicular fluid and *most* of the oestrogen released from the follicle to the blood results from cell cooperation.

The production of steroids and the increase in size of antral follicles are intimately interlinked. It has become clear recently that the steroids, in addition to their release systemically via secretion into the blood, also have important *local intrafollicular roles*. The *androgens* (the so-called 'male hormone': Chapter 3) play a key role here. First, as

we saw above, they serve as substrates for conversion to oestrogens. Second, acting with FSH, they stimulate *the proliferation of granulosa cells and thereby follicular growth.* Third, they stimulate *aromatase activity*, thereby promoting oestrogen synthesis. Thus, the rising thecal output of androgens fuels a massive increase in oestrogen biosynthetic potential. This is further enhanced by the ability of the oestrogens themselves to *stimulate granulosa cells to proliferate.* Thus, a powerful *positive feedback* system is operating. As described in Chapter 3, positive feedback culminates in a surge, in this case *a surge of circulating oestrogens* towards the end of antral expansion from the *most advanced follicle(s).* Daily monitoring of the rise in urinary oestrogen levels therefore provides a good guide to the state of maturity of the most mature follicles (Table 5.2). Not surprisingly, in females carrying mutations that prevent oestrogen synthesis or binding to receptors, follicular development arrests in the antral stages.

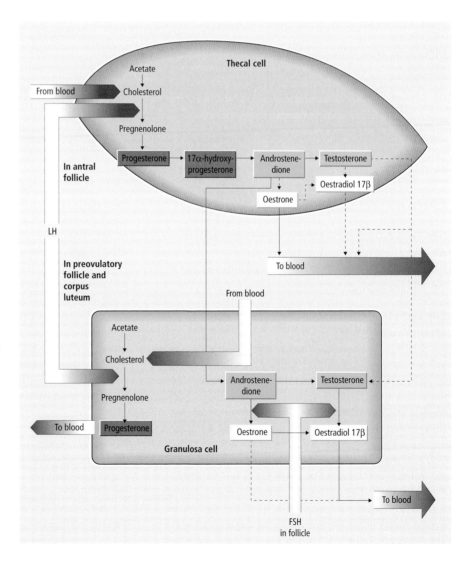

Fig. 5.4 Scheme outlining the principal steroidogenic pathways and gonadotrophic stimuli in cells of the antral follicle—theca above and granulosa below—as well as the LH stimulated pathway in the preovulatory follicle and corpus luteum. In the corpora lutea, the oestrogenic synthetic capacity of thecal cells only persists in those species in which the thecal cells become incorporated into the corpus luteum. Where alternative pathways exist, the minor pathway is indicated by a dashed line.

Table 5.2 Human follicular development.

Morphology	Day of menstrual cycle	Diameter (mm)*	FSH/LH receptors present?	Oestrogen in peripheral blood (pmol/L)
Preantral	Throughout	<0.5	–	NA
Very early antral	Throughout	<2	–	NA
Early antral	1–6	2–7	+	<20
Expanding antral†	6–10	7–10	+	100–200
Expanded antral	10–12	10–20	+	200–400
Preovulatory	13–14	20–25	+	800+§

*Recent advances in ultrasound technology now make it possible to monitor these final stages of follicular growth in the conscious subject, and thereby to ascertain how near the follicles are to ovulation. See Fig. 15.9.
NA, not applicable.
†In naturally cycling women a single dominant follicle emerges at this point and only it grows thereafter.
§10^3–10^4 higher oestrogen concentrations within the follicular fluid itself.

Table 5.3 Duration of phases of follicular development in the non-pregnant animal.

Species	Preantral phase (days)	Antral phase (days)	Preovulatory phase (hours)	Luteal phase (days)
Mouse	6–10	3–4	11	2
Human	77–85*	8–12	30–36	12–15
Sheep	NK	4–5	22	14–15
Cow	NK	c.10	40	18–19
Pig	NK	c.10	41	15–17
Horse	NK	c.10	40	15–16

*Also includes very early antral development (see Table 5.2).
NK, not known.

Androgens and oestrogens are particularly important for follicular growth and maturation, but progesterone assumes major significance only as ovulation approaches, and so its role will be considered shortly.

FSH and LH also stimulate and interact with intrafollicular cytokines

Steroids are not the only *paracrine* actors within the antral follicle. The production and activity of several cytokines are also stimulated by the gonadotrophins during the antral phase and then mediate and/or modulate the actions of steroids and gonadotrophins. Some of these cytokines are summarized together with their local actions in Table 5.3, amplified by comments in the text that follows. The full details of the different cytokines, when and where they act and interact, and what controls them, are still being unravelled. However, it already seems clear that there is a *balance* between cytokines (such as IGFs, inhibins, SCF) that in general *support follicular progression*, acting mostly in cooperation with FSH and androgens, and cytokines that *depress or restrain follicular development* or *promote atresia* (such as MIH, TNFα, leptin and IGFBPs).

We should note in particular the secretion patterns of the two inhibins, the significance of which will become clear in Chapter 6. Both are produced by granulosa cells. However, whereas inhibin B production is stimulated by FSH, inhibin A is stimulated by *both* FSH and LH. Thus, the ratio of inhibin A:B rises as the follicle expands to peak at ovulation. The ratio thus acts as a marker for follicular expansion, in addition to the rising oestrogen output noted above (see Chapter 6 for significance).

Summary

Follicular growth and maturation is partly regulated endogenously and partly by exogenous gonadotrophins. The latter pick up preantral follicles and stimulate their antral development through actions involving both cytokines and sex steroids. However, some of the latter (notably sex steroids and inhibins) act not only paracrinologically within the follicle, but also have more widespread endocrinological actions, as we will see in Chapters 6–10.

However, before moving to endocrine actions, one further and critical paracrine action of oestrogens, in conjunction with FSH, is exerted within the expanded antral follicle. Together these hormones stimulate the *appearance of LH-binding sites* on the *outer layers of granulosa cells*, which hitherto lacked them. These LH-binding sites are critical for successful entry of the expanded antral follicle into the preovulatory phase of follicular growth.

Ovulation

Just as late preantral and early antral follicles trickling through the first, hormone-independent, phase of follicular growth will become atretic unless exposed to tonic levels of FSH and LH, so the expanding antral follicles will also die unless a *brief surge of high levels of LH* coincides with the appearance of LH receptors on the outer granulosa cells. If an LH surge occurs when *both* the granulosa and thecal cells can bind LH, then entry into the preovulatory phase of growth occurs. If it does not, the expanded antral follicle dies.

The surge of LH affects these advanced follicles in two ways. First, it causes major changes in both the oocyte and the follicle cells, which results in the oocyte's expulsion from the follicle at *ovulation*. Second, it changes the whole endocrinology of the follicle, which becomes a *corpus luteum* at ovulation. Thus, although this preovulatory phase of follicular growth is the shortest (see Table 5.3), it is also the most dramatic.

The oocyte undergoes major preovulatory changes

Within 3–12 h of the beginning of a surge of LH (depending on the species), dramatic changes occur in the oocyte. The nuclear membrane surrounding the dictyate chromosomes breaks down, and the arrested meiotic prophase is at last ended, many years after its initiation. The chromosomes progress through the remainder of the first meiotic division (see Fig. 1.1 for details of meiosis), culminating in an extraordinary cell division in which *half* the chromosomes, but almost *all* the cytoplasm, go to one cell: the *secondary oocyte* (Fig. 5.5). The remaining chromosomes are discarded in a small bag of cytoplasm called the *first polar body*, which dies subsequently. This unequal division of cytoplasm conserves for the oocyte the bulk of the materials synthesized during earlier phases.

The chromosomes in the secondary oocyte immediately enter the second meiotic division and come to lie on the second metaphase spindle. Then, suddenly, meiosis arrests yet again. The oocyte is ovulated in this *arrested metaphase state*. We do not know the biological significance of this second meiotic arrest, but we do know that it is caused by

the presence of a protein complex called *cytostatic factor*. One component of this complex is a specific protein called c-Mos. How c-Mos causes arrest is considered in more detail in the context of fertilization (Chapter 9).

The termination of the dictyate stage and the progress of *meiotic maturation* through to *second metaphase arrest* and ovulation are accompanied by *cytoplasmic maturation* of the oocyte (Fig. 5.5). The intimate contact between the oocyte and the granulosa cells of the cumulus is broken by withdrawal of the cytoplasmic processes. The Golgi apparatus of the oocyte synthesizes lysosomal-like granules, which migrate towards the surface of the oocyte to assume a subcortical position as *cortical granules*. Remarkably, *centrioles are lost* at pachytene, and thereafter only pericentriolar material (PCM) organizes microtubules (contrast spermiogenesis, where PCM is lost, and reduced centrioles remain: Chapter 4). Protein synthetic activity continues at the same rate, but new and distinctive proteins are synthesized. This activity prepares the oocyte for fertilization (see Chapter 9). If an oocyte is shed from its follicle prematurely, or removed surgically before the completion of these cytoplasmic maturational events, then its fertilizability is much reduced. For this reason, in clinical *in vitro* fertilization programmes, human oocytes aspirated from preovulatory follicles may be cultured for a few hours before addition of spermatozoa. This procedure improves the chances of a complete maturation by the oocyte.

Meiotic and cytoplasmic maturation of the oocyte is stimulated by the surge of LH, yet it is clear that LH cannot, and does not, bind to the oocyte itself. Therefore its effect must be mediated via the cumulus cells of the follicle, where it is thought to act by suppressing cAMP levels.

Preovulatory growth of follicle cells is associated with a major endocrine switch

In addition to acting on follicle cells in order to generate signals to the oocyte, LH also affects directly the growth and endocrinological activity of the follicle cells themselves. A final and considerable increase in follicular size occurs (reaching 25 mm or more in diameter in humans; Table 5.2), almost exclusively due to a rapid expansion of the volume of follicular fluid. This expansion is accompanied by a loosening of the intercellular matrix between the more cortical layers of granulosa cells and an increase in total blood flow to the follicle.

The preovulatory growth in follicular size is matched by changes in the pattern of steroid secretion. Within 2 h or so of the beginning of the LH surge, there is a transient rise in the output of follicular oestrogens and androgens, followed by a decline. This rise coincides with distinctive changes in the thecal layer, which appears transiently stimulated and hyperaemic. The outer cells of the granulosa layer also show a marked change in their properties. First, they cease

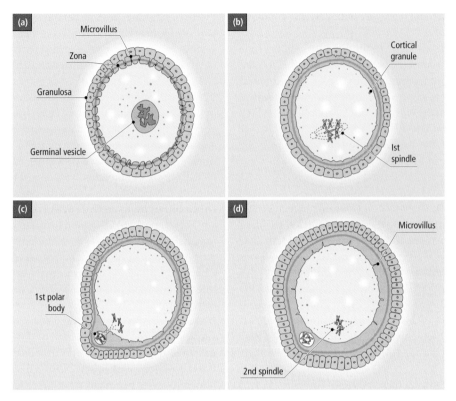

Fig. 5.5 Reactivation of arrested prophase of the first meiotic division in the preovulatory oocyte. A few hours after LH stimulation (a → b), the germinal vesicle breaks down, and the chromosomes complete prophase and arrange themselves on the first meiotic spindle. Meanwhile, cytoplasmic contact between oocyte and granulosa cells ceases and cortical granules made by the Golgi apparatus migrate to the surface. Subsequently, the first meiotic division is completed with expulsion of the first polar body (b → c). The oocyte chromosomes immediately enter the second meiotic division but arrest at second metaphase. The cytoplasm around the eccentrically placed spindle is devoid of cortical granules and the overlying membrane lacks microvilli in some species (c → d). The oocyte is ovulated in this arrested state (except in dogs and foxes in which the oocyte is ovulated at metaphase 1, and the first polar body is extruded after ovulation).

dividing and no longer convert androgen to oestrogen, but instead *synthesize progesterone*. Second, LH *stimulates this synthesis of progesterone* via the newly acquired LH receptors. Third, the cells have lost, or reduced, their capacity to bind oestrogen and FSH, but *gained the capacity to bind progestins*. This acquisition of the capacity to respond to LH by synthesizing progesterone (and then to be self-stimulated by it—positive feedback) results in an exponential release of progesterone from the follicle, which becomes significant in the human several hours before ovulation, although in most species only just before or immediately after ovulation.

This rising progestin output has three important functional consequences. First, it depresses growth in the less mature developing follicles. Second, it is essential for ovulation itself. Thus progesterone inhibitors such as mifepristone (RU486) suppress ovulation, and females genetically null for progesterone receptors do not ovulate. Third, it promotes the transition to the progestagenic phase of the ovarian cycle.

The process of ovulation involves protease activity

By the end of the preovulatory phase of follicular growth, the rapid expansion of follicular fluid has resulted in a relatively thin peripheral rim of mural granulosa cells, basement membrane and thecal cells, to which the oocyte, with its associated cumulus cells, is attached only by a tenuous and thinning stalk of granulosa cells. The increasing size of the follicle and its position in the ovarian cortex causes it to bulge from the ovarian surface. At one point, the *stigma*, this bulging wall becomes even thinner and avascular, the connective tissue breaks down, and the follicle ruptures. The follicular fluid flows out carrying with it the oocyte and its surrounding mass of cumulus cells. The biochemistry of ovulation involves proteolytic enzymes, notably members of a large family of *matrix metalloproteinases (MMPs)* and their natural *tissue inhibitors (TIMPs)*, and also serine proteases such as plasmin and plasminogen activator. Under LH influence, directly and/or indirectly via progesterone and/or prostaglandins, *collagenase* and *gelatinase* activities (both MMPs) increase, especially in the stigma, as do those of *plasminogen activator* (which cleaves procollagenase to generate active collagenase), while those of its inhibitor reach a nadir. The experimental inhibition of collagenase prevents ovulation. Proteases are also much involved in other follicular remodelling activities during conversion to a corpus luteum (see later).

In many species, including humans, the ovarian surface is directly exposed to the peritoneal cavity, but in some (e.g. the sheep, horse and rat) a peritoneal capsule or bursa encloses the ovary to varying degrees and acts to retain the oocyte cumulus mass(es) close to the ovary. There they are collected by cilia on the *fimbria* of the oviduct, which sweep the cumulus mass into the *oviducal ostium* (see Fig. 5.1). The residual parts of the follicle within the ovary collapse into the space left by the fluid, the oocyte and the cumulus cells, and within this cavity a clot forms. Thus, the postovulatory follicle is composed of a fibrin core, surrounded by several collapsed layers of granulosa cells, enclosed within a *fibrous outer thecal capsule.*

The corpus luteum is the postovulatory 'follicle'

The fate of the oocyte we will follow later in Chapters 8 and 9. For now we continue to focus on the remains of the postovulatory follicle.

The corpus luteum produces progestagens

The collapsed follicle now transforms into a *corpus luteum* (Fig. 5.2c). Within the follicular antrum, the fibrin core undergoes fibrosis over a period of several days; the membrana propria between the granulosa and thecal layers breaks down and blood vessels invade. Both granulosa cells and cells from the theca interna contribute to the corpus luteum, although many thecal cells also disperse to the stromal tissue. The granulosa cells have now ceased dividing and hypertrophy to form *large lutein cells*, rich in mitochondria, smooth endoplasmic reticulum, lipid droplets, Golgi bodies and, in many species, a carotenoid pigment, lutein, which may give the corpora lutea a yellowish or orange tinge. This transformation is referred to as *luteinization* and is associated with a steadily increasing secretion of progestagens. The thecal cells form *smaller lutein cells*, produce progesterone and androgens, and seem to be richer in LH receptors. After LH stimulation, these smaller cells can serve as a stem cell population for the more endocrinologically active, large lutein cells in some species.

In most species, the principal progestagen secreted from the large lutein cells is progesterone, but secretion of significant quantities of 17α-hydroxyprogesterone in primates and of 20α-hydroxyprogesterone in the rat and hamster also occurs. In a few species, notably the great apes and

humans, and to a lesser extent the pig, the corpus luteum also secretes oestrogens, particularly oestradiol 17β. Its source also seems to be the large luteal cells, using as substrate androgens derived from the small luteal cells (a hangover from granulosa function in preovulatory follicles?). In most species (e.g. the monkey, sheep, cow, rabbit, rat and horse), however, the corpus luteum secretes only trivial amounts of oestrogen.

The corpus luteum also secretes two other hormones. Inhibin A is secreted in large amounts in higher primates. It acts to promote production of progesterone (see also Chapter 6). The second hormone is oxytocin (see Fig. 3.7), which comes from the large lutein cells and the importance of which will become evident soon (see 'Luteolysis' below).

Luteotrophins: endocrine support of the corpus luteum varies for different species

The endocrine support of the corpus luteum, like its cellular composition and secretory pattern, shows considerable variation among species. The conversion of a follicle to a corpus luteum requires that high surge levels of LH both provoke ovulation and initiate luteal conversion. This gonadotrophin is then also required, albeit at lower levels, for the maintenance of the corpus luteum. However, in some species prolactin and/or progesterone also form an important component of the so-called *luteotrophic complex*. In those species (Table 5.4), appropriate receptors can be detected on granulosa cells from the preovulatory stage onwards.

Luteolysis: death of the corpus luteum may be active or passive depending on the species

The life of the corpus luteum in the non-pregnant female varies among species from 2 to 14 days (Table 5.3 & Chapter 11). Luteal regression or *luteolysis* involves a collapse of the lutein cells, ischaemia and progressive cell death with a consequent fall in the output of progestagens. The whitish scar tissue remaining, the *corpus albicans*, is absorbed into the stromal tissue of the ovary over a period that varies from weeks to months, depending on the species. Luteolysis can be caused by withdrawal or inadequacy of the luteotrophic complex. However, in many species, it is not primarily a failure of luteotrophic support, but active production of a *luteolytic factor* that brings about normal luteal regression. Thus, in these species, *both luteotrophic support and antiluteolytic support* are required to sustain the corpus luteum.

Most mammals studied, *with the notable exception of higher primates*, come into this latter category, and *the uterus* has been identified as the source of the luteolysin. Thus, luteal life can be prolonged by *hysterectomy* (removal of the uterus), but if the endometrium of the excised uterus is

Table 5.4 Hormones luteotrophic/antiluteolytic for the non-pregnant corpus luteum of different species.

Species	LH*	Prolactin	Oestrogen	FSH†	Progesterone
Human	++	+?	Luteolytic?	–	+++
Cow	++	+?	Luteolytic?	–	+
Sheep	++	+	–	–	?+
Pig	+	+?	+	–	+
Rabbit	+	?	+++	+	1st 3 days only
Rat/mouse	+	+++	–	–	–
Dog	+	+	?	?	±
Hamster	+	+	?	+	?

*LH is essential to stimulate the initiation of luteinization in all species. Here its role subsequently is assessed. It may be directly luteotrophic, but in species in which follicles are growing through the luteal phase, the LH may also stimulate some oestrogen synthesis locally.
†FSH may only be luteotrophic indirectly by stimulating oestrogen.

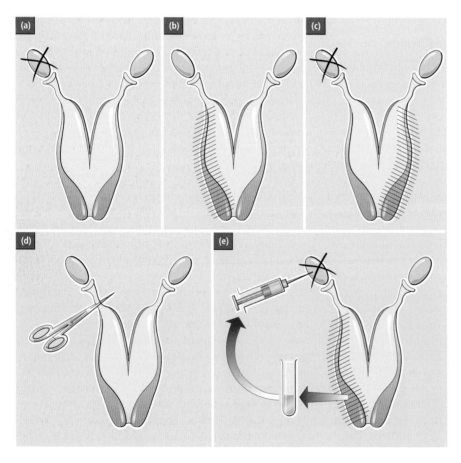

Fig. 5.6 Non-pregnant sheep uterus and ovaries. (a) A single corpus luteum present in the left ovary regresses, indicated by a cross. (b) Removal of the ipsilateral uterine horn (hatched) prevents regression. (c) Removal of the contralateral horn does not prevent regression. (d) Clamping the blood supply between the horn and ovary prevents regression. (e) If the endometrium of the removed ipsilateral horn is homogenized and re-injected into the ovarian artery, the corpus luteum regresses (compare b with e).

homogenized and injected, then luteolysis occurs (Fig. 5.6e). Luteal prolongation can also be achieved by ligating the tissues, including the blood vessels, between the uterus and the ovary (Fig. 5.6d). The results of these classical experiments led to the suggestion that a humoral factor passes from the endometrium to the ovary, and causes luteolysis. Two observations on the ewe suggested that this humoral factor was highly labile. First, if instead of removing the whole uterus, which in the ewe has two separate horns, only one horn was removed, then only the corpus luteum on the opposite side regressed (Fig. 5.6b,c). Second, if the whole uterus was transplanted elsewhere in the body, luteolysis was prevented unless the ovaries had also been transplanted with the uterus as a unit.

The identity of the endometrial substance responsible has now been established as *prostaglandin $F_{2\alpha}$* ($PGF_{2\alpha}$; see Fig. 3.4). $PGF_{2\alpha}$ is secreted in a series of pulses at roughly 6-h intervals from epithelial and glandular cells in the mid to late luteal phase. It passes from the endometrium into the uterine vein. From the vein, it passes by a local countercurrent transfer to the ovarian artery, and thence to the ipsilateral ovary. Corpus luteum regression follows shortly thereafter. Antibody neutralization of $PGF_{2\alpha}$, or inhibition of its synthesis, prevents luteolysis. Conversely, injections of exogenous $PGF_{2\alpha}$ 1 or 2 days in advance of its endogenous output leads to premature luteolysis; indeed, $PGF_{2\alpha}$ will cause regression of luteinized cells *in vitro* (see also Box 5.2).

The control of luteolysis in *higher primates*, including humans, unlike that for other species, does *not* involve uterine prostaglandins. The levels of prostaglandins secreted rise in the late luteal phase, but neither hysterectomy nor antibodies to prostaglandins prolong luteal life. Moreover, injections of prostaglandins are without effect on the corpus luteum, unless very high doses are used when a transient drop in progesterone output occurs. What then causes luteal decline in humans? It seems that it is *loss of adequate luteotrophic support* rather than the genesis of an active luteolytic agent that occurs in higher primates. Thus, the more extended preovulatory LH surge seen in higher primates followed by the relatively low sustained levels of LH during the luteal phase of primates are sufficiently luteotrophic for a normal length luteal phase. However, in order to extend the life of the corpus luteum for longer than 10–12 days, a *second exponential rise of LH activity* is required—a point that we return to in Chapter 11. Without this second surge in LH activity, the corpus luteum simply regresses slowly and spontaneously.

BOX 5.2 Molecular mechanisms underlying luteolysis by $PGF_{2\alpha}$

- *Luteal oxytocin regulates the production of $PGF_{2\alpha}$ via a receptor-regulatory mechanism.* Why does the endometrium release $PGF_{2\alpha}$ during the latter part of the luteal phase? It turns out that the timing mechanism is complex and hinges on oxytocin. Oxytocin, which is secreted from the corpus luteum (and possibly also the pituitary), can be shown to be an essential player, as its neutralization delays luteolysis. Moreover, $PGF_{2\alpha}$ itself stimulates oxytocin release from the corpus luteum, thereby effecting a *positive feedback loop*—in this case to luteal destruction, a neat symmetry with the positive feedback loop involving progesterone that drives luteal formation after ovulation!

- *However, we still have a problem*, because oxytocin is released from the corpus luteum well before the latter part of the luteal phase, so why does it not stimulate $PGF_{2\alpha}$ secretion earlier? The answer seems to be that *oxytocin receptors* in the endometrium are absent until late in the luteal phase, and so the tissue is blind to oxytocin's presence. Why? We do not know, but it may depend on two distinct and paradoxical actions of progesterone on the uterine epithelium. Thus, progesterone *stimulates* $PGF_{2\alpha}$ production but *depresses oxytocin receptor* production (receptor regulation). However, *prolonged elevation* of progesterone *depresses* progesterone receptor production (auto receptor regulation—Chapter 8), allowing escape of oxytocin receptor gene expression as the luteal phase progresses. $PGF_{2\alpha}$ release then occurs, followed by the precipitate decline of the corpus luteum. Epithelial oestrogen receptors also rise as progesterone receptors fall (Chapter 8), and the oxytocin receptor promoter has a binding motif for activated E2-receptor, so oestrogen has also been implicated in facilitating oxytocin-mediated $PGF_{2\alpha}$ release.

- *A role for endothelins in luteolysis?* How $PGF_{2\alpha}$ causes luteal regression is uncertain. One likely contributory factor is the adverse impact that it has on blood flow. The corpus luteum is highly vascularized and an early sign of luteolysis is reduced blood flow. Levels of *endothelin 1*, a potent vasoconstrictor peptide that is synthesized both by capillary endothelial cells and large and small luteal cells, rise during the mid–late luteal phase, in parallel with rising $PGF_{2\alpha}$. Moreover, premature $PGF_{2\alpha}$ injections lead to earlier and higher levels of endothelin 1 synthesis and premature luteolysis. This peptide reduces luteal blood flow *in vivo* and depresses progesterone production by bovine luteal cells *in vitro*. It also stimulates the production of $PGF_{2\alpha}$ by luteal cells, thereby setting up a *second luteolytic positive feedback loop*. Endothelial receptors are detectable on luteal cells, and receptor blockers specific for endothelin 1 reduce the antiprogesterone effects of $PGF_{2\alpha}$ *in vivo* and *in vitro*. Taken together, these results suggest that at least part of the luteolytic action of $PGF_{2\alpha}$ involves endothelin 1.

Further reading

Milvae RA (2000) Inter-relationships between endothelin and prostaglandin $F_{2\alpha}$ in corpus luteum function. *Reviews of Reproduction* 5, 1–5.

Spencer TE, Bazer FW (2004) Conceptus signals for establishment and maintenance of pregnancy. *Reproductive Biology and Endocrinology* 2, 49 doi:10.1186/1477-7827-2-49.

What controls the number of follicles ovulating?

The number of follicles ovulating in any one cycle is characteristic for each species and ranges from one to several hundred. There appear to be two points during follicular maturation at which this number can be regulated, and in both cases it is the balance between survival and atresia that is critical.

The balance between FSH and its receptors influences numbers of antral follicles surviving

In humans about 7–10 early antral follicles in each ovary are rescued from atresia and *recruited* for development at the start of each menstrual cycle. FSH is the crucial hormone for follicular rescue, although of course LH is necessary for fully functional follicles. Thus, the number of follicles recruited can be increased if endogenous FSH levels are augmented by exogenous FSH or can be reduced if FSH levels are sufficiently diminished. This observation must mean that a delicate interplay between the levels of circulating gonadotrophins and the follicular levels of FSH receptors determines the number of follicles recruited from the early antral pool. If appropriate hormone levels and acquisition of sufficient receptors coincide, then follicular development continues. If hormone levels are inappropriate when the receptors develop, then follicular atresia ensues.

The selection of dominant follicles to ovulate may be controlled by cytokines

Of the 15–20 follicles recruited in the human, usually only one emerges as *dominant* during the later stages of follicular growth. It is only this one dominant follicle that subsequently undergoes preovulatory growth, develops LH receptors on its granulosa cells, and is competent to ovulate in response to a surge in LH. This follicle is also the dominant source of oestrogen as ovulation approaches, as can be shown by selectively removing it, when the surge levels of oestrogen decline abruptly. We do not know why one follicle emerges, but it is possible that cytokines are involved. FSH stimulates the production of *insulin-like growth factor 1* or *2* (IGF-1 or -2 depending on the species; see Table 5.1) and the IGF appears to mediate both the stimulation by LH of androgen output by the thecal cells and its FSH-dependent aromatization to oestrogen by granulosa cells. If IGF activity is neutralized, the effectiveness of FSH in stimulating oestrogen output is reduced. FSH is also involved in the regulation of ovarian production of the endogenous IGF-binding proteins (IGFBPs) described in Chapter 3 (see section on 'Binding proteins'). These are also produced by the follicle, but FSH

suppresses their synthesis. It also promotes production by granulosa cells of a protease, called *pregnancy-associated plasma protein A* (PAPP-A), which cleaves the IGF from its IGFBP, thereby releasing it for action. PAPP-A expression is markedly elevated in the dominant follicle. Overall, therefore, FSH stimulates the availability of IGF to promote follicular development. It is possible therefore that among growing follicles, IGFBPs are produced preferentially by those follicles with the *least good* supply of FSH and/or the *fewest FSH receptors*. The capture of IGF by its binding protein, especially in the absence of its cleaving protease, would further impair the effectiveness of FSH and so promote a downward spiral of the follicle to atresia. In contrast, those follicles best able to respond to FSH would spiral upwards to expansion and ovulation. Interestingly, it has been shown that BMP15, produced in the oocyte, *inhibits PAPP-A production by FSH*. Might the oocyte itself have an input into which follicle gets to be dominant and indeed how many dominant oocytes there are?

Once a dominant follicle has been selected, inhibin may also be involved in its maintenance. Inhibin A is produced in the late antral phase in dominant follicles under the influence of LH (Table 5.1). Inhibin A then stimulates both thecal androgen production and its granulosa aromatization and so sets up a positive feedback loop leading to the oestrogen surge from the dominant follicle. In contrast, retarded follicles show low levels of inhibin but higher levels of activin, which attenuate androgen output by the theca and so suppress both inhibin synthesis and oestrogen output. Thus, dominant follicles are characterized by high ratios of both inhibin:activin and IGF:IGFBP. Retarded follicles show the reverse.

Oocytes are active players in folliculogenesis

Thus far, follicles may appear to be simply 'oocyte-carriers and supporters', which implies a passive role for the oocyte. However, this is far from the case. We saw in Chapter 1 that a deficiency of oogonia/oocytes during fetal development of the ovary led to follicular regression and 'streak' ovaries. In the adult ovary too, oocytes remain very active partners, producing cytokines with multiple roles (see Table 5.1). During primordial follicle recruitment, oocytic FGF2 is implicated in the stimulation of SCF activity in granulosa cells. During preantral follicular growth, a deficiency of oocytic GDF9 results in follicular arrest due to reduced granulosa cell proliferation. This defect can be rescued by restoring the absent cytokine, which acts cooperatively with IGF, FSH and androgens. During the antral phase, GDF9 may drive the changing pattern of the mural granulosa cell activity. Thus, the granulosa cells lining the follicle wall become increasingly different from the *cumulus granulosa cells* surrounding the oocyte. Whereas cumulus cells produce hyaluronic acid to provide the matrix that carries the egg out of the follicle at ovulation, mural cells express higher levels of LH receptor the further from the oocyte they are located. This granulosa heterogeneity is regulated by the oocyte through locally acting cytokines such as GDF9 that antagonize FSH stimulation locally. The depression of LH receptor forms an important role in the prevention of premature luteinization of the follicle by delaying progesterone synthesis in granulosa cells until the oocyte has left the follicle. Remarkably, if oocytes from expanding antral follicles are transplanted surgically into primordial follicles, the time for the primordial follicles to mature is halved, leading to the suggestion that the oocyte orchestrates the rate of development. This intimate and interactive partnership between oocyte and follicular cells resembles that seen for spermatogenic cells and Sertoli cells in Chapter 4. In both cases, the system has evolved exquisitely to maximize the chance of gamete fertility.

Follicular development and the ovarian cycle

In the previous sections, we have described the development of an *individual follicle* through either to ovulation and luteinization, or (for most of them) to atresia *en route*. But each of the two ovaries has many primordial follicles, and we must now consider the relationships between the various follicles developing at different times, and in both ovaries, in order to obtain an overall picture of ovarian function and cyclicity.

The ovarian cycle is the interval between successive ovulations and comprises follicular and luteal phases

One complete *ovarian cycle* is the interval between successive ovulations, where each ovulation is preceded by a period of oestrogen dominance. As the oestrogens are derived from the follicles, the period preceding ovulation is often called the *follicular phase of the cycle*. Correspondingly, the period after ovulation is often called the *luteal phase*, because progesterone is derived from the corpus luteum. The duration of the ovarian cycle and its constituent follicular and luteal phases in various species is summarized in Table 5.5. It is immediately clear that there are major differences between species in both the absolute length of the ovarian cycle and in the relative duration of its follicular and luteal components. These apparent major differences mask a fundamentally similar organization, and result only from minor but significant modifications to a basic pattern. First, we will discuss the human ovarian cycle, as it is the easiest to understand. We will then relate that pattern to those of other species.

The ovarian cycle of the human

Fig. 5.7a shows a basic outline of two sequential human ovarian cycles. The pattern of measured blood steroids and gonadotrophins is indicated below, and the activities of the four follicular stages are indicated above. A continuous trickle of developing primordial, preantral and early antral follicles occurs throughout the cycle; growth of these follicles does not require gonadotrophic support, and the follicles do not secrete significant levels of steroids, and so do not affect blood steroid levels. As we saw earlier, the early antral follicles so formed are doomed to atresia unless rescued by FSH and LH, which take them through full antral expansion. One (or two) of these rescued follicles will survive to become the dominant antral follicle, secreting high levels of oestrogens at maturity 8–12 days later: witness the rising blood oestrogen levels. This advanced follicle is then converted to a preovulatory follicle by the

Table 5.5 Ovarian cyclicity in different species.

Species	Length of cycle (days)	Follicular phase (days)	Luteal phase (days)
Human	24–32	10–14	12–15
Cow	20–21	2–3	18–19
Pig	19–21	5–6	15–17
Sheep	16–17	1–2	14–15
Horse	20–22	5–6	15–16
Mouse/rat* (+infertile male)	13–14	2	11–12
Rabbit* (+infertile male)	14–15	1–2	13
Mouse/rat	4–5	2	2–3
Rabbit	1–2	1–2	0

*See text for discussion.

transient high levels of LH that are measured in the blood at this time. The other antral follicles become atretic. The successful ovulatory follicle forms a corpus luteum, which secretes progesterone and oestrogen, until luteolysis 14 or so days later. During the luteal phase, LH and FSH levels are comparatively low and are insufficient to maintain antral development, which is also suppressed by elevated progesterone levels, so follicular atresia occurs. After luteolysis, a new cycle then begins as tonic gonadotrophin levels are elevated and progesterone is low.

Two important features emerge from this description of the human ovarian cycle: first, we need to understand what controls the fluctuating levels of gonadotrophin output (this will be discussed in detail in the next chapter); second, the complete antral expansion phase, ovulation and the complete luteal phase occupy one complete ovarian cycle. This second feature distinguishes humans from the cow, pig, sheep and horse.

The ovarian cycles of the cow, pig, sheep and horse have a shorter follicular phase

In these species, as indicated for the pig in Fig. 5.7b, significant antral expansion occurs during the luteal phase of the previous crop of follicles to have ovulated. This growth is possible because *FSH and LH in these species do not fall to such low levels during the luteal phase* (see Chapter 6 for an explanation of why this should be). Thus, in these species the complete antral expansion phase, ovulation and the complete luteal phase *occupy longer than one*

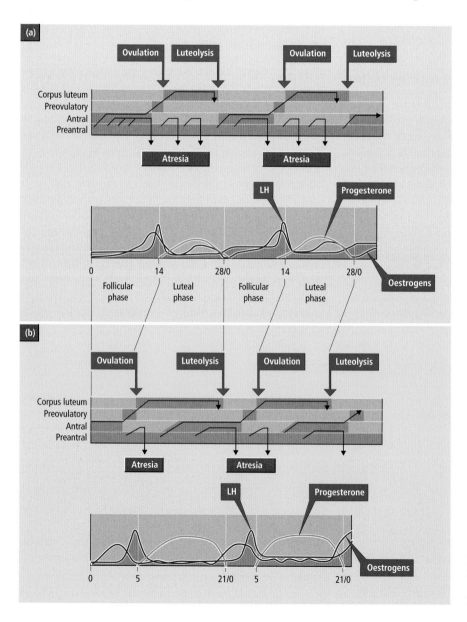

Fig. 5.7 Summary of follicular activity in two sequential ovarian cycles in: (a) the human; and (b) the pig. The presence of the different follicular stages is indicated by darker shading within each bar. Relative blood hormone levels are also indicated. The history of an ovulatory follicle from the preantral stage to luteolysis or atresia is indicated by the black lines marked with closed arrows. Note that the pig cycle is shorter than that of the human and this is due to a shorter follicular phase as indicated by the oblique arrows linking the human (a) and pig (b) panels: antral follicular growth occurs during the preceding luteal phase in pigs but not humans (see the difference in darker shading in the antral bars of human and pig).

complete ovarian cycle (follow and compare the black lines in Fig. 5.7a,b). It is almost as though in these species, the human cycle has been 'telescoped' by 'pushing' the follicular part of one cycle backwards into the luteal half of the previous cycle.

The ovarian cycles of most other species can be understood quite simply in terms of the above discussion. We will examine those of the rat, mouse and rabbit because they exhibit a certain distinctive feature of great importance in understanding the ovarian cycles of humans and the large farm animals.

The ovarian cycles of the rat and mouse can have abbreviated follicular and luteal phases

The ovarian cycles of the rat and mouse are basically of the 'telescoped' sort seen in large farm animals. They show, however, a curious and distinctive feature: the cycle differs in length, depending on whether or not the female mates. If the female has an infertile mating at the time of ovulation, for example with a vasectomized male, her luteal phase is 11–12 days in duration (often called a *pseudopregnancy*), and the ovarian cycle resembles that of the pig. However, if she fails to mate at the time of ovulation the luteal phase is only 2–3 days long. In the latter case the corpora lutea become only transiently functional in producing progestagens, secreting a small amount of progesterone, but mainly 20α-hydroxyprogesterone.

The explanation for this curious phenomenon lies in the *mechanical stimulus to the cervix* provided naturally by the penis at coitus. The presence of such stimulation is relayed via sensory nerves from the cervix to the central nervous system (CNS), and activates the release of *prolactin* from the pituitary in twice daily surges that last for about 10 days. This hormone, as pointed out earlier (Table 5.4), is an essential part of the luteotrophic complex in the rat and mouse, and without it luteal life is abbreviated from the 'normal' extended pattern characteristic of the large farm animals. Not surprisingly therefore, if the prolactin surges are blocked, pseudopregnancy does not occur.

Why such a complex cycle? The rat and mouse derive increased reproductive efficiency from this evolutionary modification, as without the abbreviating device they would only be fertile every 13 or 14 days instead of every 4 or 5. As their pregnancy only lasts 20–21 days, this is a highly significant economy. Evolutionary pressures for such a truncation of the luteal phase would not apply to the cow, pig, sheep and horse where pregnancy is a very extended event compared with the luteal phase.

This neat neural device, which shortens the luteal phase, introduces an important new concept into our discussion. It illustrates how the CNS can influence ovarian function. The following two chapters will discuss this topic in detail.

We will first look, however, at one other type of modification to the ovarian cycle that re-emphasizes the role that the CNS can play.

The ovarian cycle of the rabbit is reduced to an extended follicular phase

A female rabbit caged alone shows little evidence of a cycle: blood levels of oestrogens are high; progestagens are low; she is always on heat and ready to mate, but ovulation cannot be detected. Yet her ovary contains waves of expanding antral follicles. It is as though she is in a continuous follicular phase. If she is mated with a vasectomized buck, or if her cervix is stimulated mechanically, she ovulates 10–12 h later and has a luteal phase, or pseudopregnancy, of 12 or so days. If the vasectomized buck is left in with her, she will show a 14-day cycle with a 2+12-day follicular+luteal pattern, similar to the porcine pattern.

As in the rat, cervical stimulation in the rabbit is the source of a sensory input to the CNS, which, in this case, induces a surge of LH, high levels of which rescue any expanded antral follicles from atresia and ovulate them. In essence, the rabbit has abbreviated her cycle even more than the rat or mouse by eliminating the luteal phase completely. This phenomenon is known as *induced ovulation*, and is seen in a number of species (e.g. the rabbit, cat, ferret, camel and llama).

Our discussion on different ovarian cycles is summarized in Fig. 5.8.

Interstitial glands

We have discussed at length the activities of the maturing follicles composed of primordial follicles and accreted stromal cells: the thecal layers. However, within the stroma, and between the developing follicles, lie the interstitial glands. Do they have a role to play in ovarian function and cyclicity?

The interstitial glands show considerable variation among different species, and little is known of their activity. Interstitial glands are composed of aggregates of steroidogenic-like cells that contain extensive smooth endoplasmic reticulum and lipid droplets. In the rabbit, in which these cells are well developed, they synthesize progesterone and 20α-hydroxyprogesterone, and are sensitive to the LH activity observed after coitus. In the rat, the interstitial glands are also stimulated by the surge of LH to form progestagens. Interstitial cells have also been implicated in the synthesis of androgens in the human, rat and rabbit ovaries, and it is possible that this tissue serves as an additional source of androgens for both secretion and aromatization in the follicles.

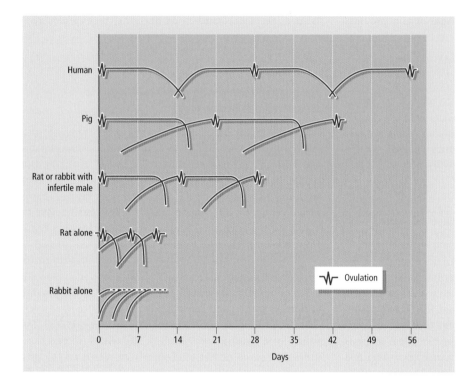

Fig. 5.8 Schematic comparison of ovarian cycles of the human, the pig, the rat or rabbit caged with an infertile male and the rat or rabbit caged alone. In this figure, day 0 indicates the day of the first ovulation. Each continuous line represents a complete and successful sequence of growth of one crop of antral follicle(s) through preovulatory follicle(s) to corpora lutea and ultimately luteolysis. Note cycle lengths and the proportions within each cycle vary (see text for explanation).

Summary

The ovarian cycle: a recap

Follicular growth and differentiation from a primordial follicle through to a functional corpus luteum is a complex process that is only completed successfully by less than 0.1% of follicles. Most become atretic at some point during the process. The resumption of development by primordial follicles is hormone independent. During this phase the oocyte undergoes its major growth, and the follicle acquires receptors for FSH and oestrogen (granulosa cells) and for LH (thecal cells). During the much shorter phase of antral expansion, growth of follicular cells occurs with a rising output of oestrogens and androgens. Adequate levels of LH and FSH are required for this phase to be completed successfully, and the higher the level of FSH, the more follicles are likely to survive. Towards the end of this phase, oestrogen output increases from the dominant antral follicles, and their outer mural granulosa cells acquire LH receptors.

During the short preovulatory phase, a large surge of LH gives a sudden stimulus via the LH receptors on both granulosa and thecal cells. This surge of LH first stimulates, and then stops, the endocrine activity of the thecal cells, and also switches off the aromatizing activity of mural granulosa cells and diverts them to the production of progestagens. This dramatic switch in endocrine activity

is accompanied by the renewed meiotic and cytoplasmic maturation of the oocyte and culminates in ovulation. During this phase the granulosa cells of most species acquire prolactin and progesterone receptors. This phase culminates in ovulation.

The final luteal phase of follicular development is characterized by a rising output of progestagens, on which may be superimposed, in primates and pigs, a rise in oestrogen output. A luteotrophic complex of LH plus some or all of the three hormones, prolactin, progesterone and oestrogen, supports the luteal phase. During this phase, oxytocin output increases and receptors for it develop in the endometrium towards the end of the luteal phase. The oxytocin stimulates prostaglandin production, at least in non-primates. The whole sequence terminates with luteolysis, due either to the production of the uterine luteolytic hormone $PGF_{2\alpha}$ or to inadequacy of luteotrophic support.

The ovary is like the testis in producing both gametes and steroids. However, whereas in the male the gametes and the androgens are produced continuously and concurrently, in the female the ovarian output is cyclic and shows two distinct phases separated by the ovulatory release of one or more oocytes. The follicular phase, before ovulation, is dominated by a rising output of oestrogen and some androgens, whereas in the luteal phase, after ovulation, progestagens predominate. In many species the follicular phase is brief, and the major part of follicular growth occurs during the luteal phase of the previous cycle. In humans, however, the follicular phase is more extended.

The ovarian cycle in relation to the oestrous and menstrual cycles

We have considered the cyclicity of reproduction in the female from the viewpoint of the ovary. However, the cyclic output of ovarian steroids imparts cyclicity to the anatomy and physiology of the whole female as we will see in more detail in Chapter 8. This external manifestation of the internal ovarian cycle can be recognized in many mammals by a behavioural characteristic. Female mammals of most species are only receptive to males (*on heat*), and therefore willing to mate, around the time of ovulation. This period of heat is conditioned by the hormonal milieu of the preovulatory phase, and can be accompanied by marked changes in behaviour patterns. The frisky state observed in some species, particularly in horses, was given the name *oestrus* (or 'attacked by gadflies'), and thus the internal ovarian cycle is manifested externally in the so-called *oestrous cycle* (Fig. 5.9a). Day 1 of each oestrous cycle

is generally considered to be *the day of first appearance of oestrous behaviour*.

Higher primates show little evidence of oestrus and thus it is inappropriate to speak of their oestrous cycle. However, in these primates, another external manifestation of ovarian cyclicity is observed: the shedding of bloody endometrial tissue via the vagina at the end of the luteal phase. This hormonally conditioned event is called *menstruation* (i.e. monthly event), and is used as the external basis for the measurement of the *menstrual cycle* in which the *first day of menstruation* is considered day 1 of the cycle, as may be observed in Fig. 5.9b. Although both the oestrous and menstrual cycles reflect ovarian cyclicity, *the starting days for each cycle occur at different points in the underlying ovarian cycle*.

We have seen in this chapter that the levels of gonadotrophins critically affect the successful completion of the ovarian (and thus of the oestrous/menstrual) cycle, and that the circulating levels of gonadotrophins vary naturally during the cycle. Moreover, we have observed that the CNS can affect the levels of circulating gonadotrophins. In the next chapter we will examine how gonadotrophin levels are regulated, and how the CNS exerts its effects.

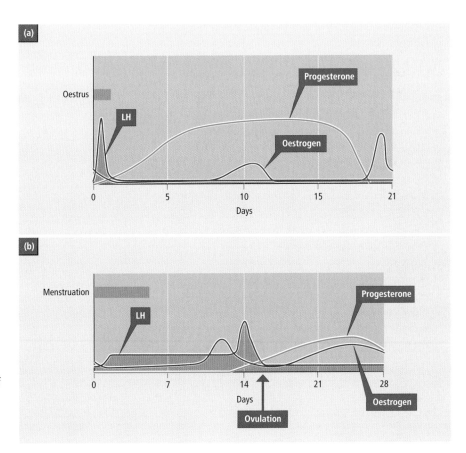

Fig. 5.9 Schematic views of the ovarian cycles in (a) the cow; and (b) the human, expressed as oestrous and menstrual cycles. The first day of the cycle coincides with the beginning of either oestrus or menstruation (plasma concentrations not to scale).

- The adult ovary produces oocytes and endocrine hormones: oestrogens, androgens, inhibins and progestagens.

- The follicle is the source of all of these and is the functional unit of the ovary.

- The follicle is an interactive partnership between oocyte and follicular cells.

- Primordial follicles mature to preantral follicles in a constant trickle throughout adult reproductive life: this maturation does not require external hormonal support but is enhanced by GH and does involve paracrine action by cytokines such as IGF1, SCF and FGF2.

- This maturation involves oocyte growth, secretion of the ZP glycoproteins and their assembly into the zona pellucida around the oocyte, granulosa cell proliferation, and the deposition of interstitial cells on the outer membrana propria to form the theca interna and externa.

- The late preantral and early antral follicles develop FSH receptors on their granulosa cells and LH receptors on their theca interna cells.

- LH stimulates thecal cells to produce androgens.

- Androgens are aromatized by granulosa cells to produce oestrogens in an FSH-dependent process.

- FSH also stimulates the production of follicular fluid, expansion of the follicle and the appearance of the follicular antrum.

- Production of growth factor(s) by the follicle is stimulated by FSH, and mediates some of its intrafollicular effects.

- A high IGF:IGFBP ratio and expression of oocytic BMP15 characterizes the dominant follicle(s).

- Production of inhibin by the follicle is stimulated by FSH and LH, and the ration of inhibin A to inhibin B rises as ovulation approaches.

- Under the influence of FSH and LH, the dominant antral follicle(s) produce(s) rising oestrogen levels culminating in a surge of oestrogen.

- Under the influence of LH, the dominant follicle(s) is induced to enter the preovulatory phase.

- The preovulatory phase is characterized by rising progesterone output from mural granulosa cells and the appearance of prolactin and progesterone receptors.

- During the preovulatory phase, the follicular antrum expands rapidly to protrude from the surface of the ovary, the granulosa cells form a thin rim lining the follicle with a stalk of cells connecting to the oocyte surrounded by cumulus cells, the cytoplasmic links between oocyte and cumulus cells are severed, and the oocyte resumes meiosis.

- The oocyte extrudes a first polar body in an unequal cytoplasmic division and then arrests in second meiotic metaphase in which state it is ovulated.

- The oocyte is ovulated through the ruptured apex of the follicular protrusion at its stigma.

- The rupture is due to the action of proteases on the follicle wall.

- The ovulated oocyte(s) is released onto the surface of the ovary.

- The empty follicle collapses, becomes fully vascularized and undergoes the process of luteinization to form the corpus luteum.

- Granulosa cells contribute large luteal cells and thecal cells contribute small luteal cells.

- Large luteal cells synthesize progestagens.

- Hormonal support of the corpus luteum is species variable: LH is required for luteinization; prolactin, oestrogen and progesterone may be involved in luteal maintenance.

- Luteolysis in most species is caused by prostaglandin $F_{2\alpha}$.

- Release of $PGF_{2\alpha}$ from the endometrium into the local circulation is stimulated by oxytocin produced by the corpus luteum and acting on endometrial oxytocin receptors that develop under the influence of sustained progesterone.

- Luteolysis in higher primates is caused by inadequate luteal LH support.

- Fertility in females is episodic: ovulation is preceded by a period of follicular/oestrogen dominance and followed by a period of luteal/progestagen dominance.

- The ovarian cycle is the time between ovulations.

- In humans the follicular and luteal phases of the cycle are of approximately equal length, and luteolysis is followed by menstruation which signals the initiation of a new ovarian cycle.

- In humans, we speak of the menstrual cycle, day 1 of which is the first day of menstrual flow.

- In most other species, the follicular phase is short as most follicular growth occurs during the preceding luteal phase; there is no menstruation but there is a visible external change in behaviour around the time of ovulation.

- In these species, we speak of the oestrous cycle, in which day 1 is the beginning of oestrus.

- In some species, neural mechanisms resulting from penile stimulation of the cervix during coitus influence the pattern and length of oestrous cycles.

FURTHER READING

General reading

Armstrong DG, Webb R (1997) Ovarian follicle dominance: the role of intraovarian growth factors and novel proteins. *Reviews of Reproduction* **2**, 139–146.

Bromsel-Helmreich O (1985) Ultrasound and the preovulatory human follicle. *Oxford Reviews of Reproductive Biology* **7**, 1–72.

Choi Y, Rajkovic A (2006) Genetics of early mammalian folliculogenesis. *Cellular and Molecular Life Sciences* **63**, 579–590.

Cupps PT (ed.) (1991) *Reproduction in Domestic Animals*, 4th edn. Academic Press, London.

Drummond A (2006) The role of steroids in follicular growth. *Reproductive Biology and Endocrinology* **4**, 16 doi:10.1186/1477–7827-4-16.

Elvin JA *et al.* (2000) Oocyte-expressed TGF-β superfamily members in female fertility. *Molecular and Cellular Endocrinology* **159**, 1–5.

Erickson GF, Shimasaki S (2001) The physiology of folliculogenesis: the role of novel growth factors. *Fertility and Sterility* **76**, 943–949.

Freeman ME *et al.* (2000) Prolactin: structure, function and regulation of secretion. *Physiological Reviews* **80**, 1523–1631.

Guigon CJ, Magre S (2006) Contribution of germ cells to the differentiation and maturation of the ovary: insights from models of germ cell depletion. *Biology of Reproduction* **74**, 450–458.

Matzuk M *et al.* (2002) Intercellular communication in the mammalian ovary: oocytes carry the conversation. *Science* **296**, 2178–2180.

McIntush EW, Smith MF (1998) Matrix metalloproteinases and tissue inhibitors of metalloproteinases in ovarian function. *Reviews of Reproduction* **3**, 23–30.

McNatty KP *et al.* (2004) The oocyte and its role in regulating ovulation rate: a new paradigm in reproductive biology. *Reproduction* **128**, 379–386.

Muttukrishna S *et al.* (2004) Activin and follistatin in female reproduction. *Molecular and Cellular Endocrinology* **225**, 45–56.

Skinner MK (2005) Regulation of primordial follicle assembly and development. *Human Reproduction Update* **11**, 461–471.

Stouffer RL (2003) Progesterone as a mediator of gonadotrophin action in the corpus luteum: beyond steroidogenesis. *Human Reproduction Update* **9**, 99–117 (primate corpus luteum function and the role of progesterone).

Webley GE, Hearn JP (1994) Embryo–maternal interactions during the establishment of pregnancy in primates. *Oxford Reviews of Reproductive Biology* **16**, 1–32.

More advanced reading (see also Boxes)

Diaz FJ *et al.* (2002) Regulation of progesterone and prostaglandin $F_{2\alpha}$ production in the CL. *Molecular and Cellular Endocrinology* **191**, 65–80.

Eppig JJ *et al.* (2002) The mammalian oocyte orchestrates the rate of ovarian follicular development. *Proceedings of the National Academy of Sciences of the USA* **99**, 2890–2894.

Erickson GF, Shimasaki S (2001) The physiology of folliculogenesis: the role of novel growth factors. *Fertility and Sterility* **76**, 943–949.

Fortune JE *et al.* (2004) Follicular development: the role of the follicular microenvironment in selection of the dominant follicle. *Animal Reproduction Science* **82–83**, 109–126.

Hull KL, Harvey S (2001) Growth hormone: roles in female reproduction. *Journal of Endocrinology* **168**, 1–23.

Juengel JL *et al.* (2004) Physiology of GDF9 and BMP15 signalling molecules. *Animal Reproduction Science* **82–83**, 447–460.

Matsui M *et al.* (2004 Pregnancy-Associated Plasma Protein-A (PAPP-A) production in rat granulosa cells: stimulation by follicle stimulating hormone and inhibition by the oocyte-derived bone morphogenetic protein-15. *Endocrinology* **145**, 3686–3695.

Pangas SA, Matzuk MM (2005) The art and artifact of GDF9 activity: cumulus expansion and the cumulus expansion-enabling factor. *Biology of Reproduction* **73**, 582–585.

Peluso JJ (2006) Multiplicity of progesterone's actions and receptors in the mammalian ovary. *Biology of Reproduction* **75**, 2–8.

Wang Y *et al.* (2005) Gonadotropin control of inhibin secretion and the relationship to follicle type and number in the *hpg* mouse. *Biology of Reproduction* **73**, 610–618.

6 Regulation of Gonadal Function

In Chapters 4 and 5 we saw how follicle-stimulating hormone (FSH), luteinizing hormone (LH) and prolactin regulate the cellular and endocrine functions of the ovary and testis. In this chapter, we will discuss the mechanisms by which secretion of these pituitary hormones themselves is regulated. Pituitary hormone secretion is influenced by the central nervous system (CNS), in particular the *hypothalamus*, which mediates hormonal and environmental influences on reproduction.

The hypothalamic–pituitary axis controls gonadal function

The pituitary secretes gonadotrophins, prolactin and oxytocin

The pituitary gland lies in the *hypophyseal fossa* of the *sphenoid bone*, overlapped by a circular fold of dura mater, the *diaphragma sellae*, which has a small central opening through which the pituitary stalk, or *infundibulum*, passes (Fig. 6.1). The gland has an extremely rich blood supply derived from the internal carotid artery via its superior and inferior hypophyseal branches. Venous drainage is by short vessels that emerge over the surface of the gland and enter neighbouring dural venous sinuses.

There are two main lobes of the pituitary gland in humans. The anterior lobe (*adenohypophysis*) is derived embryologically from a small diverticulum (*Rathke's pouch*) pinched off from the dorsal pharynx. It is closely apposed to a distinct and smaller posterior lobe (*neurohypophysis*), which is derived embryologically from neurectoderm. This origin is reflected in its connection by a stalk of nervous tissue, the infundibulum, to the overlying hypothalamus in the region of the *median eminence* (Figs 6.1 & 6.2). In rats and many other mammals, an *intermediate lobe* (the *pars intermedia*, a small subdivision of the adenohypophysis)

Fig. 6.1 A sagittal section through the human brain with the pituitary and pineal glands attached. Note the comparatively small size of the hypothalamus and its rather compressed dimensions ventrally. The pineal is attached by its stalk to the epithalamus (habenula region) and lies above the midbrain colliculi. The third ventricle is a midline slit-like structure, which has been opened up by the midline cut exposing the medial surface of the brain. The thalamus (above) and the hypothalamus (below) form one wall (the right in this view) of the third ventricle, which is best viewed in Fig. 6.3.

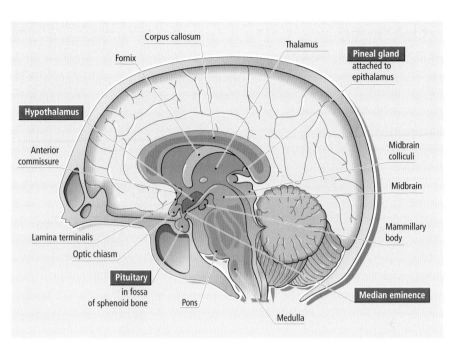

lies between the two, but it is vestigial in humans except in the fetus and the pregnant woman.

The anterior lobe of the pituitary contains a variety of cell types, among them the *gonadotrophs* (basophilic cells containing granules of FSH or LH) and *lactotrophs* (acidophilic cells containing prolactin). In addition to FSH, LH and prolactin, the anterior pituitary secretes *growth hormone* (GH or *somatotrophin*) from *somatotrophs*, *adrenocorticotrophic hormone* (ACTH or *corticotrophin*) from *corticotrophs*, and *thyroid-stimulating hormone* (TSH or *thyrotrophin*) from *thyrotrophs*. The posterior lobe of the pituitary secretes two nonapeptide hormones: *arginine vasopressin* (AVP or *antidiuretic hormone*—ADH) and *oxytocin*. Both lobes of the pituitary are connected anatomically and functionally to the overlying hypothalamus.

The hypothalamus contains groups of neurons with specific functions

The hypothalamus is a relatively small region at the base of the brain. It is part of the *diencephalon* and lies between the midbrain (caudally) and the forebrain (rostrally, see Fig. 6.1). The boundaries of the hypothalamus are conventionally described as being: (1) superiorly the *hypothalamic sulcus* separating it from the *thalamus*; (2) anteriorly the *lamina terminalis*; and (3) posteriorly a vertical plane immediately behind the *mammillary bodies* (see Fig. 6.1). The hypothalamus is split symmetrically into left and right halves by the *third ventricle*, containing cerebrospinal fluid and lying in the midline so that the hypothalamus forms its floor and lateral walls (Figs 6.1 & 6.3). The hypothalamus has

many neuroendocrine, behavioural and autonomic functions, which include the regulation of sexual and ingestive behaviours, the control of body temperature and the integration of the cardiovascular and hormonal responses to stress. Each function is associated with various *hypothalamic areas or nuclei* (Figs 6.2 & 6.3). The *supraoptic, paraventricular, arcuate, ventromedial* and *suprachiasmatic nuclei*, and also two less easily defined areas, the *medial anterior hypothalamic* and *medial preoptic areas*, are particularly concerned with reproductive functions and have either direct neural or indirect vascular connections with the pituitary gland.

The hypothalamus also has rich interconnections with widespread areas of the brain, in particular with the *autonomic areas* and *reticular core* of the *brainstem* (especially monoaminergic cell groups) and also areas of the *limbic forebrain*, such as the *amygdala, hippocampus* and *septum and orbitofrontal cortex*. Of major importance is the photic input from the *retina* to the *suprachiasmatic nuclei*, as this is the route by which the hypothalamus is made aware of the cycles of light and dark that can, in turn, affect reproductive function.

The hypothalamus has both neural and vascular connections with the pituitary

The hypothalamic magnocellular neurosecretory system secretes oxytocin and vasopressin from the posterior pituitary

Magnocellular neurons are located in the supraoptic and paraventricular nuclei (Figs 6.2 & 6.4a), and are the site of synthesis of the two major hormones of the posterior pituitary

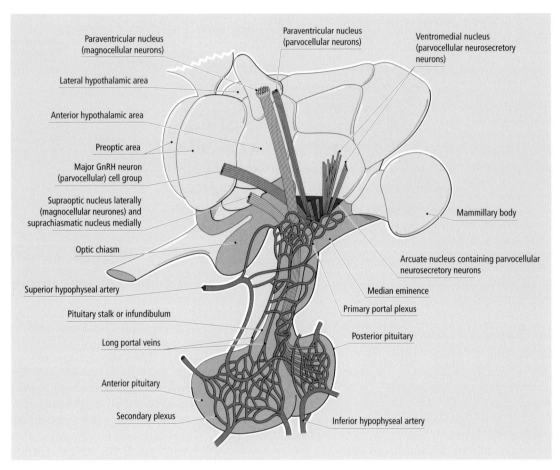

Fig. 6.2 A highly schematic and enlarged view of the human hypothalamus and pituitary. Note the portal capillary system (red) derived from the superior hypophyseal artery and running from the median eminence/arcuate nucleus region of the hypothalamus above to the anterior lobe of the pituitary below. The anatomically and functionally well-defined paraventricular, ventromedial and arcuate nuclei contain the cell bodies of parvocellular neurons whose axons (blue) terminate in close association with the portal capillaries. Parvocellular neurons also arise in the less well-defined anterior hypothalamic/preoptic areas continuum and send axons to the portal plexus. Magnocellular neurons (green) are also located in the paraventricular nuclei, with a second group in the supraoptic nuclei, and send axons along the infundibulum to the posterior pituitary.

(vasopressin and oxytocin; see Fig. 3.7). Each hormone is synthesized in a distinctive subset of neurons, and each is packaged by associating specifically with a binding protein (*neurophysin*). The cell bodies project axons directly to the posterior lobe of the pituitary via the hypothalamo–hypophyseal tract. The bound hormones pass by a process of axoplasmic flow to be stored in the posterior lobe (see Fig. 3.7c), from where release of hormone into the bloodstream occurs. This system of neurons in the hypothalamus is called the *magnocellular* (i.e. large-celled) neurosecretory system.

The hypothalamic parvocellular neurosecretory system controls anterior pituitary hormone secretion

In contrast to the direct neural connections linking the hypothalamus and posterior pituitary, the hypothalamus communicates with the anterior lobe indirectly by a vascular route (see Fig. 6.2). A variety of small neuropeptide hormones is synthesized in hypothalamic neurons, designated the *parvocellular* (i.e. small-celled) neurosecretory system. Several hypothalamic areas contain parvocellular neurons. Some are clustered in nuclei around the third ventricle—called from anterodorsal to more posteroventral the paraventricular (PVN, Fig 6.3a), ventromedial (VMN or periventricular) and arcuate nuclei (see Fig. 6.3b). Others are more diffusely located in the medial preoptic and anterior hypothalamic areas (Figs 6.2 & 6.4b). The axons of these neurons project to and terminate in the pericapillary space of the *primary portal plexus* of vessels in the median eminence. These capillaries are derived from the superior and inferior hypophyseal arteries and pass from this area of the hypothalamus down to the anterior pituitary. The neurohormones

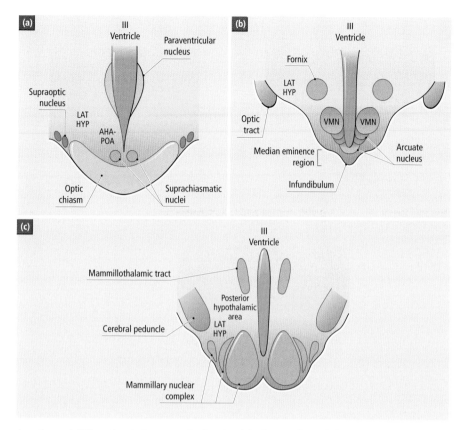

Fig. 6.3 Three coronal sections at different anterior–posterior levels of the human hypothalamus (consult Fig. 6.2 to construct the planes of sections). (a) Through the optic chiasm, note the third ventricle in the midline flanked by the anterior paraventricular (magnocellular) nuclei, which, together with the laterally placed supraoptic nuclei, synthesize oxytocin and vasopressin. The latter are then transported along the hypothalamo–hypophyseal tract (axons of neurons with cell bodies in these nuclei) to the posterior pituitary. The region of the suprachiasmatic nuclei and the anterior hypothalamic–preoptic area (AHA–POA) are also shown. (b) Through the infundibulum and median eminence, and showing the relationship between the parvocellular arcuate and ventromedial nuclei (VMN). The capillary loops of the portal plexus are found in this region. (c) Through the level of the mammillary bodies and showing the mammillary nuclear complex. The area labelled LAT HYP in all three sections is the lateral hypothalamus, and is composed of many nerve fibres ascending (largely aminergic) from the brainstem and descending from the rostral limbic and olfactory areas. This pathway represents a major input/output system for the more medially placed hypothalamic nuclei.

are released into the portal blood and pass to the anterior pituitary to act on the gonadotrophs, thyrotrophs, corticotrophs, somatotrophs and lactotrophs in order to regulate the synthesis and release of their various hormones.

Hypothalamic pulsatile secretion of GnRH controls gonadotrophin secretion

The glycoprotein hormones LH and FSH are secreted by gonadotrophs in the anterior pituitary. Immunocytochemical studies have revealed that each hormone is generally elaborated in a different cell type, but occasionally both may be found in the same cell. The synthesis and secretion of both FSH and LH depend on a hypothalamic decapeptide, gonadotrophin-releasing hormone (GnRH; see Chapter 3 & Fig. 3.6). Histochemical techniques have localized GnRH mRNA, GnRH itself and its precursor peptide to

two major subsets of the parvocellular neurons: a diffuse group of neurons within a continuum centred on the *medial preoptic* and adjacent *anterior hypothalamic* areas and a smaller cluster in the *arcuate nucleus* (Fig. 6.4b). Nerve terminals containing GnRH are particularly common in association with portal capillaries of the lateral palisade zone of the median eminence (Fig. 6.5a), which is the primary site of GnRH neurosecretion into the portal vessels.

GnRH is the most important final common mediator of all influences on reproduction conveyed through the CNS. Any abnormality in GnRH synthesis, storage, release or action will result in partial or complete failure of gonadal function. Destruction of GnRH-producing neurons in the hypothalamus, generation of genetically null GnRH mice, or immunization against the peptide, all prevent gonadotrophin function and result in gonadal atrophy. In the first

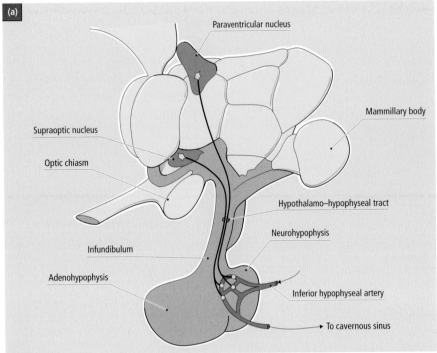

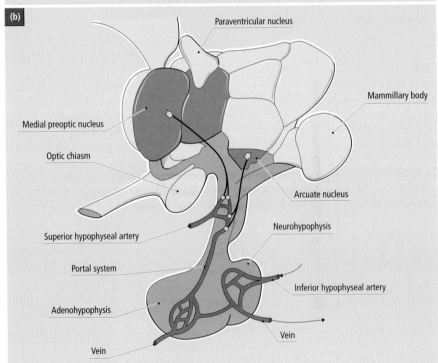

Fig. 6.4 (a) Schematic representation of the magnocellular neurosecretory system. Neurons in the supraoptic and paraventricular nuclei send their axons via the hypothalamo–hypophyseal tract and infundibulum to the neurohypophysis, where terminals lie in association with capillary walls, the site of neurosecretion. (b) Schematic representation of the parvocellular GnRH neurosecretory system. Neurons in the medial preoptic and anterior hypothalamic areas, and in arcuate nucleus send axons down to the portal vessels in the external layer (palisade zone) of the median eminence, where neurosecretion occurs.

two cases, this can be reversed by appropriate treatment with intravenous synthetic GnRH.

Concurrent sampling of portal blood to measure GnRH secretion and of peripheral blood to measure gonadotrophins has established the nature of the relationship between GnRH and gonadotrophin secretion. Both are secreted in a pulsatile manner, approximately one pulse being measured about every hour or so and therefore called *circhorial pulses*. Each peripheral LH peak coincides with a GnRH pulse (Fig. 6.6), but each GnRH pulse is not necessarily followed by an LH pulse. This GnRH pulse generator, or *circhorial clock*, controlling GnRH secretion seems to reside in the hypothalamus. Thus, in rhesus monkeys in which the hypothalamus and pituitary are isolated surgi-

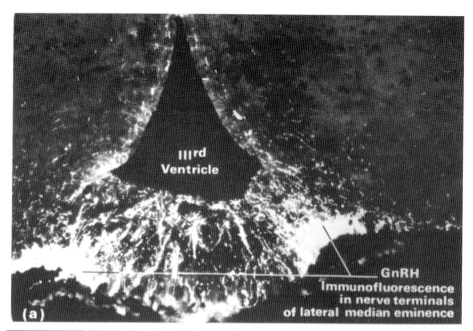

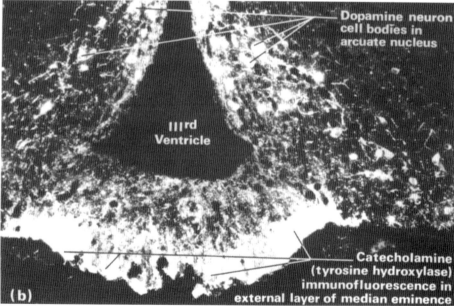

Fig. 6.5 (a) GnRH detected by immunofluorescence in the median eminence (middle region). Note the very dense network of GnRH neuron terminals in the lateral region (lateral palisade zone), but no fluorescent cell bodies are visible. (b) Tyrosine hydroxylase immunofluorescence in an adjacent section through the median eminence. The dense terminal fluorescence in the external layer largely represents mainly dopamine (although noradrenaline-containing terminals will also be labelled by this procedure). Large dopamine-containing cell bodies are clearly visible in the arcuate nucleus.

cally from the rest of the brain, the pulsatile secretion of LH and FSH is preserved. Moreover, electrophysiological recording in the mediobasal hypothalamus has revealed a marked increase in multiunit neuronal activity in synchrony with each peripheral LH pulse. Individual GnRH+ve neurons isolated *in vitro* also show a pulsatile release of GnRH, which thus seems to be a property intrinsic to them. However, whether the pulsing of many GnRH neurons together *in vivo* is coordinated by the GnRH neurons themselves or by an exogenous pulse generator that synchronizes their secretory activity is uncertain.

This pulsatile mode of GnRH secretion is crucially important for gonadotrophin secretion. Thus, after removal of endogenous GnRH by destruction of the mediobasal hypothalamus, LH and FSH secretion can be restored by use of an intravenous infusion pump programmed to deliver exogenous GnRH *in pulses* at a frequency approximating that seen naturally. Continuously infused GnRH does not restore regular menstrual cycles in females (Fig. 6.7). This critical requirement for pulsatile GnRH secretion can be understood in terms of the regulation by GnRH of its receptors on the gonadotrophs. Thus, the response to a first GnRH pulse is an initial release of stored LH and FSH occurring within minutes and lasting for 30–60 min. Associated with this release is the movement of secretory granules into a zone beneath the plasmalemma and a decrease

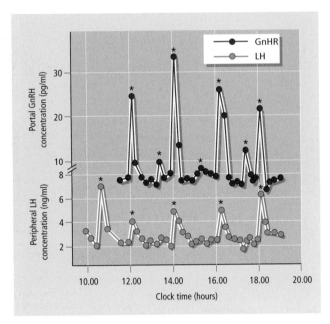

Fig. 6.6 Concentrations of GnRH in portal plasma (red line) and LH in jugular venous plasma (green line) of four ovariectomized ewes. Asterisks indicate secretory episodes (pulses) of GnRH and LH.

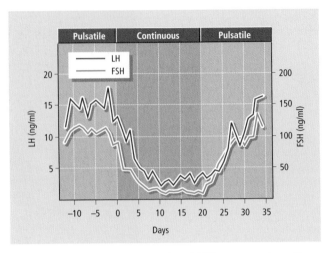

Fig. 6.7 Suppression of plasma LH and FSH concentrations after initiating (day 0) a continuous GnRH infusion (1 mg/min) in an ovariectomized, hypothalamically lesioned rhesus monkey in whom pulsatile gonadotrophin secretion had been re-established by pulsatile GnRH infusions (1 mg/min for 6 min once per hour). The inhibition of gonadotrophin secretion was reversed by reinstating the pulsatile pattern of GnRH administration on day 20.

in their size, perhaps indicating maturation of their contents. In consequence of this mobilization of granules (the *self-priming effect*), a second exposure to GnRH results in a much larger 'primed' release of LH. Over a period of hours to days with exposure to pulsatile GnRH, gonadotrophin biosynthesis is also stimulated. After binding, some GnRH–receptor complexes remain on the cell surface while others are internalized via coated pits to lysosomal structures where degradation of the peptide can occur. Continuous exposure of gonadotrophs to GnRH, or infusion of a long-acting GnRH analogue, results in maintained occupancy of the receptors and is followed eventually by their wholesale internalization—receptor downregulation (see Chapter 3)—and a reduction in pituitary LH and FSH content and secretion.

Summary

Hypothalamic GnRH neurons regulate the synthesis and secretion of FSH and LH by the anterior pituitary. The GnRH is released as a series of pulses into the portal vessels; it reaches and binds to receptors on the gonadotrophs, and drives gonadotrophin secretion in a similar, pulsatile manner. Alterations in the output of LH and FSH could be achieved therefore (1) by increasing or decreasing either the amplitude or the frequency of these pulses of GnRH, or (2) by modulating the response of the gonadotrophs to the pulses. As we shall now see, both mechanisms are employed.

Ovarian hormones regulate gonadotrophin secretion in females

In the last chapter, we saw that during the menstrual cycle, the dynamics of follicular maturation and ovulation were mainly orchestrated by the output of gonadotrophins. Now we will see that the output of gonadotrophins is regulated mainly by the secretory products of the ovary. There is thus a dynamic relationship between pituitary and ovary, and to understand it two phenomena must be examined: (1) *a depressant effect* on gonadotrophin output induced by elevation of the plasma concentrations of oestrogens, progestagens and inhibins (negative feedback); and (2) an increase, or *surge*, of LH and FSH secretion induced principally by oestradiol (positive feedback). Throughout our discussion we will use data from the primate as a model, referring to other species where corroborative evidence or species differences exist.

Oestradiol regulates FSH and LH secretion

Plasma concentrations of circulating FSH and LH increase markedly after ovariectomy or the menopause (Fig. 6.8b). This rise is largely attributable to removal of oestradiol, as infusion of this hormone results in the rapid decline of FSH and LH levels. The important characteristics of this oestrogen action are: (1) only low circulating levels of oestradiol are required to exert a marked effect; and (2) the effect is

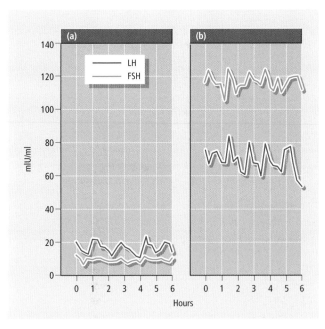

Fig. 6.8 Circulating FSH (green) and LH (red) levels in: (a) a woman at day 7 in the (early) follicular phase; and (b) a postmenopausal woman. The difference between the two represents the negative feedback effect of oestradiol. Note: (1) the reversal of LH and FSH levels between (a) and (b), which may reflect preferential inhibition of FSH secretion in (a) due to inhibin (see text); and (2) the changes in pulsatility of FSH and LH between (a) and (b).

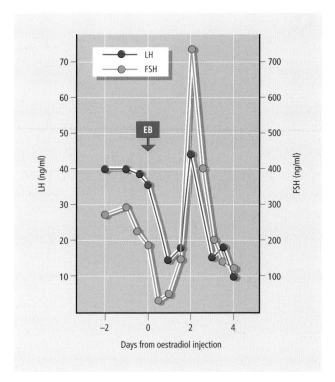

Fig. 6.9 The negative and positive feedback effects of a large injection of oestradiol benzoate (EB) in a female rhesus monkey. Note the early action of oestrogen is to decrease FSH and LH levels (negative feedback, maximal at 6 h or so). But if oestradiol levels are of sufficient magnitude and duration, a surge of the gonadotrophins occurs after 36–48 h (positive feedback). Note that one effect naturally follows the other and each is critically dependent on different time–dose effects of the steroid.

very rapid in onset, detectable within 1 h and maximal by 4–6 h. As oestradiol is acting to suppress gonadotrophin levels, the process is termed *negative feedback*.

In contrast, if plasma concentrations of oestradiol increase greatly, for example 200–400% above those seen in the early follicular phase of the cycle, and remain at this high level for 48 h or so, then LH and FSH secretion is enhanced, not suppressed (Fig. 6.9). Under these conditions we speak of a *surge* of LH and FSH. The term *positive feedback* is often used to describe the relationship whereby high levels of oestradiol increase the secretion of gonadotrophins, and thereby of oestradiol.

Thus, oestradiol has a dual function in regulating gonadotrophin secretion. At low circulating levels, it exerts rapidly expressed, negative feedback control over FSH and LH. At higher, maintained circulating levels, positive feedback becomes the dominant force and a (relatively) delayed LH and FSH surge is induced.

Progesterone also regulates FSH and LH secretion

Progesterone also has two effects. First, the high plasma concentration of progesterone, such as is seen in the luteal phase (4–8 ng/ml in humans) enhances the negative feed-

back effects of oestradiol, FSH and LH secretion being held down to a very low level. Second, the positive feedback effect of oestradiol is blocked. Thus, injection of oestradiol into women during the progesterone-dominated phase of the menstrual cycle (luteal phase) is not followed by an LH surge.

The inhibins regulate only FSH secretion

In the last chapter, we identified a number of autocrine and paracrine factors that appear to influence follicular and luteal development and function (see Table 5.3). The inhibins A and B (see Fig. 3.5) also act *endocrinologically* to influence FSH secretion selectively. Thus, intravenous administration of inhibin into ewes prevents the rise in FSH, which usually follows ovariectomy and blocks the FSH, but not the LH, response to a GnRH agonist (Fig. 6.10). Infusion of antibodies to inhibin during the late antral phase of the rat causes an increase in FSH, but not LH, concentrations in plasma (Fig. 6.11). In primates too, inhibin administration causes FSH to decline selectively. Clearly,

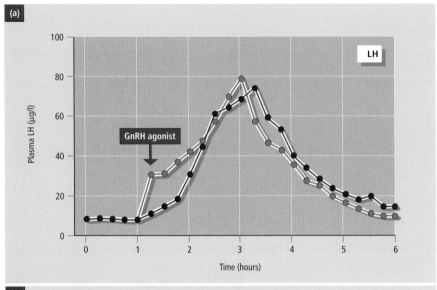

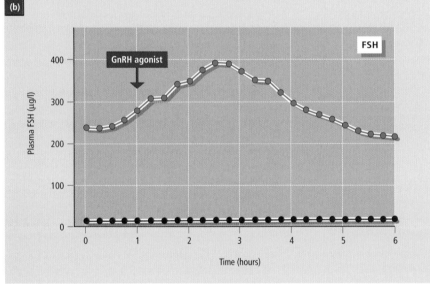

Fig. 6.10 Changes in plasma (a) LH and (b) FSH concentration following an injection of a GnRH agonist, in control ovariectomized ewes (green line) and ovariectomized ewes treated with inhibin (red line). Note the complete absence of an FSH response to GnRH in the inhibin-treated ewes in (b).

these experimental data indicate a role for inhibin in the negative feedback regulation of FSH secretion.

Feedback by steroid hormones and the inhibins regulates the menstrual cycle

Let us now re-examine the blood levels of steroids, inhibins and gonadotrophins during a normal human menstrual cycle, and interpret them in the light of positive and negative feedback.

The follicular phase of the cycle

By convention, the menstrual cycle begins with the first day of menstruation (M in Fig. 6.12). Menstruation is initiated by the preceding luteolysis, which results in falling levels of luteal oestrogen, progesterone and inhibin A. In consequence, *negative feedback inhibition is relaxed*, and both FSH and LH levels rise. These rises permit antral growth to proceed, resulting in first the rising output of inhibin B followed by androgens and oestrogens. In consequence, negative feedback is gradually re-exerted and so FSH levels fall and LH levels plateau. The fall in FSH may in part be due to an increased turnover rate, as more of the less acidic, and thus less stable (Chapter 3), FSH isoforms are secreted during the later follicular phase. What regulates the preferential secretion of short-lived isoforms is not known. The selection of a dominant follicle leads to a further rise in oestrogen (together with their biosynthetically associated androgens), culminating in an oestrogen (and androgen)

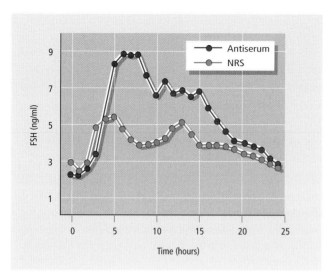

Fig. 6.11 The effect of intravenous infusion of normal rabbit serum (NRS) (green line) or inhibin antiserum (red line) on plasma FSH levels during the late antral phase. Note the marked rise in plasma FSH concentrations in the female rats immunized passively against inhibin.

surge and a switch from inhibin B to inhibin A output under the combined stimulation of LH and FSH. This output of oestrogen and inhibin A reflects the development of only the *most advanced* follicle(s), and is thus a measure of nearness to ovulation. During the preovulatory phase, the surge in oestrogens triggers a rapid rise in LH and FSH levels *via its positive feedback effect*, and ovulation follows. As a result of follicular collapse, androgen and thus oestrogen outputs fall, and progesterone levels rise. The LH and FSH levels now fall equally precipitously because, at least in part, they lack a continuing positive feedback stimulus. The first half of the cycle is complete.

The crucial role of the oestrogen surge in triggering the LH surge has been shown in female rhesus monkeys by actively immunizing them against oestradiol, when neither an LH surge nor ovulation occur. However, if a replacement synthetic oestrogen, not neutralized by the antiserum, is given, the neutralization of endogenous oestradiol is bypassed and the synthetic oestrogen reinstates an LH surge. Thus, the pattern of FSH, LH, inhibin and steroid secretion during the first half of the cycle is explicable largely in terms of the positive and negative feedback effect of oestrogens (primarily oestradiol) and inhibin B on gonadotrophin secretion. The length of the follicular phase appears to be determined by the rate at which the principal preantral follicle matures, since it is the main source of oestrogen and thereby a major arbiter of cycle length. It is therefore sometimes described as an *ovarian* or *pelvic clock*.

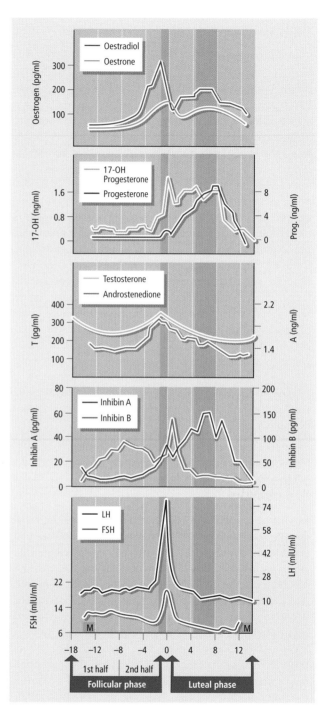

Fig. 6.12 Serum hormone levels during the human menstrual cycle. Note the units of measurements; FSH and LH are expressed in milli-international units/ml; testosterone (T), oestradiol and the inhibins in pg/ml; 17α-hydroxyprogesterone (17-OH), progesterone and androstenedione (A) in ng/ml. M, menstruation.

The luteal phase of the cycle

The luteal phase of the cycle is characterized by rising concentrations of plasma progesterone and 17α-hydroxyprogesterone, which peak around 8 days after the LH surge. In higher primates (but not in most other species), the luteinized cells of the corpus luteum also make large amounts of oestrogen and inhibin A (Fig. 6.12). In all species, progesterone depresses levels of both gonadotrophins (negative feedback), a depression particularly marked in higher primates in which inhibin A is also active in suppressing FSH (compare lower levels of gonadotrophins in the human than pig in Fig. 5.7). Growth of antral follicles is therefore suppressed and so androgens are also at a low level. Although in primates oestrogens from the corpus luteum may rise to levels that previously induced positive feedback, they fail to induce an LH surge. This failure reflects the effects of the uniquely high levels of progesterone found during the luteal phase of the cycle that *inhibit positive feedback by oestradiol.* At the end of the luteal phase, if conception has not occurred, oestrogens, progesterone and inhibin A decline at luteolysis, the negative feedback effect of these hormones is relaxed and LH and FSH levels start to rise, thereby permitting the rescue of preantral follicles and the initiation of another cycle.

Positive and negative feedback are mediated at the level of both hypothalamus and pituitary

Having described how the ovarian hormones influence gonadotrophin output during the menstrual cycle, we now consider the sites at which these hormones exert their regulatory influences. There are two obvious candidates. First, the anterior pituitary: the hormones might regulate FSH and LH secretion by a direct action on the gonadotrophs, decreasing (negative feedback) or increasing (positive feedback) their sensitivity to hypothalamic GnRH pulses of invariant frequency and magnitude. This might be achieved through regulation of the GnRH receptors. There are abundant receptors for oestrogens, progestagens and inhibins in the anterior pituitary, emphasizing the potential importance of this site.

Second, the hypothalamus: the ovarian hormones might change the GnRH output signal either directly by affecting the GnRH neurons in the hypothalamus, or indirectly by changing the activity of other neural systems that exert a modulatory influence on GnRH release. Large regional concentrations of receptors for oestradiol and progesterone exist in a continuum between the medial preoptic and anterior hypothalamic areas and also in the ventromedial hypothalamus (particularly the arcuate nucleus and median eminence). In contrast, there is no evidence to support a hypothalamic site of action of inhibin.

Of course, these two potential sites of feedback are not mutually exclusive, and a third possibility is therefore that ovarian hormones alter *both* the GnRH output signal *and* the response of the anterior pituitary to it.

The anterior pituitary can mediate feedback effects of steroids and inhibins

The most convincing demonstration that the pituitary can respond to both the negative and positive feedback effects of oestradiol comes from experiments on ovariectomized rhesus monkeys. Large lesions of the mediobasal hypothalamus, which destroy the arcuate and ventromedial nuclei and a large part of the median eminence (see Fig. 6.2), result in abolition of GnRH output, and a decrease in serum FSH and LH to undetectable levels. Hourly pulses of exogenous GnRH delivered by a programmable intravenous infusion pump restore pulsatile LH and FSH secretion. The subsequent injection of oestradiol, so as to reach surge levels, results first in a fall, and then in a dramatic rise (surge) in serum FSH and LH levels. In the presence, therefore, of GnRH pulses of invariant amplitude and frequency, oestradiol can exert both its negative and positive feedback effects on gonadotrophin secretion. Clearly, this action can only have been mediated via the anterior pituitary. Clinical studies on postmenopausal or hypogonadal women point to the same conclusion.

Studies on the pituitary sensitivity of women undergoing normal cycles provide further support for this conclusion. These experiments were performed by measuring the change in plasma levels of LH and FSH induced by pulses of exogenous GnRH administered on different days of the menstrual cycle (similar results have been obtained during the oestrous cycles in rats). The results in Fig. 6.13 show that secretion of FSH and LH by the pituitary, in response to constant GnRH pulses, increases during the follicular phase, reflecting an increased sensitivity of the secretory response with rising levels of plasma oestradiol. However, notice that the responsiveness of the pituitary to GnRH *remains* very high in the luteal phase of the cycle, a time when FSH and LH levels are normally at their lowest, and when it is impossible to induce an LH surge with an oestrogen surge (see above). This must mean that oestradiol and/or progesterone, which are both high at this time, exert an important component of their negative feedback action on FSH and LH secretion somewhere other than the pituitary. This site is the hypothalamus as we will see in the next section. The demonstration that inhibin is able to reduce the FSH secretory response to GnRH (see Fig. 6.10) strongly indicates that its effects are mediated by actions on the anterior pituitary.

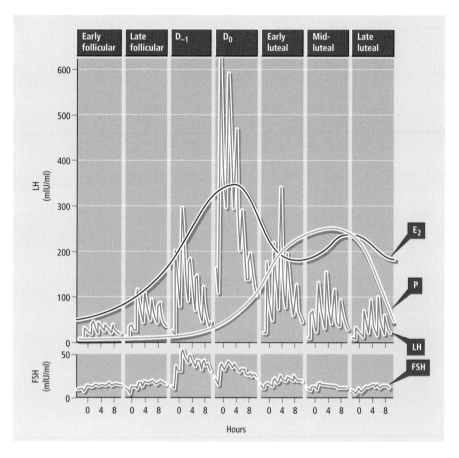

Fig. 6.13 The release of LH and FSH (green) in response to 'pulse injections' of GnRH (10 mg at 5 × 2-h intervals) during various phases of the menstrual cycle. The magnitude of the LH and FSH responses can be measured against the naturally changing circulating levels of oestradiol (purple) and progesterone (orange). Note the correlation between oestrogen levels and increasing pituitary responsiveness to the injected GnRH during the follicular phase. Note also that this responsiveness remains high in the early and mid-luteal phases, at times when further LH/FSH surges cannot be elicited by oestrogen injections (see text). D_{-1} and D_0, the day before, and the day of, the spontaneous LH surge.

Taken together, these findings imply that modulation of pituitary sensitivity to GnRH pulses can and does occur, but is not in itself sufficient to explain all the changes observed in a normal cycle. Steroid-dependent alterations in the amplitude and frequency of the GnRH signal also play an important role.

The hypothalamus mediates steroid hormone feedback only

The pattern of LH and FSH pulses varies during the menstrual cycle. Thus, during the follicular phase, LH is secreted in a series of high-frequency, low-amplitude pulses occurring approximately once every hour. By contrast, the luteal phase of the cycle is characterized by a pattern of high-amplitude, low-frequency, irregular LH pulses, often with long intervals between them of up to 6 h (Fig. 6.14). As these gonadotrophin pulses reflect underlying GnRH secretory episodes, it is likely that the different steroid hormone environments are influencing the GnRH output. The experimental manipulation of the steroid environment confirms this suspicion. Thus, *progesterone acts primarily to reduce pulse frequency* while *oestrogen acts to reduce pulse amplitude*.

More direct information on the modulation of GnRH secretory activity by steroids requires measurement of the peptide in portal blood or (by microperfusion studies) within the median eminence itself. Obviously this is impossible in humans and, even in experimental animals, presents considerable methodological difficulties. However, it has been achieved in experiments on rats, sheep and rhesus monkeys, and the data show clearly that *GnRH secretory activity is subject to modulation by steroid feedback* during the menstrual and oestrous cycles, so confirming the indirect evidence described above. Thus, in rats, GnRH secretion is increased on the afternoon immediately before the LH surge. Similarly, the LH surge induced by exogenous oestradiol administration in rhesus monkeys and ewes is associated with elevated concentrations of GnRH in portal blood (Fig. 6.15), indicating a hypothalamic site of positive feedback. In contrast, direct evidence for a hypothalamic site of negative feedback by oestradiol is less clear, as it is difficult to measure with confidence reductions in the already low levels of GnRH.

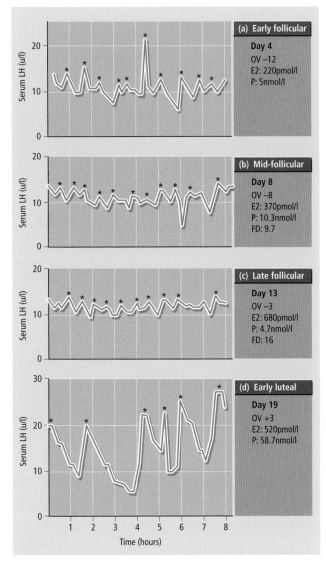

Fig. 6.14 LH pulsatility at different points during a human ovulatory cycle (ovulation occurred on day 16) in 10-min serum samples: (a) early follicular phase; (b) mid-follicular phase; (c) late follicular phase; (d) early luteal phase. Note the unique high-amplitude, low-frequency pulses characteristic of the luteal phase when progesterone plasma concentrations are high. *, LH peaks; OV, ± number of days after/before ovulation; E2, 17β-oestradiol; P, progesterone; FD, follicular diameter (mm).

Specific hypothalamic sites mediate steroid feedback effects

Where in the hypothalamus do steroids act? The problem of defining sites of steroid feedback has been approached using the classical techniques of neurobiology, namely the intracerebral implantation of sex steroids and other substances, or the localized lesioning of the suspected sites of steroid action.

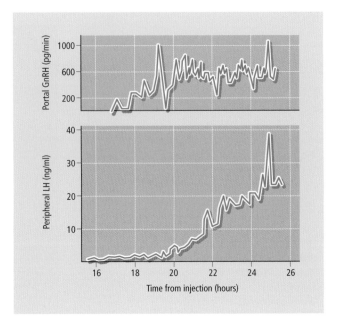

Fig. 6.15 GnRH concentration in portal blood and peripheral plasma LH levels in an ovariectomized ewe given an injection of 50 mg oestradiol monobenzoate to induce an LH surge. Note the increased frequency of GnRH and LH pulses during the LH surge.

Experiments in which oestradiol has been placed into the hypothalamus have consistently implicated the arcuate nucleus as a site of negative feedback influence on GnRH secretion. Thus, in rats, oestradiol infused into the arcuate nucleus suppressed gonadotrophin secretion without detectable amounts of the steroid reaching the anterior pituitary. Similar experiments in female rhesus monkeys showed that oestradiol, in amounts 1000-fold less than those administered systemically, exerted marked negative feedback actions when infused into the arcuate nuclei (Fig. 6.16). These actions of oestradiol seem not to involve GnRH-containing neurons directly, but to be mediated indirectly through other neural systems with convergent effects on GnRH neurosecretion (see Box 6.1 on p. 117). In addition, the negative feedback actions of progesterone during the luteal phase of the cycle appear to operate in the arcuate region, where oestradiol-induced progesterone receptors are found in considerable number.

What about positive feedback? In rats and primates, implantation of oestradiol in the anterior hypothalamic–preoptic area continuum has been shown to induce an LH surge without evidence of diffusion of the steroid into the anterior pituitary. Moreover, if GnRH levels are monitored mid-cycle, GnRH levels rise in the anterior hypothalamic area. Whether existing neurons make more GnRH in response to high oestrogen or a new subset of neurons is

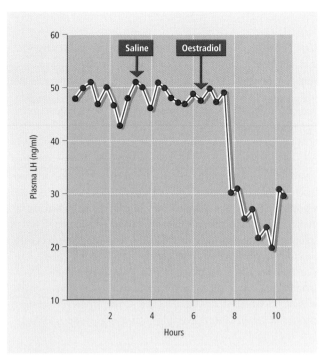

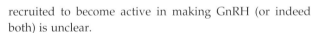

Fig. 6.16 The negative feedback effect of oestradiol (800 pg) on plasma LH when infused into the hypothalamic arcuate nucleus of ovariectomized rhesus monkeys. Note the lack of response to earlier, control injections of saline and the decline in LH concentrations within a short time after oestradiol injection.

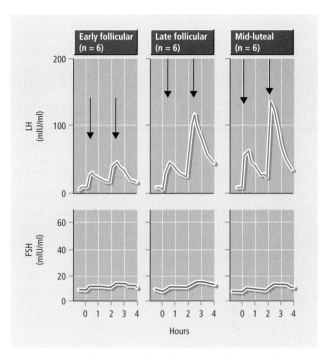

Fig. 6.17 The 'self-priming' effect of GnRH and its dependence on steroid hormone levels. The figure shows the enhanced response to a second injection of GnRH during three stages of the menstrual cycle (arrows indicate GnRH injection). Note the large increase between the early and late follicular phases, which correlates well with the rise in oestradiol secretion and, furthermore, how this effect remains pronounced in the mid-luteal phase when oestradiol, as well as progesterone, secretion is high.

recruited to become active in making GnRH (or indeed both) is unclear.

Taken together, these data indicate that while oestradiol and progesterone can act directly on the anterior pituitary to exert feedback effects on gonadotrophin secretion, the hypothalamus is also an important site for these effects via the modulation of GnRH secretion. Inhibin appears to exert its effects on FSH secretion primarily in the anterior pituitary.

The cellular mechanisms by which feedback control is achieved

Finally, we consider the nature of the *cellular* mechanisms by which negative and positive feedback are exercised. What does oestradiol do to gonadotrophs to increase or decrease their sensitivity to GnRH? How does oestradiol induce a GnRH surge? How does progesterone decrease the frequency of GnRH pulses during the luteal phase?

The anterior pituitary

Within the anterior pituitary, oestradiol appears to exert its positive feedback effects by inducing and maintaining GnRH receptors and by sensitizing the self-priming process whereby GnRH induces its own receptors. Small-amplitude GnRH pulses, which do not by themselves cause an LH pulse (see Fig. 6.6), may prime a full LH response to the next adequate GnRH pulse. Figure 6.17 shows that the presence of oestradiol enhances this interaction between GnRH and its receptor, perhaps thereby contributing to the magnitude of the oestradiol-induced LH surge. There is less information on the ways in which oestradiol might cause a decrease in gonadotrophin secretion to mediate its negative feedback. Nor is there detailed information on the way that inhibin exerts its selective depressant effect on FSH secretion. A possible clue comes from the observation that the GnRH-receptor has two *N*-linked glycosylation sites. Both oestrogen and inhibin increase glycosylation at one site, while prolonged oestrogen induces gylcosylation at both. Since the stability of the intramembranous receptor is reduced by glycosylation, a potential negative feedback control mechanism is evident, but this possibility remains speculative.

The hypothalamus

The arcuate nuclei and preoptic/anterior hypothalamic areas are rich in oestradiol receptors, and the GnRH content of neurons in this area changes in response to oestradiol. However, use of double-staining techniques has shown that GnRH+ve neurons do not express progesterone or oestradiol-α (ERα) receptors, and express ERβ only weakly. These findings indicate that steroid effects on GnRH secretion must be mediated indirectly via other steroid-sensitive neural systems, which then converge onto GnRH neuronal cell bodies or terminals (Fig. 6.18). The problem is that the GnRH+ve neurons receive, directly or indirectly, hundreds if not thousands of synaptic contacts from elsewhere in the brain, many modulated by glial cell activity—a complex network of potential neural influences. Many neurochemical systems thus impinge on GnRH-releasing neurons and,

unsurprisingly, many neurotransmitters and pharmacological agents can be shown to influence the output of GnRH pulses. The daunting task therefore is to identify the key controlling pathways that seem to be steroid sensitive and to establish some sort of hierarchy of importance among them. In particular, it is assumed that different pathways are likely to mediate negative and positive feedback effects.

Among the hypothalamic neural systems most strongly implicated in the regulation of GnRH secretion, key players having steroid receptors are the amino acid γ-aminobutyric acid (GABA), glutamate, opioid peptide β-endorphin, and noradrenaline (norepinephrine) systems (see Box 6.1). Among the many other transmitters and peptides that have been suggested to influence GnRH secretion, the recently studied peptide kisspeptin seems of particular interest in the context of feedback (Box 6.2). However, it remains a puzzle as to how these various neural mechanisms, which can affect GnRH secretion and are sensitive to steroid hormones, interact under physiological circumstances to regulate the cyclic changes in GnRH output.

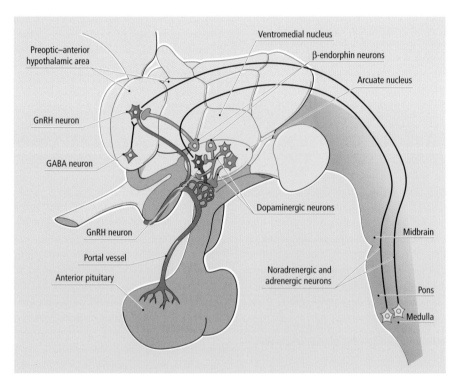

Fig. 6.18 Schematic diagram to show some of the postulated neurochemical interactions that may control GnRH secretion. GnRH neurons (blue) lie in the medial preoptic area and arcuate nucleus in primate species. They project to the portal vessels in the median eminence, especially to the lateral palisade zone. Dopamine neurons (purple) in the arcuate nucleus modulate prolactin release (and may affect GnRH output but this is controversial). Neurons within the hypothalamus that contain β-endorphin (green) also modulate anterior pituitary secretion, perhaps by modulating GnRH neuron activity in the medial preoptic area. Noradrenergic and adrenergic neurons in the medulla oblongata project to the medial anterior hypothalamus and preoptic area and may also participate in the regulation of GnRH secretion (see Boxes 6.1 & 6.2).

BOX 6.1 **Neuropharmacological systems and the regulation of GnRH output**

Negative or inhibitory regulators?

Some 70–80% of neurons containing γ-aminobutyric acid (GABA) in the preoptic and mediobasal hypothalamic areas (yellow in Fig. 6.18) bind oestradiol. Moreover, systemic surge levels of oestradiol are associated with decreased GABA release in the mediobasal hypothalamus. Might oestradiol release GABA-mediated inhibition on GnRH output? Using *in vivo* microdialysis to measure extracellular transmitter levels in small regions of the brain, fluctuations in hypothalamic GABA release are found to inversely correlate with LH pulses in the peripheral circulation. Additionally, GABA receptor antagonists such as bicuculline promote LH release. Conversely, progesterone enhances GABA release, which may mediate its negative feedback effects during the luteal phase. Thus, GABAergic neurons do seem to play a key inhibitory role in suppressing the LH surge.

β-endorphin is found in a subset of arcuate nucleus neurons that richly innervate the medial preoptic area GnRH-containing neurons (green in Fig. 6.18). Hypothalamic β-endorphin concentrations fluctuate during the cycle, with luteal highs and follicular lows. When given intraventricularly, β-endorphin suppresses pulsatile LH release and its preovulatory surge, whereas its antagonist naloxone accelerates LH pulses and elevates serum LH. Thus, these β-endorphin-containing neurons may mediate

part of the negative feedback effects of gonadal steroids, particularly progesterone.

Positive or facilitatory regulators?

Glutamate levels in the vicinity of the GnRH cell bodies (but not terminals) increase around the time of the LH surge, and the GnRH neurons express glutamate receptors and respond electrically to stimulation by glutamate analogues such as NMDA. Moreover, glutamate receptor antagonists interrupt the GnRH pulsing and block the LH surge. Might oestrogen activate the glutaminergic cells to promote GnRH release mid-cycle? There is an abundance of glutaminegric fibres within the median eminence, but at present it is unclear where these terminals originate and how their activity is regulated.

Noradrenergic neurons in the brainstem medulla oblongata (black in Fig. 6.18) richly innervate the hypothalamus and synapse directly on both preoptic and median eminence GnRH+ve cell bodies, which express both α and β adrenergic receptors. Microdialysis studies suggest that noradrenaline is released in pulses at these sites. In monkeys, α-adrenergic stimulation seems to facilitate GnRH pulsatility permissively, and after ablation of noradrenergic tone GnRH pulses decline. Noradrenergic neurons express oestrogen α-receptors, and an increase in noradrenergic transmission is observed mid-cycle as the ovulatory surge of GnRH occurs. Overall, this system may facilitate oestradiol positive feedback.

Testicular hormones regulate gonadotrophin secretion in males

The neuroendocrine mechanisms that govern testicular function are fundamentally similar to those that regulate ovarian activity. In males, hypothalamic GnRH, acting on the pituitary via pulsatile secretion into the portal system, is responsible for the secretion of gonadotrophins, which regulate the endocrine and spermatogenic activities of the testis (see Chapter 4). The major difference between the sexes is the absence of positive feedback in the male, arising from the non-cyclic nature of male reproduction, and thus the absence of any abrupt change in male gamete or hormone output that might underlie it.

Testosterone regulates the pituitary–Leydig cell axis

In Chapter 4, we saw that testosterone secretion by the testis is the result of LH stimulation of the Leydig cells. It is now accepted that testosterone is, in turn, the principal hormone responsible for regulating LH secretion. Thus neutralization of testosterone by immunization results in

increased circulating levels of LH in rhesus monkeys. Conversely, administration of exogenous testosterone causes an abrupt decline in LH levels in castrate males of all species including humans (Fig. 6.19). Even in intact men, synthetic androgens will depress LH output, as will synthetic progestagens, the basis for a possible male contraceptive (Chapter 15). The negative feedback effect of steroids is achieved largely by decreasing the frequency of episodic LH peaks via an effect on the hypothalamus, but there is also some change in pulse amplitude, reflecting a changing responsiveness of the pituitary to GnRH. Androgen receptors are found in abundance in both the hypothalamus and pituitary, and implantation of testosterone in the mediobasal, periarcuate hypothalamus of castrate male rats causes a significant fall in circulating LH levels. At least in rodents, 5α-dihydrotestosterone has some effect on LH secretion, whether given systemically or implanted in the hypothalamus. Testosterone also inhibits FSH secretion, but its effects are less than on LH. A more complete suppression of FSH comes from the combined action of androgens and the second testicular hormone, inhibin, which, as in the female, acts entirely at the level of the pituitary.

BOX 6.2 Kisspeptin and the control of GnRH secretion in mice

Kisspeptin (also known as metastin) is a 54 amino acid peptide product of the *KiSS-1* gene that is widely conserved across species. It binds to a G-protein-coupled receptor called GPR54, mutations of which lead to failure of puberty and hypogonadotrophic hypogonadism in humans. The GPR54 receptor is co-expressed in GnRH neurons, and kisspeptin is a potent stimulator of GnRH secretion and thereby of gonadotrophin secretion. GnRH antagonists block its effect on LH and FSH blood levels. Thus, kisspeptin-GPR54 seems to be an essential part of the GnRH secretion control pathway. *KiSS-1* mRNA-expressing neurons are found in both the arcuate and anteroventral periventricular (AVPV) nuclei, the latter making synaptic contact with GnRH neurons via projections to the medial preoptic area.

Steroid hormones and kisspeptin

KiSS-1+ve neurons are direct targets of oestrogens, nearly all expressing oestrogen receptor α (ERα), and some 30% expressing ERβ. Levels of *KiSS-1* mRNA in the arcuate nucleus, increase after gonadectomy and decrease with sex steroid replacement, an effect blocked by targeted deletion of the ERα. Thus, changes in arcuate kisspeptin synthesis follow a pattern to be expected for negative feedback, and its neurons thus appear well placed to mediate the hypothalamic negative feedback effects of steroids on GnRH secretion. Conversely, in the AVPV nuclei, castration depresses expression of *KiSS-1* mRNA, but steroid replacement increases it. As the AVPV nucleus projects to the preoptic area implicated in generating the preovulatory GnRH/LH surge, kisspeptin neurons might mediate the positive feedback loop involved. Moreover, the AVPV nucleus is sexually dimorphic in mice, being larger and having more KiSS-1+ve neurons in females— and mouse brains are known to show functional dimorphism with only females capable of eliciting a positive feedback response.

Further reading

Smith JT *et al.* (2006) Regulation of the neuroendocrine reproductive axis by kisspeptin-GPR54 signaling. *Reproduction* **131**, 623–630.

Inhibin regulates the pituitary–seminiferous tubule axis

Inhibin levels in testicular lymph, rete testis fluid and semen are some 100-fold lower than the level in follicular fluid. The inhibin is produced by the Sertoli cells, mostly inhibin B in humans (inhibin A in rams), and the blood levels reflect the number of functional Sertoli cells. Since FSH stimulates Sertoli cells directly, a negative feedback loop is postulated, especially during puberty, as a way of regulating Sertoli cell function. An increased output of tes-

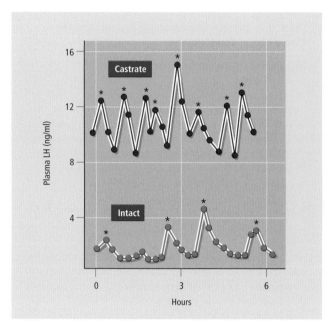

Fig. 6.19 The negative feedback effect of testosterone on plasma LH levels in male red deer. Upper part: levels in the castrate male. Lower part: levels in the intact male. Note the increased frequency of pulses (*) after castration.

ticular inhibin also appears to be related to the successful completion of spermiogenesis, and failure to complete spermatogenesis in man is correlated with depressed inhibin levels and elevated serum FSH levels. Conversely, stimulation of spermatogenesis in hypospermatogenic men is accompanied by a rising output of spermatozoa and inhibin and by declining serum FSH levels. As Sertoli cells are implicated in the support of spermatogenesis (see Chapter 4), as well as being the site of inhibin production, such a negative feedback mechanism makes biological sense.

The hypothalamic–pituitary–gonadal axis may be sexually dimorphic

We have seen that females exhibit both a negative feedback regulation by sex steroids and inhibins, and a positive feedback response to oestradiol. Does this represent a fundamental difference between males and females, or can males also show a gonadotrophin surge if given an oestradiol injection? The answer depends on the species studied, because of the different effects of fetal or neonatal hormones on the physiology of the developing brain.

If adult male rats are castrated and receive ovarian transplants, they fail to show any cyclic changes. In contrast, ovaries transplanted into recipient male rats *castrated at birth* undergo cyclic ovulation. Clearly, the presence of the testis at birth has prevented subsequent support of ovarian cyclicity. Testicular androgens are responsible for this effect. Thus, female rats injected with testosterone during the first few days after birth do not show oestrous cycles in adulthood. Their ovaries contain follicles that secrete oestrogens (they are said to be in constant oestrus), but as ovulation does not occur there are no corpora lutea.

Neonatal androgen causes acyclicity by suppression or modification of the oestradiol positive feedback mechanism. Thus, if male or female rats are castrated in adulthood and are subsequently injected with oestradiol, only the females show a surge of gonadotrophins (Fig. 6.20). If the same experiment is undertaken with female rats given testosterone during the first few days of life, no surge is observed. Does neonatal testosterone act on the ovary, pituitary or hypothalamus to suppress the positive feedback response? The ovaries or the pituitaries of androgenized females are quite capable of secreting surge levels of oestrogen or LH if transplanted into normal females, so their functional capacity does not seem to be grossly

impaired. The 'masculinizing' effect of neonatal testosterone is exerted on the hypothalamus, although precisely where is not firmly established.

This 'masculinization' of the brain occurs in most species (rodents, sheep and some carnivores), although the critical period of sensitivity to the effects of androgens varies considerably. For example, guinea-pigs have a gestation period of 68 days, compared to 21 days in the rat, and are born in a state of relative maturity. The critical period during which androgens exert their effects on the brain is pre- and not postnatal. Similar considerations apply to the large domestic animals and carnivores.

In contrast, experiments on primates indicate that 'masculinization' of the hypothalamus does not occur in the same way, and that the capacity for positive feedback exists in normal male monkeys and men. Thus, in castrated male monkeys (as well as in hypogonadal and castrated men) an administered oestrogen surge reliably induces a gonadotrophin surge (Fig. 6.21). Indeed, ovaries transplanted into castrated male monkeys undergo apparently normal monthly ovulatory cycles, a marked contrast to the results of similar experiments in rats. However, the positive feedback action of oestradiol cannot be elicited in *intact* male monkeys for reasons that are not clear. Female rhesus monkeys exposed to high levels of testosterone during fetal life are also able to show menstrual cycles as adults, although puberty occurs slightly later than usual. Indeed, in some of these monkeys the external genitalia are so

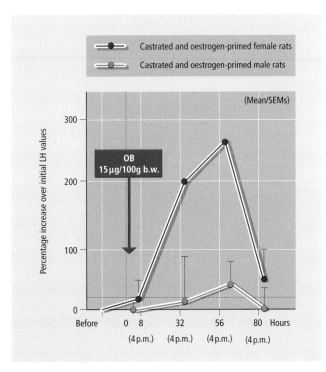

Fig. 6.20 The positive feedback effect of oestradiol in castrated male and female adult rats. The LH response, measured as a percentage change from resting values, to a single large injection of oestradiol benzoate (OB) is shown to be present only in the female (red) and not in the male (green). This is taken to be evidence of sexual differentiation of the hypothalamus, neonatal androgens in the male preventing the ability to respond to an oestrogen surge with an LH surge in the adult.

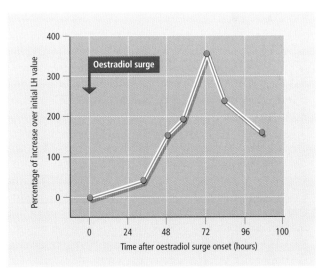

Fig. 6.21 Positive feedback effects of oestradiol in a castrate male talapoin monkey. Unlike the results in Fig. 6.20, the normal male monkey is able to respond to an oestradiol surge with an LH surge similar to that seen in the female. This suggests that exposure of the primate's brain to testosterone *in utero* does not 'masculinize' the hypothalamus as has been demonstrated in non-primate mammals.

'masculinized' that menstruation occurs through a penis-like phallus. Similarly, human females exposed to high levels of androgens during gestation, for example as the result of the adrenogenital syndrome, also have menstrual cycles as adults, often after a somewhat delayed puberty.

Clearly, 'masculinization' of the hypothalamic mechanism underlying positive feedback does not occur in normal male primates, including men, and thus, by these criteria, there are no enduring hypothalamic endocrine consequences in female primates, including women, exposed to high levels of androgens *in utero*. This conclusion is reminiscent of the less overt effects that neonatal androgens appeared to have on sexual behaviour in adult primates, as compared to their more dramatic effects on sexual behaviour in rats and other non-primate species (see Chapter 2).

Prolactin has reproductive functions

Prolactin is made in the pituitary lactotrophs, which are distributed evenly throughout the anterior pituitary. It is stored in secretory granules and released in a pulsatile manner, which probably reflects the pulsatile release of controlling hypothalamic hormones.

The hypothalamus controls prolactin secretion

Unlike other pituitary hormones, prolactin is secreted spontaneously in large amounts when the vascular links between the pituitary and hypothalamus are *disconnected*. This observation means that regulation of secretion is mainly by *inhibition*, and has led to the search for the hypothalamic factor or factors involved (*prolactin inhibitory factor, PIF*). Although several hypothalamically derived factors can induce acute or transient pulses of prolactin release experimentally, only one is essential for normal prolactin physiology.

Dopamine is the prolactin inhibitory factor

The catecholamine, dopamine (see Fig. 3.9a) is PIF. Dopamine is found in neurons of the arcuate nucleus, the axons of which project to the portal capillaries in the medial and lateral palisade zones of the external layer of the median eminence (Fig. 6.5b & 6.18). It is secreted into the portal blood from the terminals of this tuberoinfundibular dopamine (TIDA) system and carried to the lactotrophs, which express the D_2-like subtype of dopamine receptors. Agonists of either dopamine or D_2 dopamine receptors (*bromocriptine*) suppress prolactin secretion (Fig. 6.22), while dopamine D_2 receptor antagonists (e.g. *haloperidol, metoclopramide* and *domperidone*) increase prolactin secretion by direct actions on the lactotrophs. Binding of prolactin to D_2-like receptors activates coupled G-proteins,

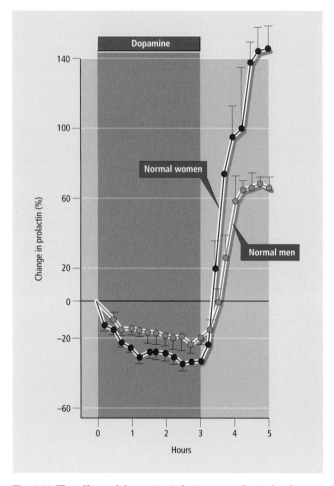

Fig. 6.22 The effects of dopamine infusion on prolactin levels in normal men (green) and women (red). Note the rapid onset of effect of dopamine and the rebound increase in prolactin levels on stopping the infusion. In women with hyperprolactinaemia, bromocriptine, a dopamine-receptor agonist, will cause serum prolactin concentrations of 80–100 ng/ml (normally they are less than 18 ng/ml) to fall to below 10 ng/ml within 5 or 6 h.

resulting in several functional consequences. Acute prolactin release is inhibited, transcription of its RNA is reduced, and lactotroph mitosis is suppressed. The overall outcome is reduced prolactin release.

What regulates the activity of TIDA neurons? It appears that the answer to this question is prolactin itself. Increases in circulating prolactin levels result in an increase in dopamine turnover within TIDA neuron terminals of the median eminence and a reduction therefore in prolactin secretion. The increase in dopamine turnover is related to an increase in tyrosine hydroxylase activity, the enzyme that is rate-limiting in the intraneuronal synthesis of dopamine (see Fig. 3.9). This so-called 'short-loop' feedback control of hypothalamic TIDA neuron activity, and hence dopamine release, by circulating prolactin is illustrated in Fig. 6.23.

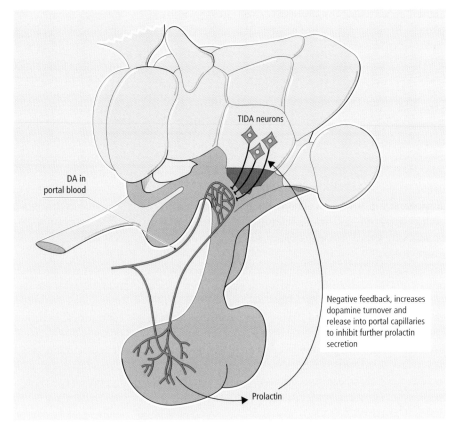

Fig. 6.23 Schematic summary of the proposed negative feedback relationship between prolactin and dopamine. Prolactin is believed to accelerate dopamine (DA) turnover in the arcuate nucleus neurons (tuberoinfundibular dopamine (TIDA) neurons), and the catecholamine is then released into the portal capillaries and thereby reaches the lactotrophs. Hyperprolactinaemia could be caused by a failure either of prolactin inhibitory factor (PIF) activity at the dopamine receptor level in the anterior pituitary, or a reduction of TIDA neuron activity in the hypothalamus.

Labels within figure: TIDA neurons; DA in portal blood; Negative feedback, increases dopamine turnover and release into portal capillaries to inhibit further prolactin secretion; Prolactin

Oestrogen stimulates prolactin release

Oestrogens induce hyperprolactinaemia by binding to ERα in the lactotrophs and stimulating prolactin synthesis. Increased spontaneous output of prolactin occurs. Chronic oestrogen exposure results in increased lactotroph numbers, which are therefore more numerous and larger in females, who also have higher ambient prolactin levels than males. An oestrous rhythm of prolactin secretion is observed in some animals, such as the rat, with a mid-cycle prolactin surge coincident with LH. This appears to result from the preovulatory surge oestrogen, and is associated with a decline in dopamine receptor level and thereby a diminished inhibitory influence of DA. Blocking the oestrogen surge, blocks the prolactin surge. However, in women, there seems to be no clear menstrual rhythm in serum prolactin levels, and prolactin secretion does not alter significantly after the menopause. During pregnancy, when oestrogen levels rise, prolactin output also rises (at least initially; see Chapter 11).

Prolactin has diverse functions

Prolactin is essential for lactation (see Chapter 13). During the luteal phase in the rat, sheep and goat, where prolactin is an essential part of the luteotrophic complex (Chapter 5),

it acts by increasing the number of oestradiol receptors in the corpus luteum. Few of these actions have been established in women. There is some evidence that prolactin may facilitate steroidogenesis in ovarian follicles, and assist in preventing premature progesterone secretion in the early stages of follicular growth and enhancing it in the luteal phase. In addition, prolactin appears to be able to modulate the number of ovarian receptors for LH and so affect steroidogenesis indirectly.

In males, most of the information concerning prolactin comes from experiments on rodents. It has been shown that, while exerting little effect on its own, prolactin may increase the number of LH receptors and potentiate the steroidogenic effect of LH on Leydig cells; testicular prolactin receptors seem to be confined to the interstitial tissue of the testis. Similarly, prolactin increases the uptake of androgen and increases 5α-reductase activity in the prostate, acting synergistically with testosterone, which maintains the prolactin receptors. Prolactin also potentiates the effects of testosterone on the seminal vesicles.

In general, prolactin seems to function as an ancillary hormone, promoting the activities of other hormones. Its non-reproductive functions in mammals are numerous, and include such diverse examples as regulation of kidney and adrenocorticotrophic activity (these tissues having higher prolactin-binding activity even than mammary tissues), in addition to the synergistic actions with ovarian and testicular steroids and gonadotrophins described above.

Hyperprolactinaemia suppresses fertility

Pathological elevation of serum prolactin, particularly a transition to a less episodic, more continuous output, is associated with reproductive pathology. High levels in men are associated with impaired fertility, decreased circulating levels of testosterone, impotence and loss of libido (Chapter 15). In women, the syndrome is characterized by amenorrhoea, and hence infertility (Chapter 15), with or without galactorrhoea (abnormal milk secretion, see Chapter 14) and loss of libido. Clearly, prolactin, in such circumstances, exerts profound effects on reproductive function. The causes of hyperprolactinaemia are multiple and varied. They may of course be 'physiological', for example in pregnancy and during the first few months of breast-feeding. They can be iatrogenic, due for example to psychiatric use of dopamine receptor-blocking neuroleptic drugs that increase prolactin secretion, as can oestrogens in some oral contraceptives. Prolactin elevation also may result from an underlying pathology. Pituitary tumours that are prolactin-secreting (so-called prolactinomas) are not uncommon, some 20% of postmortem samples showing evidence of microadenomas. Not surprisingly, in light of the oestrogen stimulatory effects, these are more common in women than in men.

The high prolactin levels are largely due to absence of the fall in prolactin secretion normally seen in the morning on awakening (Fig. 6.24), the high-amplitude prolactin pulses occurring abnormally during the daytime set against an elevated baseline level. The syndrome is more common in women than in men. The endocrine profile of women with hyperprolactinaemia is characterized by an absence of pulsatile LH secretion, a reduced pituitary LH response to injected GnRH, a failure of positive feedback, and hence chronic anovulation and amenorrhoea. Contrary to earlier opinion, it is now clear that the ovarian responsiveness to FSH and LH is not necessarily impaired and does not underlie the amenorrhoea; indeed, normal cyclicity can be maintained in the presence of high prolactin levels if exogenous gonadotrophins are administered. Exactly how elevated prolactin levels cause these changes is unclear. The decrease in pituitary sensitivity to GnRH might reflect an indirect effect of prolactin via decreased ovarian oestradiol secretion, rather than an effect exerted directly on the pituitary.

Treatment of hyperprolactinaemia has become relatively effective and simple. Dopamine D_2 receptor agonists, such as bromocriptine, are now used to lower serum prolactin concentrations immediately, and daily treatment results in the return of ovulation and cyclicity in the vast majority of women within 2 months. In the case of prolactin-secreting tumours, dopamine receptor agonists have an antimitotic action and, in addition to lowering plasma prolactin concentrations, reduce tumour size. However, in the majority of cases, cessation of treatment is followed by a resumption of prolactinoma activity and surgical removal may be necessary. The loss of libido in men and some women with hyperprolactinaemia is unexplained. The suggestion that this represents a direct action of prolactin in the brain remains to be demonstrated.

The environment influences reproduction

The foregoing discussion has established a major role for the CNS, and the hypothalamus in particular, in the provision of a GnRH and dopamine supply and as a target for steroid modulation. The CNS also mediates the effects of environmental factors, such as coital stimuli, olfactory stimuli and light, on the regulation of reproductive activity in many species. In addition, factors arising from social interactions, including anxiety or other forms of emotional distress, can have profound effects on cyclicity and fertility in men and women, and are also mediated by the CNS.

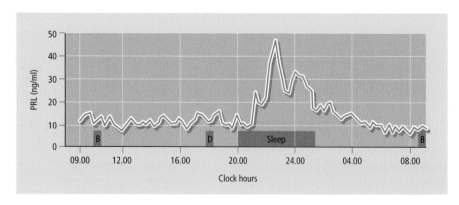

Fig. 6.24 Daily variation of prolactin (PRL) secretion. Note the onset of sleep is associated with the rise in serum prolactin concentrations, which then begin to fall towards the period of wakening. B, breakfast; D, dinner.

Although the effects of these social factors are readily observed in humans, the study of causal relationships depends, in large part, on careful analysis of animals living in social groups, where both behavioural and endocrine variables may be controlled experimentally. We now examine the way in which these various environmental influences on reproduction are mediated.

Daylight affects fertility

Reproduction is only one of a host of activities in which an individual may engage. To ensure that reproductive activity occurs effectively and with minimum interference from other processes, its appropriate timing is important. There are two levels at which control over timing is evident.

Circadian rhythms control reproductive function in some species

The temporal control of reproductive activity in females is complicated because the production of a viable oocyte is itself a cyclical event that must be matched to other cyclical events occurring within the life of an animal. In a nocturnally active rodent, for example, potential encounters with mates will be restricted to the hours of darkness. This selection pressure has led to the development of an oestrous cycle that is tightly locked to the best indicator of external time, the daily light–dark cycle. As we saw in Chapter 5, the oestrous cycle of rats is much shorter than the menstrual cycle of primates, but the temporal relationships of oestradiol, LH and FSH secretion are remarkably similar (Fig. 6.25). The really dramatic differences are: (1) the surge of progesterone secretion accompanying the LH surge, which is very important in the cyclical control of sexual behaviour in rats (see Chapter 8 for details); and (2) the LH surge itself, which is precisely timed to occur between 5 and 7h before darkness. This ensures that ovulation occurs 12h later during the night when the female is nocturnally active and behaviourally receptive (see Chapter 8). The likelihood of conception is therefore maximized. In intact animals, the LH surge occurs only every 4 or 5 days because it is dependent on the trigger of rising oestrogen production. However, the neural signal that determines the *time* of the LH surge is present every day. In ovariectomized females having a constantly high level of oestrogen delivered from a subcutaneously implanted capsule, an LH surge occurs every day at precisely the same time. By controlling oestrogen levels, the ovary therefore determines *the day* of ovulation, but a neural timer, controlling a critical period of sensitivity to oestrogen, determines *when*, during that particular day, the LH surge and thus ovulation will occur.

Reversal of the light–dark cycle causes a 12-h shift in the timing of the critical period of sensitivity to oestrogen,

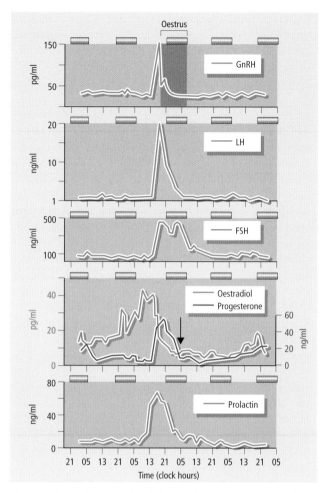

Fig. 6.25 Serum hormone levels during the oestrous cycle in the rat. The orange bars represent dark periods (18.00–06.00 h) centred around midnight, and the arrow denotes the time of ovulation. Also shown are the levels of GnRH measured in portal vein blood, which show a clear surge just before the FSH and LH surges. Note that the surge in prolactin is coincident with the gonadotrophin surges.

the LH surge and ovulation, demonstrating the essential role of information about light in setting the neural timer. However, even in constant light or dark, daily LH surges will continue, given the appropriate oestrogen environment, indicating that the timing mechanism is a *self-sustaining biological clock* (or oscillator). Under these constant conditions, the oscillator and the rhythm it controls are said to *free-run* with a period of approximately 24 h, which is therefore termed *circadian* (circa = approximately, diem = day). It is important to realize that the circadian system controls a wide range of other behavioural and endocrine rhythms, both reproductive and nonreproductive, which are held in a very strict, temporal relationship to each other.

The majority of these rhythms are driven by the *suprachiasmatic nuclei* of the hypothalamus. This cluster of neurons, located above the optic chiasm adjacent to the third ventricle (see Fig. 6.3a), has the ability to generate a circadian signal even when isolated from the rest of the brain. In life, this approximately 24-h signal is converted to a precise period of 24h by the *entraining* effect of photic stimuli, which reach the suprachiasmatic nuclei via a direct retinal input, the *retinohypothalamic tract*. Lesions of the suprachiasmatic nuclei disrupt many circadian functions, including the LH surge, and thereby cause a condition of permanent anoestrus. The SCN projects axons to the arcuate nuclei, which thus seems to be the site of integration of oestrogen level and circadian input in timing the mid-cycle GnRH surge. It is unclear whether there is a circadian rhythm in GnRH secretion, normally peaking in the afternoon, which is amplified by the oestrogen surge, or whether the circadian input leads to a transient increase in the sensitivity of GnRH to the positive feedback effects of oestrogen.

In female primates, patterns of reproductive activity are much more flexible than in rodents. The primate has a menstrual cycle in which ovulation may occur at any time of day; there is not a tightly restricted period of sexual receptivity or 'heat', and the circadian system makes little contribution to the control of reproductive function. However, you will recall that in primates including humans a daily variation in plasma prolactin levels is observed, being high during the nocturnal sleep period. However, reversal of the sleep–waking cycle results in reversal of the daily rhythm of prolactin secretion, demonstrating that the pattern is *sleep-entrained* rather than *light-entrained* (Fig. 6.24). In a normal sleep–waking cycle, prolactin release begins to increase 1–1.5h after sleep onset and is achieved by progressive increases in pulse amplitude. Plasma concentrations are elevated during the remaining hours of sleep and fall in the early morning, shortly before awakening. Lowest concentrations are found between about 10 a.m. and 12 noon. Interestingly, the bursts of prolactin secretion seem to occur during slow-wave, or 'non-rapid eye movement' (non-REM) sleep, whereas REM (or paradoxical) sleep is associated with the smallest episodic prolactin pulses. These diurnal (but non-circadian) patterns in prolactin output seem to be mediated through modulation of dopamine output, but exactly how remains to be determined.

Circannual rhythms control reproductive function in seasonal breeders

In seasonal environments, where adverse climate and the availability of food are major determinants of offspring survival and therefore of the reproductive success of the parents, it is adaptive to ensure that young are born in the equable, productive conditions of spring or early summer.

This tight control over birth season, apparent in many domestic and wild species, is achieved by a precise regulation of the *month(s)* of fertility and hence the timing of conception. In species with short gestation times, such as hamsters and birds, winter is a time of infertility with gonadal development suspended until spring. In species with longer gestation times, such as sheep and deer, the anticipation of spring must begin much earlier and seasonal changes in autumn act as a stimulus to reproductive function. This leads to the dramatic spectacle of the *rut* when animals that have been reproductively quiescent for the entire year suddenly become sexually active. Males may develop pronounced secondary sexual features, such as antlers, become fertile, aggressive and territorial, and spend their whole time engaged in an intense competition for access to females. Females come into heat and actively show interest in males, accepting their attempts to copulate. In a third group, which includes marsupials, mustelids and seals, the total length of the gestation period can be varied because of delayed implantation and embryonic diapause (see Chapter 10). These processes are sensitive to environmental influences and provide a second level of control over the timing of the birth season. For reproductive physiologists, these seasonal phenomena offer an important opportunity to investigate the central mechanisms that regulate the fertility of an individual.

In some species, such as deer and ground squirrels, there is good evidence that seasonal cycles are under the control of an endogenous *circannual oscillator*, a biological clock with a period of approximately 1 year. In other species, there is no endogenous rhythmicity and the seasonal rhythms observed in the field are triggered by cyclical stimuli within the environment. Of these, photoperiod is by far the most important; this is exemplified in the laboratory, where artificial manipulation of day lengths can be used to drive all of the components of the annual reproductive cycle. For example, exposure of Syrian hamsters to less than 12.5h of light per day (pseudowinter) leads to gonadal atrophy and the loss of sexual behaviour. In contrast, these short photoperiods stimulate gonadal activity in species, such as sheep, that normally mate in the autumn. All of these effects are mediated by changes in the frequency of the GnRH pulse generator in the hypothalamus, which then determines the level of secretion of gonadotrophins and steroids (Fig. 6.26).

Photic circannual information obviously has access to the GnRH neurons, but does it use the same pathways that are involved in the circadian control of reproduction? Certainly, the suprachiasmatic nuclei have an important role to play because lesions of these structures completely block photoperiodic sensitivity. However, the pathways involved are not exclusively intrahypothalamic. It is now well recognized that the *pineal gland*, which sits over the dorsal

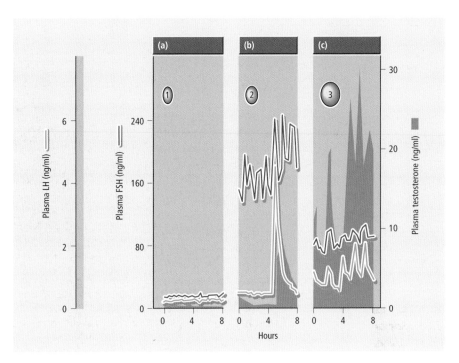

Fig. 6.26 The seasonal sexual cycle of a Soay ram. Changes in the plasma concentration of FSH (red), LH (green) and testosterone (shading) are shown at three times of the year. Testis size (blue) is shown inset at each time: (a) in the non-breeding season, when the testes are fully regressed, and LH, FSH and testosterone levels are all low; (b) towards the onset of the breeding season, when the testes are redeveloping and, associated with this process, FSH concentrations are very high; (c) during the mating season, when testosterone levels are very high and this reflects the marked increase in the frequency of pulsatile LH discharge.

midbrain, attached to the *epithalamus* in the posterior–dorsal third ventricle (see Fig. 6.1), is the mediator of photoperiodic time measurement. Removal of the gland or interruption of its sympathetic innervation leaves animals insensitive to changing day length. The primary pineal hormone, *melatonin* (see Fig. 3.9b), is synthesized and released into the bloodstream only in the hours of darkness, exhibiting a true circadian rhythmicity driven by the suprachiasmatic nuclei. At night, the circadian signal increases sympathetic activation of the gland, resulting in a dramatic rise in the activity of the enzyme, *N-acetyl transferase*, the rate-limiting step in melatonin biosynthesis.

The crucially important feature of the circadian melatonin signal is that it provides a precise representation of the length of the night, so that as days shorten and nights lengthen in autumn, the duration of the nocturnal melatonin peak is increased. Conversely, after the winter solstice, the photoperiod increases and the duration of the melatonin signal falls (Fig. 6.27a,b). The changing shape of the rhythm of circulating melatonin is detected within the hypothalamus and somehow leads to alterations in GnRH secretion. The melatonin signal is such a powerful regulator of neuroendocrine state that in pinealectomized animals the entire reproductive axis can be turned on or off by repeated nightly administration of programmed infusions of melatonin, which mimic the pattern of its secretion typical of either long or short photoperiods (Fig. 6.27c,d,f). The same melatonin signal leads to opposite neuroendocrine responses in spring-breeding species, since a progressive decrease in the duration of the night-time melatonin signal results in reproductive activation as days lengthen in the spring.

Coitus affects fertility in some species

In humans and other primates, sheep, rats and many other mammals, ovulation is said to occur 'spontaneously'. Thus, it depends on an endogenous event timed by the ovary, the oestradiol surge, which results in an ovulatory discharge of LH that may or may not be subject to additional, circadian controls. The neurally mediated variable controlling ovulation, to be discussed next in this chapter, concerns the *induced* or *reflex ovulators*, such as cats, rabbits and ferrets. These animals remain in behavioural oestrus for long periods of time without ovulating until they copulate with a male (see Fig. 5.8). Stimulation of the cervix and vagina during coitus evokes the reflex release of an ovulatory surge of LH via afferent, sensory pathways, which gain access to the GnRH release mechanism. Even in these species it seems that the hypothalamic–pituitary axis must be primed with high levels of oestrogen for the neural input to be effective.

Although the data supporting it are less than convincing, there are several reports of reflex ovulation in women. Ovulation has variously been observed to follow coitus very early in the follicular phase (even during menstruation), while termination of abnormally long follicular phases has sometimes been ascribed to coitus-induced, acute LH release. However, the subject has not been studied systematically, and these reports should therefore be viewed sceptically.

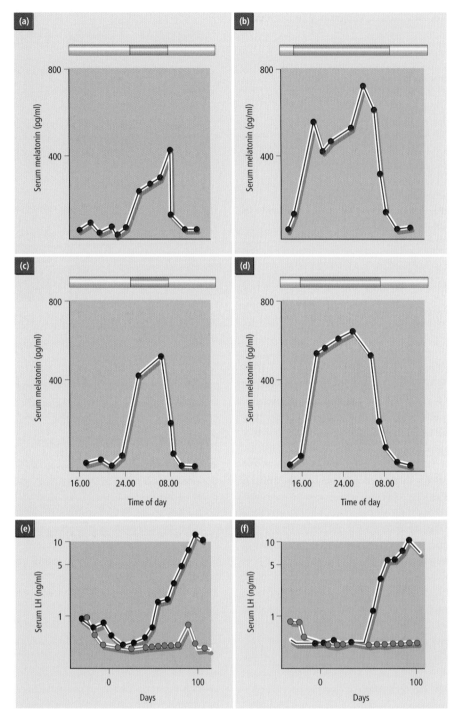

Fig. 6.27 The effects of melatonin on LH secretion in ewes in relation to the light–dark cycle (darkness is indicated by the orange bar over each graph). (a,b) Serum melatonin profiles of ewes with intact pineals exposed to artificial long (a) and short (b) photoperiods. Note the increased duration of the melatonin signal during the longer night of (b). (c,d) Serum melatonin profiles of pinealectomized ewes receiving programmed infusions of melatonin designed to mimic the patterns of long and short photoperiods (shown in a and b). (e) Reproductive response (LH secretion) of pineal-intact ewes to the artificial long (green line) or short (red line) photoperiods shown in (a) and (b) (remember that the ewe is an autumn, or 'short-day' breeder). (f) Reproductive response of pinealectomized ewes to programmed infusion of melatonin mimicking long (green line) or short (red line) photoperiodic profiles in serum shown in (c) and (d). Clearly, this is virtually identical to the pattern in (e).

Similarly, in the rat and mouse, pregnancy and pseudo-pregnancy (i.e. prolongation of luteal life; Fig. 5.8) are also dependent on coitus. In this case, cervical stimulation influences prolactin secretion patterns. It does so by adding a *diurnal* (during the day) peak in prolactin secretion to that normally occurring nocturnally. Thus, two daily peaks in prolactin concentration are measurable in the blood and are essential for corpus luteum formation, the polypeptide being an essential component of the luteotrophic complex. Changes in prolactin secretion also occur in response to suckling stimuli and are discussed in Chapter 14. These environmental influences seem to be exerted through modulation of dopamine output, but exactly how remains to be determined.

Social interactions and stress can affect fertility

Studies of primates living in social groups have revealed that the social context in which individuals interact can change their endocrine and fertility status. For example, if plasma testosterone levels are measured in male talapoin monkeys in the absence of females, all males, whether single or together as a group, have very similar testosterone levels. However, when oestrogen-treated females are introduced to an all-male group, one male becomes dominant, displays sexual activity with the females and is aggressive to subordinate males, and his plasma testosterone levels rise significantly. None of these changes is seen in the subordinate male(s) (Fig. 6.28).

That the behavioural interactions determine the change in plasma testosterone and not vice versa is apparent if all the males are taken out of the group and each replaced alone in turn with the females. In this situation, each male is sexually active and shows a significant rise in plasma testosterone. Addition of the dominant male to a group consisting of the subordinate male alone with females results in the latter male's plasma testosterone declining. These data have been interpreted to suggest that subordination, especially being on the receiving end of aggression, causes the decrease in testosterone levels. Conversely, being aggressive and/or displaying sexual behaviour, as in the dominant male, is associated with increased plasma testosterone. The significance of the elevated testosterone levels in the dominant male, and the mechanism by which it is achieved, are not entirely clear. As we will see in Chapter 8, testosterone levels have a tenuous relationship to sexual motivation in gonadally intact male primates and even subordinate males have sufficient levels of the hormone to maintain sexual behaviour. It has been suggested that testosterone may enhance the attractiveness of the dominant male to females by behavioural (e.g. posture) and/or non-behavioural (e.g. coat quality and odour) means.

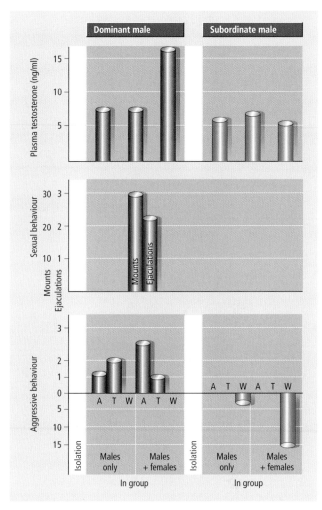

Fig. 6.28 Changes in sexual and aggressive behaviour and plasma testosterone levels in dominant and subordinate male talapoin monkeys following a 12-week period in isolation when placed for a 6-week period in an all-male group, and a 7-week period in a social group with oestradiol-treated females. Note that only the dominant male's plasma testosterone increases in the social group, and that only he is sexually active and being aggressive towards, but not receiving aggression from, other males. The subordinate male receives, but does not give, aggression and withdraws more frequently, especially when females are in the group. A, attacks; T, threats (both measures of aggressive behaviour); W, withdrawals (a measure of submissive behaviour). (Mounts and ejaculations are both measures of sexual behaviour.)

A similar consequence of the dominance hierarchy is seen in the females of the group. The dominant female receives more sexual attention from the dominant male than does the subordinate female(s), and hardly any aggressive behaviour from other members of the group (Fig. 6.29). An intriguing consequence of this state of affairs is seen if both the dominant and subordinate females are challenged

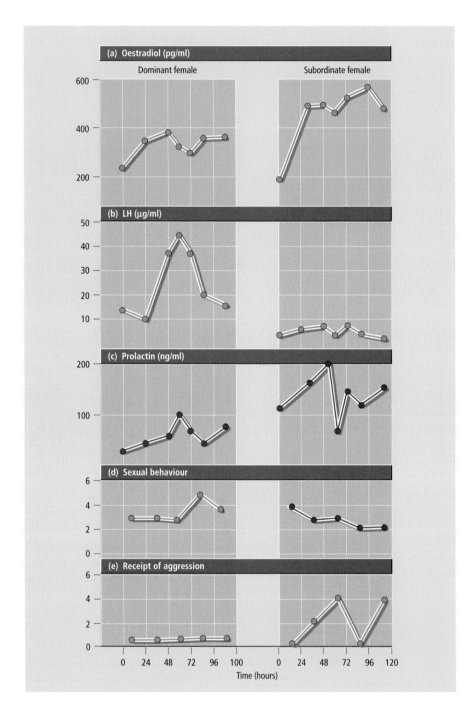

Fig. 6.29 Sexual and aggressive behaviour received by the dominant and subordinate female talapoin monkeys in a social group, and changes in plasma LH and prolactin levels when challenged with an oestradiol surge. (a) Increase in plasma oestradiol concentrations following the oestradiol surge. (b) Changes in plasma LH concentrations, which follow the oestradiol surge. (c) Plasma prolactin concentrations in the females. (d) Sexual interaction with males indicating mounts without ejaculation (red line) and mounts with ejaculations (green line). (e) Level of aggressive behaviour received by the females. Note that the dominant female receives high levels of sexual behaviour and low levels of aggression, has low plasma levels of prolactin and shows a surge of LH in response to an oestradiol surge. The converse is true of the subordinate female.

with an oestradiol surge, since only dominant females display an LH surge. If plasma prolactin levels are measured, it is seen that they are much higher in the subordinate females (hyperprolactinaemia). Thus, it seems likely that dominant females have the capacity for positive feedback, show normal menstrual cycles and are therefore potentially fertile. Not so subordinate females, who appear to lose the capacity to respond to an oestrogen surge with an LH surge, therefore having anovulatory and irregular cycles

and probably amenorrhoea. This is clearly reminiscent of the situation seen in some women with hyperprolactinaemia. That prolactin is the key to this change in positive feedback capacity was demonstrated by lowering plasma prolactin concentrations in subordinate females using a dopamine D_2 receptor agonist, and raising it in dominant females using a dopamine D_2 receptor antagonist. These treatments effectively reversed the LH response to an oestradiol surge in the two types of female. These two examples emphasize the important and far-reaching consequences of social interaction in determining levels of sexual activity as well as endocrine and reproductive status.

Summary

The critical event underlying ovulation in the menstrual or oestrous cycle is an oestradiol-induced gonadotrophin surge. The oestradiol surge is not preceded by an obvious endocrine or neural trigger, and appears to arise spontaneously within the ovary, being determined by the dynamics of follicular growth. This leads to the conclusion that the ovary, and not the hypothalamus or pituitary, determines cycle length. However, the oestrogen surge from the ovary acts on both the pituitary and the hypothalamus to induce the release of an ovulatory surge of LH (Fig. 6.30).

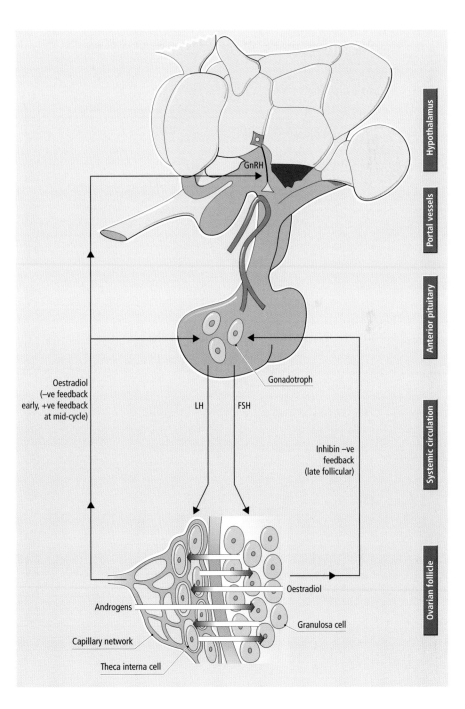

Fig. 6.30 Summary of hypothalamic–pituitary–ovarian interactions during the follicular phase of the cycle.

This capacity to respond to an oestradiol surge with an LH surge is lacking in male non-primate species. However, in both males and females, similar negative feedback effects of gonadal hormones on the pituitary and hypothalamus are observed (Figs 6.31 & 6.32). The feedback effects of gonadal hormones are adequate, in themselves, to explain all the basic features of the reproductive patterns in both males and females. However, the hypothalamic–pituitary–gonadal axis is not a closed system. External factors clearly modulate its activity to render the basic reproductive pattern susceptible to environmental influences, such as the time of day or year, and proximity of a potential reproductive partner or rival. By such mechanisms, the efficiency of the reproductive process is increased and the survival of the species promoted.

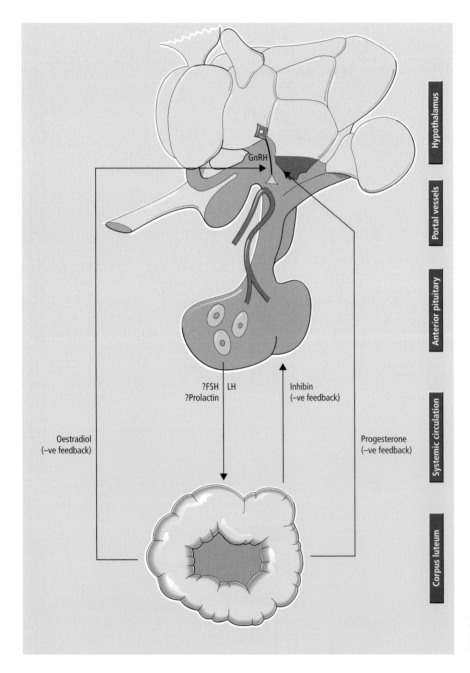

Fig. 6.31 Summary of hypothalamic–pituitary–ovarian interactions during the luteal phase of the cycle.

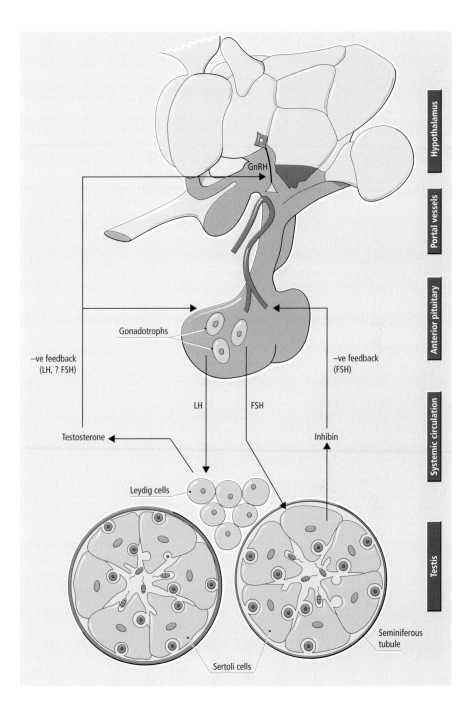

Fig. 6.32 Summary of hypothalamic–pituitary–testis interactions in the male.

FURTHER READING

General reading

Arendt J (1998) Melatonin and the pineal gland: influence on mammalian seasonal and circadian physiology. *Biology of Reproduction* **3**, 13–22.

de Kretser DM *et al.* (2004) The role of activin, follistatin and inhibin in testicular physiology. *Molecular and Cellular Endocrinology* **225**, 57–64.

Evans NP *et al.* (1997) Estradiol requirements for induction and maintenance of the gonadotropin-releasing hormone surge: implications for neuroendocrine processing of the estradiol signal. *Endocrinology* **138**, 5408–5414.

KEY LEARNING POINTS

- The anterior lobe of the pituitary makes and secretes LH, FSH and prolactin.

- The posterior lobe of the pituitary secretes the peptide hormones oxytocin and vasopressin.

- The hypothalamus contains groups of neurosecretory neurons and other neuronal groups that have reproductive functions.

- The parvocellular neurosecretory system consists of neurons in the preoptic/anterior hypothalamic areas and arcuate nuclei that synthesize GnRH, which is secreted into the portal vessels in the median eminence and is carried in the blood to the anterior pituitary where it controls LH and FSH secretion.

- The magnocellular neurosecretory system consists of neurons in the paraventricular and supraoptic nuclei that synthesize oxytocin (and vasopressin), which is packaged with a neurophysin and transported by axoplasmic flow to the posterior pituitary, which is the site of secretion into the blood.

- Hypothalamic GnRH secretion is pulsatile and thereby controls the pulsatile secretion of gonadotrophins.

- Oestradiol and progesterone secreted by the ovary exert feedback control over GnRH, FSH and LH secretion by actions within both the hypothalamus and the anterior pituitary.

- Oestradiol, in addition to negative feedback effects on LH and FSH secretion, has a unique ability to induce the ovulatory surge of LH secretion by what is called a 'positive feedback' action.

- Ovarian inhibin controls FSH secretion by negative feedback actions in the anterior pituitary.

- The pattern of hormone secretion during the menstrual cycle is determined by these feedback interactions between ovarian hormones and GnRH, LH and FSH secretion.

- Ovarian steroid feedback regulation of GnRH secretion is mediated indirectly by a variety of neural mechanisms within the hypothalamus.

- In males, GnRH also controls the pulsatile secretion of LH and FSH.

- Testosterone exerts negative feedback control over LH secretion.

- These effects are mediated through both the hypothalamus and the anterior pituitary.

- Testicular inhibin exerts negative feedback control over FSH secretion by actions in the anterior pituitary.

- Prolactin is secreted by the anterior pituitary.

- Prolactin secretion is regulated by the release-inhibiting hormone dopamine, released from tuberoinfundibular dopamine (TIDA) neurons into the portal blood.

- Prolactin can regulate its own secretion via short-loop negative feedback effects on TIDA neuronal activity.

- Oestradiol stimulates lactotrophs and increases prolactin secretion.

- Hyperprolactinaemia can result in infertility in males and females. It can be treated with dopamine D_2 receptor agonist drugs that mimic the actions of dopamine in the anterior pituitary and thereby reduce prolactin secretion.

- Environmental light can affect reproductive neuroendocrine integration.

- There is a circadian regulation of the time of ovulation during the oestrous cycle of some species, such as nocturnal rodents, which ensures that ovulation and behavioural oestrus are coordinated so as to maximize conception.

- In seasonal breeders, the change in day length throughout the year underlies a circannual rhythm of reproductive activity which is mediated by the night-time secretion of melatonin from the pineal gland.

- Coitus itself may induce ovulatory discharges of LH by a neural mechanism in species therefore known as reflex ovulators.

- Social subordination and stress can affect fertility in socially living species such as primates.

Everitt BJ *et al.* (1992) The organization of monoaminergic neurons in the hypothalamus in relation to neuroendocrine integration. In: *Neuroendocrinology* (ed. C.B. Nemeroff), pp. 87–129. CRC Press, Boca Raton, FL.

Groome NP *et al.* (1996) Measurement of dimeric inhibin B throughout the human menstrual cycle. *Journal of Clinical Endocrinology and Metabolism* **81**, 1401–1405.

Herbison AE (1997) Noradrenergic regulation of cyclic GnRH secretion. *Reviews of Reproduction* **2**, 1–6.

Kalra SP (1993) Mandatory neuropeptide–steroid signalling for the preovulatory luteinizing hormone-releasing hormone discharge. *Endocrine Reviews* **14**, 507–538.

Rispoli LA, Nett TM (2005) Pituitary gonadotropin-releasing hormone (GnRH) receptor: structure, distribution and regulation of expression. *Animal Reproduction Science* **88**, 57–74.

More advanced reading (see also Boxes)

Laven JSE, Fauser BCJM (2004) Inhibins and adult ovarian function. *Molecular and Cellular Endocrinology* **225**, 37–44.

Macklon NS *et al.* (2006) The science behind 25 years of ovarian stimulation for *in vitro* fertilization. *Endocrine Reviews* **27**, 170–207.

CHAPTER 7

7 Puberty and the Maturation of the Hypothalamic–Pituitary–Gonadal Axis

In earlier chapters, we have seen how the gonads and genitalia develop during fetal life and how they function in the adult. The regulation of adult function is complex, as we saw in the previous chapter. Now we return to examine the transition from a sexually immature individual to a sexually mature adult. This involves a consideration of the subject of puberty.

Puberty

Puberty is a state of transition: a collective term that encompasses all the physiological, morphological and behavioural changes that occur in the growing individual during the transformation from a juvenile to a potentially fertile adult. In humans, puberty (the *adolescent* stage) is preceded sequentially by *infancy* (from birth to weaning), *childhood* (a period of dependence on adults for survival) and the *juvenile* stage (when survival without adults is possible). All mammals undergo puberty, but primates including humans uniquely do so a long time after birth. Thus, whereas in most human females the first evidence of fertility occurs between 12 and 14 years of age, in non-primate species it occurs much earlier: 6–7 months in the ewe, 12 months in the cow, 7 months in the pig and 30–35 days in the mouse. Prepubertal development is prolonged in higher primates, and we focus on the primates in this chapter.

A fairly definitive sign of puberty's occurrence in girls is *menarche*, the first *menstrual bleeding*. An indication of a similar stage of maturity in boys is the first *ejaculation*, which often occurs nocturnally and is thus much more difficult to date precisely. The first menstruation and ejaculation do not signify fertility. Indeed, in early puberty the ovary does not ovulate and the ejaculate consists of small quantities of seminal plasma lacking spermatozoa. Rather, these two dramatic events are signs that the gonads have been awakened and are beginning to assume adult levels of activity.

Some 2–4 years before these obvious signs of sexual maturation, a series of other changes in most of the organs and in the structure of the body is initiated. These changes are dependent on, and orchestrated by, the increasing level of sex steroids from the gonads (*gonadarche*) and also, uniquely in humans and the great apes, from the adrenal glands (*adrenarche*). However, only gonadarche seems to be essential for fertility. A key point to grasp is that the sequence of maturational changes does not begin at the same chronological age or take the same length of time to reach completion in all children, even though the sequence in which these changes occur varies but little.

Growth hormone and sex steroids underlie the physical changes during puberty

The *adolescent growth spurt* is an acceleration, followed by a deceleration, of growth in most skeletal dimensions, and can be divided into three stages: (1) the *time of minimum growth velocity* (or 'age at take-off'); (2) the time of *peak height velocity* (PHV); and (3) the time of decreased growth velocity and cessation of growth at *epiphyseal fusion*. Fig. 7.1 shows that boys begin their growth spurt about 2 years later than girls on average. They are therefore taller at the age of take-off and reach their PHV 2 years later. The height gain of boys and girls between take-off and cessation of growth is similar, about 28 cm and 25 cm, respectively, indicating that the 10 cm difference in mean height between adult men and women is due more to the height difference at take-off than gain during the spurt. Age at take-off and PHV are poor indicators of adult height and, in addition, they show a poor correlation with the rate of passage through the various stages of puberty described below. Virtually every muscular and skeletal dimension is involved in the adolescent growth spurt; however, sex differences in the growth rates of different regions occur, which enhance sexual dimorphism in the adult, in, for example, the shoulders (greater in boys) and hips (greater in girls). This dynamic phase of growth is dependent not only on sex steroids but also on *growth hormone* from the *anterior pituitary*. Thus, patients with poorly functional pituitaries (*hypopituitarism*) must be given both growth hormone and steroids if a pubertal growth spurt is to occur.

As well as growth, considerable changes in body composition occur during puberty. Lean body mass and body fat are virtually identical in prepubertal girls and boys, but in adulthood, men have about 1.5 times the lean body mass of women, while women have twice as much body fat as men. In addition, the skeletal mass of men is 1.5 times that of women. These alterations in body mass commence at about 6 and 9 years of age in girls and boys, respectively, and represent the earliest changes in body composition at

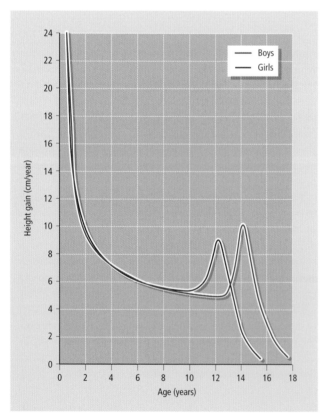

Fig. 7.1 Growth velocity curves for boys and girls. Note the later time of 'take-off' in boys, which generally ensures a greater height at the start of the adolescent growth spurt. Also note that average peak height velocity is 9 cm/year for girls and 10 cm/year for boys.

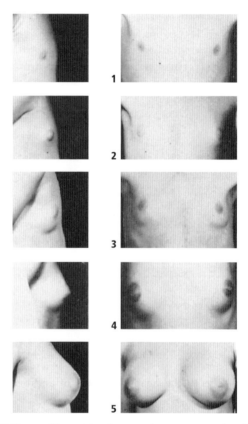

Fig. 7.2 Stages of breast development (oestrogen regulated): 1, preadolescent stage during which the papilla (nipple) alone is elevated; 2, breast bud stage in which the papilla and breast are elevated as a small mound and the areolar area increases; 3, continued enlargement of the breast and areola, but without separation in their contours, and pigmentation increases; 4, further breast enlargement but with the papilla and areola projecting above the breast contour; 5, mature stage in which the areola has become recessed, and forms a smooth contour with the rest of the breast—only the papilla is elevated. Classification of this stage is independent of breast size, which is determined principally by genetic and nutritional factors.

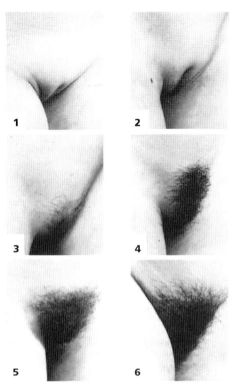

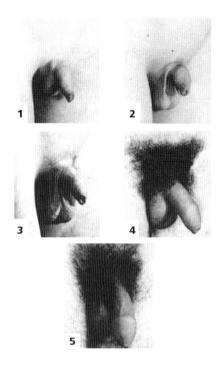

Fig. 7.4 Stages of external genitalia development in boys: 1, preadolescent stage during which penis, testes and scrotum are of similar size and proportion as in early childhood; 2, scrotum and testes have enlarged; texture of the scrotal skin has also changed and become slightly reddened; pubic hair is at the base of the penis and downy; 3, testes and scrotum have grown further but now the penis has increased in size: first in length and then in breadth; facial hair appears for the first time on upper lip and cheeks, and pubic hair is longer and more extensively distributed; 4, further enlargement of the testes, scrotum (which has darkened in colour) and penis; the glans penis has now begun to develop; 5, adult stage; facial hair has now extended to lower lip and chin. Hair on the chest, back, abdomen and more of the face is genetically variable and starts appearing 3 or so years after stage 5 is achieved.

Fig. 7.3 Stages of pubic hair development in girls (adrenal androgen regulated): 1, no pubic hair is visible; 2, sparse growth of long, downy hair which is only slightly curled and situated primarily along the labia; 3, appearance of coarser, curlier and often darker hair; 4, hair spreads to cover labia; 5, hair spreads more over the junction of the pubes and is now adult in type but not quantity; no spread to the medial surface of the thighs; 6, adult stage in which the classical 'inverse triangle' of pubic hair distribution is seen, with additional spread to the medial surface of the thighs. Pubic hair maturation is accompanied by apocrine odour development, and skin oiliness and acne.

puberty. The greater average strength of men compared to women reflects a greater number of larger muscle cells, which is due to the anabolic effects of androgens (see Chapter 8 for details).

Gonadal activation underlies the development of secondary sexual characteristics

In addition to growth and changes in body composition, development of the *secondary sexual characteristics* occurs at puberty, for example breasts (Fig. 7.2), genitalia and pubic hair (Figs 7.3 & 7.4), and beard growth and voice change. Ovarian oestrogens regulate growth of the breast and female genitalia, but *androgens* from both the ovary and the adrenal gland control the growth of female pubic and axillary hair. Testicular androgens not only control develop-

ment of the genitalia and body hair in boys, but also, by enlarging the *larynx* and *laryngeal muscles*, lead to *deepening* of the voice.

These various characteristics develop at very different chronological ages in different individuals (see for example Fig. 7.5). However, the *sequence* in which the changes occur is quite characteristic for each sex. This is important for the clinician, who has *staging criteria* (summarized in Figs 7.2–7.4) by which abnormalities can be detected and comparisons made between individuals, populations and cultures. For example, a boy with advanced penile and pubic hair growth but small testes must have a non-gonadal source of excess androgen, such as congenital adrenal hyperplasia or an adrenal tumour.

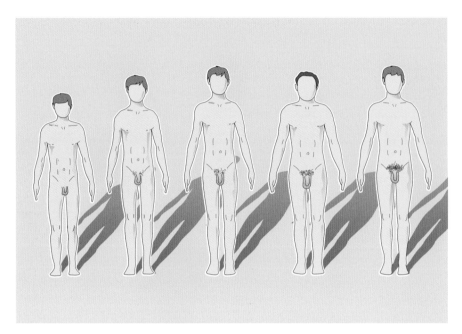

Fig. 7.5 Five boys all aged 14 years illustrating marked individual differences in physical maturation at the same chronological age.

There is a distinctive pattern of hormonal changes at puberty

In Fig. 7.6, the physical changes occurring through puberty are summarized. They are largely controlled by gonadal and adrenal steroids, together with some direct involvement of pituitary hormones. We will now examine the endocrinology of the process of gonadal activation, which results in the adult pattern of regulation described in Chapter 6.

Plasma levels of gonadotrophins may be in the adult range soon after birth, rising and falling intermittently for the first year or two of life. This may reflect the acute drop in maternally derived steroid levels at parturition and suggests that negative feedback is capable of operating at this early stage. Moreover, there is evidence of endocrine circhorial pulsing at this time. These observations suggest that a steroid-sensitive pulse-generating system is competent at birth, although it seems less well developed in females than males. In both sexes, gonadotrophin output then declines and blood levels remain very low during childhood and juvenile stages, until the initiation of events leading to puberty (Fig. 7.7). From this time, mean levels of follicle-stimulating hormone (FSH) and luteinizing hormone (LH) rise gradually to reach adult levels and pulsing becomes obvious (Figs 7.7 & 7.8). Prolactin concentrations also increase in late puberty in girls, but not in boys, in whom the plasma levels of this hormone are already similar to those seen in men. This sex difference may be attributed to the rising oestradiol that enhances prolactin secretion in females (see Chapter 6).

Probably the most intriguing and dramatic change in gonadotrophin secretion occurs in early puberty at night during sleep. In men and women, there is no evidence of a circadian rhythm of FSH and LH secretion (Fig. 7.9d). The same is true in prepubertal juveniles (Fig. 7.9a), who have low plasma levels and evidence of very depressed circhorial pulsing. From early to mid-puberty, however, a striking increase in the magnitude, and possibly also the frequency, of nocturnal LH pulses occurs, which reflects a sleep-augmented LH secretion (Fig. 7.9b). In late puberty, daytime LH pulses also increase (Fig. 7.9c), but are less than those still occurring at night, until the adult pattern of higher basal levels with no daily pulsing variation is achieved.

Testosterone levels in plasma follow the gonadotrophins. Thus, they are less than 0.1 ng/ml in boys and girls (except during the first 3–5 months after birth in boys when levels similar to those at puberty are found). In early puberty, testosterone levels in boys rise at night when LH secretion becomes elevated (Fig. 7.9b). Later in puberty, blood samples taken during the day also show increases, the greatest changes appearing during pubertal stage 2, when testosterone concentrations may change from 0.2 to 2.4 ng/ml. There are smaller, but nonetheless consistent, increases in plasma testosterone concentrations in girls between pubertal stages 1 and 4.

Oestrogen plasma concentrations are extremely high in both male and female fetuses at birth (5000 pg/ml) because

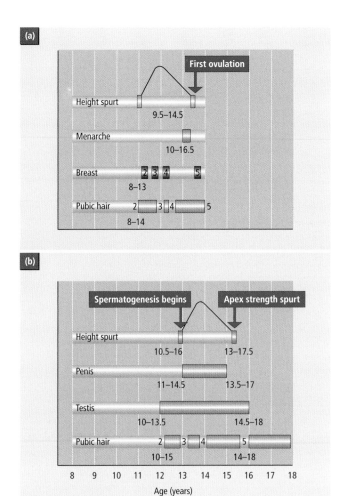

Fig. 7.6 Summary of the sequence of events during puberty in (a) girls and (b) boys. The figures below each symbol represent the range of ages within which each event may begin and end. The figures within each symbol refer to the stages illustrated in Figs 7.2–7.4.

of the conversion of fetal and maternal C_{19} steroids by the placenta (see Chapter 11). Indeed, newborn infants may display breast budding and even milk secretion ('*witches' milk*') as a consequence of these high oestrogen levels. Oestradiol and oestrone levels soon drop to 7 and 20 pg/ml, respectively, and remain low until puberty. In girls, oestradiol levels rise consistently through the stages of puberty to reach the concentrations seen in mature women (see Fig. 7.8a). In boys, plasma concentrations of oestrone are higher than oestradiol, but both are considerably lower than in girls at comparable stages of puberty. In males, about half the oestradiol is derived from extraglandular aromatization of testosterone, and a quarter, or less, from testicular secretion.

Surprisingly, the earliest detectable endocrine change, preceding those of gonadotrophins and gonadal steroids, is a progressive increase in the plasma concentration of adrenal androgens, notably dehydroepiandrosterone and its sulfate. This adrenal maturation is selective, in that glucocorticoid and mineralocorticoid secretion does not increase at the same time. It is called *adrenarche*, and starts around 8 years of age (6–8 years skeletal age), continuing until 13–15 years. The circulating levels of these weak androgens are orders of magnitude higher than those of the gonadal sex steroids, yet their significance in relation to hypothalamic–pituitary–gonadal activation is obscure. The only clear somatic function of these adrenal androgens appears to be the promotion of pubic and axillary hair growth. The adolescent growth spurt does not depend on them. Neither hypersecretion nor hyposecretion of adrenal androgens seems to be associated consistently with either early or delayed puberty, and there is little evidence to suggest that these hormones are concerned with timing the onset of puberty in normal children.

In summary, the peripubertal period is associated with the activation of the gonads (and adrenals), which results in elevated steroid secretion. These events are, in turn, dependent on increased trophic stimulation by FSH and LH. In the next three sections, we will examine the control of these trophic stimuli, the neuropharmacological regions of the central nervous system (CNS) involved, and the nature and timing of the trigger that induces them.

Activation of pulsatile hypothalamic GnRH secretion is a key event in the onset of puberty

The distinctive postnatal pattern of gonadotrophin and presumptively GnRH output (elevated in infants, depressed in children and juveniles, and then rising in adolescents) suggests a *central maturational role for the CNS* and, in particular, the hypothalamus, at puberty. Is there evidence to support this view?

Activation of hypothalamic GnRH secretion is the driving force behind pubertal development

Experimental evidence supporting the view that puberty is driven by a primary change in the hypothalamic output of GnRH comes from experiments in young rhesus monkeys castrated at birth. Thus, like their intact controls, they show pulsatile LH and FSH secretion and levels that vary within the adult range for the first 10–20 weeks of infant life (see Fig. 7.7). Thereafter, concentrations fall and remain at low or undetectable levels for the next 2.5 years or so (see Fig. 7.7). Following this period of gonadotrophic quiescence, the pulsatile secretion of LH and FSH recommences and

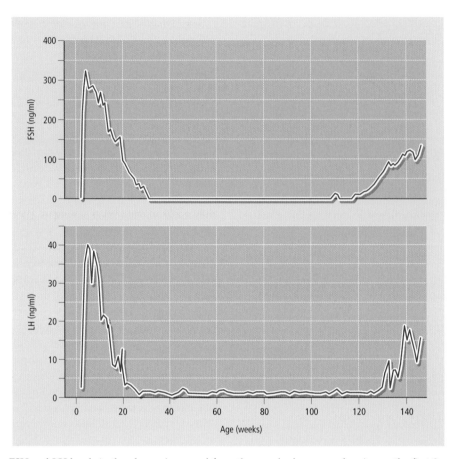

Fig. 7.7 Circulating FSH and LH levels in the plasma (averaged from three male rhesus monkeys) over the first 3 years of life (0, day of birth). These data actually came from monkeys that were bilaterally orchidectomized at approximately 1 week of age, but intact animals show very similar patterns (see text). Blood samples were collected at weekly intervals for 142 weeks. LH and FSH pulses occur during the first 20 weeks or so of life when plasma levels are in the adult range. Thereafter secretion ceases and levels remain low or undetectable through childhood and juvenile stages until about week 120. The first visible change is an increase in FSH secretion followed soon after by increasing pulsatile secretion of LH. It is important to emphasize that these changes occur whether or not testosterone is present in the circulation. Thus, altered gonadotrophin secretion is a function of altered hypothalamic GnRH output independent of any alteration in steroid feedback regulation of this hypothalamic–pituitary system.

levels rise to the adult range, thereby heralding the onset of puberty. As we have established in Chapter 6, pulsatile gonadotrophin secretion is driven by pulsatile GnRH secretion. Therefore, the search for the mechanisms underlying puberty must inevitably focus on why the GnRH pulse generator becomes inactive during the juvenile hiatus and what overcomes it at the time of onset of pulsatile GnRH secretion.

Complementary experiments in intact juvenile female rhesus monkeys (about 2 years old) make a similar point. They were provided with an externally situated pump, which delivered pulses of GnRH intravenously at 1–1.5-h intervals (as described in Chapter 6). As can be seen in Fig. 7.10, ovulatory menstrual cycles, complete with oestradiol surges, LH surges and luteal progesterone peaks, were initiated and maintained in these females. Similar experiments on male juveniles give a comparable male maturational outcome.

These data suggest that the most important event in the initiation of puberty is activation of the hypothalamic mechanism, which delivers GnRH pulses to the anterior pituitary. Once this has occurred, the pituitary and ovary are able to respond instantly, and maintain their steroid-mediated negative and positive feedback interactions with the GnRH and gonadotrophin secretory mechanisms. All that the pituitary–gonadal unit requires for an adult pattern of functioning is the pulsatile secretion of GnRH from the hypothalamus. Figure 7.10 also shows rather dramatically that switching off the GnRH pump is followed by re-entry into the immature, prepubertal state. This reversibility

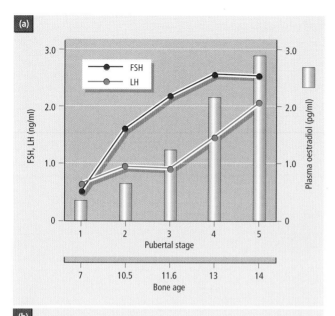

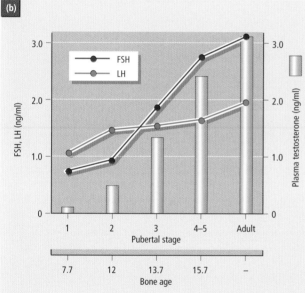

Fig. 7.8 Plasma concentrations of gonadotrophin and steroid hormones during various pubertal stages in (a) girls and (b) boys. Bone age is assessed by examining radiographs of hand, knee and elbow, and comparing them with standards of maturation in a normal population. It is an index of physical maturation, and better correlated with the development of secondary sexual characteristics than chronological age.

indicates that simply exposing the hypothalamus to adult levels of circulating steroids does not contribute to the attainment of a 'mature' pattern of functioning. These experiments provide a convincing demonstration that puberty arises solely as a consequence of a maturational event within the CNS, translated to the pituitary–gonadal system as a stream of GnRH pulses.

The outcome of clinical studies confirms these experimental results. Thus, in human infants, the first 6 months or so of life are associated with fluctuating, often high, plasma levels of FSH, LH, testosterone (in boys) and oestradiol (in girls, see above). By about 1–2 years of age, the system has quietened down and gonadotrophin and steroid concentrations are very low prepubertally. Gonadotrophin levels in agonadal children, for example those with Turner's syndrome (see Chapter 1), increase around the expected time of puberty in the absence of gonadal steroid influences, similar to the observations on immature castrate monkeys (see Fig. 7.7). Furthermore, precocious puberty may occur in children as young as 2 years of age. Here it is also apparent that the pituitary and gonads can function in an adult manner when activated pathologically, often as a result of a CNS tumour (see Table 7.1).

Thus, it is clear that the hypothalamus is capable of synthesizing GnRH during the prepubertal period, and indeed does so at a low level. Likewise the anterior pituitary can respond to GnRH stimulation by secreting gonadotrophins, as can the ovary and testis to LH and FSH. The genesis of puberty must therefore be sought within the CNS. How is a GnRH secretion restrained or damped during childhood and juvenile years? And what triggers its reactivation at the onset of adolescence?

Neural mechanisms regulating GnRH secretion at puberty initiation

The neural sites mediating puberty initiation must involve the hypothalamus, given that the GnRH neurons are the final common effector pathway. Clinical pathology provides us with limited information on areas of the CNS concerned with puberty. Thus, cases of advanced or delayed puberty may be associated with an underlying neuropathology (Table 7.1), but understanding the mechanisms by which lesions affect puberty onset is not simple. Generally, lesions of the anterior hypothalamic area are associated with delayed puberty, whereas more posterior lesions, from the median eminence to the mammillary bodies, are associated with precocious puberty. The problem is that the lesions are often large, of complicated and widespread origin, and variably secrete gonadotrophins or prolactin, which may have direct effects on gonads, so accurate interpretation of the lesion significance is difficult.

Neuropharmacological studies are more informative. We have seen that GnRH synthesis and even release are detectable at very low levels throughout the juvenile period. Moreover, premature activation of GnRH output can occur pathologically to drive early puberty. Can pharmacological manipulations also stimulate GnRH output and thereby give us clues as to CNS sites of control?

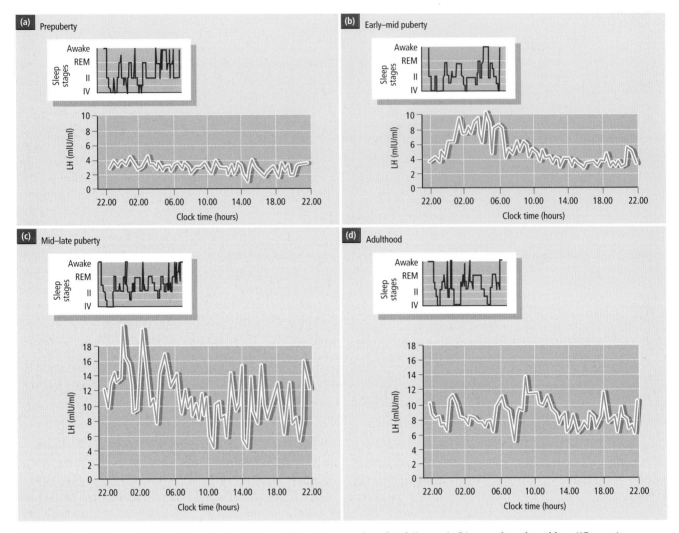

Fig. 7.9 Plasma LH concentrations throughout a 24-h period in: (a) a prepubertal girl (9 years); (b) an early pubertal boy (15 years); (c) a late pubertal boy (16 years); and (d) a young adult male. The sleep pattern for each nocturnal sleep period is depicted in the top left-hand corner of each graph (REM, rapid eye movement or 'paradoxical' sleep). Note the marked daily rhythm in (b), with sleep-augmented LH secretion, and the overall higher LH concentrations in (d) compared with (a), but no clear daily rhythm in either.

We saw in Chapter 6 (Box 6.1) that two neuropharmaco-logical systems exercised depressant effects on GnRH and gonadotrophin output: opioids and γ-aminobutyric acid (GABA). Might they be responsible for suppressing GnRH output before puberty? The use in juveniles of opioid antagonists such as naloxone has not, under a range of conditions, led to increased GnRH pulsing. In contrast, GABA has been clearly implicated in pubertal activation. Thus, microdialysis experiments in the rhesus hypothala-mus showed that GABA release became depressed as GnRH output rose. In addition, premature juvenile dis-charge of GnRH can be achieved either by down-regulating GABA synthesis or by blocking its interaction with its receptor using bicuculline. In humans, treatment of

childhood premature gonadarche with a GABA agonist decreased gonadotrophin output and regressed the puber-tal changes. Agonist use has also been reported to delay puberty. Thus, release of GABAergic inhibition is impli-cated in puberty initiation.

What about a role for neuropharmacological systems that promote GnRH release in adults? Hypothalamic gluta-mate (Box 6.1) release becomes elevated at puberty initia-tion, and the sustained pulsatile administration of the glutamate analogue NMDA prepubertally results in increased GnRH pulsing and precocious puberty. In addi-tion, we noted in Chapter 6 that puberty failed to occur in patients with null mutations of the receptor for kisspeptin (Box 6.2). *KiSS-1* gene expression rises as puberty is initi-

Fig. 7.10 Induction of ovulatory menstrual cycles in an intact immature female rhesus monkey by the infusion of GnRH (1 mg/min for 6 min once every hour). The period of GnRH infusion is shown by the horizontal bar (day 0–110); levels of LH, FSH, oestradiol and progesterone were undetectable in blood samples prior to GnRH infusions. Note that the first oestradiol surge did not elicit a full LH surge (c.day 30). However, subsequent oestradiol surges induced both LH surges and evidence of corpus luteum formation (progesterone peaks). These LH surges, as well as ensuring menstrual periods (M), occurred at 28-day intervals. Cessation of GnRH infusions (immediately after the LH surge, c.day 112) was followed by prompt re-entry into a non-cyclic, prepubertal state. Implantation of an oestradiol-containing silastic capsule subcutaneously (between 140 and 150 days, as indicated by bar) to produce surge levels of oestradiol in blood, did not induce an LH surge in the absence of exogenous GnRH.

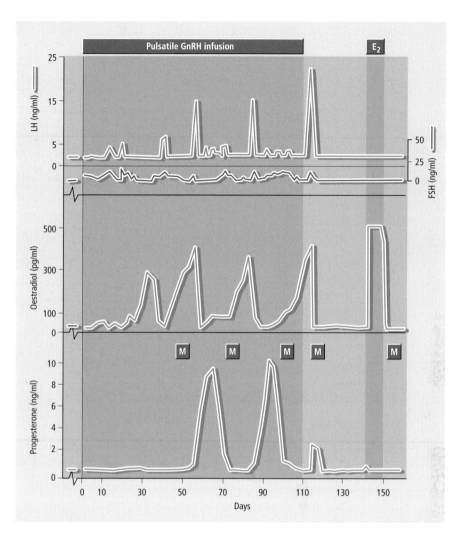

Table 7.1 Neurological lesions associated with advanced or delayed puberty in humans.

| Site of lesion | Puberty | | Type of lesion |
	Precocious	Delayed	
Hypothalamus			
Anterior		X	Hamartoma (hyperplastic nerve cells, fibres and glia)
Middle and posterior (including mammillary bodies)	X		Germinoma (germ cell tumour); teratoma (embryonic tumour); third ventricle cyst
Pineal gland*			
Parenchymatous		X	Glandular tissue tumour (rare)
Non-parenchymatous	X		Non-glandular tissue tumour
Pituitary gland*			
		X	Craniopharyngioma/chromaphobe adenoma
	X		Gonadotrophin-producing

*Pineal gland tumours were thought to affect puberty onset indirectly by mechanical compression of the underlying hypothalamus (see Fig. 6.1), but probably in fact secrete gonadotrophins (particularly teratomas) or melatonin (glandular tumours of the pineal). Chromaphobe adenomas (hyperplastic lactotrophs) producing high levels of prolactin. Craniopharyngioma: tumour of Rathke's pouch originating from the pituitary stalk; chromaphobe adenoma: prolactin-secreting tumour of the anterior pituitary.

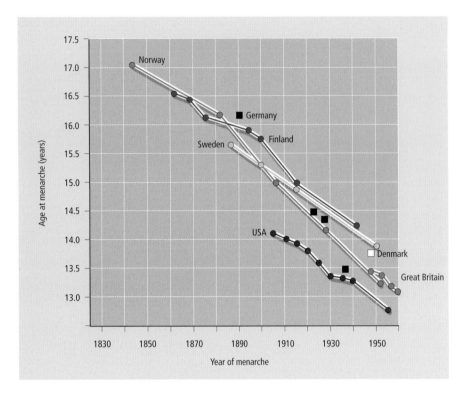

Fig. 7.11 Secular trend towards an earlier age at menarche in girls from Western Europe and the USA.

ated in monkeys, and the administration of exogenous kisspeptin to juvenile monkeys activates GnRH output and advances puberty.

These studies suggest that puberty initiation is associated with both the lifting of inhibitory restraint by GABA and the activation of glutamate and kisspeptin systems. They do not, however, establish whether there is a hierarchy of controls, or the precise level(s) of control within that hierarchy. Furthermore, although these studies provide possible mechanisms for pubertal activation, they do not address the activating signal itself. We now consider what is known of how puberty timing might be triggered via these neuropharmacological systems.

The timing of puberty is linked to the attainment of a critical body weight

The factors responsible for triggering and timing the onset of puberty have proved elusive. Is there a clock built into the brain, or is the brain monitoring responsively some parameter of ageing or growth? One phenomenon that suggests the latter mechanism is illustrated in Fig. 7.11. Thus, although the age at which girls first menstruate shows a considerable range within the population, there has been a clear secular trend towards an earlier menarche in girls and puberty in boys in Western Europe and the USA over the past century. What factors

have changed that might have contributed to the earlier attainment of sexual maturity, and do they give any insight into the mechanisms controlling the initiation of puberty?

Clearly, there may be more than one answer to this question. Health care and personal health have improved during this time, along with living conditions and socioeconomic standards. Clinical and experimental studies implicate two factors in this secular trend to earlier puberty, and in the mechanisms underlying pubertal onset. These are photoperiod and nutrition, of which the second does indeed seem to be important in humans.

Photoperiod influences reproductive activation in some mammals—but not in humans

In Western society, we are able to control our physical environment, for example by using electricity to artificially extend the length of the day. Indeed, daily dark periods may be consistently as short as 7 h all the year round, as if we were in constant 'long days' or a summer photoperiod. As we discussed in Chapter 6, in non-primate species, such changes in day length may have a major impact on reproductive status. However, the intensity of domestic lighting is probably not high enough to influence photosensitive neural mechanisms that might regulate GnRH secretion. Moreover, there is little direct evidence that photoperiod affects either reproductive maturation or adult reproductive activity in the human.

Nutritional factors influence sexual maturation

It seems reasonable to suggest that nutritional factors might have important effects on sexual maturation. Indeed, examination of cultures, such as the nomadic Lapps, that have not experienced such major improvements in living standards and nutrition, show that between 1870 and 1930 there was little or no trend towards an earlier menarche. Experimental studies that emphasize the importance of nutrition on reproduction in the adult are abundant. For example, maintenance of female rats on a low-protein diet, such that their body weight is held consistently at 80% of normal, results in the cessation of oestrous cycles. Subsequent sudden exposure of these animals to high-protein food restores the ability to discharge LH after oestradiol challenge. The practice of 'flushing' sheep, exposing them to rich pasture, increases the ovulation rate and also induces an earlier onset of oestrus and lambing, a phenomenon exploited by farmers. These examples suggest that food intake, or some reflection of it such as body weight or relative adiposity, is correlated with reproductive efficacy in the adult. Is it similarly associated with the onset of puberty?

Body weight appears to be a critical determinant of pubertal activation

In Fig. 7.12, it can be seen that although age at menarche has changed considerably during the past 100 years, the body weight at menarche has remained surprisingly constant at about 47 kg for females. Similar constancy is seen in the weight at onset of the adolescent growth spurt. These data have led to the suggestion that, at least in girls, a critical weight must be attained before the hypothalamic–pituitary–gonadal axis is activated and the growth spurt can occur. According to this view, body weight or, more correctly, a critical metabolic mass related to body weight, may trigger and therefore time the onset of puberty. A similar suggestion for a critical weight of 55 kg underlying sexual maturation in boys has also been made. The earlier occurrence of puberty today, compared to a century ago, may therefore be explained by earlier attainment of a critical weight, resulting from improvements in nutrition, health care and social living conditions. Evidence in support of this view is, at first sight, abundant. Moderately obese girls experience an earlier menarche than lean girls. Malnutrition is associated with delayed menarche. Primary amenorrhoea is extremely common in ballet dancers at professional schools who are in the very low range of weight for height and relative fatness for their age. Adolescent girls with the complex syndrome of anorexia nervosa, who have a very low food intake (particularly carbohydrate) and body weight, show primary amenorrhoea and/or delayed puberty. Moreover, the amenorrhoea is associated with a body weight below 47 kg, while in some anorexic girls who begin to refeed, the recurrence of menstruation is associated with attainment of a 47 kg body weight.

This impressive array of supportive data relating body weight to menarche also seems commonsensical. Thus, the attainment of a body size sufficient to cope with the

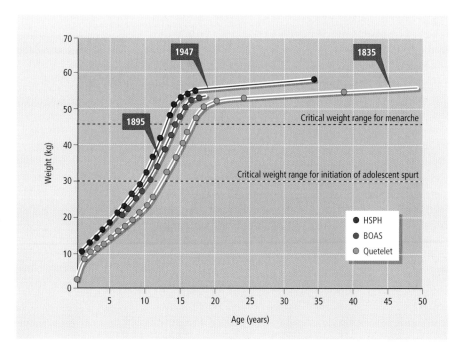

Fig. 7.12 Age plotted against body weight in three populations of girls in 1835, 1895 and 1947. Note the constant weights at initiation of the growth spurt (30 kg) and at menarche (47 kg). (Populations: Belgian girls in 1835 from data of Quetelet, 1869; American girls in 1895 adapted from data of BOAS; and in 1947 adapted from data of Reed and Stuart, 1959).

demands placed on it by adult reproductive activities such as pregnancy (some 50000 kcal) would be a logical signal for the onset of puberty. However, whether it is simply a total body weight threshold that is monitored is controversial. Thus, the time of onset of puberty might be related causally to other parameters, such lean body weight, absolute or proportionate body fat, or total body water. Indeed, it is quite difficult to predict age of menarche from knowledge of an individual's body weight and weight gain. Secondly, many anorexic girls who reattain their critical body weight do not begin having menstrual cycles, although this may simply reflect the fact that anorexia nervosa is a far more complicated syndrome than just a disorder of food intake and consequent weight loss. Thirdly, menarche is a rather late event in puberty, and may therefore be much removed from the critical factors that determine the onset of those endocrine changes described above, even if menarche itself is often related to body weight. Recent studies in molecular endocrinology have explored the triggering signals that might reflect some aspect of body weight.

Hormonal involvement in the activation of puberty?

Several hormones have been investigated for a possible role in monitoring some aspect of body growth and thereby triggering puberty initiation. Most recently, leptin (see Table 3.6) has been a focus of attention. Leptin is a cytokine secreted by adipocytes, its levels being a measure of fat mass. It acts on the hypothalamus to regulate feeding behaviour, energy expenditure and body weight. Leptin is the product of the *obese* gene, mutations in which increase food intake and lower body temperature, leading to obesity. Homozygous mutant mice are also infertile, a feature reversed by treatment with leptin. Could leptin be involved in the control of the hypothalamic–pituitary–gonadal axis at puberty?

Leptin does indeed rise during puberty. However, it is not at all clear from studies in humans and monkeys that the rise precedes, and could therefore drive, puberty initiation. What about premature induction of puberty by leptin? In juvenile monkeys or in children being treated for leptin deficiency the evidence for premature GnRH pulsing, LH elevation or puberty induction or advancement is thin and very mixed. Genetic studies in humans do suggest some sort of role for leptin in puberty, although not necessarily in its initiation. Thus, in one family, three obese sisters were homozygous for a splice mutation in the leptin receptor, leading to a truncated form of the receptor with no signalling function. Two of the sisters (aged 13.5 and 19 years) showed no sign of pubertal development and no GnRH secretion was detected. In a second family, a homozygous mutation of the leptin gene resulted in low circulating levels of plasma leptin and morbid obesity in three affected family members. Two of these, a 22-year-old man and a 34-year-old woman, had clearly failed to go through puberty, again with good evidence of a failure of hypothalamic GnRH activation of pituitary gonadotrophin secretion.

Thus the evidence linking leptin to the activation of hypothalamic GnRH secretion at puberty leaves unresolved the precise role that it plays. Leptin seems unlikely to be a trigger for GnRH secretion, but perhaps does provide some form of permissive or background presence that is essential if another as yet unidentifed trigger is to initiate pulsatile GnRH secretion.

Studies on melatonin, growth hormone and corticosteroids have likewise proved inconclusive, and none of these hormones seems a likely trigger for puberty.

Summary

Puberty is a crucial transition for reproduction. In humans and higher primates there is a particularly prolonged period between birth and puberty initiation, which may mean that the features by which the timing in higher primates is controlled are unique. It is clear that a reactivation of GnRH pulsing to levels seen immediately postnatally is involved and that the CNS provides the route by which reactivation is mediated. There is clear evidence linking some aspect of body weight increase and growth to the triggering of puberty, but as yet we have not identified the exact link between these two processes.

In the next chapter, we leave consideration of the development and maturation of the hypothalamic–pituitary–gonadal axis and its regulation, and begin our examination of its impact functionally on the rest of the body.

FURTHER READING

General reading

Conway GS, Jacobs HS (1997) Leptin: a hormone of reproduction. *Human Reproduction* **12**, 633–635.

Ebling FJP (2005) The neuroendocrine timing of puberty. *Reproduction* **129**, 675–683.

Hughes IA (1983) Precocious puberty and its management. *British Medical Journal* **66**, 664–665.

Plant TM, Barker-Gibb ML (2004) Neurobiological mechanisms of puberty in higher primates. *Human Reproduction Update* **10**, 67–77.

Plant TM, Witchel SF (2006) Puberty in non-human primates and humans. In: *The Physiology of Reproduction*, Vol. 2 (ed. J.D. Neill), 3rd edn, pp. 2177–2230. Academic Press, New York.

O'Rahilly S (1998) Life without leptin. *Nature News and Views* **392**, 330–331.

Smith JT *et al.* (2006) Regulation of the neuroendocrine reproductive axis by kisspeptin-GPR54 signaling. *Reproduction* **131**, 623–630.

KEY LEARNING POINTS

- Puberty is a state of transition (adolescence) between the juvenile and adult states.

- In primates it is preceded by infancy (from birth to weaning), childhood (a period of dependence on adults for survival) and the juvenile stage (when survival without adults is possible).

- In higher primates, the onset of puberty is considerably delayed postnatally compared with other mammals.

- Puberty involves gonadarche in all mammals and adrenarche in great apes and humans.

- Physical changes include sexually dimorphic growth differences and differences in lean muscle and fat mass.

- Secondary sexual characteristics develop at puberty under the influence of the rising output of gonadal steroids.

- Adrenal androgens stimulate the appearance of pubic and axillary hair.

- Characteristic increases in the secretion of GnRH, gonadotrophins and gonadal steroids occur during pubertal activation.

- Activation of pulsatile hypothalamic GnRH secretion is the key and primary event underlying gonadal activation.

- One of the first endocrine changes to occur is an increase in gonadotrophin secretion at night.

- Pubertal activation is associated with reduced GABAergic inhibition and increased glutaminergic and kisspeptin stimulation of GnRH output.

- Lesions in the CNS can be associated with advanced or delayed puberty, but are difficult to interpret mechanistically.

- There is a secular trend towards an earlier age of onset of puberty.

- This secular trend is primarily linked to attainment of a critical body weight at progressively earlier ages during the last century.

- Attainment of a critical body weight, or some related feature such as a critical body fat content, seems to be a key trigger to the onset of puberty.

- Endocrine markers of body development such as leptin are implicated in the onset of puberty, but are unlikely to be causally involved as its trigger.

Terasawa E, Fernandez D (2001) Neurobiological mechanisms of the onset of puberty in primates. *Endocrine Reviews* **22**, 111–151.

More advanced reading

Carel J-C *et al.* (2004) Precocious puberty and statural growth. *Human Reproduction Update* **10**, 135–147.

Clément K *et al.* (1998) A mutation in the human leptin receptor gene causes obesity and pituitary dysfunction. *Nature* **392**, 398–401.

Frish RE *et al.* (1972) Weight at menarche: similarity for well-nourished and under-nourished girls at differing ages and evidence for historical constancy. *Pediatrics* **50**, 445–450.

Frisch RE *et al.* (1973) Components of weight at menarche and the initiation of the adolescent growth spurt in girls: estimated total water, lean body weight and fat. *Human Biology* **45**, 469–483.

Hull KL, Harvey S (2001) Growth hormone: roles in female reproduction. *Journal of Endocrinology* **168**, 1–23.

Reed RB, Stuart HC (1959) Patterns of growth in height and weight from birth to eighteen years of age. *Pediatrics* **24**, 904–921.

Tanner JM (1978) *Foetus into Man; Physical Growth from Conception to Maturity*. Open Books, Wells.

Tanner JM (1986) *Growth at Adolescence*. Blackwell Scientific Publications, Oxford.

8 Actions of Steroid Hormones in the Adult

In the foregoing chapters we have established the pivotal role of the gonads and their steroid secretions in reproductive events. We have been concerned mainly with steroid action in two areas: (1) in the generation and maintenance of sexual differentiation during fetal, neonatal and pubertal life; and (2) in the regulation of gonadotrophin secretion by the hypothalamic–pituitary axis. In this chapter, we will examine in more detail those remaining actions of the steroids in the adult male and non-pregnant female that ensure the attainment of full reproductive capacity both physically and behaviourally.

The effects of sex steroids may conveniently be thought of as falling into two broad categories: some steroid actions are *determinative*, others are *regulatory*. *Determinative actions* involve essentially qualitative changes, which are irreversible or only partially reversible. Examples of this type of action are provided by the effect of androgens on the development of the Wolffian ducts and the generation of male external genitalia, the mild enhancement of these sexually distinct features by the low prepubertal androgen levels in males, and the changes in hair pattern, baldness, depth of voice, penile and scrotal size and bone growth that occur at puberty, as well as those in brain structure and function in non-primates. These actions constitute part of a progressive androgenization, which establishes a clear and distinc-

tive male phenotype. It represents the completion of a process initiated with the expression of the *SRY* (sex-determining region on the Y chromosome) gene. In females, an active determinative role for steroids first occurs during the prepubertal and pubertal period, when body growth, changes in size and shape, and growth of secondary sex hair are stimulated.

In contrast, the *regulatory actions* of steroids are reversible, and can involve both quantitative and qualitative changes to established accessory sex organs and tissues. These actions are not concerned with establishing the individual as a male or a female. They are concerned with ensuring that their reproductive tracts and genitalia function effectively in the reproductive process. In males, the regulatory actions of testicular steroids influence the activity of the accessory sex glands, metabolism, erectile capacity and, in some species, the more exotic secondary sexual characteristics, such as antlers in deer. These actions may be continuous or show seasonal variation. In females, it is the regulatory action of oestrogens and progestagens that results in the external manifestations of the menstrual and oestrous cycles. These external changes are accompanied by cyclic changes in the vagina, cervix, uterus and oviducts and, in some species, for example the ferret, swelling of the vulva or, in various female primates, the perineal sexual skin.

Androgens regulate the functional activity of the male reproductive system

In Chapter 4, we saw that testosterone was essential for the maintenance of spermatogenesis. Neutralization of testosterone by an antibody, or by synthetic antiandrogens, blocks or reduces spermatozoal production. Testosterone deprivation also has profound and immediate effects on the accessory sex glands of the male's genital tract (Fig. 8.1). After castration, the prostate, seminal vesicles and epididymides (or their equivalents in various species: Table 8.1), involute, their epithelia shrink and secretory activity ceases (Fig. 8.2). Direct measurement of their metabolic and synthetic activity shows a dramatic fall, and seminal plasma is no longer produced. If castrated animals are provided with exogenous testosterone, the involuted organs are fully restored, in both size and secretory activity. This reversible regression of accessory sex gland activity occurs naturally in seasonally active males, such as sheep and deer. The seasonal appearance of secondary sexual characteristics, such as antlers, and the behavioural interactions during which they are used, are similarly dependent on the actions of androgens. This androgen reaches its targets in blood, lymph and, in the case of the epididymus, in the fluids carrying the spermatozoa (Chapter 4).

Not surprisingly, these target organs for androgen activity are found to possess both androgen receptors and the enzyme 5α-reductase, so androgenic stimulation is

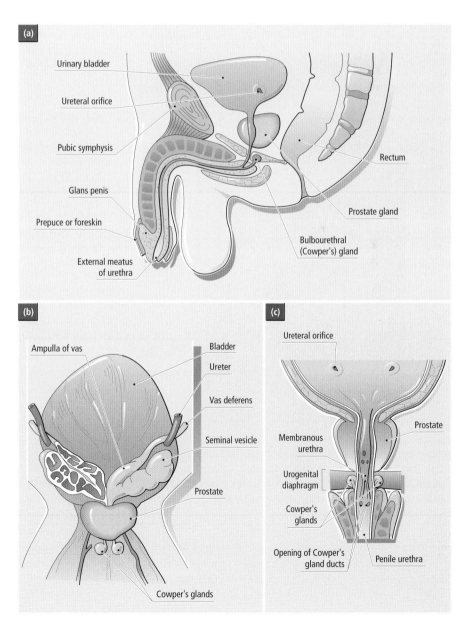

Fig. 8.1 View of human male accessory sex glands: (a) midsagittal section through pelvis; (b) posterior view of dissected pelvic contents; (c) coronal section through (b) viewed anteriorly.

Table 8.1 Relative size of principal male accessory sex glands.

Species	Prostate	Seminal vesicle	Ampulla	Cowper's or bulbourethral glands
Human	+++	++	+	±
Bull	+	+++	++	±
Dog	+++	–	–	–
Boar	++	+++	–	++
Stallion	++	+	++	±
Ram	++	+	++	++

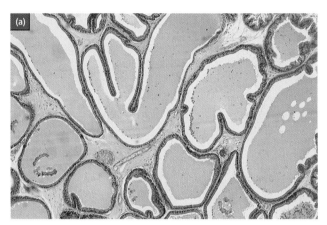

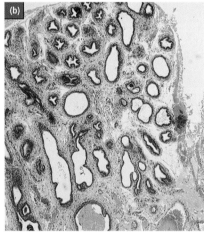

Fig. 8.2 Sections through prostate from: (a) intact rat; and (b) rat 18 days after castration (both same magnification). Note that after castration there is a reduction in luminal size and secretory content, a reduced height of the luminal secretory epithelium and a relative expansion of the proportion of connective tissue.

provided by both testosterone and its more potent derivative 5α-dihydrotestosterone. In Chapter 6, we mentioned that the local activity of androgens is enhanced by prolactin. This relationship is reciprocated, as androgen-dependent prolactin receptors are present in both prostate and seminal vesicles, and prolactin itself is detectable in seminal plasma at higher levels than in blood.

In addition to their effects on secondary sex organs, androgens also have distinctive anabolic or myotrophic effects, a reflection of which is the characteristically more muscular appearance of males that becomes progressively established after puberty. Androgens also increase kidney and liver weight, depress thymus weight, affect fat metabolism and distribution and stimulate erythropoiesis. The behavioural effects of androgens are addressed later. Pharmacologists have devised a range of synthetic androgens with different relative androgenic and anabolic potencies for use medically and abuse socially (Box 8.1).

Oestrogens and progestagens cyclically regulate the functional activity of the female reproductive system

In females, the shifting balance of hormones during the ovarian cycle affects oviducal, uterine, cervical and vaginal activity, as well as exerting more generalized physiological actions. The effects of steroids on these target organs may be studied by correlating changes in a normal cycle with changing steroid levels or experimentally by observing the consequences of injection of exogenous steroids into intact or castrate females.

Oestrogen and progesterone affect gamete transport by actions on the oviduct (Fallopian tube)

The oviduct is a thin muscular tube covered externally with serosal tissue and peritoneum. A ciliated, secretory, high columnar epithelium overlies the stromal tissue internally. The oviduct is the site of fertilization and therefore the oocyte passes along it from the fimbriated ostium towards the spermatozoa, which pass in the opposite direction from the isthmic junction with the uterus (see Fig. 5.1). A few days later, the fertilized zygote reverses the path taken by the spermatozoa to enter the uterus (see Chapters 9 & 10). Clearly then, the oviduct has a role in gamete transport. It

BOX 8.1 Anabolic effects of steroids: uses and abuses of anabolic-androgenic steroids (AASs)

- *What are AASs?* A range of synthetic testosterone derivatives has been developed with different relative anabolic and androgenic potencies, solubilities (and thus routes of administration) and metabolic stabilities (variable hepatic degradation or tissue conversion to oestrogens and 5α-dihydrotestosterone) (see Table 3.7 for some commonly used examples).

- *The anabolic actions* increase lean body mass, and muscle size, strength, repair and exercise tolerance, arising from increased muscle protein synthesis and possibly reduced degradation. Muscle fibre hypertrophy, increased myonuclear number, and muscle pennation (to give improved high-force, low velocity contractions) are observed. In addition, anabolic enhancement of collagen synthesis and of bone density (by osteoclast suppression) improves the mechanical effectiveness of the musculoskeletal system. AASs achieve this effect in part through direct binding to androgen receptors, but also perhaps by increasing the numbers of the receptors. GH and IGF1 stimulation may also assist anabolic impact.

- *AASs have been used medically* to treat muscle repair or wasting (age-, immobility- or HIV-related), as well as male hypogonadism, and, more controversially, for treatment of the 'male menopause' and erectile dysfunction (testosterone replacement therapy: Chapter 15). They have also been used to improve repair in elderly women suffering hip fractures.

- *Epidemiology of 'recreational use'.* Some 3% of young American adults (roughly equal numbers of men and women), around 20% of weight trainers, and, worryingly, 3–12% of adolescents (1–3% in Europe) have taken an AAS at least once in their lives for competitive or cosmetic muscle-building purposes. Lifetime prevalence usage data may exaggerate, as it is sustained use that is undesirable (see below). In general, supraphysiological doses of the more anabolic analogues such as stanozolol (30× more anabolic than testosterone) are used, but at such high levels that androgenic effects are also marked. Also, in an attempt to enhance anabolic effects, self-administration of multiple analogues occurs in combination (so-called 'stacking').

- *Health side effects of AAS use* are rarely serious in adults and probably are all reversible without long-term damage, but may be compounded by physical damage from excessive exercising, exacerbation of any psycho-sociological damage which may in part underlie AAS use in the first place, and, perhaps related to this, use of other performance-enhancing and self-esteem-boosting drugs at supraphysiological doses (adrenaline, amphetamines, growth hormone, diuretics, thryroxine, etc.). Minor and reversible adverse effects common to most users include acne, infection, hepatotoxicity, elevated blood pressure, temperamental instability; in men testicular atrophy, impotence, gynaecomastia; and in women hirsutism, voice deepening, clitoral enlargement and menstrual irregularities. For pubescent/immature users, longer-term problems associated with premature puberty and epiphyseal closure arise. For women, the long-term effects on fecundity are uncertain. Long-term administration to animals is associated with cardiovascular disease, hepatic tumours and infertility.

- *Ethico-legal aspects of AAS use* for the clinician include counselling about self-harm and psychological support and acute awareness of the dangers for adolescents. The professional consequences of detection for athletes are potentially severe. Legally, AASs are prescription-only drugs under the Medicines Act (UK), and thus only a doctor can legally prescribe them. They are classed as Schedule III Controlled Substances (USA) and Class C (UK, Misuse of Drugs Act; unlawful to possess or supply, although in practice possession purely for personal use is rarely pursued by the police).

Further reading

Bahrke MS, Yesalis CE (2004) Abuse of anabolic androgenic steroids and related substances in sport and exercise. *Current Opinion in Pharmacology* **4**, 614–620.

Cafri G *et al.* (2005) Pursuit of the muscular ideal: physical and psychological consequences and putative risk factors. *Clinical Psychology Review* **25**, 215–239.

Carson JA *et al.* (2002) Steroid receptor concentration in aged rat hind-limb muscle: effect of anabolic steroid administration. *Journal of Applied Physiology* **93**, 242–250.

Evans NA (2004) Current concepts in anabolic-androgenic steroids. *American Journal of Sports Medicine* **32**, 534–542.

Livermore CT, Balzer DG (eds) (2004) *Testosterone and Aging: Clinical Research Directions.* Institute of Medicine Committee on Assessing the Need for Clinical Trials of Testosterone Replacement Therapy. National Academies Press, Washington, DC.

Thiblina I, Petersson A (2004) Pharmacoepidemiology of anabolic androgenic steroids: a review. *Fundamental & Clinical Pharmacology* **19**, 27–44.

Vermeulen A (2001) Androgen replacement therapy in the aging male: a critical evaluation. *Journal of Clinical Endocrinology and Metabolism* **86**, 2380–2390.

---

must also provide a suitable environment for fertilization and the earliest development of the conceptus.

After ovariectomy, oviducal cilia are lost, secretion ceases and muscular activity declines, indicating an important steroidal influence on the oviduct. Subsequent injections of oestrogen restore both the ciliated, high columnar epithelium and secretory activity, and increase spontaneous muscle contractions. When progesterone is imposed on this oestrogen background, the numbers of cilia decline and the quantity of the oviducal secretion also declines, the small volumes of fluid that are produced having a lower sugar and protein content. Raising the progesterone:oestrogen ratio may also exert a mildly depressant effect on oviducal musculature, particularly relaxing the sphincter-like muscle at the uterotubal junction (although data on this are somewhat conflicting; see Box 8.2 for more discussion).

Oestrogen and progesterone cause cyclic changes in the uterus to support gamete transport and implantation

The uterus shows even more prominent steroid-dependent cyclic changes in structure and function than the oviduct (Fig. 8.3). During each cycle, the uterus first prepares to receive and transport the spermatozoa from the cervix to the oviduct (Chapter 9), and subsequently prepares to receive the conceptus from the oviduct and nourish it through to term (Chapters 10–13). The uterus consists of an outer peritoneal and serosal investiture, over a thick *myometrium* of smooth muscle arranged in distinctly orientated layers, which show spontaneous *fundo-cervical, cervico-fundal* and *isthmo-fundic peristaltic activities* throughout the cycle, but the balance of each varies (see below). Internally, the endometrium consists of a *stromal matrix* over which lies a simple low columnar *luminal epithelium* with *glandular epithelial* extensions penetrating into the stroma (Fig. 8.4).

BOX 8.2 The oviduct, hormones, emergency contraception, tobacco and cannabis

- *Can sudden changes in the oestrogen:progesterone ratio cause disturbances in gamete and conceptus transport?* When high doses of the synthetic oestrogen stilboestrol were taken within 72 h of fertilization, the pregnancy rate was reduced. This reduction was thought to be due to either *defects in sperm or oocyte transport*, and thus reduced fertilization, or *premature expulsion* of the conceptus from the oviduct. The drug was also associated with an increased incidence of *ectopic oviducal pregnancy*, leading to the suggestion that in these cases the embryo had became 'tube-locked'—perhaps due to spasm of the oviducal musculature *preventing* passage of the conceptus to the uterus.

- *Modern hormonal emergency contraception* (the 'morning-after pill') uses two doses of pills containing either a mix of synthetic high-dose progestagen AND oestrogen (the so-called *Yuzpe method*: levonorgestrel plus ethinylestradiol; see Table 3.7; prevents 57% of pregnancies), or high-dose progestagen-only (levonorgestrel—prevents 85% of pregnancies). In both cases, the first tablet should be taken within 72 h of intercourse and the second 12 h later, and efficacy declines with time since coitus. A double-strength single tablet is now also available. The progestagen-only preparation has fewer side effects, such as dizziness, nausea and vomiting (which itself may adversely affect efficacy by drug expulsion), and is thus preferred.

- *So how does levonorgestrel act?* The answer to this question has ethical implications for those who place a higher moral value on a fertilized than an unfertilized oocyte. The balance of evidence suggests that the absence/reduction of oestrogen reduces oviducal motility dysfunction as the underlying contraceptive mechanisms by a mix of ovulatory suppression, cervical mucus thickening, and perhaps endometrial dysfunction. Thus, the high dose of progestagen reduces sperm transport to the oviduct (see below and Chapter 10) and impairs terminal preovulatory maturation (Chapter 5). Together these actions would reduce fertilization rates, although this has not been measured directly in women. However, for women who are close to ovulating at the time of tablet-taking might there be a postfertilization action? Some indirect and inconclusive evidence suggests that endometrial sensitivity to the embryo may be reduced, but animal studies do not support any postfertilization effects. Thus, the cases of contraceptive failure may be due to the fact that the women had already been fertilized. Effective *postfertilization emergency contraception* (within 5 days of fertilization) can be achieved by inserting a copper intrauterine device (see Chapter 15).

- *Tobacco, cannabis and tubal function?* Recent evidence has suggested that cannabinoids can induce abnormalities of gamete/conceptus transport through an action on noradrenergic release, raising the question: might use of cannabis influence ectopic oviducal pregnancy rates? Similarly, tobacco smoking is associated with effects on tubal motility and higher ectopic rates.

Further reading

Croxatto HB *et al.* (2003) Mechanisms of action of emergency contraception. *Steroids* **68**, 1095–1098.

Faculty of Family Planning and Reproductive Health Care Clinical Effectiveness Unit (2006) Emergency contraception. *Journal of Family Planning and Reproductive Health Care* **32**, 121–128.

Gemzell-Danielsson K, Marions L (2004) Mechanisms of action of mifepristone and levonorgestrel when used for emergency contraception *Human Reproduction Update* **10**, 341–348.

Piaggio G *et al.* (1999) Timing of emergency contraception with levonorgestrel or the Yuzpe method. *Lancet* **353**, 721.

Talbot P, Riveles K (2005) Smoking and reproduction: the oviduct as a target of cigarette smoke. *Reproductive Biology and Endocrinology* **28**, 3:52.

Task Force on Postovulatory Methods of Fertility Regulation (1998) Randomised controlled trial of levonorgestrel versus the Yuzpe regimen of combined oral contraceptives for emergency contraception. *Lancet* **352**, 428–433.

Wang H *et al.* (2004) Aberrant cannabinoid signaling impairs oviducal transport of embryos. *Nature Medicine* **10**, 1074–1080.

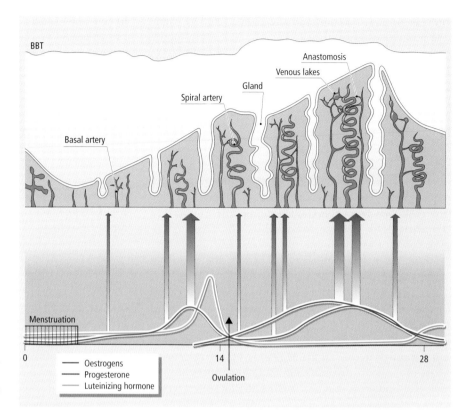

Fig. 8.3 Changes in human endometrium during the menstrual cycle. Underlying steroid changes are indicated below and basal body temperature (BBT) is indicated above. Thickness of arrows (oestrogens, red; progestagens, blue) indicates strength of action.

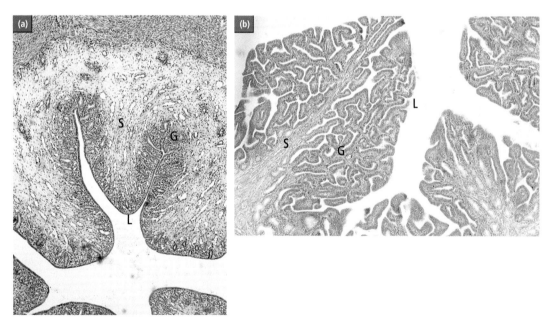

Fig. 8.4 Sections through rabbit endometrium during: (a) the late follicular phase (oestrus); and (b) the progestational phase. Note the dramatic increase in invaginations of the glandular epithelium (G) from the luminal surface epithelium (L) into stromal tissue (S).

After ovariectomy, all uterine tissues hypotrophy and the blood supply is reduced. Administration of oestrogen reverses this effect, with massive increases in mRNA and protein synthesis, cellular division and growth. In the normal cycle, the period of rapid oestrogen rises coincides with the latter half of the follicular phase of the menstrual cycle or, in non-primates, with the whole of the abbreviated follicular phase. During this phase a similar *uterotrophic* effect of oestrogen is observed. The myometrium increases both its contractility and its excitability, and cervicofundal peristalsis comes to dominate as ovulation approaches. Meanwhile in the endometrium, stromal thickening occurs, partly due to stromal cell proliferation. Reflecting this, the *uterine cycle* equivalent of the ovarian *follicular* phase is often called the *proliferative phase*. Stromal oedema also contributes to the thickening. The surface epithelium increases in surface area and metabolic activity. In primates and large farm animals, this also involves an increase in the numbers, and size, of the glandular invaginations of the stroma; this is less marked, however, in rabbits and rats. The oestrogen-primed epithelial cells secrete a fluid of a characteristically watery constitution, which contains a range of proteins, including proteolytic enzymes. These changes reach a maximum at the time of the oestrogen surge.

The oestrogens act by binding to oestrogen receptors (mainly the α receptor) present in abundance in uterine tissue. One of the most crucial actions of oestrogens over this period is to induce the synthesis of intracellular receptors for progesterone. At the beginning of the oestrogenic phase of the cycle, progesterone-binding receptors are at a low level, and progesterone therefore has little effect on the uterus. However, by the time of ovulation, the uterus is primed to bind progesterone, and so begins the progestagenic phase. In the rabbit and mouse, there is a rapid extension of the epithelial proliferation into glandular regions at this time (Fig. 8.4b).

Progesterone stimulates the synthesis of secretory material by the glands of most species so that they become distended with a thick secretion rich in glycoprotein, sugars and amino acids. In some species, the release of this glandular secretion into the lumen requires, or is facilitated by, a secondary peak of luteal-phase oestrogen imposed upon the progesterone background (see Chapter 10). For this reason, the luteal phase of the ovarian cycle corresponds to the *secretory phase* of the uterine cycle. Stromal proliferation also increases under the influence of progesterone, the stromal cells becoming larger and plumper, particularly so in rodents and primates. Within the stromal tissues of primates, characteristic spiral arteries become fully developed (see Fig. 8.3). Curiously, but importantly (see Chapters 10 & 11), prolonged progesterone exposure of the uterine epithelia (but *not* of the stroma) causes down-regulation of progesterone receptors and a corresponding rise in oestrogen receptors, indicating that luteal oestrogen may act primarily through epithelial cells. Progesterone also acts on the myometrium causing further enlargement of cells but, in contrast to oestrogens, progesterone *depresses* the overall excitability of the uterine musculature such that the fundus is quiescent, and only limited range peristalsis occurs from cervical and isthmic

foci. It is important to re-emphasize that these actions of progesterone will only occur in an oestrogen-primed uterus, another example of receptor regulation (see Chapter 3).

With the withdrawal of steroid support at the end of the luteal phase of the cycle, the elaborate secretory epithelium collapses, with evidence of apoptotic cell death. In most mammals, the endometrium is resorbed and a thin stromal layer overlain with epithelium replaces it, ready for entry into a new uterine cycle as oestrogens rise. In humans, apes and Old World monkeys, the endometrial tissue is shed via the cervix and vagina, together with blood from the ruptured arteries, as the menses. The spiral arteries contract to reduce bleeding.

The properties of the cervix show steroid-dependent changes during the cycle that affect gamete transport

The cervix is traversed by the spermatozoa at coitus and the neonate at parturition (see Chapters 9 & 13). In many species, including humans, the spermatozoa must actively swim through the cervix, which also acts as a storage reservoir for them (see Chapter 9). The properties of the cervix show marked steroid-dependent changes during the cycle and these can be crucial for fertility. During exposure to oestrogen in the follicular phase, the muscles of the cervix relax and the epithelium becomes secretory. However, during the luteal phase, when progesterone levels are elevated, secretion is reduced and the cervix is firmer.

Cervical mucus may be collected for examination during the human cycle and tested in a variety of ways for its steroid-dependent properties. The test of greatest functional significance is that of sperm penetration, in which the capacity of spermatozoa to swim into and through a smear of mucus on a slide is assessed. Characteristically, sperm penetration is low in the early follicular and in the luteal phases of the cycle, and reaches a maximum around the time of ovulation (Fig. 8.5). These effects can be mimicked by administration of exogenous steroids: oestrogens enhance sperm penetration while progesterone, even in the presence of oestrogens, depresses penetration. Thus, continuous administration of progestagens throughout the cycle, or the local release of progestagens from capsules placed in the uterus, suppresses sperm penetration even at the time of ovulation and the oestrogen surge. Use is made of this property in the morning-after pill (Box 8.2) and low-dose progestagenic contraceptives (Chapter 15).

The steroids act via an effect on the amount and nature of the glycoproteins secreted by the cervical epithelium. Rising oestrogens stimulate the production of Muc5B and Muc4, both hydrophilic mucins which may form an aqueous

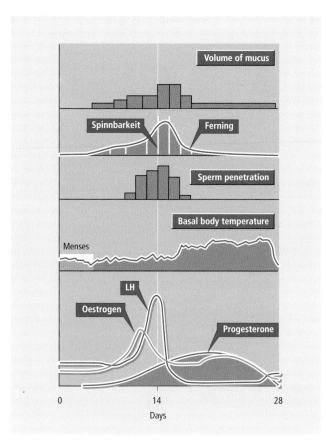

Fig. 8.5 Schematic view of changes in properties of cervical mucus at various days of the human cycle (blood hormone levels and basal body temperature shown). Parameters changing under the influence of high oestrogen and low progesterone are: volume of mucus; spinnbarkeit of mucus (bar height illustrates relative length to which mucus thread can be stretched before snapping); ferning (curve illustrates proportion of crystallized mucus that shows a ferning pattern when dried on a slide); and *in vitro* tests of the ability of spermatozoa to penetrate mucus. Note luteal oestrogen does not induce changes due to elevated progesterone at the same time. Progestagenic contraceptives, including the emergency 'morning-after' pill, prevent or reduce normal periovulatory changes. LH, luteinizing hormone.

matrix through which spermatozoa can swim, and which also may trap pathogens. The mucinous gel matrix may also hold the cervical canal patent. If mucus from oestrogenic cervices is allowed to dry on a slide, its distinctive molecular composition results in a characteristic pattern known as *ferning* (Fig. 8.5). Under progestagen dominance, secreted mucin levels decline precipitously, and strands of mucus can only be stretched a short length before the threads snap: a low *spinnbarkeit* (Fig. 8.5). These simple tests of cervical mucus are important, because a hostile, impenetrable cervix will reduce the progress of the sperm towards the oviduct and thus fertility.

Oestrogen and progesterone cause cyclic structural changes in the vagina

The vagina is the initial site of sperm deposition and also vulnerable to infection (Chapter 9), and it must distend sufficiently for parturition (Chapter 13). It shows marked structural changes during the cycle in some species. In the guinea-pig, for example, a membrane completely closes the vaginal os throughout most of the cycle, and only breaks down under the influence of rising plasma oestrogen concentrations at oestrus. In many mammals, including humans, oestrogens induce an increased mitotic activity in the columnar epithelium of the vagina, with a tendency to keratinize. This change is particularly marked in rodents, in which the stages of the oestrous cycle can be assessed reliably by examination of the different cell types present in daily smears from the vaginal epithelium (Fig. 8.6). The fluids within the vagina also change during the cycle, and one effect of this is to vary the metabolic substrates available to the bacterial flora there. Cyclic changes in the vagina, induced by oestrogen and progesterone, result in the generation by bacteria of differing proportions of volatile aliphatic acids. These give distinctive odours to vaginal secretions and may have marked behavioural consequences, as will be seen later in this chapter. The leukocyte population of the vagina is also steroid sensitive, an influx of polymorphonuclear neutrophilic leukocytes (PNLs) occurring under progesterone domination (Fig. 8.6).

Steroids, immune function and the female genital tract

The female tract has evolved to receive and transmit spermatozoa. This function exposes it to pathogens—particularly dangerous given the patent continuity between vaginal and peritoneal cavities. However, spermatozoa and the conceptus itself differ antigenically from the mother. There is thus a potential immune conflict for the uterus, the resolution of which is not yet fully understood. In addition, immune cells play roles in tissue remodelling, which is substantial during the menstrual cycle. It is clear that a dynamic, steroid-dependent population of immune cells and molecules characterizes the endometrium, some 7% of its cells being leukocytes. Chemokines that attract immune cells are synthesized in the uterus in patterns that vary with the steroid balance. Macrophages peak in the late secretory phase, and are thought to be involved in tissue breakdown associated with menses. Neutrophils are present in small numbers through most of the cycle, increasing massively as menstruation approaches because of progesterone withdrawal. During the secretory phase, uterine-specific natural killer cells (uNK cells) predominate in close contact with glands and blood vessels. Progesterone may stimulate uNK cells indirectly via stromal cells,

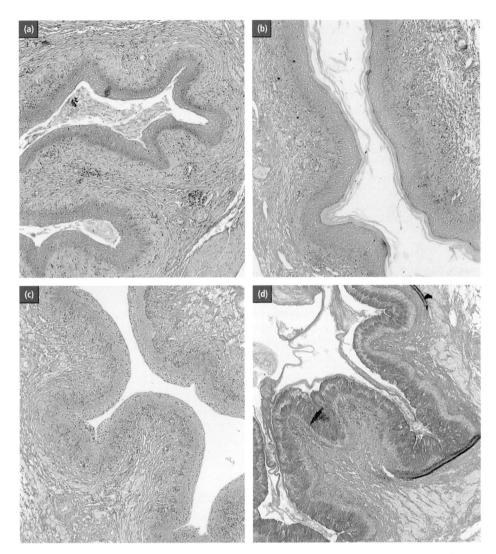

Fig. 8.6 Sections through the rat vagina to illustrate changes in the vaginal epithelium in response to changing hormones during the reproductive cycle. (a) Rising oestrogen during the follicular phase leading up to oestrus (*pro-oestrus*) causes nucleated cells (small dark spots) to be shed into the lumen and a keratin layer starts to develop on the surface epithelium. (b) This process is completed at oestrus with a heavily keratinized layer (yellow), some of which desquamates into the lumen. (c) During the short transition from oestrogen to progesterone dominance immediately after ovulation (the pregestational phase of *dioestrus*), the epithelial cells are nucleated and non-keratinized, and leucocytes are visible in the epithelium and pass into the lumen. (d) Under progesterone dominance during pregnancy, the surface epithelium is glandular and secretory (blue).

which possess progesterone receptors and secrete interleukin 15 (IL-15) and prolactin (which in turn stimulates IL-2 production). We return to the vexed question of maternal immune function in Chapter 12.

Other tissues

Many other features of a female's anatomy and physiology may change with the ovarian cycle. Oestrogens have general effects on the cardiovascular system and metabolism that may be revealed cyclically or in women taking oral contraceptives. Thus, oestrogens depress appetite, are mildly anabolic and maintain bone structure. They also appear to be involved in the reduced capillary fragility and higher levels of low- and high-density lipoproteins, and thus in the ability to bind cholesterol and the reduced incidence of thrombosis seen in premenopausal women when compared to men. Oestrogens may also increase the ability of the cardiovascular system to withstand high blood pressures. The mechanisms by which oestrogens act in this way are unclear. However, maintained elevated levels of oestrogens, such as occur in pregnancy or during treatment with *some* contraceptive pills, may in some women actually cause hypertension and, via effects on lipid metabolism, an increased blood-clotting rate (see Chapter 15).

Progesterone, in contrast to oestrogens, is mildly catabolic in humans. It has two major sorts of systemic action that may become manifest during the menstrual cycle. The first is on the central nervous system (CNS): so-called neuroactive effects. Progesterone elevates basal body temperature (Fig. 8.5) by a direct action on hypothalamic areas concerned with thermoregulation. The rise in temperature occurs only *after* ovulation and thus is only useful as a basis for establishing the regularity of a woman's cycle if the rhythm method of contraception is contemplated (see Chapter 15). Progestogenic steroids, such as progesterone, pregnenolone, dihydroepiandrosterone (DHEA) and 5α-reduced pregnenolone (*allopregnenolone*) also have anxiolytic effects, and the fall in progestagens towards the end of the menstrual cycle can result in the loss of this property and the development of anxiety, excitability and disturbances of mood (premenstrual tension).

Second, progesterone shows some affinity for aldosterone receptors in the kidney, presumably because of similarities of stereochemical structure. However, after binding by progesterone, the receptor is not activated and, in consequence, progesterone acts as an inhibitor such that natriuresis ensues. A compensatory rise in aldosterone output occurs to restore sodium (Na$^+$) retention. Retention of Na$^+$ in women may also be enhanced in the luteal phase by a direct stimulatory effect of luteal oestrogen on angiotensinogen production. The consequence of these events may be a net retention of Na$^+$ and water towards the end of the luteal phase, which contributes to some symptoms characteristic of the premenstrual period, for example, heavy, tender breasts.

These examples of the widespread cyclic changes in structure and function of many of the somatic tissues of a female, and not just her reproductive organs, show how the ovary and its secretions play such a dominant part in day-to-day physiology. Ovarian steroids also have profound and cyclic effects on the behaviour and mood of the females of some species and this, together with comparable effects of testicular hormones in males, is the subject of the next section.

Androgens and oestrogens are not exclusively male and female hormones

Before we leave peripheral tissues, a final reminder that whilst the concept of 'steroid hormone dimorphism' is broadly correct, it is also simplistic. For example, we have already encountered the androgen dependence of secondary sex hair in females (see Androgen Insensitivity Syndrome in Chapter 2). Likewise, in males, oestrogens play

an essential role in the transport of spermatozoa out of the testis, and genetic knockout of the oestrogen α-receptor renders males infertile (see Chapter 9 for details). Such observations affirm the view that oestrogen and testosterone should not be considered as simply 'female' or 'male' hormones: both have important roles in each sex.

Hormones regulate sexual behaviour in many species

We have already discussed in Chapter 2 how hormones may affect the developing brain and so influence or even determine the types of sexually dimorphic behaviour observed later in life. These same hormones can also influence how and whether these types of behaviour are actually expressed in adulthood.

Stimuli capable of eliciting sexual behaviour surround most of us most of the time, but sexual interaction occurs only sporadically. What determines when these sexual stimuli induce sexual activity? The answers to this question, particularly in primates and humans, are complex, but if we examine non-primate species we see rather clearly that hormones are very important. A castrated male or female rat, cat or dog does not display sexual activity when placed with a member of the opposite sex. Treatment with the appropriate hormones results in the activation of sexual behaviour, that is, sexual stimuli become effective again in inducing sexual responses. In these species, therefore, hormones increase the probability that an appropriate set of sexual stimuli will elicit sexual activity. In primates, including humans, this profound controlling influence of sex hormones has been modified considerably, such that social, experiential and volitional factors become increasingly important. Undoubtedly, this is one reflection of the increasing size and complexity of the brain, particularly the neocortex. We will first discuss the ways in which hormones affect sexual behaviour in various species, and then go on to consider how and where they exert their effects. Although much remains to be discovered, an important message will become apparent. Hormones alter the expression of sexual behaviour by acting *both* within the *brain* and on the *genitalia*.

Masculine sexual behaviour

Testosterone controls the expression of sexual behaviour in male non-primates

In adult non-primate males, sexual behaviour is clearly hormone dependent. It declines after castration and this decline is reversed by treatment with testosterone (Fig. 8.7). However, one feature of this relationship between testicular androgens and sexual behaviour remains difficult to explain. Although plasma testosterone is virtually undetectable within hours of castration, the decline in sexual behaviour takes several weeks to reach its nadir (Fig. 8.7). Similarly, treatment with testosterone after long-term castration will restore sexual behaviour, but does so with a relatively long latency (Fig. 8.7). Moreover, if the interval between castration and the initiation of testosterone replacement therapy is short, sexual behaviour is more readily restored than if several weeks elapse (Fig. 8.8). Furthermore, not all elements of masculine sexual behaviour are equally affected by removal of testosterone. Thus, mounting persists long after the cessation of intromission and ejaculation.

These results suggest that a 'memory trace' of the presence of testosterone lasts for some time in the target tissue(s) after castration, that sexual behaviour is only slowly restored, and that perhaps there are varying degrees of 'dependence' of different sexual responses on testosterone. What are these target tissues and do different tissues influence different responses and also have different sensitivities to testosterone? Clearly, the brain might be one important target, affecting the male's motivational state *directly*. But so also might be the genitalia, the peripheral effects of testosterone on their sensitivity to tactile stimuli or on the capacity for penile erection contributing *indirectly* to changes in sexual behaviour.

Some insight has been gained into this complicated problem as a result of the fortuitous finding in rats that testosterone exerts its *behavioural effects on the brain* only after aromatization to oestradiol (see Chapters 2 & 3). After castration, therefore, small amounts of oestrogen administered to male rats *will reverse the central or motivational deficits*, such as reduced mounting behaviour, but regression of seminal vesicles, prostate and cornified spines on the penis persists as do the attendant deficits in related sexual responses, such as erection and intromission. Conversely, when dihydrotestosterone, which cannot be aromatized to oestrogens in the brain, is given to castrate male rats, it has *potent stimulatory effects on sex accessory glands, penis and erectile responses*, but little or no effect on mounting behaviour. Combining extremely small amounts of oestradiol with dihydrotestosterone results in identical effects on behaviour and on genitalia to those seen after testosterone treatment. These findings suggest that in rats testosterone serves as a *prehormone*. Its androgenic effects on somatic structures depend on reduction to dihydrotestosterone and its effects on the brain depend on aromatization to oestradiol. Unfortunately, this precisely worked-out chain of events is far from universally applicable; for example, in primates aromatization does not seem to represent an obligatory event for the central actions of androgens, so the same dissection of behaviour cannot be applied.

Testosterone affects the sexual behaviour of male primates, including men

Chemical castration of male monkeys or men is usually followed by a reduction in sexual activity after weeks, months or years, but with considerable interindividual

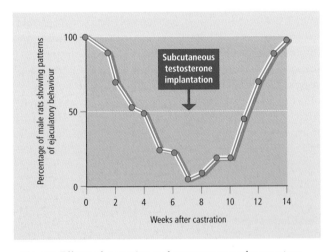

Fig. 8.7 Effects of castration and testosterone replacement on patterns of ejaculatory behaviour in the male rat. (Ejaculatory behaviour consists of a prolonged intromission and a characteristic manner of terminating the intromitted mount.) Note that appreciable levels of the behaviour persist for some weeks after castration and that a comparable time was required for restoration of the behaviour following the subcutaneous implantation of testosterone.

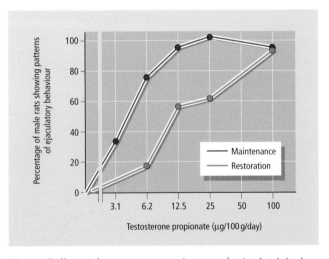

Fig. 8.8 Differential testosterone requirements for 'maintaining' ejaculatory behaviour in newly castrated rats and 'restoring' the same behaviour in long-term castrates. Note that more testosterone propionate was required in the latter group; treatment, as in Fig. 8.7, was given for several weeks to cause this change.

variability, and it is rarely complete. Even in monkeys, there are enormous individual differences in the types of response to castration. For example, a male monkey that has a history of separate sexual interactions with each of two females may, after castration, continue copulating more or less unchanged with one female, but lose his sexual interest completely in the other. Clearly, while testosterone has an important influence on sexual activity, its presence is not obligatory and other factors are also important in maintaining sexual interest, arousal and behaviour. Testosterone treatment effectively restores sexual interest to precastration levels, but the level of androgen required is much less than pretreatment levels, suggesting that normally testosterone levels are well above threshold for behavioural effects.

The same conclusion comes from the study of a different male population. Testosterone therapy has been used successfully to treat low levels of sexual arousal and activity in *hypogonadal or agonadal* men, and withdrawal of the hormone is followed reliably by a reduction in arousal and activity (Fig. 8.9). The same situation is occurring naturally at puberty. Thus prepubertal boys experience sexual arousal and erections, but at much lower levels than do pubescing and postpubescent adolescents. These situations can be contrasted with the testosterone treatment of intact (i.e. *eugonadal*) men, which generally does *not* result in an increase in sexual activity. Testosterone is not an aphrodisiac. It seems that treatment is only beneficial at restoring or stimulating sexual activity and interest *in men (or boys) with low testosterone levels*. There is a critical range of low plasma testosterone concentrations over which a clear positive sexual response to treatment can be expected. But once the adult range of testosterone levels is reached, that relationship is lost. The situation may be different in female primates, including women, as will be discussed further below. Conversely, antiandrogens, such as cyproterone, may reduce indices of sexual arousal in eugonadal men,

which has led to their use clinically to treat individuals with antisocial patterns of sexual behaviour, such as exhibitionism or paedophilia.

If the nature of the processes affected by androgens in these studies of hypogonadal men is to be elucidated, it is important to measure more than just the frequency of sexual acts. In the study summarized in Fig. 8.9, the frequency of sexual thoughts has been measured and this has proven to be a sensitive index of the effects of testosterone in hypogonadal men. Penile erections, whether spontaneously during rapid eye movement (REM) sleep (*nocturnal penile tumescence* or NPT) or in response to sexual stimuli, have also been measured. Only nocturnal erections are clearly testosterone dependent, an observation that has led to the differential diagnosis of organic and psychogenic impotence. Thus, preservation of NPT in men who lose erectile ability during sexual interactions is strongly indicative both of psychogenic impotence and of the likely ineffectiveness of testosterone therapy. Moreover, while it is the case that the low levels of plasma testosterone seen in hypogonadal men are highly correlated with low frequencies of sexual thoughts and erections induced by sexual fantasy (internal stimuli), erections in response to external stimuli, such as erotic films, do not appear to be so testosterone dependent (Fig. 8.10). However, their rigidity tends to be less and they are more likely to detumesce as soon as the external stimulus is removed.

As with studies on animals, the nature of the stimulus and the response must be considered carefully when interpreting these data. An interesting issue in studies of sexual behaviour in men is whether erections occur as a result of sexual arousal, or whether they also contribute to its development. Is penile erection a response or a stimulus? Erections may be such an important indicator to men of sexual excitement that a decrease in erectile ability may contribute to a much higher threshold for sexual arousal and hence decreased sexual activity. A clear separation of genital and

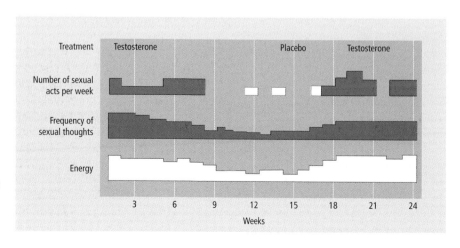

Fig. 8.9 The effects of testosterone replacement in a hypogonadal man aged 40, castrated 1 year earlier for testicular neoplasm. Sexual activity, ejaculation, sexual thoughts and energy all decline about 3 weeks after stopping testosterone treatment. There is no response to placebo, but a rapid response within 1 or 2 weeks of restarting testosterone treatment.

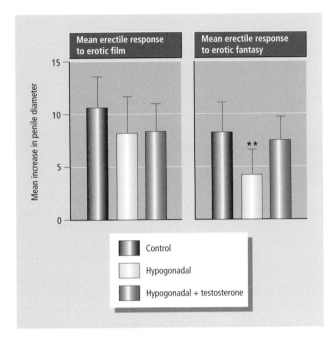

Fig. 8.10 Erectile response (measured as increase in penile diameter) to erotic film and fantasy in hypogonadal men with and without testosterone replacement. The hypogonadal men did not differ from controls in their response to the film, but their response to fantasy was significantly lower than controls when they were androgen deficient but improved with testosterone replacement. The latency of their erectile response was significantly reduced after hormone replacement. $**P < 0.01$.

motivational responsiveness to androgens in hypogonadal men has simply not been achieved, but actions at each site are probable.

Feminine sexual behaviour

Oestrogen and progesterone are critical for oestrous behaviour in female non-primates

In Chapters 5 and 6, we described how sexual receptivity or 'heat' occurs cyclically, and is closely coordinated with the period of ovulation, which ensures that copulation occurs at a time when fertilization is most likely. (Reflex ovulators such as the cat, rabbit and ferret have a somewhat different mechanism for achieving this end: the female comes into heat and stays in that state until she copulates, and this event itself triggers ovulation; see Chapters 5 & 6.) Ovariectomy in these species is followed by a prompt and usually complete abolition of *receptivity* (they will no longer accept mounts by the male) and *proceptivity* (they no longer 'solicit' males). Restoration of these elements of feminine sexual behaviour is achieved equally rapidly by treatment with oestradiol and, in some species, progesterone, which must be given by injection in appropriate sequence with

oestradiol so as to mimic the hormonal events seen during the oestrous cycle (see Fig. 6.25 for an example of the progesterone surge at oestrus in the rat). These behavioural events may be affected additionally by a circadian rhythm (e.g. in the rat, oestrus occurs in the dark phase of the day–night cycle) and/or a seasonal rhythm (e.g. in the ewe, oestrous cycles begin in the autumn), events discussed in more detail in Chapter 6.

Similarly, dramatic changes in behaviour are seen in large domestic animals, like the sheep and pig. Thus, the active nudging, blocking and nibbling responses displayed by oestrous ewes, or the immovable lordosis posture displayed by sows in heat, disappear after ovariectomy. Reinstatement of oestrous levels of these behavioural responses follows appropriate treatment with ovarian hormones, for example, progesterone followed by oestradiol in the ewe, mimicking the end of the luteal phase and the short follicular phase leading up to oestrus in the natural cycle.

So as in non-primate males, sexual behaviour in female non-primates seems to be totally dependent on their hormonal state. But, as for male primates, the situation for female primates is more complex.

Oestradiol and progesterone in female non-human primates do affect sexual behaviour—but in males

The strict relationship between ovarian hormones and sexual behaviour seen in non-primate female mammals is largely lost, or at least takes a rather different form, in female primates. Superficially, this does not appear to be the case since, if sexual interaction between a male and female monkey is observed, it is often seen to follow a cyclic pattern (Fig. 8.11a). Ovariectomy is followed by a major reduction in sexual interaction, which is restored by treating females with oestradiol. However, careful measurement of the sexual responses of males and females shows that it is mainly the *male's behaviour* that declines markedly after ovariectomy and increases after oestradiol treatment of ovariectomized females. Oestradiol is somehow changing the sexual 'attractiveness' of females to males. How?

Numerous experiments have pointed to the vagina as the site where oestradiol exerts these effects (Fig. 8.11b(D)), and have shown that it affects the odour of a female's vaginal secretions. Male rhesus monkeys rendered reversibly anosmic fail to discriminate between oestrogen-treated and untreated ovariectomized females. They copulate with the latter until their anosmia is reversed, at which point they usually cease promptly until oestrogen treatment (systemic or intravaginal) is resumed.

Analysis of vaginal secretions using gas chromatography and mass spectrometry has revealed the presence of a mixture of simple aliphatic acids (acetic, propionic, isobutyric, butyric and isovaleric), the concentrations of which

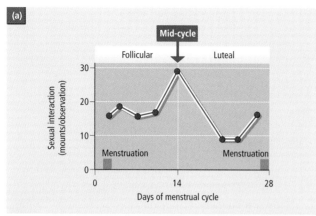

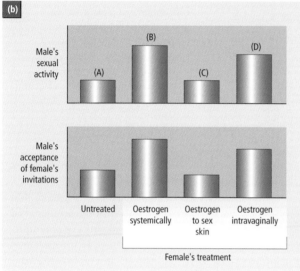

Fig. 8.11 (a) Sexual interaction, measured as mounts by the male, between pairs of male and female rhesus monkeys during the menstrual cycle. Note the high follicular-phase levels of interaction, which peak at mid-cycle and fall in the luteal phase. The premenstrual rise is characteristic. This pattern of interaction seems to be more due to fluctuating interest in the female by the male than vice versa, as is revealed more clearly in (b). (b) A block diagram summarizing the results of experiments which demonstrate that: (A) ovariectomy of females depresses the males' sexual activity and reduces their acceptance of sexual invitations by females; (B) treating females with oestradiol, by subcutaneous injections, increases both these parameters of the males' behaviour; (C) the effect is lost if the oestradiol is smeared, as a cream, on the female's perineum; (D) if it is placed in the vagina, an effect identical to that seen in (B) occurs. These data indicate that oestradiol increases sexual attractiveness by an action on the vagina.

vary during the menstrual cycle, which disappear after ovariectomy and are restored after oestrogen treatment. Vaginal lavages taken from oestrogen-treated female monkeys and placed on the perineum of untreated females

stimulate the sexual interest of males, as indeed do vaginal secretions from women and other species of monkey. Not surprisingly, therefore, the same aliphatic acids have been found in human vaginal secretions and they also vary in concentration during the menstrual cycle. Proof of the involvement of the aliphatic acids comes from the observation that a synthetic mixture in the correct proportions placed intravaginally in females can activate the same sexual interest of males (Fig. 8.12). The effectiveness of this mixture can be enhanced by the addition of phenolic compounds (phenylpropanoic and parahydroxyphenylpropanoic acids), which are also present in vaginal secretions, but are ineffective when applied alone. Thus, a female monkey's vagina clearly produces odour cues that are dependent on oestradiol. The acids are not a glandular product, but result from microbial action on vaginal secretions, and can be blocked by use of penicillin.

Progesterone can decrease the sexual attractiveness of female monkeys and does so by reducing the sex-attractant properties of vaginal secretions. This observation explains the decrease in sexual interaction during the luteal phase of the menstrual cycle. Clearly vaginal secretions can both 'turn on' and 'turn off' a male's sexual interest in a female.

Finally, it must be emphasized that these effects of odours on the sexual activity of males are not all or none. Some males are oblivious to changes in a female's odour, others seem to have their sexual activity completely regulated by them. This situation differs enormously from the stereotyped behavioural responses of other mammals, and particularly insects, to *pheromones*. These highly species-specific substances 'release' patterns of aggressive or sexual (and other) behaviour in an invariant way, very different from the effects of aliphatic acids in primates.

Androgenic steroids affect sexual activity in female non-human primates

As we have seen, oestrogen-treated, ovariectomized female monkeys are both attractive to males and willing to solicit and accept their attempts to copulate. However, removal of the remaining source of circulating androgens (by suppression or removal of the adrenal cortex) or passive immunization against testosterone results in a marked reduction in proceptive and receptive behaviours (Fig. 8.13), despite the continuing presence of oestradiol. These changes in the sexual behaviour of females are reversed by treatment with testosterone (Fig. 8.13) or an androgen not bound by the testosterone antiserum, such as androstenedione. Although the decreases in sexual behaviour in female monkeys deprived of androgens are considerable, it should be emphasized that they may still accept mounting attempts by males (Fig. 8.13), just as androgen-deprived males may continue to display sexual interest in females. It is the

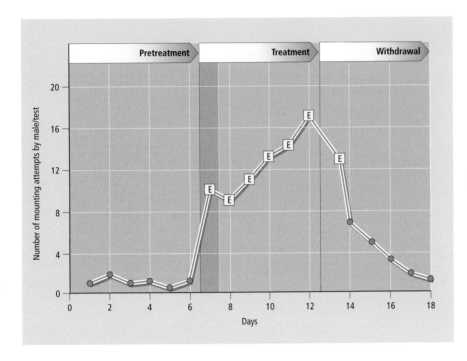

Fig. 8.12 Summary of effects on three male rhesus monkeys of a synthetic mixture of aliphatic acids applied to the perineal region (sexual skin) of an ovariectomized female rhesus monkey. Mounting behaviour is markedly stimulated during treatment, and ejaculations (E) occur consistently. Withdrawal of the mixture is followed by a reversal of these changes in the males' sexual behaviour.

incidence of such acceptances and interest that is reduced. Thus, the strict dependence of sexual behaviour on steroid hormones seen in female non-primates has no obvious parallel in primates.

Steroid hormones in women may affect human sexual behaviour patterns

It is generally accepted that ovariectomy in women does not usually result in loss of libido, although oestrogen replacement therapy may be necessary to prevent a decline in sexual activity by ensuring vaginal lubrication and preventing atrophic changes in the reproductive tract, as occur after the menopause. As with males, then, direct effects of sex steroids on the genitalia in maintaining levels of sexual activity must be taken into account before making assumptions about changes to motivational states.

However, there is now an accumulation of reports suggesting that coital activity varies during the menstrual cycle. For example, a prospective diary study on 68 women aged 25–35, all of whom were infertile because of IUCDs or ligated tubes, indicated a significant increase in coital activity as the mid-cycle ovulation approached (Fig. 8.14). Why? Other studies have reported diary records of both increased female libido and increased male partner initiation of sexual interaction just before ovulation. The latter could reflect a response to female behaviour or some physical indicator such as pheromones. There is some evidence that pheromones in women attract sexual interest by men, but no direct evidence that vaginal odours are involved. At present, the possibility of pheromonal communication in

humans as a mechanism for ovarian hormones to affect sexual interaction remains unproven.

Anecdotal evidence from clinical studies suggests that androgens may affect sexual activity in some women, but interindividual variability is again high. For example, women taking low-dose combined oestrogen–progestagen oral contraceptives have reduced androgen levels and a substantial minority report reduced sexual interest and enjoyment. Antiandrogen treatment for female acne and hirsutism was followed by reduced sexual satisfaction in most women. Controlled studies of the effects of androgens and oestrogens on sexual behaviour in bilaterally ovariectomized women, in whom androgens fall substantially and immediately, has also provided inconsistent evidence, one study implicating androgens in sexual interest, fantasy and arousal (Fig. 8.15) but not in sexual activity or orgasm, another reporting the exact opposite, namely increased sexual activity and orgasm, but not desire or arousal! However, at least a positive impact of androgens on some aspects of sexual function was detected in both studies. These data suggest that androgen may play a role in sexual functioning in women, perhaps especially after the menopause or after ovariectomy, but still emphasizes how other variables are influential.

The finding that androgens increase measures of sexual arousal and interest in women, but only do so in hypogonadal men, has led to the suggestion that males are 'overdetermined' and females 'underdetermined' so far as androgenic influences on sexual behaviour are concerned. Fig. 8.16 illustrates the notion that the normal range of

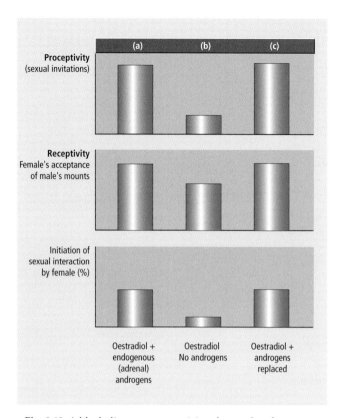

Fig. 8.13 A block diagram summarizing the results of experiments on adrenal androgens and proceptive and receptive behaviour in ovariectomized female rhesus monkeys receiving oestradiol benzoate throughout the experiment to ensure their attractiveness to the males. (a) Controls. (b) Removal of endogenously secreted androgens from the adrenal by suppression with dexamethasone or adrenalectomy with glucocorticoid replacement, caused large decreases in proceptive behaviour and initiation of sexual interaction by the female, and smaller decreases in receptive behaviour. (c) These decreases were reversed by treatment with testosterone propionate or androstenedione.

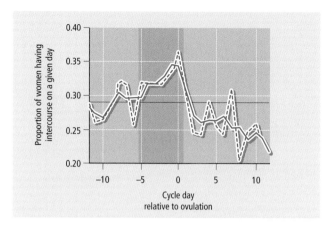

Fig. 8.14 Plot of intercourse frequency relative to day of menstrual cycle (Day 0 = ovulation). Solid line shows 3-day moving average and dashed line shows mean values for each day. Horizontal line shows mean overall frequency. N = 68, 171 cycles, all women 24–35 and having ligated tubes or IUCDs. (Redrawn from Wilcox AJ *et al.* (2004) *Human Reproduction* **19**, 1539–1543.)

plasma testosterone levels in men exceeds the range within which there is a clear relationship between the hormone and indices of sexual activity. Only when starting from a low baseline, as in hypogonadal men, is this relationship seen. However, in women, it is hypothesized that the range over which testosterone can influence sexual responsiveness overlaps and exceeds the normal range of plasma levels.

Summary

This account of steroid hormones and sexual behaviour should reveal two important points. First, it is clear that gonadal hormones are not essential for sexual interactions in humans (and other primates), and they thus exert a less dramatic controlling effect than in other mammals. Second, there is evidence that ovarian (or adrenal) and testicular hormones may influence sexual behaviour in primates, but it is also profoundly modified by the dynamics of the social group in which primates live (see also Chapter 6, subordinate male monkeys tend not to engage in sexual interactions, yet their plasma levels of testosterone are clearly adequate for them to do so). In the case of human sexual behaviour, social, environmental and emotional factors are also important. We now turn our attention to a brief investigation of the possible sites of hormone action in the brain where the expression of sexual behaviour might be controlled or influenced.

Sex steroids act in the brain to control sexual behaviour

The techniques available to study the neuroendocrine mechanisms underlying sexual behaviour include the stereotaxic placement of lesions, hormones and also drugs at discrete neural loci; electrical stimulation in these areas; and autoradiographic methods designed to localize the target neurons bearing receptors for behaviourally active hormones. Although these techniques are sophisticated, each brings with it particular sorts of interpretational problems. For example, electrolytic lesions destroy not only the neuronal cell bodies in a part of the brain, but also axons traversing that area. Changes in sexual behaviour that follow such lesions may therefore be independent of damage to the neuronal population under study and reflect instead incidental damage to the passing fibre

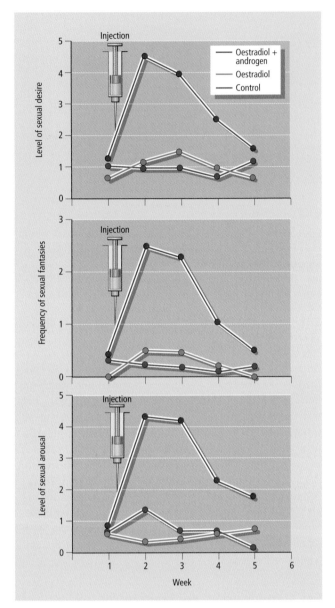

Fig. 8.15 The effects on women who had undergone ovariectomy of treatment with oestradiol, oestradiol plus androgen or no hormone. Levels of sexual desire, the frequency of sexual thoughts and level of sexual arousal are all significantly greater in the combined treatment group, indicating the impact of androgenic steroids on sexuality in women.

system. Implanted or injected hormones may diffuse away from the site at which they were placed (although this can be controlled). Although advances in techniques and their application have increased our understanding of some neuroendocrine mechanisms controlling sexual behaviour, it should be borne in mind that sex hormones are taken up in many areas of the brain, but it is not clear whether they are all involved in reproductive functions there and,

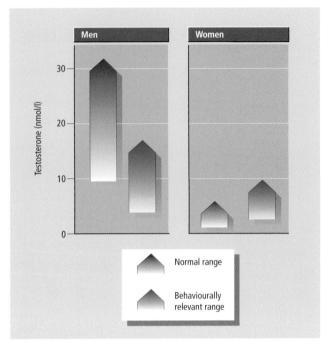

Fig. 8.16 The hypothetical relationship between the normal circulating levels of testosterone and the levels between which changing testosterone can affect sexual behaviour in men and women (behaviourally relevant range). It is postulated that the behaviourally relevant range is lower than the normal range in men, which explains why clear sexual effects of testosterone are only seen in hypogonadal men and not in intact eugonadal men. By contrast, the behaviourally relevant range is higher than the normal range in women and this may explain why administration of testosterone to women more readily results in changes in sexual behaviour, such as those illustrated in Fig. 8.15.

if not, what functions they may serve at such a wide variety of sites.

Testosterone or its metabolites act primarily within the medial preoptic area to control masculine sexual behaviour

It has been a consistent finding that lesions, including those specific to neuronal cell bodies, placed in the medial preoptic area (including the sexually dimorphic area, see Chapter 2) and adjacent anterior hypothalamus of males of many non-primate and some primate species, severely impair the ability to copulate. The testes do not atrophy as a result of these lesions, indicating that the pituitary–gonadal axis is unaffected, and the behavioural changes are not simply secondary to a decrease in testosterone secretion. Indeed, treatment with testosterone does not restore sexual behaviour in males with lesions in the preoptic area.

Conversely, implantation of testosterone into the preoptic–anterior hypothalamic areas, which are rich in androgen receptors, restores sexual behaviour in castrate male rats (Fig. 8.17). These dramatic effects of testosterone in the anterior hypothalamus (which in rodents depend on aromatization to oestradiol) argue strongly that this area is of primary importance in the hormonal regulation of sexual behaviour. This does not in any way minimize the important peripheral effects of androgens, but instead points to the fact that neuroendocrine integration in this behavioural system requires the actions of the hormone at different levels. Thus, copulation in males requires the action of testosterone not only in the hypothalamus but also in the periphery (and in the spinal cord), presumably to facilitate the transduction and transmission of sensory stimuli to behaviourally relevant areas of the CNS or to enable the motor responses to these stimuli.

It has become clear that, while both preoptic area lesions and removal of testosterone by castration decrease the display of sexual behaviour, they do so in different ways. Castrate male rats do not copulate and show no interest in females in heat. By contrast, male rats with preoptic area

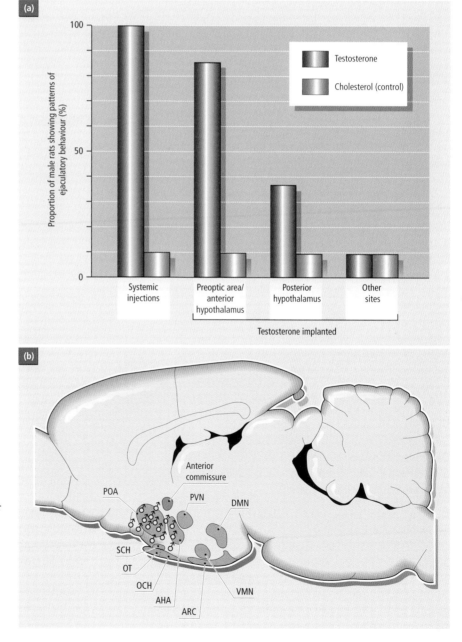

Fig. 8.17 (a) The effects of testosterone implanted in the CNS on the sexual behaviour of castrated male rats. Testosterone placed in the preoptic–anterior hypothalamic continuum induced high levels of ejaculatory patterns, comparable to those observed following systemic treatment with the hormone. Testosterone placed in the posterior hypothalamus or elsewhere in the brain had no significant effect. Important controls were provided by the fact that cholesterol had no effect on sexual activity in any site, so arguing for some degree of hormonal specificity. More recently it has been shown that, at least in rats, oestradiol has similar effects. (b) Sites (♂) in the hypothalamus at which testosterone induced increases in sexual behaviour in male rats. AHA, anterior hypothalamic area; ARC, arcuate nucleus; DMN, dorsomedial nucleus; OT and OCH, optic tract and chiasm; POA, preoptic area; PVN, paraventricular nucleus; SCH, suprachiasmatic nucleus; VMN, ventromedial nucleus.

lesions show high levels of interest in oestrous females and make repeated attempts to mount. However, these mounting attempts are often ill-directed and are not associated with pelvic thrusting, and these males are unable to intromit. This observation suggests a dissociation of the neural substrates underlying the appetitive behaviour that precedes copulation (behaviour that serves the purpose of bringing a male and a female into close proximity) from that influencing the performance of copulatory reflexes. The preoptic area would appear to be especially important for the latter and also provides the key site of action for steroids in facilitating the appearance of these reflexes in sexual contexts. A similar conclusion follows the fascinating observation that male rhesus monkeys with lesions in the preoptic area make little attempt to copulate with females, but masturbate to ejaculation at other times. Clearly, the capacity for sexual arousal and the performance of copulatory reflexes are separable neurally in primates as well.

This pattern of results leaves open some important questions. For example, where does testosterone exert its motivational effects? As castrate males show low levels of sexual interest in females, but males with lesions in the preoptic area retain their interest, it follows that the medial preoptic area is unlikely to be the only site at which testosterone exerts effects on sexual behaviour. An extrahypothalamic site central to the regulation of appetitive behaviour, including precopulatory behaviour, is the dopamine-dependent area of the nucleus accumbens. Dopamine receptor antagonists, for example, when infused directly into this site can selectively impair appetitive aspects of sexual behaviour, but leave the ability to copulate unaffected. Much remains to be learned about the neural mechanisms underlying the different elements of the integrated pattern of sexual behaviour, for example gender preferences, as well as the complexities of sexual feelings and pleasure. However, it seems to be the case that the multiple levels and sites capable of influencing sexual behaviour in the male are ultimately integrated through the medial preoptic area

Oestradiol and progesterone act primarily within the ventromedial hypothalamus to control sexual behaviour in female non-primates

In female non-primate mammals, notably the rat, it is the ventromedial nucleus of the hypothalamus that is the principal site of action of oestradiol (see Fig. 6.3b). Implanting hormone in this area, sufficient to saturate a proportion of the oestrogen receptors there, increases markedly the receptive behaviour of ovariectomized females. This treatment is quite adequate as a background 'priming' for the subsequent actions of progesterone in those species, such

as the rat, which require it together with oestradiol to induce oestrous levels of proceptive and receptive behaviour. The site of action of progesterone has proved more elusive to define, but a number of studies now point to the ventromedial hypothalamic area as most likely. It is rich in progesterone receptors, which are actually induced by prior treatment with oestradiol. This probably explains why the sequence of oestradiol followed by progesterone is so critical in this species for oestrous behaviour to occur.

As we have seen, androgens rather than oestrogens seem to underlie proceptivity in female monkeys and they also seem to act within the anterior hypothalamus. Thus, implanting testosterone in an area extending from the ventromedial nucleus to the preoptic area reverses the decrease in sexual activity that follows androgen deprivation in female monkeys (Fig. 8.18). No comparable effects of intrahypothalamic oestradiol have been reported in monkeys.

How do hormones affect behaviour?

Relatively little is known about the ways in which hormones alter neural activity to bring about changes in sexual behaviour. Experiments on rats have revealed that oestradiol, for example, exerts its effects on receptivity after a delay of 26–48h. The finding that inhibitors of protein synthesis completely prevent these actions of oestradiol has led to the widely held view that the hormone, which is clearly accumulated in neuronal nuclei, modulates neural activity via an action involving gene expression. However, the nature of the products of this action has not been determined, although they may include progesterone receptors in females. Nor is it clear whether the passage of time between exposure to oestradiol and its behavioural effects is necessary for materials synthesized in the neuronal cell body (e.g. enzymes, receptor molecules or peptidergic transmitters themselves) to be transported to other regions of the neurone (e.g. terminals, dendrites).

There is considerable interest in the nature of the neurochemical mechanisms in the hypothalamus with which sex steroids interact when exerting their behavioural effects. Hypothalamic neurons containing gonadotrophin-releasing hormone (GnRH) have been suggested to be one indirect target of steroid action (see Chapter 6). Thus, GnRH infused into the dorsal midbrain, a site to which preoptic GnRH neurons project, enhances the display of receptive lordosis postures in the female rat. Conversely, GnRH antibodies infused into the same site have the opposite effect. However, despite some early positive demonstrations, GnRH generally has little or no effect on the sexual behaviour of male rats or monkeys of either sex, so its precise importance remains uncertain.

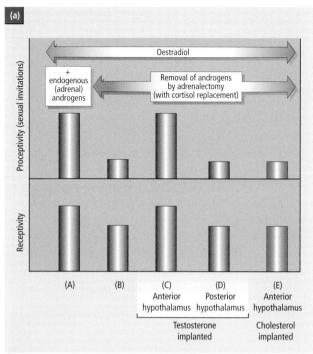

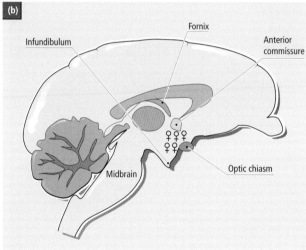

Fig. 8.18 (a) A block diagram summarizing the results of experiments in which testosterone propionate was implanted in the CNS of androgen-deprived female rhesus monkeys. All females were ovariectomized and received injections of oestradiol benzoate throughout the experiment, so that they remained attractive to males. Adrenalectomy was followed, as shown in Fig. 8.14, by decreased levels of proceptive and receptive behaviour (compare A with B). These changes in sexual activity were reversed by placing testosterone in the anterior hypothalamus (C) but not in the posterior hypothalamus (D). Cholesterol in the anterior hypothalamus was without effect (E). (b) Diagram of a sagittal section of the rhesus monkey's brain to show sites in the anterior hypothalamic area where testosterone implants reversed the behavioural effects of adrenalectomy in females (C).

Neurons in the arcuate nucleus containing pro-opiomelanocortin-derived peptides, particularly β-endorphin, richly innervate the medial preoptic area (see Fig. 6.18), and infusion of β-endorphin into the latter site profoundly inhibits copulation in male rats. Levels of β-endorphin in the preoptic area vary markedly with the steroidal environment, suggesting that this neural system may be important in mediating some of the behavioural effects of testosterone withdrawal. The fact that the same peptide reduces GnRH secretion in both males and females (Box 6.1) has been taken to indicate that it may have an important, pivotal role in mediating the inhibition of reproduction in a number of different situations, for example during stress, which is known to activate this population of neurons and increase intracerebral levels of β-endorphin. The monoamine transmitters noradrenaline, dopamine and serotonin have also been shown to be involved in the neural mechanisms underlying sexual behaviour. Drugs that increase noradrenaline and dopamine transmission, or reduce serotonin, can all—in quite specific ways—increase sexual responses in males and females. Drugs with opposite effects tend to reduce sexual activity. However, specific interactions between these neural systems and the sex steroids that exert such powerful controls over the expression of sexual behaviour in males and females remain incompletely understood; they may in fact represent different levels of neural control over sexual responses.

Summary

A great deal is known about the strict, controlling role of hormones in the sexual behaviour of non-primate species and about the hypothalamic sites where their actions are exerted. But even in these species, many aspects of the neural regulation of sexual behaviour are not understood: for example, what are the functions of structures in the limbic forebrain, such as the amygdala and septum, which bind large amounts of steroid hormones in males and females and are well known to be concerned with the control of emotional behaviour? In primates, although the effects of hormones and their sites of action in males and females have been described to some extent, it is clear that much remains to be understood about the ways in which social interactions modify, and are modified by, these basic neuroendocrine mechanisms. Clearly, gonadal hormones are not the only determinants of sexual activity. Furthermore, social interaction, as we have seen in Chapter 6, may profoundly influence the activity of the hypothalamic–pituitary–gonadal axis and hence fertility. If such factors are complicated and poorly understood in non-human primates, it is hardly surprising that we have only limited information concerning the interactions between hormones (which do influence human sexual activity), social environment and individual

KEY LEARNING POINTS

- Steroids have determinative and regulatory actions.

- Testosterone, and its reduced metabolite 5α-dihydrotestosterone, maintain spermatogenesis and the functional integrity of the accessory sex glands.

- Androgens also have anabolic effects, and some synthetic androgens emphasize this property for use clinically and abuse recreationally.

- Oestradiol and progesterone regulate cyclic changes in the oviduct, uterus, cervix and vagina that are critical for gamete transport, fertilization and implantation.

- Oestrogens and progesterone have other effects on, for example, appetite, bone metabolism, vascular function, body temperature regulation, mood and water/mineral balance.

- Testosterone critically controls the sexual behaviour of male non-primate mammals.

- The effects of testosterone on masculine sexual behaviour are mediated by actions on both the brain and the genitalia.

- In some species (e.g. rodents) oestradiol is the active metabolite of testosterone, mediating its actions on sexual behaviour in the brain. Dihydrotestosterone is the active metabolite maintaining the integrity of the genital periphery.

- In male monkeys testosterone, clearly greatly influences sexual behaviour. However, sexual activity can persist in castrates.

- In men, testosterone clearly affects sexual motivation, behaviour and fantasies, but only in hypgonadal males are androgens of (variable) benefit.

- The tight control exerted by testosterone over sexual responses in non-primate males is not seen in male monkeys and men, where social and other factors are also important determinants of sexual activity.

- Oestradiol and progesterone are critical determinants of sexual receptivity and proceptivity in female non-primates. Ovariectomized females are sexually inactive; appropriate sequential treatment with oestradiol and progesterone reinstates oestrous behaviour.

- In female monkeys, oestradiol and progesterone may affect sexual behaviour, but ovariectomized animals remain sexually receptive and proceptive.

- Ovarian steroids may profoundly affect sexual interaction between males and females by effects on the odour of females' vaginal secretions.

- Androgens, of adrenal and ovarian origin, affect sexual proceptivity and receptivity in female monkeys.

- In women, ovariectomy does not generally affect libido.

- Androgen treatment in women improves sexual function, but with interindividual variation.

- There is variation in coital activity through the menstrual cycle, but what causes it remains uncertain.

- The medial preoptic area is a critical site for the effects of testosterone, or its metabolites, on sexual behaviour in males.

- The ventromedial hypothalamus is a critical site for the effects of oestradiol and progesterone on sexual behaviour in female non-primates.

- The anterior hypothalamus is an important site mediating the effects of androgens on sexual behaviour in female monkeys.

- Other neural systems, including monoaminergic systems, influence the expression of sexual behaviour in males and females.

variables (such as personality, mood and early history) which determine patterns of human sexual behaviour.

FURTHER READING

General reading

Bancroft J (1989) *Human Sexuality and its Problems*, 2nd edn. Churchill Livingstone, Edinburgh.

Bancroft J (2005) The endocrinology of sexual arousal. *Journal of Endocrinology* **186**, 411–427.

Britton KT, Koob GF (1998) Premenstrual steroids? *Nature* **392**, 869–870.

Everitt BJ (1990) Sexual motivation: a neural and behavioural analysis of the mechanisms underlying appetitive copulatory responses of male rats. *Neuroscience and Biobehavioural Reviews* **14**, 217–232.

Everitt BJ, Bancroft J (1991) Of rats and men: the comparative approach to male sexuality. In: *Annual Review of Sex Research*, Vol. 2 (ed. J. Bancroft, C.M. Davis & H.J. Ruppel, Jr), pp. 77–118. Society for the Scientific Study of Sex, Allentown, PA.

Hess RA *et al.* (1997) A role for oestrogens in the male reproductive system. *Nature* **390**, 509–512.

Jabbour HN *et al.* (2006) Endocrine regulation of menstruation. *Endocrine Reviews* **27**, 17–46.

Pfaus J, Everitt BJ (1995) The psychopharmacology of sexual behaviour. In: *Psychopharmacology: The 4th Generation of Progress* (ed. F.E. Bloom & D. Kupfer), pp. 743–758. Raven Press, New York.

Sharpe RM (1997) Do males rely on female hormones? *Nature* **390**, 447–448.

van Gestel I *et al.* (2003) Endometrial wave-like activity in the non-pregnant uterus. *Human Reproduction Update* **9**, 131–138.

More advanced reading (see also Boxes)

Gipson IK (2001) Mucins of the human endocervix. *Frontiers in Bioscience* **6**, D1245–1255.

Kayisli UA *et al.* (2004) Endocrine–immune interactions in human endometrium. *Annals of the New York Academy of Sciences* **1034**, 50–63.

Kunz G, Leyendecker G (2001) Uterine peristaltic activity during the menstrual cycle: characterization, regulation, function and dysfunction. *Reproductive BioMedicine* **4** (Suppl. 3), 5–9.

Sherwin BB, Gelf MM (1987) The role of androgen in the maintenance of sexual functioning in oophorectomized women. *Psychosomatic Medicine* **49**, 397–409.

Stern K, McClintock MK (1998) Regulation of ovulation by human pheromones. *Nature* **392**, 177–179.

Weller A (1998) Communication through body odour. *Nature* **392**, 126–127.

Wilcox AJ *et al.* (2004) On the frequency of intercourse around ovulation: evidence for biological influences. *Human Reproduction* **19**, 1539–1543.

9 Coitus and Fertilization

In the foregoing chapters, we have considered reproductive function in the male and the non-pregnant female. A central concept underlying all of our discussion is the coordinating role played by the gonadal hormones in the production of mature gametes and the conditioning of reproductive function and sexual behaviour. In this way the chance of fertilization is maximized. Reproduction requires fertilization to be successful. If it is, then a dramatic change must ensue for both reproductive partners but particularly for the female. Her whole anatomy and physiology must change from cyclic fertility patterns to pregnancy and nidatory patterns. In this chapter, we will consider how the oocytes and spermatozoa travel from their sites of production to the site of fertilization in the oviduct. Then we will consider the critical events of fertilization itself.

The transport of spermatozoa to the oocyte is hazardous and most do not arrive

In Chapter 4, we left the spermatozoa in the lumina of the seminiferous tubules. Human spermatozoa, a few microns in length, must travel through some 30–40 cm of male and female reproductive tract, or more than 100 000 times their own length, to reach the oviduct. During this long and hazardous journey, several major obstacles must be overcome, including *transport between individuals at coitus*. Fewer than one in a million of the spermatozoa produced ever complete the journey. It is not just that the journey itself is difficult, but also that the spermatozoa must successfully undergo a series of changes in both the male and female genital tracts before they gain full fertilizing capacity. These changes are termed *maturation* in the male tract, and *capacitation* and *the acrosome reaction* in the female tract.

Spermatozoa require a period of epididymal maturation

Spermatozoa are released from their close association with the Sertoli cells into a fluid secreted by these cells such that a continuous flow rich in spermatozoa washes towards the *rete testis* (see Fig. 1.9). As the fluid passes through the rete testis, the composition of its ions and small molecules changes, probably mainly by diffusional equilibration through the tubule walls, since the absence of inter-Sertoli cell junctions renders the blood–testis barrier much less complete. The spermatozoa are then carried through the short and delicate *vasa efferentia*, which come together within the *initial segment* of the *epididymis* (Fig. 9.1). The vasa efferentia *absorb over 90% of the fluid* carrying the spermatozoa, and, if they are ligated, the seminiferous tubules literally 'blow up' with accumulating fluid, and spermatogenesis ceases as a result of pressure atrophy. The absorption is *dependent on oestrogen*, which is carried in the fluid at high concentrations, having been synthesized in both

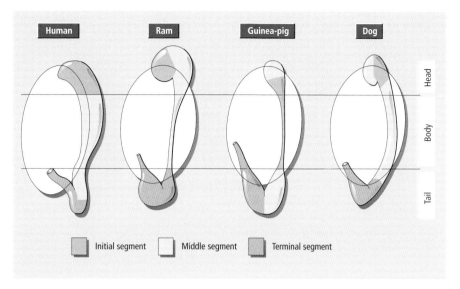

Fig. 9.1 Excurrent ducts of the human, ram, guinea-pig and dog to illustrate anatomical variation. Vasa efferentia (varying in length and from 10 to 20 in number between the species) connect the rete testis to a long, highly convoluted tube: the epididymis. Anatomically, the coils of the tube form a head (caput, which also contains the termini of the vasa efferentia), body (corpus) and tail (cauda). Three histological segments, which usually do *not* correspond with the anatomical divisions, are present: an initial segment of high, ciliated epithelium and smallish lumen; a middle segment with wider lumen and shorter cilia; and a wide terminal segment of low cuboidal, relatively poorly ciliated epithelium with more smooth muscle in the underlying stroma. Micropinocytosis and fluid absorption occur mainly in the vasa efferentia and initial segment, with secretion in the middle and terminal segments, which also store spermatozoa at a high density in the lumen (see also Fig. 1.9).

Leydig cells and the developing spermatozoa themselves. The dependence on oestrogen of the absorbtive epithelium of the vasa efferentia is seen dramatically in mice genetically lacking in the α oestrogen receptor. At puberty, fluid secretion begins, but it is not absorbed, and so back-pressure builds and pressure aspermatogenesis and infertility results—a sort of 'genetic ligation'

The fluid absorbtion continues in the epididymis to concentrate the spermatozoa some 100-fold, and their further onward transport becomes dependent on the activity of epididymidal musculature. In addition, the epididymis adds secretory products (both exocrine and apocrine), including carnitine, glycerophosphorylcholine, fructose and glycoproteins, the latter coating the surface of the spermatozoa. Passage through the vasa efferentia takes about a day and through the epididymis a further 5–11 days depending on the species and affects spermatozoal behaviour profoundly. Thus, spermatozoa entering the vasa efferentia are quite incapable of movement (beyond an infrequent twitch) and, when inseminated into females, cannot attach to and fertilize an oocyte. However, by the time they arrive in the cauda epididymidis, spermatozoa have acquired the potential to fertilize oocytes and to swim progressively (although they do not swim actively *in vivo*, but only after their release from the male tract). These maturational changes in functional capability are accompanied by changes in the biochemistry and morphology of the spermatozoa (Table 9.1). This whole process of *maturation* is crucially dependent on adequate stimulation of the epididymis by androgens.

If the androgens are removed by castration, the epididymis hypotrophies. Injection of testosterone restores activity. Most of the androgens which stimulate epididymidal function are derived not from the circulation but from the lymph and the fluid entering from the vas efferentia. Thus, ligation of the vasa efferentia to impair these flows results in considerable functional and structural regression of the epididymis. Within this fluid, testosterone is bound to androgen-binding protein and reaches concentrations approaching those of testicular venous blood (between 30 and 60 ng/ml; dihydrotestosterone is also present at about half this level). Within the epididymis, intracellular receptors take up the androgens, and 5α-reductase converts testosterone to dihydrotestosterone to yield very high tissue levels of this more active androgen. There is some evidence to suggest that the epididymis may even engage in a little androgen synthesis itself.

In some species, spermatozoa may be stored for several weeks in the cauda, but in humans storage seems to occur for a few days only. After leaving the tail of the epididymis, spermatozoa enter the *vas deferens* as a very densely packed mass. Ligation of the vas deferens (*vasectomy*) does not

Table 9.1 Maturational changes to spermatozoa in the epididymis.

Property	Details of changes
Concentration	100-fold; 50×10^6/ml entering suspended in fluid; dense packed 50×10^8/ml on leaving
Completion of sperm modelling	Nuclear condensation and acrosomal shaping completed
	Cytoplasmic drop 'squeezed' down tail and shed
Metabolism	Cholesterol and phospholipids selectively metabolized, shifting lipid balance towards diacylglycerol, unsaturated fatty acids and desmosterol
	Increased dependence on external fructose for glycolytic energy production; little oxidative metabolism
	pH rises
Mobility	Increase in disulfide linkages between proteins in outer dense fibres of tail, yielding a more rigid flagellum with a stronger potential beat
	cAMP content of tail rises
	Acquires capacity for forward motion
Membrane	Coated with glycoproteins
	Rise in surface charge (due to sialic acid increase) and change in profile of surface proteins
	Membrane fluidity increases

accumulate masses of fluid behind the ligature, as occurs with ligation of the vasa efferentia, and so there is no pressure atrophy within the seminiferous tubule. However, spermatozoa do build up behind the vasectomy ligature and these must be removed either by phagocytosis within the epididymis or by leakage through the epididymidal wall. The normal non-ligated vas deferens serves as a storage reservoir for spermatozoa. In the absence of ejaculation, spermatozoa dribble through the *terminal ampulla* of the vas deferens into the urethra and are washed away in the urine.

Semen is made up of spermatozoa and seminal plasma

Ejaculated spermatozoa are carried to the female tract in *seminal plasma*; the two together are called *semen*. Seminal plasma is derived largely from the major accessory sex glands (see Fig. 8.1), with only a small contribution from the epididymis. Different species have bewilderingly different patterns of accessory sex gland structure (see Table 8.1) and function (Table 9.2). Knowledge of the origin of some of the main constituents of seminal fluid, as shown in Table 9.2, can help to diagnose deficiencies of function in particular accessory sex glands. Seminal fluid cannot be essential for effective sperm function, as spermatozoa taken directly from the vas deferens can fertilize oocytes in the test-tube. However, *in vivo*, spermatozoa require a 'fluid vehicle' for their normal transport and the seminal plasma supplies this, either exuberantly in half-litre volumes in the boar, or with a more conservative 3 ml or so in the human. In addition to providing a transport medium, the seminal plasma also provides nutritional factors such as fructose or sorbitol, buffering capacity to alkalinize the acid pH of

vaginal fluids, and reducing agents such as ascorbic acid, hypotaurine and ergothioneine to protect against potential oxidation following exposure of spermatozoa to atmospheric oxygen. It has been proposed that prostaglandins in semen might stimulate muscular activity in the female tract.

Semen does not only carry spermatozoa and substances to assist the maintenance of sperm fertility. Large numbers of leucocytes may be present in seminal plasma, as well as potentially infective agents. Sexual interaction between individuals provides one occasion when these genitourinary infectious agents can be transmitted. Of particular concern is the presence of hepatitis B or C virus, human immunodeficiency virus (HIV, the cause of AIDS) and genital human papillomavirus (HPV, associated with genital warts and cancers) in the semen of infected men, as these agents cause seriously debilitating and/or potentially fatal diseases. The chance of transmitting these viral infections during ejaculatory vaginal intercourse depends on: the virulence of the viral strain; the viral load within the seminal plasma of the infected individual; concurrent infections or inflammatory conditions in the genital tracts of either sexual partner; and whether or not safe sex is practised. In general, rates of transmission of hepatitis B virus are about 10 times those of HIV, and there is an increasing risk of transmission with oral, vaginal and anal intercourse. Potential transmission is, of course, not unidirectional, although infected females seem to transmit to males during vaginal intercourse at about half the reciprocal rate. Effective prophylactic vaccination is available only against hepatitis B, although anti-HPV immunization is being developed. Proper use of the right type of condom, lubricant and viricide (see Table 15.3) can provide effective pro-

Table 9.2 Composition of ejaculate* of man and domestic animals.

Constituent	Species	Concentration range (mM)	Principal source	Function
Spermatozoa (concentration expressed as no./nl; ejaculate volume in ml in brackets)				
	Boar (150–500)	20–300	Testis	
	Bull (2–10)	300–2000		
	Dog (2–15)	60–300		
	Man (2–5)	50–150		
	Ram (1–2)	2000–5000		
	Stallion (30–300)	30–800		
Fructose				
	Man, ram, bull	8–37	Seminal vesicle and ampulla	Anaerobic fructolysis (sorbitol also used in ram)
	Boar, dog, stallion	<0.5		
Inositol				
	Man, bull, stallion, ram	1–3	Testis and epididymis (seminal vesicle in bull, boar)	Preserves seminal osmolarity
	Boar	28		
Citric acid				
	Bull, ram	15–45	Seminal vesicle and prostate (stallion, ram, boar, bull); prostate (man, dog)	Ca^{2+} chelator (limits rate of Ca^{2+}-dependent coagulation to prevent seminal 'stones'?)
	Man	5–73		
	Stallion	0.5–2.5		
	Boar	2.5–10		
Glycerylphosphorylcholine				
	Man, stallion	2–3	Epididymis	See below
	Ram	58–73		
	Bull	4–18		
	Dog, boar	5		
Acid phosphatase (expressed in activity units/mL)				
	Man	2470	Prostate	Cleaves choline from glycerylphosphorylcholine for use in phospholipid metabolism
	Bull	6		
	Boar	2		

*pH = 7.2–7.8; also contains significant amounts of various prostaglandins (PGs), especially 19-hydroxylated PGE_1 and PGE_2 (humans, monkeys); PGE_1 and PGE_2; and 19-OH PGFs and $PGF_{1\alpha}$ and $PGF_{2\alpha}$ (humans). Role unclear.

tection against viral transmission—if, of course, a pregnancy is not desired.

Coition involves genital reflexes and sexual responses

In mammals, fertilization is internal and the male gametes must be deposited in the female tract at coitus. Coitus itself is of variable duration (minutes in man, hours in the camel) and is accompanied by extensive physiological changes not just in the genitalia but also in the body as a whole.

It is only since the mid-1960s that research into human sexual physiology has become an accepted part of the study of reproduction. Masters and Johnson, from their studies on human heterosexual interaction and masturbation, proposed a widely accepted model for sexual responses in men and women. Their so-called 'EPOR' model describes: (1) an initial *excitement phase* (E) during which psychogenic or somatogenic stimuli raise sexual arousal; (2) the *plateau phase* (P) during which arousal becomes intensified; (3) the *orgasmic phase* (O), which is reached if the level of stimulation is adequate and entails the few seconds of involuntary *climax* in which sexual tension is relieved, usually in an explosive wave of intense pleasure; and (4) the *resolution phase* (R) during which sexual arousal is dissipated and pelvic haemodynamics resolve to the unstimulated state. The specific physiological changes occurring during these phases will be discussed below. In the male, an *absolute refractory period* occurs after orgasm during which time sexual re-arousal and orgasm are impossible. Its duration depends somewhat on age, being abbreviated in boys, and also on a variety of situational factors, such as novelty of partner or context. Women may not generally experience an absolute refractory period, although relevant data are relatively sparse.

The male

Penile *erection* can be elicited by *psychogenic stimuli*, such as visual cues and erotic imagery. These are integrated in the brain, presumably involving mechanisms within the *limbic system*, which is then able, via descending projections to the spinal cord, to influence somatic and autonomic efferents to the genitalia. These same efferents can be activated reflexly by tactile stimulation of the penis and adjacent perineum, this being a most effective means of inducing erection. Data from animals and from men with spinal cord transection reveal that the afferent limb of the reflex is carried by the *internal pudendal nerves*. Three efferent outflows influence erection: (1) the *pelvic nerve* (parasympathetic outflow) promotes erection; (2) the *hypogastric nerve* (sympathetic outflow) carries fibres that depress erection and possibly some also that promote it; and (3) the *pudendal nerve* (somatic) promotes erection. In man, erection is achieved entirely by *haemodynamic changes*, which in other species may be complemented by the relaxation of a retractor muscle which pulls the penis back into the prepuce in the flaccid state (e.g. the bull and macaque) and/or by a penile bone or *os penis* attached to the capsule of the corpora cavernosa (e.g. the dog, macaque, mink and sea lion). It is the two *corpora cavernosa* (trabeculated sinus spaces surrounded by a tough fibrous capsule: Fig. 9.2) that provide the main erectile tissue.

The sequence of events underlying the change from *flaccidity* through *tumescence* to *erection* and then *detumescence* of the penis is as follows. In the flaccid state, *myogenic tone* within the smooth muscle fibres of the cavernous trabeculae and of the arteries supplying the penis is maintained by the sympathetic outflow of the hypogastric nerve (*adrenergic tone*). During a natural erection, this sympathetic effect is countered by stimulation of the parasympathetic outflow to reduce myogenic tone in the arterial smooth muscle (causing arterial dilatation and an increased blood flow into the corpora cavernosa) and in the cavernous trabecular muscle (decreasing intracavernous resistance

and expanding cavernous volume). Additionally, arteriovenous shunts, which bypass the sinuses of the corpora cavernosa when the penis is flaccid, now direct blood into them. Finally, the venous outflow from the corpora cavernosa is reduced by compression of the subtunical venous plexus resulting from the rapidly developing turgor. This sequence of events changes the intracavernous space from a low-volume, low-pressure system into a large-volume, high-pressure one. In man, all this is achieved by increasing the *inflow* of arterial blood but reducing its *through flow*, such that in a fully rigid state in- and outflow are almost absent. Prolonged erection (*priapism*) thus endangers the oxygenated blood supply to the penis (*ischaemic priapism*), and may need to be relieved pharmacologically. The *corpus spongiosum* (Fig. 9.2) also increases in turgor, but not as much as the corpora cavernosa, thereby avoiding compression of the urethra.

Several neurotransmitters have been implicated in erection, both facilitatory (dopamine, acetycholine, oxytocin, VIP, prostanoids, nitric oxide) and inhibitory (noradrenaline, encephalins, angiotensin II), but the most important locally is *nitric oxide* (NO), production of which by *nitric oxide synthase* (NOS) leads to vasodilatation through the production of cGMP within the vascular smooth muscle cells. The *initiation* of erection seems to depend on release of *neuronal* NOS (nNOS), but *maintenance* of erection requires further amplificatory release of NOS from the local *vascular endothelium* itself (eNOS), perhaps as a result of increased sheer pressure from blood flowing through the vessels. The parasympathetic outflow also relaxes the retractor penis muscle in those species that have one.

Erectile dysfunction (ED or *impotence*) is defined as 'the consistent or recurrent inability of a man to attain and/or maintain a penile erection sufficient for sexual activity'. ED may be caused by tears in the fibrous capsule of the corpora cavernosa, obstructions to the vessels supplying the penis, diabetes which impairs release of nNOS and eNOS, use of drugs (including alcohol) which antagonize neurotransmitters mediating tumescence, physical nerve damage (a potential side effect of prostatectomy), psychogenic factors, or a mixture of these. Smoking is a strong predictor of ED, associated as it is with several of the causative factors above. Some types of ED can be treated therapeutically by the pharmacological stimulation of erection either by the intracavernosal injection of the synthetic prostanoid prostaglandin E_1 (also called alprostadil; registered trade names Caverject, Viridal) or its injection intraurethrally (trade name MUSE). Less physically invasive are orally active agents such as sildenafil (Viagra), tadafil (Cialis) and vardenafil (Levitra). These are phosphodiesterase-5 inhibitors that enhance the action of NO by stabilizing cGMP. Side effects may include more widespread consequences of vascular relaxation, such as headaches, vasocongestion

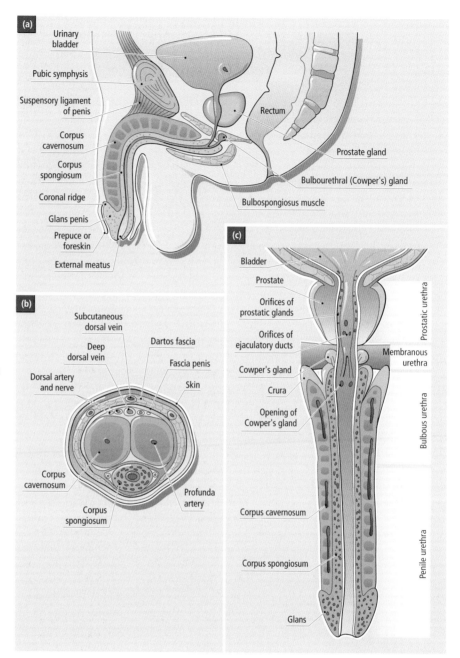

Fig. 9.2 Structure of the human adult penis: (a) midsagittal section through the pelvis; (b) transverse section through shaft of the penis: note fibrous sheaths enclosing the corpora cavernosa, which allow the generation of hydrostatic pressure required for erection; tears in the fibrous capsule lead to failure of erection; and (c) coronal section showing entry of prostatic, ejaculatory (vasa deferentia and seminal vesicles) and Cowper's (bulbourethral) gland ducts. Penile secretory glands of Littré open into the roof of the penile urethra. The internal pudendal arteries supply both the dorsal arteries to the glans and the pudendal arteries to the corpora cavernosa. There is considerable species variation in glans structure: mushroom-shaped in man, corkscrew-shaped in boar and bull, spiny in cat and rat, and having thin urethral vermiform processes in goat and ram.

(especially rhinitis) and skin flushes, as well as risk of ischaemic priapism.

The importance of testosterone in erectile function is not entirely clear. Nocturnal erections, which occur during each episode of *rapid eye movement (REM, dreaming or paradoxical) sleep* are known to be testosterone dependent, whereas erections in response to visual erotic stimuli, for example, are much less dependent on testosterone and occur readily in hypogonadal men. It has been suggested, therefore, that measuring nocturnal penile tumescence (NPT) provides a method of assessing the capacity for sexual arousal independently of the complicating cognitive factors that may compromise sexual function.

As ejaculation approaches, the turgor in the penis increases further and the penile circumference at the *coronal ridge* of the glans penis increases, largely achieved by the action of the pudendal somatic outflow to the perineal striated muscle fibres (the ischiocavernous and bulbocavernous muscles) surrounding the *corporeal crura* (see Fig. 9.2). Coincidentally, the testes are drawn reflexly towards the perineum and may increase their volume by as much as 50% as a result of vasocongestion. The scrotal skin thickens and contracts due to activity in the dartos muscle. With further stimulation, a sequence of contractions of the muscles of the prostate, vas deferens and seminal vesicle is induced, and the components of the seminal plasma, together with the spermatozoa, are expelled into the urethra. This process of *emission* is mediated largely by noradrenergic sympathetic fibres via the hypogastric plexus, and administration of drugs that interfere with the α-adrenergic system (as in treatment for hypertension) leads to '*dry orgasms*'; erection is not impaired (and may be assisted: see earlier), but emission is. The efficient emission of sperm from the vas deferens also seems to require the co-release of ATP with noradrenalin acting via *purinergic receptors* on the smooth muscle of the vas.

Ejaculation, whereby semen is expelled from the posterior urethra, is achieved by contraction of the smooth muscles of the urethra and striated muscles of bulbocavernosus and ischiocavernosus. It is usually associated with contractions of the pelvic floor musculature innervated by the pudendal nerves. The passage of semen back into the bladder is normally prevented by contraction of the vesicular urethral sphincter; failure of this can lead to *retrograde ejaculation* into the bladder. The composition of the early and late fractions of the human ejaculate reflects the sequential nature of the contractions and the relative lack of mixing of the various seminal components within the urethra. The early fraction is rich in acid phosphatase (prostate), the midfraction is rich in spermatozoa (vas deferens) and the late fraction is rich in fructose (seminal vesicle).

Concomitant with penile erection in men, erection of the nipples and increases in heart rate and blood pressure occur as sexual excitement increases. Immediately before ejaculation, skin rashes may develop over the epigastrium, chest, face and neck together with involuntary muscle spasms. At ejaculation, the cardiovascular changes, skin rash and muscle spasms intensify and are often accompanied by hyperventilation, contractions of the rectal sphincter and vocalizations. Associated with ejaculation is orgasm whereby sexual tension and arousal are released and an intense sensation of pleasure occurs. Penile detumescence occurs through the activity of the pelvic nerve sympathetic outflow restoring smooth muscle tone.

The female
At coitus, frictional stimulation of the glans penis is provided by movements against the external genitalia and vaginal walls of the female (Fig. 9.3). The human female undergoes a remarkably similar sequence of reflex responses to that observed in the male, and its elicitation is also dependent on tactile and psychogenic stimulation. Tactile stimulation in the perineal region, and in some women particularly on the *glans clitoris*, provides the primary affer-

ent input reinforced by vaginal stimulation after penile penetration. A vascular response may cause engorgement of the corpora of the clitoris, with consequent clitoral erection, although the extent of clitoral involvement varies considerably. The pharmacological agents used to treat erectile dysfunction in men may also be of use in facilitating genital sexual responsiveness in women. Vaginal lubrication occurs by *transudation* of fluid through the vaginal wall, which vasocongests and becomes purplish red. The vagina expands and the labia majora become engorged with blood. With increased stimulation, the width and length of the vagina increase further and the uterus elevates upwards into the false pelvis lifting the cervical os to produce the so-called *tenting effect* in the midvaginal plane. At orgasm, frequent vaginal contractions occur and uterine contractions beginning in the fundus spread towards the lower uterine segment.

Systemically, the female may experience increased heart rate and blood pressure and manifest skin flushes, vocalizations and muscle spasms (notably rhythmic contractions of the pelvic striated musculature), and intense sensations of pleasure. Postorgasmically, clitoral erection is lost, the labia and the vaginal os detumesce, and the uterine and vaginal walls relax to their original positions. It has not proved possible to differentiate between the orgasms that follow clitoral or vaginal stimulation in terms of their physiological manifestations.

The general descriptions of orgasm recorded by men and women are so similar as to be indistinguishable. The time course of sexual responses in the female is generally longer than in the male. Indeed, ejaculation and orgasm are the end result of coitus within minutes in men (an average of 4 min in the Western world according to one study). Proportionately fewer women appear to achieve orgasm from coitus, various surveys giving figures of 30–50%. Larger numbers achieve orgasm by clitoral stimulation, but even then a significant number, 10–20%, do not achieve orgasm despite being highly sexually aroused. It has been suggested that orgasm in women is not a reflex action, as it appears to be in men, but is learned. Cross-cultural studies suggest strong psychosocial influences; for example, women are more likely to enjoy sex and have orgasms in societies where this is expected than in societies where it is not. Phosphodiesterase-5 inhibitors such as sildenafil have been reported to improve womens' arousal, orgasm and enjoyment, but it is unclear how this improvement is achieved pharmacologically.

The ability to communicate sexually and to give and receive sexual pleasure within a relationship is very often a cornerstone of its success in modern Western society. Social and physical factors affect the capacity to respond sexually to a partner by experiencing orgasm and, when communication and the relationship itself are becoming

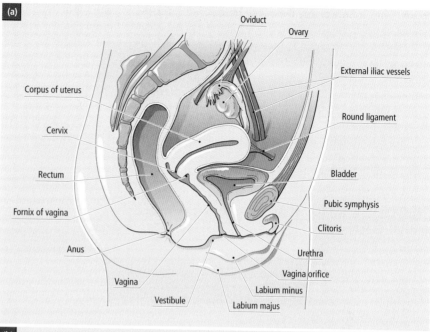

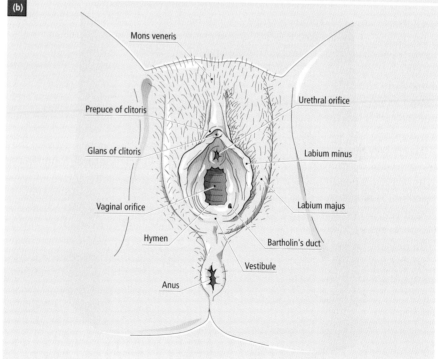

Fig. 9.3 Structure of human adult female genitalia. (a) Midsagittal section through the pelvis: note ventroflexure of the uterus, which tends to lift upwards during sexual stimulation, moving the cervical os anteriorly in the tenting effect. The smooth muscular wall of the vagina is overlain by extensive highly vascularized stroma covered in a stratified squamous epithelium. It is not a secretory epithelium; vaginal fluids are derived either by transudation, or from secretions of the cervix and Bartholin's glands, as well as minor vestibular glands at the vaginal vestibule. (b) View of genitalia from the exterior. In some species, the clitoris contains a small bony structure, the os clitoris, homologous to the os penis in the male.

poor, efforts to define at least some of these factors can have considerable value.

Semen is deposited in the vagina, cervix or uterus depending on the species

At coition, the semen is ejaculated within the vagina and onto the cervical os in the human, sheep or cow. In some other species, e.g. the pig, dog, horse, mouse and rat, there is a direct deposition into the cervix and/or uterus. In many species studied, the semen *coagulates* rapidly during or immediately after deposition. The coagulation may become gelatinous (e.g. in the human, pig and horse), fibrous (e.g. in the guinea-pig) or calcareous (e.g. in the mouse) and results from an enzyme–substrate interaction. In humans, coagulating enzymes derived from the prostate interact with a fibrinogen-like substrate derived from the seminal vesicle. The coagulum may act to retain spermatozoa in the vagina, preventing their physical loss or perhaps buffering them against the hostile acidity of the vaginal fluids (pH 5.7). In some cases of ejaculatory disorder, coagulation takes place within the urethra or (in *retrograde ejaculation*) within the bladder, and obstruction to urinary flow can result. In normal circumstances in the human female tract, the coagulum is dissolved within 20–60 min by progressive activation of a proenzyme derived from the prostatic secretion of the ejaculate.

Gametes are transported through the female genital tract

Spermatozoa are transported largely by their own activity

Spermatozoa deposited in the vagina face a journey of some 160–200 mm if they are to reach the site of fertilization. Most do not make it. Within a minute or so of mating in all species studied, some spermatozoa can be detected in the cervix or the uterus. It is not at present clear how human spermatozoa deposited in the vagina actually enter the cervix. Perhaps the ciliated surface of the cervical os wafts them towards the cervical canal. However, in the human over 99% of spermatozoa do not enter the cervix and are lost by leakage from the vagina. The few successful spermatozoa may survive for many hours deep in the cervical crypts of the mucous membrane (Table 9.3). Here they are nourished by mucoid secretions, their further progress to the uterus depending on the mucus consistency. Only in the absence of progesterone domination does the mucus permit sperm penetration (see Chapter 8), and even then morphologically abnormal spermatozoa are prevented from passing further up the female tract.

Studies on the transport of spermatozoa through the uterus to the oviduct are difficult to undertake. It seems clear that the vaginal, cervical and uterine movements often present in the preorgasmic and orgasmic phases are not *required* for effective sperm transport but may assist it. Nor is it likely that the prostaglandins present in the semen are required as stimulants to the female tract. In humans, the spermatozoa probably move through the uterus and into the ampulla of the oviduct by their own propulsion and in currents of fluid set up by the action of uterine cilia. This conclusion fits with the timescale of spermatozoal migration, since the earliest that living spermatozoa are recovered from the oviduct is 2–7 h after coition. The number of living oviducal spermatozoa detected during the early stages of fertilization can be measured in tens or hundreds, and even subsequently the total number present at any one time rarely exceeds several hundred. It is not at all clear how the flow of sperm to the oviduct is regulated. The cervical crypts may act as a reservoir, slowly releasing sperm into the uterus. Additionally, the uterotubal junction seems to regulate entry to the oviduct by its action as an intermittent sphincter.

Having reached the isthmus of the oviduct, spermatozoa linger and become immotile, binding temporarily to oviducal epithelial cells. Only at ovulation do spermatozoa reacquire motility and swim to the ampullary–isthmic junction (see Fig. 5.1) and the site of potential fertilization. This process seems to depend on the *release of chemo-attractants* by both the oocyte and the cumulus mass. The nature of the chemo-attractant(s) is unclear, although the examination of spermatozoa for potential chemo-attractant-sensing receptors has revealed the presence of *odorant receptors* that resemble those found in the olfactory epithelium. They are located in the sperm midpiece and flagellum base and are activated by small aldehyde molecules, the molecular nature of which is species specific. Receptor stimulation results in G-protein activation of an adenylate kinase, leading to cAMP-mediated stimulation of a rise in intracellular Ca^{2+}. This rise is associated with *sperm chemotaxis* and *chemokinesis* (enhanced swimming speed) and *hyperactive flagellar beating*. It remains to be proved that such a system of chemoattraction actually functions *in vivo* and, if so, what the molecular identity of the *in vivo* chemo-attractant molecule(s) is.

Oocyte transport depends on the activity of the oviduct

While the spermatozoa are moving towards the oviducal ampulla, the ovulated oocyte(s), with enclosing cumulus cells, is picked up from the surface of the ovary in the peritoneal cavity by the fimbriated ostium of the oviduct (see Fig. 5.1) to which it adheres, and is then swept by oviducal cilia along the ampulla towards the junction with the isthmus (Fig. 5.1; for videos see <*www.talbotcentral.ucr.edu/oocytemovie.htm*>). Oocyte transport is affected adversely if cumulus cells are lacking and/or if oviducal cilia are

Table 9.3 Estimates of the survival of viable fertile gametes in the female genital tract.

Species	Spermatozoa (h)	Oocytes (h)
Human	28–48	6–24
Cow	30–48	8–12
Sheep	30–48	15–25
Horse	75–120	6–8
Pig	25–50	8–10
Mouse	6–12	6–15
Rabbit	30–36	6–8

malfunctional. As for the uterus, there is no evidence that muscular activity in the oviduct is essential for transport into and along the ampulla, although smooth muscle in the mesosalpinx and tubo-ovarian ligaments may aid the ostial pick-up of oocytes. The oocytes and the spermatozoa come together in the ampulla and it is here that the final events leading to fertilization occur.

Fertilization is a protracted process taking many hours for completion

Spermatozoa gain their full fertilizing capacity in the female tract: capacitation

If mature spermatozoa recovered at ejaculation are placed with oocytes *in vitro*, fertilization either does not occur or does so only after a delay of several hours. In contrast, spermatozoa recovered from the uterus or oviduct a few hours after coitus are capable of immediate fertilization. This attainment of a full fertilizing capacity within the female tract is called *capacitation*. The process includes a stripping from the spermatozoal surface of much of the coating of glycoprotein molecules acquired during passage through the epididymis and after contact with seminal plasma, resulting in changes to the surface charge, macromolecular organization and lipid structure (especially loss of cholesterol) of the spermatozoal membrane, all of which reduce its stability and enhance its fusibility. The process is experimentally reversible; thus, if capacitated spermatozoa are re-incubated in epididymal fluid or seminal plasma, they become *decapacitated*. An oestrogen-primed uterus or oviducal isthmus is optimal for capacitation, critical features being the proteolytic enzymes and high ionic strength provided by their secretions. In addition, there is good evidence that, at ejaculation and exposure to atmospheric oxygen, reactive oxygen species form and stimulate production of hydrogen peroxide (H_2O_2), a potent capacitating agent. It is possible to mimic these conditions *in vitro* by preparation of suitable culture media of high ionic strength in atmospheric oxygen.

The capacitated spermatozoon can be distinguished by two characteristics: (1) a change in its movement pattern to a *hyperactivated motility* state in which the regular undulating wave-like flagellar beats are replaced by stronger, wide-amplitude or *'whiplashing' beats* of the tail that push the spermatozoon forwards in vigorous lurches (Fig. 9.4b); and (2) a change in the surface membrane properties that renders the spermatozoon responsive to signals encountered in the immediate vicinity of the oocyte, which themselves then induce a further change in the spermatozoa called the *acrosome reaction* (see next section). How is capacitation achieved? Several molecular events seem to underlie the process.

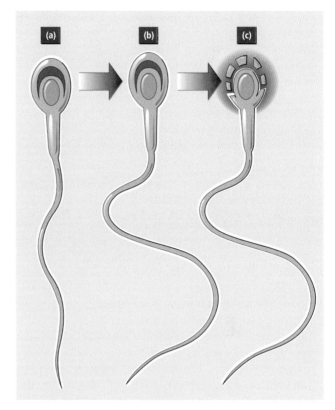

Fig. 9.4 (a) Schematized spermatozoon prior to capacitation; a consequence of capacitation is (b) hyperactivated tail movements, and development of the capacity subsequently to undergo (c) the acrosome reaction, in which multiple sites of fusion between the plasma membrane and the outer acrosomal membrane occur, first at the tip of the acrosome and then at the equatorial region. As a result of the acrosome reaction, the plasma membrane remaining in the equatorial and postacrosomal regions acquires the potential to fuse with the plasma membrane of the oocyte.

First, an increased calcium permeability of the spermatozoal membrane occurs, leading to a modest rise in internal calcium levels. This is coupled with a loss from the spermatozoal surface of calmodulin-binding proteins, which may make the spermatozoa more responsive to the effects of calcium. The development of hyperactivated motility is sensitive to calcium levels. Second, and as a result of elevated calcium, adenyl cyclase activity within the spermatozoa increases, leading to elevation of cAMP levels and increased cAMP-dependent phosphorylation of spermatozoal proteins. Sperm motility is enhanced by addition of either exogenous cAMP or inhibitors of phosphodiesterase (such as pentoxyfylline, thereby preventing destruction of cAMP). Third, the cAMP activates a spermatozoal protein kinase A (PKA) which phosphorylates tyrosine residues on both itself (autophosphorylation) and other intracellular proteins. If this autophosphorylation is prevented, the ability of spermatozoa to undergo a subsequent acrosome reaction (next section) is impaired, and thus the event seems to be a critical component of the capacitatory process. Fourth, actin polymerization occurs in the cytosol between the surface and acrosomal membranes. This F-actin may intervene to prevent a premature acrosome reaction of the now destabilized membranes.

The capacitated spermatozoon is now in a metastable state. Unless it finds an oocyte fairly rapidly, it will die.

The acrosome reaction is essential if spermatozoa are to penetrate the zona pellucida

Those capacitated spermatozoa that manage to reach the zona pellucida of the oocyte, bind to it via receptors on the spermatozoal anterior head region. The zona then induces a dramatic morphological transformation in the spermatozoa called the *acrosome reaction* (Fig. 9.4c). During this process, the acrosome swells, its membrane fuses with the overlying plasma membrane, a vesiculated appearance is created and the contents of the acrosomal vesicle and the inner acrosomal membrane both become exteriorized in a process of *exocytosis*. The acrosome reaction is associated with further large increases in intracellular calcium and cAMP. The calcium elevation seems central to the acrosome reaction as is shown by the failure of activation in the absence of calcium and by the induction of activation prematurely by use of calcium ionophore to enhance its entry. It also seems clear that a rise in intracellular pH from about 7.1 to 7.5 occurs, and may work synergistically with the calcium. A key function of the elevated calcium is the depolymerization of the recently formed F-actin in the cytosol separating the surface and acrosomal membranes, which is achieved by calcium-activated actin-severing proteins. What stimulates the calcium entry and how? A number of agents have been shown to increase calcium influx. The problem has been to discriminate which of them is biologically relevant.

It is now generally accepted that the agent responsible for the acrosome reaction *in vivo* is a constituent of the zona pellucida. The zona is made up of three glycoproteins called *ZP1, 2* and *3*. ZP1 is a minor component and is not essential for binding of capacitated spermatozoa. The evidence suggests a dominant binding role for ZP3 but only if organized structurally in conjunction with ZP2. This three-dimensional ZP2/3 molecular framework is *species specific*—mouse sperm bind mouse ZP2/3 and human sperm bind human ZP2/3—the major natural block to cross-species fertilization. What about the ZP2/3 binding site on spermatozoa? It seems likely that β*1,4-galactosyl transferase 1 (GalT 1)* located on the anterior sperm membrane overlying the acrosome is a key player, since site directed mutation or knockout of the *GalT 1* gene greatly

reduces ZP binding. The weak residual sperm binding suggests involvement of a second sperm membrane player, which may be a protein called SED1.

The sperm–ZP binding then stimulates the further calcium influx and pH elevation, via an action involving a G protein. The acrosome reaction follows. As might be expected, blocking the calcium rise prevents the acrosome-inducing effect of the zona. As much of the sperm receptor for ZP2/3 is shed on the vesiculating membrane during the acrosome reaction, spermatozoal binding to ZP3 is short lived. In addition, the acrosome releases β-*hexosaminidase B*, which digests away any local ZP3 receptor, so preventing further binding. The acrosome reaction now exposes the inner acrosomal membrane, on which are located proteolytic enzymes, such as *acrosin*. These digest a path through the zona, along which the spermatozoon passes aided by the whiplash forward propulsion of the hyperactivated tail. Penetration of the zona takes between 5 and 20 min.

It is important that the acrosome reaction occurs close to the oocyte, because acrosome-reacted spermatozoa have a very short lifespan. Herein probably lies the explanation for the rather complex series of changes that spermatozoa undergo in the female tract. Hours (or even days, in the human) may intervene between deposition of the ejaculate into the female tract and the ovulation of an oocyte. High fertility may be ensured by establishing a reservoir of spermatozoa, releasing a gradual trickle through the capacitating uterus and oviduct where their final fertilizing capacity can only be realized in the presence of an oocyte. If all spermatozoa were fully competent to fertilize immediately after their release into the female tract, much stricter time limits on fertility would operate.

Sperm–oocyte binding involves disintegrin–integrin interaction, but fusion involves additional molecules

After penetrating the zona pellucida, the spermatozoon eventually comes to lie tangential to the oocyte surface between the zona pellucida and the oocyte membrane *(oolemma)* in the *perivitelline space,* where microvilli on the surface of the oocyte envelop the sperm head (Fig. 9.5b). Two sequential events then follow, each involving distinct molecular partnerships: first sperm–oocyte *binding* and second sperm–oocyte *fusion*. It is important to note that *only capacitated spermatozoa that have undergone an acrosome reaction are capable of binding and fusion*.

Binding occurs between the surface membrane of the *oolemma* and the sperm surface membrane overlying the middle and the posterior half of the spermatozoal head (the equatorial and postacrosomal region). The binding involves an interaction between an integrin-like molecule in the oolemma and a molecule named ADAM on the sperm,

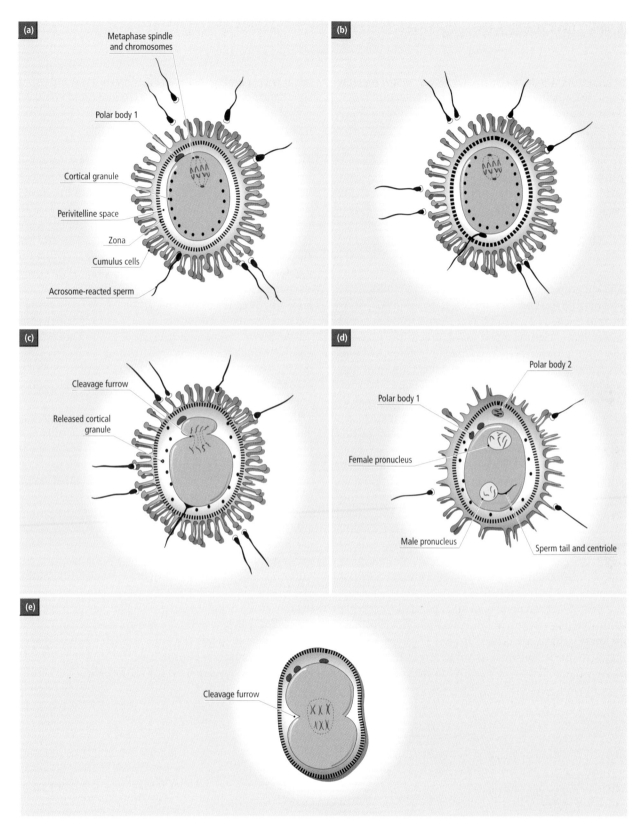

Fig. 9.5 (a) Spermatozoa approach an ovulated oocyte with its first polar body, chromosomes on the second metaphase spindle, cortical granules and perivitelline space between the oolemma of the oocyte and the zona pellucida. One capacitated spermatozoon binds to the ZP2/3 components of the zona pellucida inducing the acrosome reaction and then (b) penetrates the zona to lie in the perivitelline space, where it (c) binds to and then fuses with the plasma membrane via its equatorial and postacrosomal membrane, thus activating a series of calcium waves (see Fig. 9.6). The calcium induces a release of cortical granules and resumption of meiosis with formation of an asymmetrically located cleavage furrow. (d) Meiotic division is completed, yielding the second polar body and female pronucleus. Meanwhile the sperm nucleus decondenses and the male pronucleus forms, the sperm centriole and tail being adjacent.
(e) Chromosomes duplicate their DNA, pronuclei migrate together, their membranes break down as the first mitotic spindle forms. After its formation, chromatids separate and move apart, and a cleavage furrow develops. By this stage the cumulus cells have dispersed.

where ADAM is an acronym for **a** **d**istintegrin **a**nd **m**etalloproteinase domain-containing protein. The integrin family has many members, and several of them are expressed on the surface of the oocyte. Use of antibodies to neutralize individual integrins and of specific genetic knockouts of some integrin genes in the oocyte has not yet resolved which of the integrin αβ dimers mediate binding of the spermatozoa. In contrast, a similar approach on spermatozoa has been more successful. Three sperm ADAMS have been detected called *fertilin α*, *fertilin β* and *cyritestin*, and all three appear to be co-regulated and involved in sperm–oocyte binding. Thus, knockout of one reduces expression of the others and reduces binding to the oocyte.

The integrins form part of a multiprotein complex in the oolemma, and this complex appears to be essential *if fusion is to follow binding*. Two molecular partners in this oocyte complex have been identified as important for successful fusion. *CD9* is a large membrane-spanning protein involved in membrane fusion in several situations (viral infection, myotube fusion). Oocytes from CD9-null mice bind spermatozoa but do not fuse with them, unless rescued by injection of mRNA encoding CD9. The null oocytes can also develop if the blocked fusion is bypassed by injecting a spermatozoon directly into the oocyte cytoplasm. Similarly, antibodies to CD9 block fusion of sperm with normal oocytes. A second molecular suspect is a class of proteins called glycosylphosphatidylinositol (GPI)-anchored proteins. These are deficient in oocytes lacking a critical biosynthetic enzyme subunit of N-acetyl glucosaminyl transferase. It is not clear what the corresponding molecular partners are on the spermatozoa, although an epididymidal protein called CRISP1 that coats the sperm during maturation, has been implicated.

It is probable that a number of other molecules can influence the binding and fusion processes through interactions with these central molecular players. Calcium is again required for the fusion process, and its action may be mediated by calmodulin, as antagonists to this molecule can block sperm–oocyte fusion. Once fusion has occurred, the spermatozoon dramatically ceases to move and its nucleus (together with variable parts of the midpiece and tail contents, depending on the species) passes into the ooplasm.

Sperm phospholipase Cζ stimulates calcium waves in the oocyte

Within 1–5 min after fusion of the oocyte with the spermatozoon, there is a dramatic increase in the level of free intracellular calcium in the egg, due largely to the release of calcium from internal stores (Fig. 9.6). The rise lasts about 2–3 min and does not occur synchronously over the whole oocyte, but rather sweeps in a wave across the oocyte starting from the point of sperm entry. This first rise is followed by a series of calcium spikes, each spike being of 1–2 min duration, becoming more synchronous over the whole oocyte and occurring every 3–15 min depending on the individual oocyte (Fig. 9.6). This spiking activity can last for several hours. This calcium rise is critical for all the subsequent events of fertilization, and if it is blocked, so are fertilization and development.

Despite the importance of the calcium rise, it is still not entirely clear how the fusion of oocyte and spermatozoon triggers it. Currently, the most likely explanation is that the fertilizing spermatozoon releases a protein into the oocyte at fusion, which then initiates the release of internal calcium (Fig. 9.7). This protein has been identified as a sperm-specific enzyme called *phospholipase Cζ* (zeta). Thus, injection of either mRNA encoding PLCζ or recombinant PLCζ protein itself into oocytes is sufficient alone to activate calcium pulsing and development, whereas RNAi-mediated neutralization of endogenous PLCζ truncates calcium pulsing and blocks development. PLCζ exerts its effects by stimulating the release of the second messengers *inositol triphosphate* (IP$_3$) and *diacylglycerol* (DAG). The former then activates the calcium release, while the latter activates *protein kinase C* (PKC) to stimulate the phosphorylation of proteins essential for the further development of the conceptus.

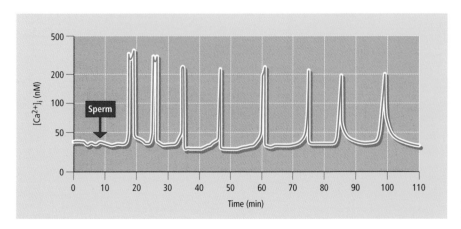

Fig. 9.6 The calcium spiking pattern of a fertilized zona-free oocyte inseminated with spermatozoa at the time indicated by the arrow. After 12 min, a spermatozoon fused with the oocyte, generating a transient 5–10-fold rise in internal calcium. Thereafter, calcium pulses followed at 3–15-min intervals (characteristic for each oocyte) and lasted for several hours.

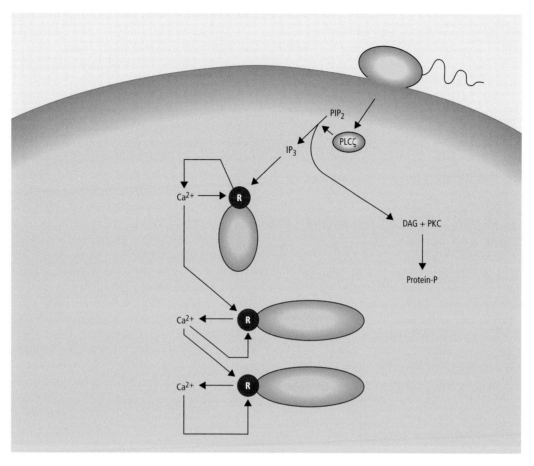

Fig. 9.7 Model for activation of the oocyte calcium waves by the fertilizing spermatozoon. After fusion, the spermatozoon introduces *phospholipase Cζ (zeta)* into the oocyte. The PLCζ stimulates the release of the second messengers *inositol triphosphate* (IP$_3$) and *diacylglycerol* (DAG). The IP$_3$ activates the calcium release, while the DAG activates *protein kinase C* (PKC) to stimulate the phosphorylation of proteins essential for the further development of the conceptus. R = IP$_3$ receptor type.

This first phase of fertilization, from entry into the cumulus mass to fusion, is completed. The oocyte is now called a *zygote*. The ensuing events of fertilization last some 20h or so and are concerned with two distinctive types of activity. First, the diploid genetic constitution of the zygote must be ensured. Second, the developmental programme of the conceptus must be initiated. The calcium and the phosphoproteins stimulated by the activity of PLCζ play critical roles in both events.

The establishment of diploidy requires a single fertilizing spermatozoon and the expulsion of the second polar body

The newly fertilized oocyte confronts two immediate problems. First, it must prevent further spermatozoa from fertilizing it (the *block to polyspermy*) as this would cause *triploidy* (for one extra sperm) or *polyploidy* (for several). Polyploidy of this sort is described as *androgenetic*, as the extra sets of haploid chromosomes are derived from the

male. Second, the oocyte was ovulated arrested in its second meiotic division. If it is to transmit only one set of chromosomes to the next generation, it must complete its second meiotic division, dispatching one set of chromosomes to the *second polar body* (Fig. 9.5c), and enter interphase of the first cell cycle. The failure to complete the second meiotic division and jettison a set of female chromosomes would lead to *gynogenetic triploidy*. The calcium pulsations resulting from gamete fusion play a key role in achieving diploidy, as can be demonstrated clearly by blocking them experimentally. The pulses probably work at least in part by activating *calmodulin-dependent protein kinase II (CamKII)*, which in turn phosphorylates several target proteins critical for the next steps in the fertilization process. Indeed, inhibition of CamKII prevents further development. So how exactly is diploidy achieved?

First, the elevated calcium results in fusion of the *cortical granules* in the cortex of the zygote with the overlying oolemma, thereby releasing their contents into the perivitelline space (*the cortical reaction*) (Fig. 9.5c). Among the contents of these granules are enzymes that act on the zona pellucida to prevent, or impair, further binding and penetration by spermatozoa (*the zona reaction*). These enzymes have at least three actions. A protease cleaves glycoprotein ZP2, and β-hexosaminidase B digests the oligosaccharide receptor on glycoprotein ZP3. In this way, the ZP sperm-binding properties are removed, and sperm binding to the zona ceases. In addition, tyrosine residues on adjacent ZPs are cross-linked, rendering the zona indissoluble to proteolytic cleavage and so impenetrable by spermatozoa. A final consequence of sperm–oocyte fusion, the mechanism for which is not yet understood, is a reduction in the sperm-binding properties of the oolemma itself. All these events occur rapidly to reduce the chances of androgenetic polyploidy.

Second, the avoidance of gynogenetic triploidy also depends on the calcium rise. At fertilization, the oocytes are arrested in the second meiotic metaphase (M phase). It is now clear that this arrest depends on the continuing presence of two types of cytoplasmic activity called *maturation promoting factor* (MPF) and *cytostatic factor* (CSF) (Fig. 9.8). MPF has been shown to consist of a complex of at least two proteins: a kinase (phosphorylating) enzyme called

cdk1 and a smaller protein called *cyclin B*, and CSF includes a key protein called *c-Mos* (working through stimulation of a MAP kinase signalling pathway). Only when MPF is present, stabilized by CSF, and active will the M phase persist. However, this complex is very sensitive to calcium, such that a rise in calcium tilts the equilibrium away from complex synthesis towards destruction. How does the calcium act? It seems possible that it interferes with CSF-mediated inhibition of another enzyme complex called *anaphase-promoting complex/cyclosome* (*APC/C*). When activated, this complex *ubiquitinates* cyclin B, stimulates its proteolysis, and leaves insufficient of it to complex with cdk1 to form MPF. As a result, the oocyte exits from the M phase and progresses through the second meiotic division.

In most species, the metaphase spindle lies just under and perpendicular to the surface (Fig. 9.5a). This means that as meiosis is completed the cleavage furrow is eccentrically placed, generating a large zygote and a small, second polar body (Fig. 9.5c). It is important to note that spermatozoa do not bind to the oocyte membrane immediately overlying the second metaphase spindle, indeed this area is devoid of integrins, CD9 and GPI-anchored proteins (Fig. 9.5b,c). This makes sense biologically, as the coincidence of a spermatozoon entering the oocyte and a second polar body being ejected could lead to mutual interference and *aneuploidy* (deviation from the normal euploid chromosomal number). There is evidence that the extrusion of the polar body requires the activity of protein kinase C in addition to the triggering calcium rise. The whole process takes about 30–45 min.

With the successful attainment of one maternal and one paternal set of haploid chromosomes, a *euploid* zygote is formed. Aneuploidy causes embryonic abnormality. Fortunately, most aneuploid conceptuses die relatively early, although a few survive to term and beyond (see Chapter 15). Others may develop into tumours, such as *hydatidiform mole* (a benign trophoblastic tumour) or *choriocarcinoma* (its malignant derivative). Thus, aneuploidy, apart from being of potential danger to the mother, is reproductively wasteful and can be distressing. Failure of the normal mechanisms for establishing euploidy is increased under certain conditions; for example, the fertilization of prematurely ovulated oocytes is associated with defective cortical granule release and poor sperm head incorporation. The fertilization of oocytes that have been ovulated and passed into the oviduct 24 h or more before sperm arrival can also be problematic (Table 9.3). In most mammalian species, in which ovulation and behavioural oestrus are closely synchronized, the problem of ageing oocytes will not be acute. In humans, however, where coitus and ovulation are not necessarily, or even usually, associated, the fertilization of old oocytes may be much commoner. There is evidence that the high incidence of genetic abnormality and early preg-

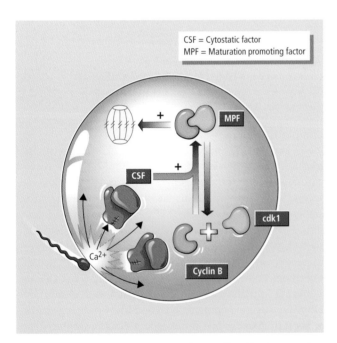

Fig. 9.8 Schematic view of the stabilizing effect (+) of maturation promoting factor (MPF) (= cyclin B + cdk1) on the second meiotic spindle (shown in yellow). MPF is in turn stabilized (+) by cytostatic factor (CSF). Raised calcium, as occurs when the spermatozoon fuses with the oocyte, destroys cyclin B and CSF. The MPF in equilibrium with cyclin B unravels and so the spindle is no longer stabilized and meiosis resumes.

nancy loss in humans reflects this dissociation of mating from fertility (see Chapter 15).

The gametes provide more than just their haploid sets of chromosomes

The establishment of diploidy is accompanied by other contributions to the zygote by each gamete. The fertilizing spermatozoon of most species also contributes another essential component to the zygote in the form of a *centrosome*. The centrosome consists of *centrioles* plus *pericentriolar material*. Although the oocyte contributes some of the latter, only the spermatozoon contributes a centriole (see Chapters 4 & 5). The centrosome is a key player in the regulation of karyo- and cytokinesis. Without it, cellular division during early development is compromised and eventually fails (see later section on parthenogenesis).

The oocyte provides the cell membrane, cytoplasm, cell organelles and macromolecular matrix in which the two sets of chromosomes and the centrosome operate: the so-called *maternal cytoplasmic inheritance*. It thus is critical for successful development, and defects in oocyte maturation lead to defects in development. In particular, although the mitochondria of the spermatozoon may enter the oocyte at fertilization, they do not survive. *All of the mitochondria in the adult are maternally derived*. Since mitochondria contain a mini-chromosome, which encodes some of the mitochondrial proteins, there is thus a small part of the total genetic inheritance that is exclusively maternally derived. Genetically based defects of mitochondrial function in a mother will therefore be transmitted to her offspring.

Gamete fusion initiates a developmental programme

During oocyte–sperm fusion and second polar body expulsion, the cytoplasmic contents of the sperm cell membrane (now fused with the oocyte membrane) pass into the oocyte cytoplasm. The sperm nuclear membrane breaks down and the highly condensed chromatin starts to swell, releasing filamentous strands of chromatin into the cytoplasm. The protamines that created such compressed chromatin are released and replaced by normal histones. This chromatin decondensation is actively induced by factors in the oocyte cytoplasm that develop in the terminal phases of intrafollicular maturation, such as high levels of the reducing agent *glutathione*.

Between 4 and 7h after fusion, the two sets of haploid chromosomes each become surrounded by distinct membranes and are now known as *pronuclei* (see Fig. 9.5d). The male is usually the larger of the two. Both pronuclei contain several nucleoli. During the next few hours, each pronucleus gradually moves from its subcortical position to a more central and adjacent cytoplasmic position. During this period, the haploid chromosomes synthesize DNA in preparation for the first mitotic division, which occurs

about 18–24h after gamete fusion. The pronuclear membranes around the reduplicated sets of parental chromosomes break down (see Fig. 9.5e), the mitotic metaphase spindle forms and the chromosomes assume their positions at its equator. The final phase of fertilization has been achieved: *syngamy* (or coming together of the gametic chromosomes) has occurred. Immediately the first mitotic anaphase and telophase are completed, the *cleavage furrow* forms, and the one-cell zygote becomes a two-cell conceptus.

Oocytes can be activated in the absence of a spermatozoon (parthenogenesis) but cannot develop to term

Although the spermatozoon induces many remarkable changes in the oocyte, it does not appear to be essential for many of them. An oocyte may be activated *parthenogenetically* by a variety of bizarre stimuli, such as electric shock, or exposure to various enzymes or to alcohol. Activation by these stimuli is especially easy in 'aged' oocytes that have been ovulated several hours previously. These stimuli have the common feature that they induce a calcium rise, thereby mimicking the act of spermatozoal fusion. As a result, cortical granules exocytose, meiotic metaphase is resumed and the oocyte's developmental programme is activated. The *parthenote* so formed may undergo some cell divisions but eventually fails in most species, including humans and the large farm animals. In a few species, such as the mouse, rat and hamster, cell division is unimpaired and a blastocyst may form, implant and develop to a stage where a beating heart, somites and forelimbs are present. However, even in these species, most parthenotes die fairly early on in this sequence and none survive to term (see also discussion on asexual reproduction in Chapter 1). There are two reasons for this lack of survival.

• First, because in most species activated oocytes lack a centriole and thus a fully functional centrosome, an early cessation of cell division occurs. In the mouse, in contrast, the cells of the conceptus appear to be able to generate their own centrosome *de novo* such that cell division is relatively unimpaired, hence its further development. However, even in the mouse parthenogenetic development fails eventually and the second reason, which applies to all species, explains why.

• Second, it seems that during the packaging of the chromosomes for transmission to the zygote, the environment in which the chromosomes find themselves influences the organization of some of their genes in a way that affects their ability to become transcriptionally active subsequently in the conceptus. It is not the actual genetic code (the base sequence) itself that is changed but the way in which the genes are chemically modified and then wrapped up in associated proteins to form chromatin (see Fig. 9.9 and Box 4.3). This process is called *imprinting*, because it leaves an imprint on the genes that is 'remembered' and affects later expression. It is described as being an *epigenetic change* to the genome, because it does not affect the genetic code itself (which would be a *genetic change*) but does affect expression of the encoded genes. The important point about this particular epigenetic change is that the genes affected by it in the spermatogenic lineage differ from those imprinted in the oogenetic lineage. In other words, the imprinting pattern is *parentally specific*. These *maternal and paternal imprinting processes* mean that, although the oocyte and the spermatozoon each contribute one complete set of chromosomes and genes to the conceptus, each set is not on its own fully competent to direct a complete programme of development. Only when a set of genes from an oocyte is combined with a set of genes from a spermatozoon is a fully functional genetic blueprint achieved. A parthenote lacks access to some crucial genetic information which, although present in its chromosomes, cannot be accessed because of the maternal imprinting to which it was subjected during oogenesis. In the normal zygote, this information would be

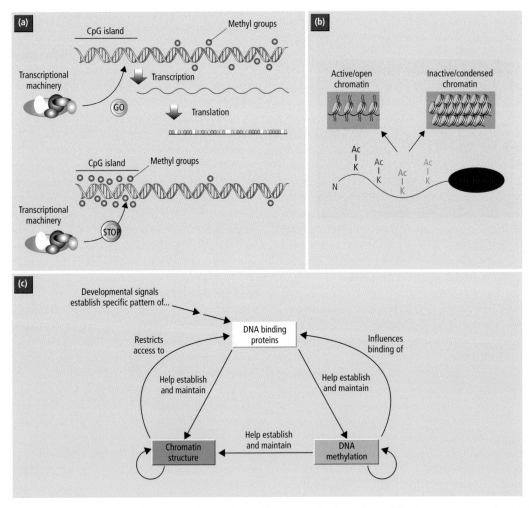

Fig. 9.9 Summary of mechanisms available for genetic imprinting. Two sorts of epigenetic modification can leave an imprint. (a) The direct methylation of some, but not all, cytosines (see CpG island in lower part of panel) within the DNA sequence itself. This methylation then blocks access to transcriptional machinery (lower part). Once initiated, this methylation pattern can be copied at each round of DNA replication as long as the maintenance methylase is present, and it is thus heritable through many mitoses. (b) A second sort of epigenetic modification is seen in the chromatin histone isotypes used in the chromatin surrounding the promoter region of the genes, as well as in their post-translational modification (me = methylation; Ac = acetylation; P = phosphorylation). See also Box 4.3 for discussion of this type of modification during chromatin reorganization during spermatogenesis. (c) Quite complex interactions may occur during development between the two types of epigenetic modification and associated transcriptional proteins. However, these are early days in the science of epigenesis and much remains to be understood (see Chapters 12, 14 and 15 for further discussion of the importance of epigenetic imprinting in health and disease).

provided by genes on the paternally derived set of chromosomes.

Parental imprinting has profound implications for mammals, because it *compels us to reproduce sexually*. There are costs to obligatory sexual reproduction, as discussed in Chapter 1. The time and energy taken up with seeking a sexual partner, courting and mating is costly. Males cannot be dispensed with, but consume resources. Asexual reproduction has many advantages for rapid and efficient propagation of the species. Sexual reproduction may be more advantageous at times of stress when maximum genetic flexibility is required for the species to survive—the more extreme the threat, then there is a greater chance of the species surviving if its genetic variability is maximized. Many organisms retain an option on asexual reproduction, even where sexual reproduction can occur, but mammals have lost that option during evolution. One of the great puzzles of mammalian biology is why?

Reproductive 'cloning' by somatic cell nuclear transfer (SCNT)

Although asexual reproduction naturally by parthenogenesis cannot occur in mammals, the ingenuity of scientists has circumvented this block experimentally. A diploid somatic nucleus, taken from an adult or fetal differentiated cell, can be placed into the cytoplasm of an oocyte from which the metaphase 2 spindle has been removed together with its chromosomes (Fig. 9.10). The reconstituted oocyte can then be activated to develop and the developing diploid conceptus placed in a uterus. Such conceptuses, can, albeit at low frequency, develop to term (so far achieved, *inter alia*, in sheep, cattle, pigs, goats, cats, dogs, mice). The individual animal produced shares all its nuclear chromosomes with the donor of the adult or fetal nucleus. This process is called *reproductive cloning* and the process leading to it is called *somatic cell nuclear transfer* or *SCNT*.

Despite examples of SCNT resulting in live young, the vast majority of cloned conceptuses die at early to midgestation stages of development. The very small percentage of conceptuses that survive to late fetal stages or birth are characterized by a high mortality rate and frequently display grossly increased placental and birthweights and respiratory distress, and the healthy lifespan of the surviving offspring may be curtailed. Why? The answer to this question is complex and the subject of continuing research, but certain explanations already seem likely.

First, although the conceptuses created by SCNT are diploid, most if not all show abnormal gene expression patterns compared with those developing from fertilized oocytes. The reason for this difference is, in part if not entirely, due to *abnormal epigenetic modification patterns*. We saw in the last section the important role of parental imprinting in forcing sexual reproduction. However, epigenetic changes to the genome also occur naturally in non-parentally determined ways as cells divide and differentiate

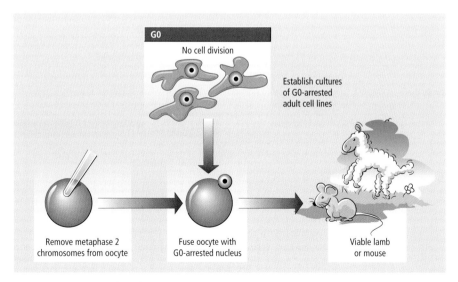

Fig. 9.10 Schematic summary of the procedure for somatic cell nuclear transfer (SCNT) in sheep or mice. A differentiated cell is cultured and its division cycle arrested by removal of nutrients (G0 stage). A karyoplast (the nucleus with a small amount of cytoplasm and cell membrane surrounding it) is then prepared from the quiescent cell. It is placed next to an M2 arrested oocyte from which the second meiotic spindle and chromosomes have been removed by suction. A fusogenic signal is then given. The nucleus and enucleated oocyte fuse and initiate cleavage. The cleaving conceptus is placed into the uterus of a ewe (or mouse) and a viable offspring can result.

to generate all the multitude of cell types making up the body—these are called *developmental epigenetic imprints*. This process ensures that the genes needed for a particular tissue are available for expression in that tissue and that other un-needed genes are closed down to expression (see Fig. 9.9 and Box 4.3). Thus, when a diploid nucleus from, say, the skin is used in SCNT it carries with it whole sets of epigenetic modifications to its genes that must be erased if it is to be able to express all the genes required to make an entire organism. Although it seems that the oocyte cytoplasm is very effective at erasing these developmental epigenetic imprints, it may not have sufficient time or capacity to erase them all. Evidence to support this explanation is shown by the greater ability of nuclei from very early developmental stages to support cloned conceptus development than nuclei from more differentiated cells. In addition, serial transfer of differentiated nuclei through one ooplasm into a second one improves the capacity of these nuclei to support development.

A second reason for the failure of the cloned conceptuses to develop may arise from the fact that although differentiated nuclei have properly parentally imprinted genes, these parental imprint patterns may also be disturbed during the process of SCNT, with further adverse developmental consequences.

Finally, it has been shown that the transferred somatic cell nuclei carry with them a coating of cytoplasm containing mitochondria and that these mitochondria, unlike those brought in by spermatozoa, survive. Thus, the cells of the cloned conceptus have a mixture of mitochondria from different sources and it is suggested that incompatibility between them and the nuclear genome may be developmentally problematic.

There is clearly a long way to go before we fully understand what happens after SCNT in animals. On safety grounds alone, therefore, the prospect of *human* reproductive cloning is unethical. However, ethical concerns go beyond safety, and these concerns have led to the legal prohibition of human reproductive cloning in many jurisdictions. However, in some countries, including the UK, non-reproductive human SCNT is permitted under strict licence for research purposes only. This research aims to understand the earliest postfertilization molecular events in humans, such as how, where and when epigenetic imprints are erased or modified and what problems mitochondrial heterogeneity may present. Such research is of particular importance if human embryonic stem cells are to be medically useful. But more of that in the next chapter!

Summary

The interval between the departure of the gametes from the gonads and the successful formation of a two-cell conceptus encompasses an extraordinarily complex sequence of events involving biochemical, behavioural, endocrine, physiological and genetic components. Not surprisingly, aspects of this process often go wrong and infertility results (see Chapter 15). Fortunately, recent biomedical advances mean that most of these events can now be carried out *in vitro*. Mature oocytes can be aspirated directly from the follicles; spermatozoa can be recovered from ejaculates or even microsurgically from the testis and epididymis, and can be capacitated and activated in defined media; fertilization and the formation of a zygote can be achieved outside the body. These techniques have provided help for many otherwise infertile couples. Considerable controversy has surrounded the ethics of using these procedures; in particular, the decisive role that fusion of an oocyte and a spermatozoon might play in the establishment of a human life has been stressed. It is important to be aware that scientific evidence does not support the view that one single event is decisive for the creation of an individual life. The process is a continuum which starts with the growth of the oocyte and the synthesis of the maternal cytoplasmic inheritance, involves distinctive epigenetic changes to the sperm and oocyte genomes, and continues with the formation and development of the zygote, the signalling by the conceptus to the mother of its presence, and the subsequent acquisition of a distinctive human form capable ultimately of independent existence. The natural losses in mammals are massive over the early events in this sequence, particularly from oocyte atresia, sperm wastage and preimplantation death. Human preimplantation losses are increased further by our changed social and sexual habits and the use of various forms of contraceptive. So biology cannot provide the answer to the question 'When does a human life begin?' because the question is based on false premises. Biologically, life is a continuum. Ethical decisions cannot therefore be taken on the basis of biological observation alone.

FURTHER READING

General reading

Aitken RJ (1997) Regulators of sperm function. *Molecular Human Reproduction* 3, 169–213.

Allen CA, Green DPL (1996) The mammalian acrosome reaction: gateway to sperm fusion with the oocyte? *BioEssays* **19**, 241–247.

Bancroft J (1989) *Human Sexuality and Its Problems*. Churchill Livingstone, Edinburgh.

Breitbart H *et al*. (1997) Regulatory mechanisms in acrosomal exocytosis. *Reviews of Reproduction* **2**, 165–174.

Cirino G *et al*. (2006) Pharmacology of erectile dysfunction in man. *Pharmacology & Therapeutics I₂* **111**, 400–423.

Creed KE *et al*. (1991) The physiology of penile erection. *Oxford Reviews of Reproductive Biology* **13**, 72–95.

KEY LEARNING POINTS

- Spermatozoa leave the testis through the rete testis and vasa efferentia carried in fluid secreted by the Sertoli cells.

- This fluid is absorbed by the vasa efferentia in an oestrogen-dependent process.

- Thereafter, spermatozoa are moved through the male genital tract by the activity of its musculature.

- Spermatozoa mature during transit through the epididymis.

- Epididymal maturation is androgen dependent and most androgen arrives via lymph and testicular fluid.

- Spermatozoa may be stored in the cauda epididymis and/or vas deferens depending on the species.

- Seminal plasma is produced in the male accessory sex glands, especially the prostate and seminal vesicle.

- Seminal plasma forms a fluid vehicle for spermatozoa and may provide buffering, antioxidant and metabolic support for them.

- Seminal plasma is also a vehicle for transfer of infection between individuals, as is vaginal fluid.

- Seminal plasma combines with spermatozoa at emission and ejaculation to form semen.

- Coition involves sexual responses and genital reflexes.

- The phases of sexual responsiveness are called excitement, plateau, orgasmic and resolution (EPOR).

- These phases are accompanied by a range of systemic and emotional manifestations.

- Erection involves haemodynamic changes to the corpora cavernosa (of the penis and clitoris) converting each to a high-volume/high-pressure system.

- In some species, retraction of the penis and a penile bone aid the erectile process.

- The haemodynamic changes depend on increased blood inflow due to vasodilatation mediated by nitric oxide which reduces sympathetic myogenic tone; vascular shunts may also be closed and turgor-induced pressure may reduce blood outflow.

- Erectile dysfunction (or impotence) may be treated with smooth muscle relaxants such as prostaglandin E_1 (alprostadil) or phosphodiesterase-5 inhibitors (sildenafil, tadafil and vardenafil).

- Semen is deposited in the vagina, cervix or uterus depending on the species.

- After vaginal deposition, most spermatozoa fail to enter the cervix and those that do may be stored there for up to 2 days.

- Spermatozoa reach the oviduct by swimming, perhaps helped by ciliary currents.

- Spermatozoa wait in the oviducal isthmus until ovulation when they move into the ampulla, possibly by chemotaxis involving odorant receptors on spermatozoa.

- The ovulated oocyte is picked up actively by the oviducal ostia and transported to the ampullary–isthmic junction.

- Spermatozoa are capacitated in the female genital tract to gain forward activated movement and the capacity to undergo the acrosome reaction.

- Capacitation involves removal of adsorbed macromolecules, destabilization of the sperm surface, entry of calcium, activation of adenyl cyclase, a rise in cAMP and phosphorylation of tyrosine kinase.

- The acrosome reaction involves fusion of the acrosome with the overlying plasma membrane and release of acrosomal contents.

- It is induced by binding to zona glycoproteins 2 and 3 involving β1,4-galactosyl transferase and SED1.

- Acrosome-reacted spermatozoa then digest a path proteolytically through the zona.

- A spermatozoon binds at its equatorial postacrosomal segment with the oolemma, probably via an integrin/ADAM molecular interaction.

- Fusion of spermatozoon and oocyte involves the further involvement of CD9 and GPI-anchored proteins.

- Fusion results in the entry of spermatozoal phospholipase Cζ into the oocyte, where it generates a series of calcium spikes, which lasts for several hours.

- The fertilized oocyte is now called a zygote.

- The calcium activates release of cortical granules which prevent polyspermy by effects on the zona and the oolemma.

- The calcium also reactivates arrested meiosis and second polar body extrusion by destroying cytostatic factor and cyclin B and thereby maturation promoting factor (MPF) activity.

- Spermatozoa also contribute their centrioles to the zygote in most species and this is essential for continuing cell division during development.

- Oocytes contribute most other cell organelles to the zygote including mitochondria, which are inherited exclusively via the maternal route.

- A male pronucleus forms and its heterochromatin decondenses, protamines being replaced by histones.

- A female pronucleus forms and is usually smaller than the male pronucleus.

- Over an 18–24-h period, the pronuclei replicate their DNA, move together, lose their nuclear membranes and form a mitotic spindle, and the male and female chromosomes come together for the first time on the spindle at syngamy.

- Oocytes can be activated in the absence of a spermatozoon but show only limited development because of the absence of a centriole (in most species) and the fact that some genes are differentially parentally imprinted (in all species) and therefore not formally equivalent on homologous chromosomes.

- Reproductive cloning by transfer of the nucleus from an adult somatic cell to an enucleated oocyte (SCNT) can result in the development of a few live young which differ genetically from the donor of the nucleus mainly in their mitochondrial DNA.

- Most cloned conceptuses die early in development, and most of those surviving have enlarged placentae or other pathologies, probably mainly as a result of epigenetic abnormalities.

D'Alessio AC, Szyf M (2006) Epigenetic tête-à-tête: the bilateral relationship between chromatin modifications and DNA methylation. *Biochemistry and Cell Biology* **84**, 463–476.

Drobius EZ, Overstreet JW (1992) Natural history of mammalian spermatozoa in the female reproductive tract. *Oxford Reviews of Reproductive Biology* **14**, 1–46.

Hoodbhoy T, Dean J (2004) Insights into the molecular basis of sperm–egg recognition in mammals. *Reproduction* **127**, 417–422.

Jones KT (2005) Mammalian egg activation: from Ca^{2+} spiking to cell cycle progression. *Reproduction* **130**, 813–823.

Johnson MH (2001) The developmental basis of identity. *Studies in History and Philosophy of Biological and Biomedical Sciences* **32**, 601–617.

Kaji K, Kudo A (2004) The mechanism of sperm–oocyte fusion in mammals. *Reproduction* **127**, 423–429.

Malcuit C, Kurokawa M, Fissore RA (2006) Calcium oscillations and mammalian egg activation. *Journal of Cell Physiology* **206**, 565–573.

Masters WH, Johnson VE (1966) *Human Sexual Response.* Churchill, London.

Masters WH, Johnson VE (1970) *Human Sexual Inadequacy.* Little, Brown, Boston.

Moore HDM (1996) The influence of the epididymis on human and animal sperm maturation and storage. *Human Reproduction* **11**, 103–110.

Palermo GD *et al.* (1997) The human sperm centrosome is responsible for normal syngamy and early embryonic development. *Reviews of Reproduction* **2**, 19–27.

Sakai RR *et al.* (2005) Cloning and assisted reproductive techniques: influence on early development and adult phenotype. *Birth Defects Research (Part C)* **75**, 151–162.

St John JC *et al.* (2004) The consequences of nuclear transfer for mammalian foetal development and offspring survival. A mitochondrial DNA perspective. *Reproduction* **127**, 631–641.

Swales AKE, Spears N (2005) Genomic imprinting and reproduction. *Reproduction* **130**, 389–399.

Swann K *et al.* (2004) The cytosolic sperm factor that triggers Ca^{2+} oscillations and egg activation in mammals is a novel phospholipase C: PLCζ. *Reproduction* **127**, 431–439 (reviews events occurring at sperm:egg fusion).

Talbot P, Riveles K (2005) Smoking and reproduction: the oviduct as a target of cigarette smoke. *Reproductive Biology and Endocrinology* **28**, 3:52 (also details oviducal transport features, with web video links).

More advanced reading (see also Boxes)

Breitbart H *et al.* (2005) Role of actin cytoskeleton in mammalian sperm capacitation and the acrosome reaction. *Reproduction* **129**, 263–268.

Dunn PM (2000) Purinergic receptors and the male contraceptive pill. *Current Biology* **10**, R305–R307 (emission control).

Eisenbach M (1999) Sperm chemotaxis. *Reviews of Reproduction* **4**, 56–66.

Ensslin MA, Shur BD (2003) Identification of mouse sperm SED1, a bimotif EGF repeat and discoidin-domain protein involved in sperm–egg binding. *Cell* **114**, 405–417.

Hess RA (2000) Oestrogen in fluid transport in efferent ducts of the male reproductive tract. *Reviews of Reproduction* **5**, 84–92.

Hess RA (2003) Estrogen in the adult male reproductive tract: a review. *Reproductive Biology and Endocrinology* **1**, 52.

Holt WV, Van Look KJW (2004) Concepts in sperm heterogeneity, sperm selection and sperm competition as biological foundations for laboratory tests of semen quality. *Reproduction* **127**, 527–535.

Hunter RHF, Rodriguez-Martinez H (2004) Capacitation of mammalian spermatozoa in vivo, with a specific focus on events in the Fallopian tubes. *Molecular Reproduction and Development* **67**, 243–250.

Hurt KJ *et al.* (2002) Akt-dependent phosphorylation of endothelial nitric-oxide synthase mediates penile erection. *Proceedings of the National Academy of Sciences of the USA* **99**, 4061–4066.

Knott JG *et al.* (2005) Transgenic RNA interference reveals role for mouse sperm phospholipase Cζ in triggering Ca^{2+} oscillations during fertilization. *Biology of Reproduction* **72**, 992–996.

Ono Y, Kono T (2006) Irreversible barrier to the reprogramming of donor cells in cloning with mouse embryos and embryonic stem cells. *Biology of Reproduction* **75**, 210–216.

Partridge JM, Koutsky LA (2006) Genital human papillomavirus infection in men. *Lancet Infectious Diseases* **6**, 21–31.

Santos F, Dean W (2004) Epigenetic reprogramming during early development in mammals. *Reproduction* **127**, 643–651.

Spehr M *et al.* (2006) Odorant receptors and olfactory-like signaling mechanisms in mammalian sperm. *Molecular and Cellular Endocrinology* **250**, 128–136.

Toda N *et al.* (2005) Nitric oxide and penile erection function. *Pharmacology and Therapeutics* **106**, 233–266.

Tulsiani DRP, Abou-Haila A (2004) Is sperm capacitation analogous to early phases of Ca^{2+}-triggered membrane fusion in somatic cells and viruses? *BioEssays* **26**, 281–290.

10 Implantation and the Establishment of the Placenta

The tiny fertilized egg sitting in the oviduct now has to perform a heroic task. It must somehow communicate its presence to the mother and convert the whole of her physiology and anatomy from a cyclic reproductive state to a pregnant one. How it does so is the subject of this and the next chapters.

The conceptus converts the maternal reproductive pattern from cyclic to pregnant

The conceptus remains at the site of fertilization for a further few days (Table 10.1, column 3). It is then transferred through the isthmus of the oviduct and enters the uterus. Transfer is facilitated by the changing endocrine milieu of the early luteal phase with its rising ratio of progesterone to oestrogen, which affects the oviducal and uterine musculature and relaxes the isthmic sphincter (see Chapter 8). It is probable, however, that the cilia rather than the musculature of the genital tract are the primary active transporters of the conceptus. Thus, if a segment of oviduct is excised, turned round and replaced such that its cilia beat away from the uterus, the conceptus moves only up to this point of oviducal reversal and then stops.

On reaching the uterus, the conceptus engages in an elaborate interaction with the mother in which several messages are transmitted in both directions. This interaction, which may be likened to a conversation, has two important and distinctive components: one short range and one long range. First, the conceptus establishes physical and nutritional contact with the maternal endometrium at *implantation*; failure to do so properly would deprive the conceptus of essential nutritional substrates and arrest its growth. The conversation operating during implantation involves short-range messages, and is the major subject of this chapter. Second, the conceptus *signals its presence* to the maternal pituitary–ovarian axis; failure to do so would result in the normal mechanisms of luteal regression coming into operation, causing a fall in progesterone levels and loss of the conceptus. Somehow the conceptus must convert the whole of the female from a cyclic pattern with oscillating dominance of oestrogens and progestagens, to a non-cyclic pregnant pattern, in which progestagens dominate throughout. The conversation operating during this *maternal recognition of pregnancy* involves long-range signals, and is the major subject of Chapter 11. Thus, pregnancy is not initiated with fertilization but only when the

Table 10.1 Times (in days) after ovulation at which various developmental and maternal events occur.

Species	Cleavage to four cells	Major burst of transcription	Conceptus enters uterus	Formation of blastocyst	Time of attachment	Luteal regression time if mating infertile	Duration of pregnancy
Invasive							
Mouse	1.5–2	2-cell	3	3	4.5	10–12	19–20
Rat	2–3	2-cell	3	4.5	4.5–5.5	10–12	21–22
Rabbit	1–1.5	8–16-cell	3.5	3.5	7–8	12	28–31
Human	2	4–8-cell	3.5	4.5	7–9	12–14	270–290
Non-invasive							
Sheep	4	8–16-cell	2–3	6–7	15–16	16–18	144–152
Pig	1–3	4-cell	2	5–6	18	16–18	112–115
Cow	2–3	8–16-cell	3–4	7–8	30–45	18–20	277–290
Horse	1.5–2	?	5–6	6	30–40	20–21	330–345

conceptus has signalled its presence successfully to the mother.

The preimplantation conceptus

The control of development switches from mother to conceptus soon after fertilization

During its period in the oviduct, the two-cell conceptus proceeds through cellular divisions at a rate characteristic for each species (Table 10.1, column 1). Each cell or *blastomere* undergoes a series of divisions, during which the total size of the conceptus remains much the same (Fig. 10.1). In consequence, with each of these so-called *cleavage divisions*, the size of the individual blastomeres is reduced progressively, restoring the high cytoplasmic/nuclear ratio of the oocyte and zygote to adult levels. The large volume of oocyte cytoplasm, distributed to blastomeres during cleavage, contains materials essential for this cleavage process, as was indicated in Chapter 9. These include: ribosomes and the full protein biosynthetic apparatus for making proteins including a vast diversity of mRNA species; the maternal mitochondria and an ATP-generating system, which is based initially on the use of pyruvate and then on glucose as a metabolic substrate; a Golgi system for production and modification of glycoproteins; and a cytoskeletal system essential for cyto- and karyokinesis. The spermatozoon has little cytoplasm when compared with the *maternal cytoplasmic inheritance of the oocyte*, and contributes, in most species, only its centriole in addition to its parentally imprinted *genetic inheritance*. It is clear that the earliest stages of development are marked by very low levels of mRNA synthesis that are not essential for proximate development. Thus, these early stages are, in effect, controlled by the products of

oogenesis, and thus by the maternal genome. This almost total dependence of the early conceptus on its maternal cytoplasmic inheritance means that any deficiency in oocyte maturation will result in impaired or failed early development and possible failure to establish pregnancy.

However, eventually the reservoir of maternally inherited cytoplasmic information ceases to be the sole controller of development. At a developmental stage that is characteristic for the species (Table 10.1, column 2), the numbers of conceptus genes being transcribed increases markedly and become essential for further development. At the same time, most of the maternally inherited mRNA is destroyed. However, despite the fact that most *newly synthesized proteins* are switched from being maternally encoded to being embryonically encoded, many proteins that were synthesized earlier on maternal mRNA templates persist until the blastocyst stage and beyond and continue to influence development. The handover of genetic control is extended.

Shortly after this major burst of gene activation, the conceptus also shows a marked quantitative increase in its biosynthetic capacity. Net synthesis of RNA and protein increases, transport of amino acids and nucleotides into the cells rises, and changes occur in the synthetic patterns of phospholipids and cholesterol. Maturational changes occur in mitochondria, Golgi and the endocytic and secretory systems of the conceptus. From this time onwards, the growth and metabolic activity of the preimplantation conceptus *in vitro* has been shown to be stimulated by a number of growth factors, which vary with species but include the insulin-like growth factors (IGF-1 and 2), transforming growth factors α and β (TGF-α, β1, β2), epidermal growth factor (EGF), and platelet-derived growth factor A (PDGF-A). Receptors for these factors have been identified on the early conceptus. Moreover, synthesis of many of these

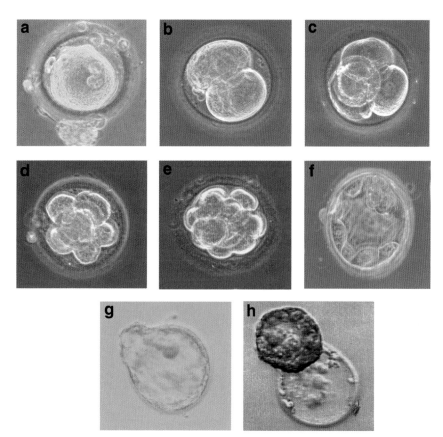

Fig. 10.1 Photographs of various stages of human preimplantation development. In each case the zona pellucida is visible. (a) Newly fertilized oocyte: note cumulus cells attached to outer surface of zona, a few non-fertilizing spermatozoa visible, two pronuclei internally and a clear second polar body to left. (b) Two-cell stage: polar bodies clearly visible between blastomeres. (c) Four-cell stage. (d) Eight-cell stage. (e) Early morula stage, approximately 16 cells: the blastomeres are smaller and are flattened on each other due to the process of compaction. (f) Early blastocyst stage: note the blastocoelic cavity and the small cluster of cells at top which is the pluriblast or inner cell mass. (g) Blastocyst hatching through the zona pellucida at top left: note that the zona is much thinner. (h) Hatched blastocyst with the empty zona lying beneath it and partially covered by it. (Photographs courtesy of Professor P.R. Braude.)

growth factors has been detected either in the conceptus itself (IGF-1 and 2, PDGF-A, TGF-α) or in maternal tissues, as a result of which they appear in uterine fluids (insulin, IGF-1, TGF-α, EGF). It is therefore reasonable to conclude that *in vivo* these factors act as *autocrine or paracrine* agents to promote early development. An at least *adequate* autocrine secretion may be indicated by the observation that oocytes fertilized *in vitro* can develop in defined media lacking the uterine cytokines.

Early differentiative events are mostly concerned with establishing extraembryonic supporting tissues for the future embryo and fetus

At around the 8- to 16-cell stage in most species studied, the cleaving conceptus changes its morphology by undergoing the process of *compaction* to yield a *morula* (Figs 10.1 & 10.2). This process involves maximizing intercellular contacts and also transforming the cell phenotype from radially symmetrical to highly polarized or epithelioid (Fig. 10.2c). This polar phenotype is important developmentally, as when each 8-cell blastomere divides to the 16-cell stage, one of the offspring may inherit its basal domain while the other inherits its apical domain. This differential inheritance then prompts these two cells to develop into different

cell types in the *blastocyst*, which forms shortly thereafter at the 32- to 64-cell stage in most species (Figs 10.1 & 10.2d,e; Table 10.1). The precise form of the blastocyst varies in different species, but in all species the blastocyst contains two distinctive types of cell: (1) an outer rim of *trophoblast* cells surrounding a *blastocoelic cavity* containing *blastocoelic fluid*; and (2) an inner group of *pluriblast* or *inner cell mass* (ICM) cells, which is eccentrically placed within the blastocoelic cavity against, or embedded within, the wall of trophoblast. The expansion of the blastocoele is stimulated by growth factors EGF and TGF-α.

The trophoblast cells constitute the first so-called *extraembryonic* tissue, as they do not contribute to the embryo or fetus itself. Instead, they give rise to part of an accessory fetal membrane called the *chorion*, which is concerned with the nutrition and support of the embryo and fetus. Indeed, the first 14–16 days of human development are concerned mainly with the elaboration within the conceptus of various extraembryonic tissues and their discrete separation from a population of cells, the *embryo*, that will give rise exclusively to a *fetus* (Figs 10.3 & 10.7). This approximately 14-day period is therefore called the *embryogenic phase* of development (generating an embryo). Before this stage the total product of fertilization is properly called the *conceptus* (also called *pre-embryo*, *pro-embryo* or *embryogen*).

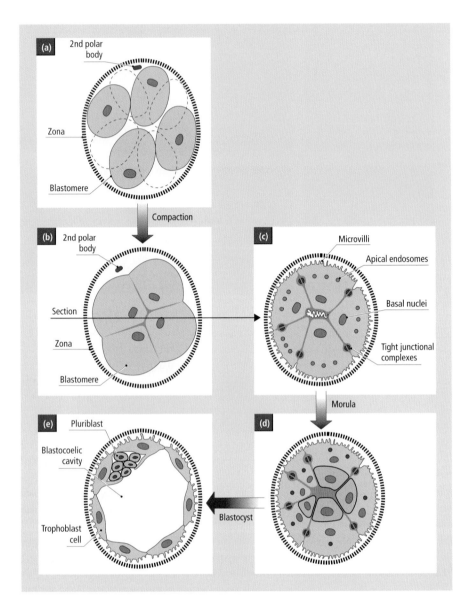

Fig. 10.2 (a–c) Compaction of eight-cell conceptus. Spherical cells (a) become wedge-shaped (b,c) and, by apposing adjacent surfaces, maximize cell contact. In cross-section (c), it can be seen that tight junctional complexes develop between the outer membranes of adjacent cells; these are punctate at first, but later become zonular, forming a barrier to intercellular diffusion between the inside and outside of the conceptus. Each cell also becomes polarized: the nucleus occupying a more basal position, endosomes and other organelles being apical and microvilli being restricted to the exposed surface and points of contact with other cells basally. (d) During cell division to the 16- and 32-cell stages (shown in section), two populations of cells form: the precursors of the outer trophoblast and inner pluriblast (blue) cells. The numbers of each cell type forming depend upon the orientation of the cleavage plane in each cell as indicated. (e) Section through a 64-cell blastocyst; fluid accumulation within the blastocoelic cavity becomes possible when the tight junctional complexes between adjacent trophoblast cells become zonular and prevent its escape. Note the eccentric position of the pluriblast or inner cell mass.

Once an embryo is generated, the *embryonic phase* is under way. It lasts about 6 weeks and during this time the various embryonic cell and tissue types differentiate, and the basic body plan is laid down such that, by its end, a tiny fetus is formed, shorter than the length of a matchstick. The transition from embryo to fetus marks the end of the *first trimester* (= 3 months or the first third of pregnancy). The *fetal phase* of development then proceeds through the second and third trimesters to term and production of a baby, whereupon the *neonatal phase* begins. A summary of the approximate lengths of each phase for selected species is given in Table 10.2.

Throughout development to the blastocyst, the conceptus remains enclosed within the zona pellucida. The zona has two functions. First, it prevents the blastomeres of the

conceptus from falling apart during early cleavage, before compaction. If the conceptus becomes divided into two distinct groups of cells at this stage, *monozygotic twins* result (derived from one zygote and therefore genetically identical, compared with *dizygotic* twins, which are derived from the independent fertilization of two oocytes from the same ovulatory episode). Second, and conversely, the zona prevents two genetically distinct conceptuses from sticking together to make a single *chimaeric* conceptus composed of two sets of cells each of distinct genotype.

It is during the transition from a morula to a blastocyst that the conceptus enters the uterus (Table 10.1, column 3), and it is therefore the blastocyst that engages in the conversations vital to its survival and future development. So next we will consider how the blastocyst and the uterine

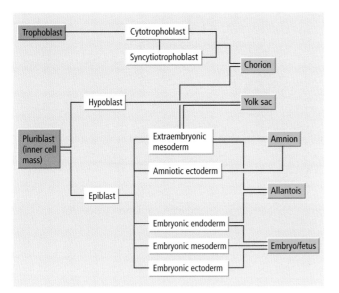

Fig. 10.3 Derivatives of the blastocyst. The trophoblast lineage is characterized by expression of *Cdx2* and *Eomes* genes. The epiblast (also called primary embryonic ectoderm) is characterized by expression of *Nanog* and *Oct 3/4* genes. The hypoblast (also called primary endoderm) is characterized by expression of *GATA6* genes (see references by Rossant, 2004 and Smith, 2006).

Table 10.2 Comparison of the durations (in days post-fertilization) of the main developmental phases in five mammals (modified from Johnson and Selwood, 1996). *Note*: the process of development is continuous, not categorical, as this descriptive system implies, so the durations of each phase are necessarily approximate, as are their beginnings and ends!

Species	Embryogenic	Embryonic	Fetal
Mouse	6	5	9
Human	14	36	220
Cow	16	25	240
Opossum	7	4.5	1.5
Wallaby	14	8	5

endometrium interact locally with one another to effect implantation.

The timing and spatial organization of the implantation events affect the form the placenta will ultimately take

The free-living blastocyst is bathed in uterine secretions from which it draws the oxygen and metabolic substrates required for continued growth and survival. Through the trophoblast

cells, it actively accumulates organic molecules and ions by specific transport mechanisms, while the exchange of oxygen and carbon dioxide is diffusional. There is a limit to the size that a free-living conceptus can attain before such exchanges become inadequate. Before this critical stage is reached, the growing conceptus develops its own blood vascular system that exchanges essential metabolites at its extraembryonic surface and distributes them throughout its tissues. Conceptuses also develop one or more anatomically distinct and highly vascularized regions of their extraembryonic surface through which the interchange of materials with maternal tissues is particularly facilitated. These vascularized regions draw on two major maternal sources of nutrition. During the initial *pre-, peri- and early postimplantation* stages of pregnancy, the conceptus utilizes almost exclusively maternal 'tissue juices' of various sorts (such as secretions or cell debris, see later for details). This sort of nutrition is called *histiotrophic* and in the human lasts until towards the end of the first trimester. However, these sources become progressively inadequate in most species, and so for the remainder of pregnancy there develops in the maternal endometrial tissue a corresponding specialized and vascularized region. This zone of adjacent and highly vascularized contact between mother and conceptus is called the *haemotrophic placenta*. In the placenta, the two discrete circulations lie sufficiently close that rapid and efficient transfer of materials between them can occur. The placenta, then, is the ultimate outcome of the primary interactions between mother and conceptus that occur at attachment and implantation, and so the form that the mature placenta takes is determined largely by the pattern and timing of the earlier events of attachment and implantation.

On entering the uterus, the conceptus is positioned to implant at a site (or sites) within the uterus that is characteristic for each species. Uterine muscular activity may be important in this process, as its inhibition leads to abnormal sites of implantation. The appropriate location and spacing of implantation sites in *polytocous species*, having several conceptuses and bicornuate uteri, is important in minimizing physical and nutritional competition between conceptuses.

Implantation involves an initial process of *attachment*. Attachment has two phases: close *apposition* is followed by *adherence* of the trophoblast cells of the blastocyst to the luminal epithelial cells of the endometrium. However, before attachment can occur, the zona pellucida interposed between these cells must be removed. The proteolytic enzymes required can come from either the trophoblast cells themselves or the uterine secretions, depending on the species (Fig. 10.4a–c). Attachment induces changes in the endometrial epithelium and the underlying endometrial stromal tissue, initiating its development as the maternal component of the placenta. How this is achieved varies

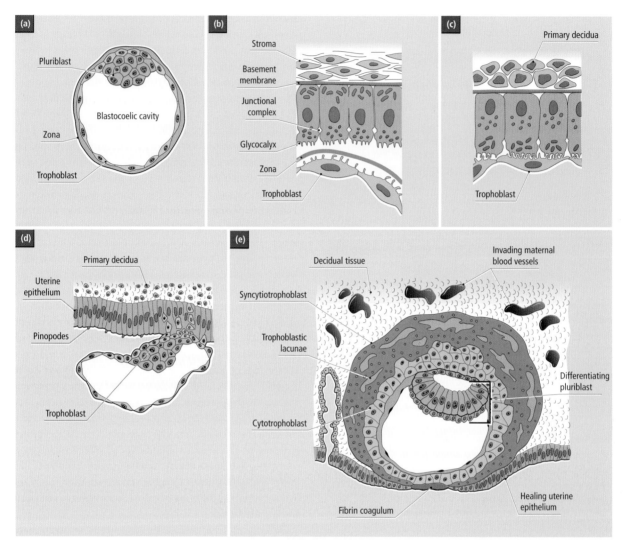

Fig. 10.4 Schema of conceptus–uterine relations during invasive implantation in the human. (a) At 4–5 days: free-living zona-enclosed blastocyst. (b) Detail of blastocyst in (a) showing microvillous trophoblast and zona interposed between blastocyst and the uterine luminal epithelial cells which are linked to each other by zonular junctional complexes, with surface microvilli interdigitating with a thick electron-dense glycocalyx. Within epithelial cells are apical pinocytotic vesicles, central nuclei, and basal lipid droplets and mitochondria. The epithelial cells rest on a basement membrane underlain by connective tissue containing spindle-shaped endometrial stromal cells in an extensive extracellular matrix abundant in collagen fibres. (c) At attachment, zona and glycocalyx have been lost, trophoblast and epithelial cells become very closely apposed and their microvilli become shorter, flatter and interdigitated. Attachment is seen to be inducing changes in the uterine epithelial and underlying stromal tissues. Epithelial nuclei assume a basal position and mitochondria are apical, with dispersed fat droplets in between. The endometrial stroma becomes oedematous due to increased vascular permeability, which is accompanied by loss of collagen fibres and swelling of stromal cells that subsequently develop extensive endoplasmic reticulum, polysomes, enlarged nucleoli, lysosomes, glycogen granules and lipid droplets, and become primary 'decidual cells'. Extensive intercellular gap junctions are also seen. Nuclei frequently become polyploid. Peripherally, sprouting and ingrowth of maternal blood vessels occurs. *Note:* in the human endometrium, some decidual-like changes may occur in stromal cells in the absence of a conceptus during the late luteal phase. These changes are often called 'predecidualization'. (d) A slightly later post-attachment lower-power schematic view in which the trophoblast is starting to penetrate the epithelium. (e) Decidualization in underlying stromal tissue spreads out rapidly from the attachment site; trophoblast rapidly erodes surface epithelium, invades and destroys adjacent primary decidual tissue, and becomes embedded. The vascularization response in the decidua is evident.

with the species. In some, implantation is *invasive*, the conceptus breaking through the surface epithelium to invade the underlying stroma. In other species, implantation is *non-invasive*, epithelial integrity being retained (or at least only breached locally, transiently or much later in gestation: see later) and the epithelium becomes incorporated within the placenta.

Invasive implantation occurs in the human, all primates except lemurs and lorises, the dog, cat, mouse and rabbit

The attachment phase

The blastocysts of these species are first nurtured by uterine secretions but, compared with species in which implantation is non-invasive, this free-living phase is relatively short lived (Table 10.1, column 5). In consequence, invasive conceptuses tend to be smaller at attachment and only a few trophoblast cells are involved in making contact with the maternal epithelium. Yet, within a few hours, an increased vascular permeability in the area of stromal tissue underlying the conceptus is observed. This is associated with an oedema, localized changes in the intercellular matrix composition and stromal cell morphology, and a progressive sprouting and ingrowth of capillaries (Fig. 10.4c–e). This *stromal reaction* is particularly marked in primates and rodents, where it is called the *primary decidualization reaction*. After 2–3 days, the decidualization spreads to give a larger *secondary decidua*, as the major endometrial component of the placenta is prepared. In other invasively implanting species the decidual reaction may be less marked but is functionally equivalent. Thus, a *primary, highly localized signal* from the small conceptus has been effectively *transduced through the epithelium* to the stroma where it is *amplified* rapidly.

The invasive (or penetration) phase

Within a few hours of attachment, the surface epithelium underlying the conceptus becomes eroded (Fig. 10.4d). Trophoblastic processes seem to 'flow' between adjacent epithelial cells, isolating and then dissolving and digesting them. Some trophoblast cells fuse together and form a syncytium (*syncytiotrophoblast*), while others retain their cellularity (*cytotrophoblast*) and serve as a proliferative source for generating more trophoblast cells stimulated by EGF (Fig. 10.4e). The uterine glandular tissue and the decidual tissue immediately adjacent to the invading trophoblast of the conceptus are destroyed, releasing primary metabolic substrates (lipids, carbohydrates, nucleic acids and proteins), which are taken up by the growing conceptus as part of the histiotrophic support. However, sustained histiotrophic support comes from the uterine glands adjacent to the implantation site, the secretions from which continue for at least the first 10 weeks of human pregnancy and which bathe the trophoblastic tissue.

The depth to which the conceptus invades maternal tissues varies with species and also in certain pathological conditions. Those species in which the conceptus invades the stroma so deeply that the surface epithelium becomes restored over it are said to implant *interstitially* (e.g. the human, chimpanzee and guinea-pig; Table 10.3 & Fig. 10.4e). In other species, the stroma is only partially invaded and the conceptus continues to project to varying degrees into the uterine lumen: so called *eccentric* implantation (e.g. the rhesus monkey, dog, cat and rat). Indeed, in these species, secondary contact and attachment by the conceptus to the

Table 10.3 Classification of implantation and placental forms in several species.

Species	Depth of invasion	Extent and shape of attachment (Fig. 10.5)	Maternal tissue in contact with conceptus (Fig. 10.6)	No. of layers of chorionic trophoblast (Fig. 10.6)	Histological type (Fig. 10.6)
Invasive					
Human	Interstitial	Discoid	Blood	1	Haemomonochorial
Rabbit	Eccentric	Discoid	Blood	2	Haemodichorial
Rat/mouse	Eccentric	Discoid	Blood	3	Haemotrichorial
Rhesus monkey	Eccentric	Bidiscoid	Blood	1	Haemomonochorial
Dog/cat	Eccentric	Zonary	Capillary endothelium	1	Endotheliochorial
Non-invasive					
Pig/mare	Central	Diffuse	Epithelium	1	Epitheliochorial
Ewe/cow	Central	Cotyledonary	Syncytium of epithelium and binucleate cells	1	Synepitheliochorial

uterine epithelium on the opposite side of the uterine lumen may result in two sites of placental development, a *bidiscoid* placenta (e.g. the rhesus monkey), or a complete 'belt' of placenta round the 'waist' of the conceptus, a *zonary* placenta (e.g. the dog and cat; see Table 10.3 and Fig. 10.5a,b).

The *invasiveness of the conceptus is influenced by the effectiveness of the decidual response.* Thus, where the decidual response is inadequate, either pathologically in the uterus, or after implantation at non-uterine *ectopic* sites, invasion is much more aggressive and penetrating. This observation has been taken by some to suggest a 'restraining' influence of the decidual tissue over the conceptus, but it could reflect an attempt by the invading trophoblast to overcome the inadequate nutritional support of a defective decidual response.

There are also species differences in the degree of proximity ultimately established between the circulations of the invasive conceptus and the mother. In some species, a relatively high degree of integrity of maternal tissue is retained, but in others, such as the human, the maternal blood vessels are eroded so that the trophoblast cells are eventually bathed in maternal blood (summarized in Table 10.3 & Fig.

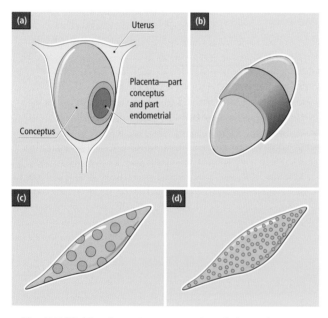

Fig. 10.5 Highly schematic representation of placental morphologies. (a) A discoid human placenta. The egg-shaped sac is the conceptus; it has a specialized disc on its surface that forms the placental component. A corresponding area on the endometrium also contributes to the placenta. Discoid placentae are also found in the mouse, rat, rabbit, bat and insectivores. Other types of placentae (uterine part is not shown) are: (b) zonary (e.g. the cat, dog, bear, mink, seal and elephant); (c) cotyledonary (e.g. the cow, sheep, giraffe, deer and goat); and (d) diffuse (e.g. the horse, pig, camel, lemur, mole, whale, dolphin and kangaroo).

10.6a–d). There is little evidence that the number of layers of tissue that ultimately lie between the circulation of mother and conceptus can in any way be related to the *efficiency of placental transfer.* However, it may well influence the *types of transport mechanism* used (see Chapter 12 for more details).

With the formation and invasion of the decidua, implantation is completed, a physical hold and an immediate nutritional source of histiotrophic glandular secretions are established, and the basis for placental development, leading to adjacent circulations and exchange of nutrients haemotrophically, is initiated.

Non-invasive implantation occurs in the pig, sheep, cow and horse

Attachment of non-invasive conceptuses is, in general, initiated relatively later than that of invasive conceptuses (Table 10.1, column 5). During the prolonged interval before attachment, the free-living conceptuses (like the invasive conceptus described above) continue to draw on rich and copious secretions from uterine glands. The conceptus utilizes these resources to grow to a much greater preimplantation size than the human or rodent invasive conceptus. The growth may be prodigious and rapid. The pig conceptus, for example, elongates from a spherical blastocyst 2 mm in diameter on day 6 of pregnancy to a membranous, highly convoluted thread some 1000 mm long by day 12. This growth is confined almost exclusively to the extraembryonic tissues of the conceptus, and establishes a vast surface area over which exchange of metabolites with the uterine milk can occur.

This large surface area of extraembryonic chorionic trophoblast also permits a much more extensive attachment to uterine epithelial cells than occurs with the invasive conceptus. In the horse and pig, attachment occurs at multiple sites over most of the external surface of the conceptus, but in ruminants attachment is limited to *uterine caruncles*, distinct areas of projecting aglandular uterine mucosa, which in sheep and goats may be up to 90 in number. As a result, the ultimate form of the placentae in these non-invasive species differs from that of invasive conceptuses, and is said to be *diffuse* (e.g. in the mare and pig) or *cotyledonary* (e.g. in the cow and sheep; see Fig. 10.5c,d). Between the sites of attachment, uterine glands continue to secrete a nutrient 'milk' for the conceptus, especially in the pig and horse. Because penetration and erosion of the epithelium does not occur at implantation in these species, the conceptus is said to implant *centrally.* This means that there are more layers interposed between the two circulations developing in the placenta (Fig. 10.6e,f). However, junctional complexes are observed between the trophoblast and the adjacent uterine epithelial cells (in the pig and sheep), and some invasion of

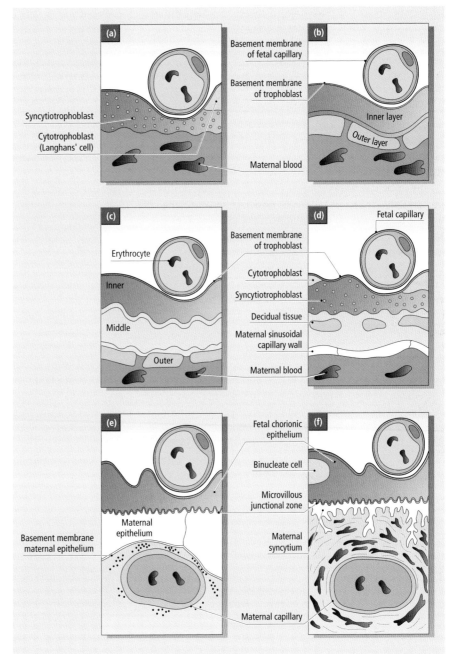

Fig. 10.6 Schematic view of microstructure at the mature placental interface of various species. (a) Human: haemomonochorial (one layer of trophoblast); (b) rabbit: haemodichorial (two layers of trophoblast); (c) rat and mouse: haemotrichorial (three layers of trophoblast); (d) dog (also bears, cats and mink): endotheliochorial; (e) mare and pig (also whales, lemurs, dolphins, deer and giraffe): epitheliochorial; (f) sheep and cow: synepitheliochorial: the maternal uterine epithelial cells fuse with binucleate cells from the fetal side to form a syncytium; the binucleate cells may also invade maternal tissues later in pregnancy.

conceptus cells into the endometrium may occur either transitorily (in the horse) or much later in development (in the sheep). No proper decidual response is induced in the underlying stroma (the epithelium acting to control invasion), but stromal vascularity increases and distinct changes in cellular morphology occur, providing evidence of the recognition of the presence of the conceptus. These changes constitute the beginnings of the formation of the placenta and mark the end of the protracted preimplantation period seen in these species.

The ovary, uterus and conceptus engage in complex conversations to control the process of implantation

Implantation depends on ovarian steroid support

The blastocyst provokes a response of considerable magnitude in the uterus. However, it can only do so over a very narrow window of time during a normal oestrous or menstrual cycle. During this time, the endometrial epithelial surface is said to be receptive to the conceptus—the so-called *window of implantation*.

The implantation window

Before this window, the endometrium is said to be *pre-receptive* and is characterized by long apical microvilli, a thick glycocalyx, which includes transmembrane mucin glycoproteins integral to the endometrial epithelial cells, and high surface charge (Fig. 10.4b): all features likely to impair attachment. Accordingly, the transition to receptivity is associated with two broad sorts of structural change: (1) the appearance over much of the epithelium of apical protrusions known as *pinopodes*, which may act to absorb uterine fluids, reduce the volume of the uterine cavity and so bring into close apposition the opposing epithelia (*occlusion*). Occlusion is assisted by a generalized oedema in the uterine stroma which further compresses the lumen; and (2) loss of surface negative charge, shortening of microvilli and thinning of the mucin coat together with changes in its molecular composition, either globally or locally in the site of attachment (Fig. 10.4c,d), changes which will facilitate close apposition of trophoblast and uterine epithelium. If this receptive phase does not lead to attachment (no embryo), then it is followed by a *refractory* phase. Uteri in both the prereceptive and refractory phases not only resist attachment by a blastocyst, but in many species are embryotoxic to any conceptus that leaves the oviduct prematurely or arrives too late (e.g. in rodents, sheep and rabbits, but not humans or monkeys). Thus, the uterus can be thought of as a primarily hostile environment able to carefully control a potentially dangerous invasive trophoblastic tissue. Clearly, for the conceptus to survive, its early development and transport must be coordinated precisely with the changing receptivity of the uterus. This coordination is achieved by the mediation of the steroid hormones.

Progestagenic domination is required if the uterus and implanting blastocyst are to engage effectively. We saw in Chapter 8 that the luteal phase of the cycle in many species was characterized by distinctive patterns of uterine secretions. Likewise, the changes in epithelial surface properties are driven by hormonal changes. However, although progesterone is indeed critical, the release of specific uterine secretions and the changes in epithelial receptivity seem to require an additional endocrine input: namely, the *superimposition of oestrogen during the luteal phase*. This is most clearly seen in female rodents, which can be deprived of this oestrogen by ovariectomy during the first 2–3 days of pregnancy while maintaining progesterone levels by daily injections. Under such conditions the conceptus enters the uterus as normal, but instead of proceeding to implant, remains free in the uterine lumen. The blastocyst may spend many days in the uterus in this quiescent state, its

metabolism 'ticking over'. If a single injection of oestrogen is then given, blastocyst metabolism increases, attachment occurs rapidly and decidualization is initiated.

Both sex steroids act mainly via their respective receptors (ERα and β and PRα and β), which are expressed in luminal, glandular and stromal cells of the endometrium (see Chapters 3 and 8), but it is the luminal epithelial cells with which the blastocyst must first engage. The oestrogen affects the epithelial cells of the uterus in two ways. First, it stimulates the release of a glandular epithelial secretion of a characteristic composition including cytokines. This secretion stimulates activation of the blastocyst. Second, the oestrogen also acts on the luminal epithelial cells to make them responsive or sensitive to a blastocyst signal, so that they can attach to the trophoblast and transmit evidence of the blastocyst's presence to the underlying stromal cells: the oestrogen opens the window of receptivity. This facility of the rat and mouse to suspend the blastocyst *in utero* for several days is called *delayed implantation*, and it provides a clear example of the uterine control over the development of the blastocyst.

Delayed implantation and diapause

Delayed implantation should not be thought of as purely an artificial or experimentally induced phenomenon. It occurs naturally in the rat, because of the suppression of endogenous oestrogen secretion in females that are suckling young of the previous litter (see Chapter 14 for details). This type of natural delay is often called *facultative delayed implantation*, as it only occurs under conditions of suckling. It is also shown by mice, gerbils, the bank vole and some marsupials, and is clearly useful to the mother since it delays the growth of her uterine litter for as long as she is suckling the previous litter. If this delay did not occur, the helpless newborn of the second litter would have to compete for milk with older and bigger siblings of the first litter.

In addition, there are many species in which an *obligatory delayed implantation* is an essential and normal part of their pregnancy (e.g. in the roe deer, badger, elephant seal, fruit bat, mink, stoat and brown bear). In these species, a prolonged period of weeks or months may be spent with blastocysts in delay (or *diapause*, as an obligatory delay is also called). Diapause confers distinct biological advantages. The roe deer, for example, mates in July and August when the adults are well fed and in their prime, ensuring effective competition for mates. The conceptus remains as a blastocyst until January when it reactivates for delivery of young in May and June when the nutritional conditions will have become optimal for the new offspring.

The oestrogen required for attachment and implantation comes from the ovary in many species, but in some, including humans, ovarian oestrogen is not required. However, oestrogen can also be synthesized *by the conceptus itself*. In the pig, for example, the luteal phase lacks a significant rise in oestrogen, but if a conceptus is present a clear oestrogen peak is detectable. Thus, the interactions between the conceptus and the uterus in these species may prove to be even more complex than those in the rodent. The conceptus may first produce oestrogens to stimulate the progesterone-primed uterus; the uterine epithelium may then respond by secreting embryotrophic factors and showing increased sensitivity to blastocyst attachment. Finally, the blastocyst may co-respond by attachment, and so initiate implantation.

There is no clear evidence for delayed implantation or diapause in humans, rabbits, pigs, guinea-pigs and hamsters.

The molecular language used by the communicating endometrium and conceptus at attachment and implantation is rich and interactive

What is the nature of the messages passing between conceptus and uterus involved in these signalling processes? The answer to this question is not fully resolved. The main players are being identified and some aspects of their roles clarified. However, there are two general points to bear in mind. First, there seem to be differences between species in some details. Second, within a species there appears to be some *redundancy* between different molecular messages, that is, several types of messenger may be able to fulfil similar functions. In what follows, a general outline of current thinking is presented with these cautions in mind.

The messages mediating attachment

Two types of linguistic exchange occur during the transition from the prereceptive to the receptive state. First, '*go away messages*' from the luminal epithelium are switched off in order to remove barriers to attachment and adhesion. Then '*come hither*' messages are sent to promote active engagement of the conceptus.

A key 'go away' message seems to be provided by a complex glycoprotein called *Muc1*. Expression of Muc1 at the epithelial surface increases during the early progestagenic phase, but it then declines during the receptive phase, either globally (mouse) or locally in the vicinity of the blastocyst (rabbit, human). In the human, it is thought that the local decline is mediated by an enzyme produced by the conceptus that cleaves carbohydrate side-chains thereby removing its repulsive properties.

A critical molecular player in the 'come hither' language is *leukaemia inhibitory factor* (LIF). LIF is an oestrogen-induced cytokine produced by the cells of the endometrial glands (Table 3.6 & Fig. 10.7). The uteri of mice genetically deficient in LIF cannot support implantation, although the blastocysts from these uteri are fully competent to attach if transferred to normal recipients. Receptors for LIF are also upregulated in both the epithelium and stroma of the endometrium around the time of implantation, as is the LIF-dependent adhesion protein *amphiregulin* in the epithelium (Fig. 10.8). LIF acts to promote luminal epithelial receptivity to attachment and the subsequent stromal decidualization.

In contrast to LIF, which elicits global responses, the earliest *localized* uterine response to a mouse blastocyst is the appearance in the endometrial luminal epithelium of several members of the EGF family. The first to appear is *heparin-binding EGF-like growth factor* (HB-EGF; see Table 3.6) This oestrogen-dependent appearance occurs *only* in epithelial cells adjacent to the blastocyst, and *precedes* dissolution of the zona pellucida, attachment and any increase in stromal vascularity (Fig. 10.7). Thus, its expression seems to be stimulated by the presence of the blastocyst. Both membrane-bound and soluble forms of HB-EGF are detected, raising the possibility that it might be able to act on the conceptus after passing through the zona pellucida. Significantly, trophoblast cells do express both *EGF receptors* and *heparan sulfate proteoglycans* (HSPG), thereby providing double binding sites for HB-EGF. Moreover, when HB-EGF binds to EGF receptors on the blastocyst, it induces receptor phosphorylation and activation of the intracellular second messenger cascade (see Fig. 3.10). This is followed by local dissolution of the zona pellucida and attachment and invasion by trophoblast. Exposure of blastocyts to inhibitors of HSPG renders them incompetent to attach.

These observations enable us to start to build a picture of the molecular language used in the conversations occurring between uterus and conceptus. In the presence of oestrogen, *either* the blastocyst is induced to send a signal *or* the local endometrium becomes sensitive to a signal being sent already. The nature of this putative signal is unknown (X in Fig. 10.7), but it induces HB-EGF production locally, and the conceptus in turn responds by shedding its zona and attaching. As we saw earlier, blastocysts produce a number of growth factors as well as oestrogen, but none is yet identified unambiguously as X. Other EGF family members in both the epithelium (and underlying stroma) may then assist the attachment process, as they too are locally upregulated following zona loss and blastocyst attachment, and include *betacellulin, epiregulin* and *neuroregulin-1*. In addition, another family member, the LIF-responsive globally elevated amphiregulin (see above), becomes *restricted* to the region of attachment at this time. Receptors for these family members (the ERB receptor family which includes the EGF receptor) are indeed expressed on trophoblast. Although this experimental work has been undertaken largely on mice, humans also upregulate HB-EGF expression over the receptive period,

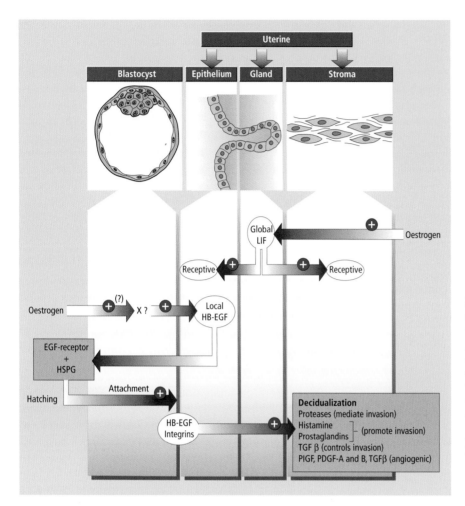

Fig. 10.7 The language of implantation between blastocyst, uterine epithelium (luminal and glandular) and stroma. + indicates a stimulatory interaction; ? indicates uncertainty; X indicates a putative blastocyst signal to the endometrium. LIF, leukaemia inhibitory factor; HB-EGF, heparin-binding epithelial growth factor; HSPG, heparan sulfate proteoglycan; TGF, transforming growth factor; PIGF, placental growth factor; PDGF platelet derived growth factor.

and HB-EGF binds to and stimulates human blastocysts. Overall, the EGF family seems to contribute the major molecular players in attachment.

Several other adhesion molecules have been implicated in attachment and adhesion, including certain *integrins*, extracellular matrix molecules such as *laminin, fibronectin* and *collagen family* members, *selectins* and the *trophinin–bystatin–tastin* complex. However, it is not yet clear whether or how they might act *in vivo*.

The messages mediating invasion (penetration)

During invasion, two types of linguistic exchange are also in play. On the one hand, there is the language of containment and control, keeping the trophoblastic invasion in check. On the other, there is the language of incitement and encouragement, promoting the invasive events. For example, *metalloproteinases* (MMPs) digest stromal components, but the action of *tissue inhibitors of MMPs* (TIMPs) holds them in check.

The precise sequence of molecular events that follows the initial attachment of the blastocyst to the luminal epithe-

lium is unclear, but somehow the epithelial cells signal to the underlying stromal tissue that invasion is imminent. The resulting stromal reaction is often described as resembling a 'pro-inflammatory endometrial reaction', because prostaglandins (PGs), key molecular players in inflammatory responses such as *hyperaemia, oedema* and *angiogenesis*, are also involved in implantation. Thus, *cycloxygenase-2* (*Cox2*), an inducible enzyme with a key role in PG synthesis by converting arachidonic acid to PGH_2 (Fig. 3.4), becomes elevated in both the luminal epithelium and the stroma over the receptive period. However, this elevation occurs *only at the site of the implanting blastocyst*, which seems to induce it locally (Fig. 10.7). Moreover, inhibitors of Cox2 or of PGs themselves (especially of PGI_2) reduce decidualization, and implantation fails in mice genetically null for Cox2, a defect at least partially overcome by the local injection of PG stabilizers. In addition, null mutants for phospholipase A_2 (PLA_2), a major supplier of arachidonic acid for PG synthesis, show delayed implantation, and PLA_2 itself rises in the luminal epithelium over the receptive period. Thus, PGs are strong candidates as molecular cheerleaders for invasion.

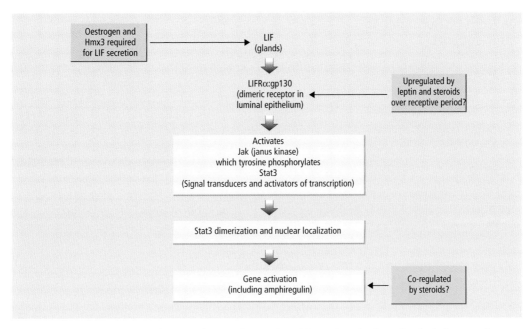

Fig. 10.8 Schematic view of the mechanism of action of LIF. LIF is produced in uterine glands under the influence of oestrogen. Gene knockout studies suggest that expression of the homeobox gene family *Hmx* (especially *Hmx3*) is required, possibly in the underlying stroma. LIF acts on luminal epithelial (and stromal) cells via a dimeric receptor, which is upregulated in the epithelium over the receptive period, probably by leptin and sex steroids. Receptor binding activates the Jak–Stat3 intracellular signalling pathway, which results in activation directly or indirectly of several genes involved in attachment and invasion.

PGs can exert their actions through both conventional cell surface PG-receptors and nuclear peroxisome proliferator-activated receptors (PPARs; Fig. 3.4). Endometrial localization and pharmacological studies suggest that it is PPARδ that is the most important mediator of the decidual response to locally produced PGs.

An important feature of the decidual response is the increased vascular permeability and the growth of new capillaries that occurs (*angiogenesis*). In addition to the role of PGs in these processes, several families of placental growth factors (and receptors to them) are also involved, namely *vascular endothelial growth factors* (*VEGFs*), the *angiopoietins* and prolactin-related proteins such as *proliferin* and *proliferin-related protein* (*PRP*).

The cellular events of decidual remodelling and trophoblastic invasion are complex, and a number of other cytokines, extracellular matrix molecules and cell surface adhesion molecules have also been implicated in the process. However, the precise patterns of interplay between all these various factors, where in the sequence of interactions between blastocyst, uterine epithelium, stroma and decidua they might act, and precisely how the endocrine milieu might influence their roles, remain to be elucidated and are the subjects of continuing research. It is clear, however, that the conversation occurring between the conceptus and the uterine tissues is complex and employs a rich molecular language.

Summary

We have seen that the earliest physical attachment of the blastocyst to the uterine endometrium shows considerable interspecies variability in timing, extent and degree of invasiveness. This variation at the earliest stage of pregnancy results, subsequently, in a correspondingly diverse pattern of placental forms that frequently confuses students of reproduction. Certain simple rules, however, help to clarify this confusion. The invasive conceptus attaches early when still small, in order to yield the prize of uterine decidual nourishment. Its placenta therefore tends to be compact and to have fewer interposed layers between the fetal and maternal circulations. The non-invasive conceptus attaches late when larger, being nourished initially by uterine secretions. Its placenta therefore tends to be extensive and to be epitheliochorial. In both cases, the maternal endocrine condition influences the effectiveness with which mother and conceptus communicate during implantation, and does so via effects on cytokines, adhesion molecules, prostaglandins and proteases.

So far we have considered only the anchoring of the conceptus to the mother. We must now consider precisely how the histiotrophic nourishment of the embryo by uterine secretory and decidual products is superseded by the more direct haemotrophic support provided by the intervascular exchange route of the mature fetoplacental unit.

The change from histiotrophic to haemotrophic support

The preimplantation conceptus derives its nutrition from endogenous reserves and via the glandular secretions of the genital tract. During invasive implantation these exocrine secretions continue to be important but are supplemented by decidual material released by the invading trophoblast. For how long does this histiotrophic route for nutritional and excretory exchange persist, and what replaces it? In order to answer these questions, we need first to examine briefly the structure of the developing conceptus and the principal routes of metabolic exchange that become available.

The extraembryonic membranes give rise to the fetal membranes

The development of the fetal membranes and the interspecies variety of their organization provide one of the most enduring confusions for students of embryology. A simplified scheme to explain the developmental route linking blastocyst, embryo, fetus and the extraembryonic membranes and fetal membranes is shown in Fig. 10.9, and this figure and its legend should be studied carefully before you read further. During the early histiotrophic phase of growth, the blastocyst takes up materials from, and excretes waste products into, the surrounding endometrial fluids. These materials pass through the thin 'shell' of trophoblast and are distributed by simple diffusion through the cavities and tissues of the conceptus itself. However, as the *mesoderm* of the conceptus forms, blood vessels develop and invade it, and then link up to form an extensive vascular network. Blood formation occurs in the yolk sac mesoderm, and a primitive heart forms in the cardiac mesoderm (Fig. 10.9f) within the developing embryo itself. Blood can thus be pumped throughout the extensive mesodermal tissue of the whole conceptus in both its embryonic and its extraembryonic parts. This blood passes throughout the chorionic mesoderm where equilibration with maternal glandular secretory and decidual fluids occurs. By this stage, it has become possible to image an implanting conceptus for the first time using ultrasound imaging, and a *clinical pregnancy* is diagnosed.

With further development, the vascularity in the conceptus becomes particularly marked in the yolk sac mesoderm and where the yolk sac and chorionic mesoderm fuse together (arrowed in Fig. 10.9e), and a corresponding vascularity develops within the endometrium adjacent to this site of fusion. Together, the two adjacent, highly vascular sites form the *yolk sac (or choriovitelline) placenta*. The yolk sac, and the yolk sac placenta to which it contributes, is a structure homologous to the yolk-containing sac found in the eggs of reptiles, birds and monotremes such as the platypus. This comparatively primitive origin is reflected in the transitory existence and function of the yolk sac placenta in most mammals. In some mammals (e.g. marsupials), the yolk sac placenta functions alone throughout pregnancy and in others (e.g. the rabbit, rat and mouse), it persists and remains functional, serving a specific subset of transport functions during pregnancy. However, in most mammals a second exchange site develops called the *chorioallantoic placenta* (arrowed in Fig. 10.9f). In higher primates (e.g. the human), the yolk sac placenta is never functional at all.

The chorioallantoic placenta forms as a result of the outgrowth of an endodermal diverticulum (the *allantois*) from the hindgut region of the developing embryo (Fig. 10.9f). Together with its ensheathing mesoderm, containing the proumbilical blood vessels, it fuses with the chorionic mesoderm and thereby determines the site (or sites) of chorioallantoic placentation. As we saw earlier, the consequence of allantoic outgrowth in species with early invading conceptuses is a restricted discoidal, bidiscoidal or zonary placenta, whereas late-attaching conceptuses acquire a more extensive cotyledonary or diffuse chorioallantoic placenta.

It is important to re-emphasize that the functional placenta incorporates a contribution not only from the conceptus, as shown developing in Fig. 10.9, but also from endometrial tissue. This is shown schematically in Fig. 10.10 for the developing human conceptus, which has a discoid, chorioallantoic placenta. Having considered the general disposition of fetal membranes, fetus and placenta, we will now take a closer look at the organization of the placental interface itself.

The placental interface is organized to facilitate exchange between maternal and fetal circulations

The chorioallantoic placenta is characterized by: (1) extensive proliferation of the chorionic tissue to give a large surface area for exchange; (2) highly developed vascularity of both fetal and maternal components; and (3) intimately juxtaposed, but physically separate, fetal and maternal blood flows. The precise anatomical arrangement of vessels in the functional placenta varies considerably, and here we describe the human (discoidal, haemomonochorial) and sheep (cotyledonary, synepitheliochorial) placentae as illustrative representatives.

The human placenta

In the mature *haemomonochorial* placenta of the human, tongues or *villi* of chorionic syncytiotrophoblast, containing cores of mesodermal tissue in which fetal blood vessels run, penetrate deeply into the maternal tissue to form an

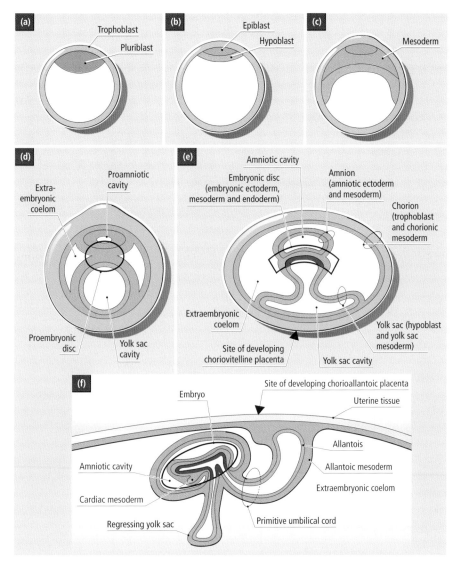

Fig. 10.9 Schematic view of the development of the extraembryonic and then fetal membranes. (a) Blastocyst with trophoblast and pluriblast. (b) Development has occurred within the pluriblast: two layers of cells have formed, namely epiblast (salmon pink, also called primary ectoderm) and hypoblast (blue, also called primary endoderm). (c) A third mesodermal tissue develops (pink) between the epiblast and hypoblast. The hypoblast spreads out over the underside of the trophoblast. (d) The hypoblast edges meet to form a hollow spherical cavity: the yolk sac cavity. Mesoderm extends between the hypoblast and trophoblast and between the epiblast and trophoblast. Cavities develop within the mesodermal tissue (the extraembryonic coelom) and within the epiblast tissue (proamniotic cavity). The proembryonic disc forms. (e) The extraembryonic coelom, proamniotic cavity and yolk sac cavity enlarge and change shape. The epiblast is now divisible into amniotic and embryonic ectoderm, the hypoblast is now divisible into yolk sac and embryonic endoderm, and the mesoderm is divisible into extraembryonic and embryonic mesoderm. Between the amniotic and yolk sac cavities, a triple cell layer structure of embryonic ectoderm, mesoderm and endoderm is now evident as the trilaminar or embryonic disc of the definitive embryo, which will eventually give rise to the fetus. All the other tissues are extraembryonic and will form the fetal membranes. Thus, the amnion develops from a layer of extraembryonic ectoderm fronting the amniotic cavity and a layer of extraembryonic mesoderm outside it. The yolk sac develops from a layer of extraembryonic endoderm fronting the yolk sac cavity and a layer of extraembryonic mesoderm outside it. The chorion develops from a layer of trophoblast fronting the uterine tissue and a layer of extraembryonic mesoderm within it. The point at which the yolk sac mesoderm and chorionic mesoderm fuse is arrowed; this is the site of formation of the yolk sac (or choriovitelline) placenta. Blood vessels develop throughout the embryonic and extraembryonic mesoderm, and the embryonic blood starts to flow through them. (f) The trilaminar embryonic disc curls up with its outer ectoderm surrounded by amniotic fluid in the amniotic cavity; the derivatives of this ectoderm will include the outer 'skin' of the fetus, as well as most of the nervous system. Within this curled-up disc, there is an endoderm-lined cavity (continuous with the yolk sac cavity) that is the primitive gut. The interposed filling of embryonic mesoderm (which will form many of the fetal tissues between the gut and the skin and their derivatives) is highly vascular and includes, at the anterior or head end of the embryo, the primitive heart (cardiac mesoderm) that pumps blood through the network of embryonic and extraembryonic vessels. A diverticulum of the endoderm, the allantoic endoderm, develops at the posterior or tail end of the embryo and it grows out surrounded by mesoderm to form the allantois. The allantoic and chorionic mesoderm (both rich in blood vessels) fuse (arrowed) and mark the site of formation of the chorioallantoic placenta. The connection that the allantois makes between the embryo and the chorioallantoic placenta will become the umbilical cord (see Fig. 10.10).

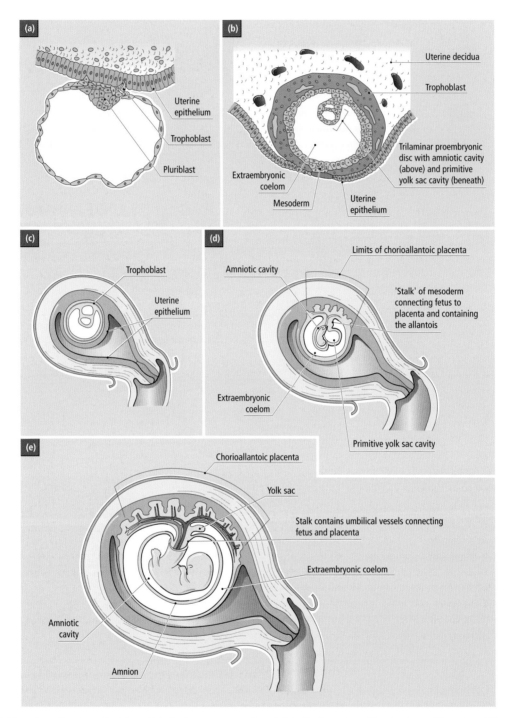

Fig. 10.10 Highly schematic views (not to scale) of a human conceptus at: (a) attachment and beginnings of invasion; (b) well-advanced invasion; and (c–e) progressively later stages of pregnancy. The general relationship of fetus, fetal membranes, placenta and maternal vessels is shown. Note how the fetus itself ends up floating in amniotic fluid and linked to the placenta by an umbilical stalk.

extensive network (Fig. 10.11b). Each villous blood vessel, by progressive branching of the main divisions of the umbilical vessels, is separated from the surface by a thin syncytiotrophoblastic layer (Fig. 10.11c). At the tips of the terminal villi, the capillaries are dilated and form tortuous loops (Fig. 10.12). Thus, fetal blood flow through the tips will be slow, allowing for exchange of metabolites with maternal blood. The branches of the villi are arranged, with a somewhat

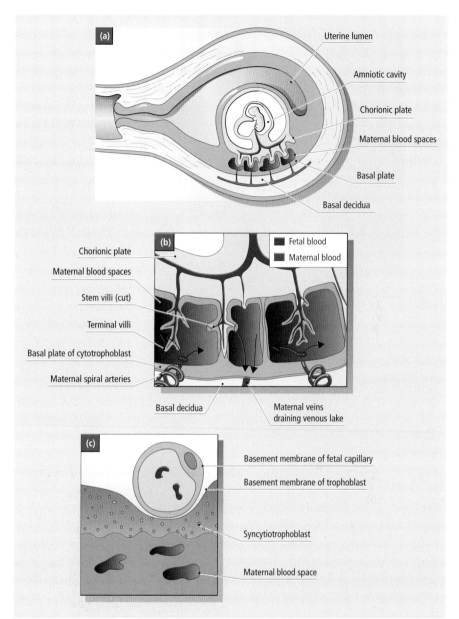

Fig. 10.11 Schematic representation of structures of the human placental interface. (a) Stem villi connect the chorionic plate to the basal plate forming a labyrinthine series of spaces. (b) From the stem villi and the chorionic plate, smaller villi ramify into the intervillous space forming a network of fine filamentous terminal villi, which are the principal sites of metabolic exchange. (c) At these sites, only a thin layer of chorionic syncytiotrophoblast separates the fetal blood vessels from maternal blood. Villi are classified as: *primary*, when composed of solid trophoblast; *secondary*, when mesoderm invades the villous core; and *tertiary*, when blood vessels penetrate the mesoderm. As a villus grows and extends, it goes through each of those stages.

variable degree of regularity, to form 'fenestrated bowls' (rather in the shape of the bowl of a brandy glass). Their terminal villi project inwards into the central space of the bowl, between the adjacent villi that form the fenestrated wall of the bowl, and outwards into the space peripheral to the bowl. Each 'bowl' unit is sometimes called a *fetal lobule*.

It is suggested that, in the human, the maternal spiral artery at the decidual base of the placenta ejects its blood into the space that forms the bowl of this lobule, filling the brandy glass as it were. The pressure of the blood causes its circulation through the fenestrated wall of the lobule over the fine terminal villi. The blood is then thought to drain back via the basal venous openings into maternal

veins (Fig. 10.11b). Up to 200 such lobular units form in the mature human placenta, which is a 'pancake' 15–20 cm in diameter and 3 cm thick. Several lobular units are grouped together to form a *lobe*, the boundaries of which may be seen grossly on the placenta, defined by fibrous septa.

This anatomical description is probably somewhat idealized, and the consistency with which such a regular arrangement of maternal vessels and villi occurs in the human placenta is perhaps questionable. The important point to understand is that maternal blood circulates across the fine terminal villi containing the fetal capillaries. The general anatomical organization of the placental interface is achieved by 3–4 weeks of pregnancy.

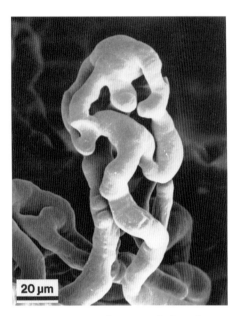
20 μm

Fig. 10.12 Low-power view of a cast made from the microvascular capillaries in a terminal villus on the fetal side of the placental circulation. Note how the terminal vessels form a convoluted knot supplied by straight capillaries. Note also the terminal dilatations of the vessels in which blood flow is slower and at which exchange of metabolites between fetal and maternal blood takes place.

The ovine placenta

The sheep placenta is *synepitheliochorial* and *cotyledonary*, having some 80–90 independent sites of close vascular proximity. Attachment occurs at each uterine epithelial caruncle, the fetal chorion at the point of attachment showing specialization as a cotyledon. The fetal cotyledon and maternal caruncle together constitute the functional unit of the placenta known as a *placentome* (Fig. 10.13). In the mature cotyledon, an ingrowth of chorionic villi indents and compresses the epithelium of the maternal caruncles. Within the villi, a core of vascularized fetal mesoderm develops. Each cotyledon receives one to three branches of the umbilical vessels. The vessels divide and ramify within the villi where they come to lie under the surface of the trophoblast at the tips of the villi (Fig. 10.13). On the maternal side, the surface epithelium of the caruncle becomes syncytial, and the underlying stroma becomes acellular and vascular. Binucleate cells form in the fetal cotyledon, and some of these contribute to this maternal syncytium (an equivalent penetration into maternal tissues may occur in other large farm animals that are nonetheless appropriately classified as non-invasive at implantation itself). Tortuous, coiling maternal arteries supply each caruncle and split into capillaries between the penetrating terminal villi of the fetal cotyledon. The capillaries then run back along the long axis of the terminal villus towards the tip, where

they drain into maternal veins (Fig. 10.13). This organization of fetal and maternal vessels means that, in the capillary beds, the blood could flow in opposite directions, which would maximize opportunities for metabolic exchange.

Blood flow in the human placenta

So much for placental structure, but what do direct measurements of blood flow tell us about the functional interpretations given above?

The chorioallantoic placenta only becomes fully functional after the embryo has formed

The general anatomical organization of the placental interface is achieved in the human chorioallantoic placenta by 3–4 weeks of pregnancy. Until recently, it was believed that the circulation of the maternal blood within the placenta was established at the same time. However, measurements of maternal blood flow and oxygenation at the placental interface suggest that, despite the apparent anatomical competence, a fully mature *maternal* blood flow does not develop until 10–12 weeks. Thus, for the first trimester of human pregnancy, the conceptus is developing in an environment of relatively low oxygen. This situation is caused by the invasion of trophoblast cells into the tips of the maternal spiral arteries that supply the developing chorioallantoic placenta (so-called *endovascular trophoblast*), partially occluding them and impeding the maternal blood flow. Indeed, the intervillous space is filled with a clear fluid made up of maternal plasma percolating through these trophoblastic plugs mixed with the secretions of the uterine glands. Because this fluid lacks an oxygen carrier, the oxygen supply within the placenta is less than 20 mmHg. Why does the placenta, having created the possibility of good oxygenation, then go to such lengths to delay it from happening?

The answer seems to lie in the two-edged sword that is oxygen. Oxygen is essential for efficient ATP production via mitochondrial oxidative phosphorylation. However, oxygen can also be highly toxic via the production of *reactive oxygen species* (ROS) such as the *superoxide anion*, which is a by-product of the less than 100% efficient mitochondrial respiratory chain. Excess superoxide anions (and active derivatives of it) are mopped up by antioxidants such as vitamins C and E and by a series of protective enzymatic reactions involving superoxide dismutase, catalase and glutathione peroxidase. However, ineffective mopping results in the ROS inflicting oxidative damage on proteins, lipids and nucleic acids with severe consequences such as cell stress, death and even carcinogenesis. It seems that the risk of ROS production affecting adversely the critical events of embryonic development, with the

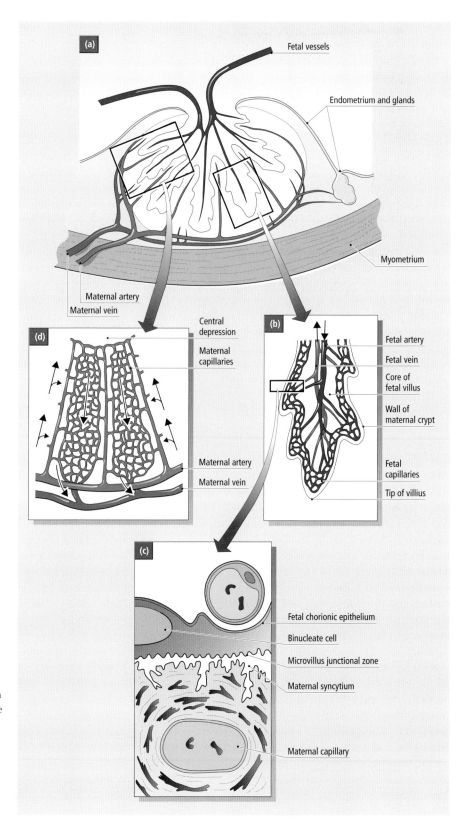

Fig. 10.13 (a) General structure of a sheep placentome. Fetal villi shown in longitudinal section in (b) interdigitate with maternal tissue giving close apposition of circulations (c). Maternal blood flows around the fetal villus, as indicated in (d). A similar interdigitation of fetal villi with maternal tissue also occurs in the horse and the cow.

potential for malformation and even embryonic death and pregnancy loss, is just too great. Thus, the placenta has evolved a mechanism to hold oxygenation levels in check until the crucial embryonic events are completed. From 10 weeks onwards, the trophoblastic plugs start to disperse and the circulation of maternal blood into villous spaces gets underway. Thus, haemochorial placentation, and haemotrophic support, in the human does not truly occur *functionally* until the second trimester. Until then, histiotrophic support reigns.

Haemotrophic support is more efficient than histiotrophic support at establishing metabolic gradients to drive diffusional and carrier-mediated exchange of metabolic substrates and excretory products. So the second trimester onwards is characterized by growth and maturation as the fetus rapidly increases in size, a counterpoint to the preceding embryonic period when the primary developmental process was the increase in complexity of form and tissues. The significance of this histiotrophic to haemotrophic transition occurring effectively and at the correct time is seen in the consequences arising from situations in which it occurs too early (pregnancy loss) or too late (placental insufficiency, fetal retardation and eclampsia).

Haemotrophic blood flow at fetal stages

The effectiveness with which gradients are established depends largely on how effectively rates of blood flow through the two sides of the placental circulation are regulated, as well as on the diffusional barriers and special transport mechanisms that might exist between them. The latter are considered in detail in Chapter 12. Here we are concerned with rates of blood flow and the factors affecting them.

Cardiac output and total blood volume are increased by up to 40% in pregnancy, in response to the additional peripheral load. Maternal blood reaches the placenta via uterine and ovarian vessels and constitutes about 25% of the mother's total cardiac output by the end of pregnancy, achieved through a threefold increase in flow due to both vascular dilation and proliferation. In the human, the uterine arteries course along the lateral walls of the uterus giving off 9–14 branches, each of which penetrates the outer third of the myometrial tissue. At this level, anastomosis of these arteries with the ovarian arteries may occur, and from the anastomosis a series of arcuate arteries runs within the anterior and posterior myometrial walls of the uterus, thereby encircling it. From this enveloping vascular network, radial arteries penetrate through the remaining myometrium into the basal endometrial tissue. Here the so-called basal arteries distribute spiral arteries to supply the endometrial decidua. This convoluted or spiral nature of terminal endometrial arteries, together with a tendency to dilate terminally and a lack of responsiveness to vaso-

constrictor transmitters and drugs, is a feature common to many species. Each of these features tends to diminish the arrival velocity of the maternal blood, which is further diminished to 0.1–10 ml/s in the primate by the extensive volume of the intervillous blood spaces.

This sluggish flow may protect the conceptus from being dislodged by 'spurts' of blood, and also gives ample time for the exchange of metabolites at the placental interface (estimated mean transit time of 15 s in the full-term monkey placenta). A similar slowing of flow occurs on the fetal side of the circulation, where the total cross-sectional area of blood vasculature increases as a result of both the profusion of vascular branching and the terminal capillary dilatations (Fig. 10.12) at which exchange occurs. This massive expansion of the fetal blood vasculature means that the fetal circulation operates at low pressure. The protection of the fetal blood vessels from collapse is assured by a corresponding low maternal perfusion pressure (4–10 mmHg) within the intervillous spaces.

The maternal arteries have a sympathetic innervation restricted to their myometrial course, which enables them to constrict in response to sympathetic nerve stimulation or sympathomimetic drugs. Reduced placental perfusion can therefore result either from local vasoconstriction or from lowered systemic pressure. Transient reductions in perfusion pressure do not seem to have adverse effects on placental exchange or fetal growth, but chronic reductions do, particularly later in pregnancy. Thus, chronic anxiety, heavy smoking and stress during pregnancy result in smaller term babies, probably caused in part by effects on placental perfusion. Similarly, administration of drugs to relieve maternal hypotension as, for example, in asthma, will cause an increase in visceral vasoconstriction, which will already be elevated reflexly, and thereby further reduce placental perfusion. During maternal exercise, some reduction in blood flow to the uterus occurs, but the conceptus itself seems to be relatively protected, unless exercise is severe and prolonged.

In addition to the adverse effects of impaired flow towards the placenta, occlusion or slowed blood flow at the placental interface will also reduce the efficiency of metabolite exchange. Such an effect occurs in conditions of increased maternal blood viscosity, for example sickle cell anaemia, or after the expansion of placental villous structures, with a consequent reduction in the intervillous space available for circulation. This occurs in conditions of increased umbilical vein pressure, such as erythroblastosis or vascular occlusion of the fetal liver, both of which cause distension of the villi. Smoking in pregnancy also exerts direct effects on the fetal vasculature in the placenta, there being fewer, narrower and less convoluted capillaries in the terminal villi. Finally, occlusion of the maternal venous drainage, as can occur during compression of the inferior vena cava when lying supine or during uterine contractions at parturition, will reduce flow through the placental interface. Engorgement of the intervillous space can then, via pressure effects, reduce fetal blood circulation and the efficiency of placental exchange.

Summary

The growing conceptus faces a hazardous few days of early life. Not only must it pass from the oviduct to uterus at exactly the right time, but it must also establish adequate nutritional support for its growth and development. It is perhaps not surprising that in human *in vitro* fertilization (IVF) programmes, the major treatment failures occur over the implantation period (see Chapter 15). Thus, a sound understanding of the dynamics of implantation, the molecular language used and the roles of steroids in influencing these processes is of profound practical importance to infertile couples and those treating them.

The days leading up to implantation are marked by little growth at all, but the rising progesterone stimulates the secretory phase of the uterus to provide a nutritious glandular fluid support. The superimposition of an oestrogenic stimulus allows attachment and implantation to occur. The conceptus can then secure a physical hold on the mother, establish its own circulation and stimulate, at adjacent endometrial sites, the establishment of special maternal circulatory changes. The prolonged transition from a histiotrophic to a more efficient haemotrophic route of metabolic exchange has been achieved via this placental structure and allows the more rapid growth seen in the last two trimesters.

However, a successful pregnancy requires more than this. The uterus will only provide a congenial environment as long as appropriate endocrine conditions persist. While the conceptus is establishing a secure physical and nutritional anchorage within the uterus, the luteal phase of the cycle is progressing. In a few species, such as the dog, the luteal phase is of the same duration as pregnancy (Table 10.1). In others, such as the rat, rabbit and mouse, coitus is equated with possible pregnancy, and so the coital stimulus neurogenically activates a pituitary secretion of luteotrophic prolactin that prolongs the normal brief luteal phase of the oestrous cycle into a pseudopregnancy, which is about half the length of pregnancy (Table 10.1, Chapters 5 & 6). In primates and the large farm animals, however, pregnancy greatly exceeds the normal life of the corpus luteum (Table 10.1), and even in the rat, rabbit and mouse, the prolonged luteal phase is not as long as pregnancy itself. As we saw earlier, a uterus dominated by oestrogen and lacking progesterone is hostile to the conceptus. The progesterone-dominated state must therefore be extended in some way. The conceptus must somehow prevent or neutralize corpus luteum regression. This achievement is all the more remarkable when considering that, in species such as the pig and cow, attachment has not even occurred by the expected time of luteal regression (Table 10.1). How does the conceptus achieve this task? How does it signal its presence to the maternal organism? This is the subject of the next chapter.

FURTHER READING

General reading

Burton GJ *et al.* (2006) Anatomy and genesis of the placenta. In: *The Physiology of Reproduction*, 3rd edn. (ed. J.D. Neill). Elsevier, St Louis.

Burton GJ, Jauniaux E (2004) Placental oxidative stress: from miscarriage to preeclampsia. *Journal of the Society for Gynecological Investigation* **11**, 342–352.

Dey SK *et al.* (2004) Molecular cues to implantation. *Endocrine Reviews* **25**, 341–373.

Hill J (2001) Maternal–embryonic cross-talk. *Annals of the New York Academy of Sciences* **943**, 17–25.

Johnson MH, Selwood L (1996) The nomenclature of early development in mammals. *Reproduction, Fertility and Development* **8**, 759–764.

Johnson MH, McConnell JML (2004) Lineage allocation and cell polarity during mouse embryogenesis. *Seminars in Cell and Developmental Biology* **15**, 583–597.

Kimber SJ (2005) Leukaemia inhibitory factor in implantation and uterine biology. *Reproduction* **130**, 131–145.

Lopes FL *et al.* (2004) Embryonic diapause and its regulation. *Reproduction* **128**, 669–678.

Lotgering FK *et al.* (1983) Maternal and fetal responses to exercise during pregnancy. *Physiological Reviews* **65**, 1–36.

Poswillo D, Alberman E (1992) *Effects of Smoking on the Fetus, Neonate and Child.* Oxford University Press, Oxford.

Rossant J (2004) Lineage development and polar asymmetries in the peri-implantation mouse blastocyst. *Seminars in Cell and Developmental Biology* **15**, 573–581.

Selwood L, Johnson MH (2006) Trophoblast and hypoblast in the monotreme, marsupial and eutherian mammal: evolution and origins. *BioEssays* **28**, 128–145.

Sharkey AM, Smith SK (2003) The endometrium as a cause of implantation failure. *Best Practice & Research Clinical Obstetrics & Gynaecology* **17**, 289–307.

Simon C (1996) Potential molecular mechanisms for the contraceptive control of implantation. *Molecular Human Reproduction*, **2**, 475–480.

Smith A (2006) The battlefield of pluripotency. *Cell* **123**, 757–760.

Steven DH (1975) *Comparative Placentation.* Academic Press, London.

More advanced reading

Caniggia I *et al.* (2000) Hypoxia-inducible factor-1 mediates the biological effects of oxygen on human trophoblast differentiation through TGFβ3. *Journal of Clinical Investigation* **105**, 577–587.

KEY LEARNING POINTS

- Development may be divided into embryogenic, embryonic, fetal and neonatal phases.

- The embryogenic phase involves the separation of a small embryonic stem cell population from the extraembryonic tissues.

- Early development involves a switch from almost exclusive use of maternally inherited molecular information to increasing use of mRNA and proteins made by the genes of the conceptus.

- Early cell divisions are cleavage divisions, which reduce the cytoplasmic/nuclear ratio, and involve no net growth.

- Compaction, blastomere polarization, blastocoele formation and the differentiation of pluriblast and trophoblast cells evident in the blastocyst characterize preimplantation development.

- The preimplantation period ends with attachment of the trophoblast to the uterine epithelium.

- Attachment marks the initiation of implantation.

- Total or focal digestion of the zona pellucida is required before this can occur.

- The length of the preimplantation period depends on the species, varying from 4 to >30 days.

- Attachment requires the imposition of oestrogen on a progestagenic background.

- The oestrogen can come from the ovary or conceptus depending on the species.

- Some species always delay oestrogen production to control the time of year at which implantation occurs; this is called obligate delay of implantation or diapause.

- In other species the oestrogen production can be delayed by the suckling of young from a previous litter; this is called facultative delay of implantation.

- Oestrogen renders the endometrium receptive.

- Oestrogen causes loss of surface negative charge, shortening of microvilli and thinning of the mucin coat together with changes in its molecular composition such as loss of Muc-1 expression to facilitate close apposition of trophoblast and uterine epithelium.

- Oestrogen stimulates leukaemia inhibitory factor (LIF) production by the endometrial glandular epithelium.

- LIF acts on uterine luminal epithelium and stroma via LIF-receptors and stimulation of the Jak–Stat3 pathway; without it implantation does not occur.

- Oestrogen stimulates heparin-binding EGF-like growth factor (HB-EGF) production by the uterine luminal epithelium adjacent to the blastocyst.

- HB-EGF binds to receptors on the blastocyst and stimulates zona hatching and attachment.

- HB-EGF, together with amphiregulin, epiregulin and other EGF family members, may also be involved in binding blastocysts to the epithelia cell surface.

- Attachment results in immediate changes to the underlying stromal tissues, which includes primary decidua formation in invasive implanters.

- The nutrition of the conceptus is initially histiotrophic (uterine secretions and/or decidua) and then haemotrophic.

- Conceptuses that implant early also tend to be invasive and form compact placentae with few layers interposed between maternal and fetal circulations.

- Conceptuses that implant late tend to be non-invasive and form diffuse placentae with multiple layers between maternal and fetal circulations.

- Invasive implantation involves prostaglandins, metallo-proteases and their inhibitors, and angiogenic growth factors.

- Extraembryonic tissues develop into fetal membranes (chorion, yolk sac, amnion, allantois).

- A primitive yolk sac (or choriovitelline) placenta is functional throughout pregnancy in marsupials, transitorily in the rabbit, rat and mouse, and not at all in higher primates.

- In most mammals, the chorioallantoic placenta assumes the sole or major role in fetal nutrition, but only becomes fully functional after the embryonic phase of development during the second and third trimesters.

- The embryonic stage of development is protected from damaging reactive oxygen species.

- The placenta is a site where the maternal and fetal circulations pass close to each other but do not mingle, and where exchange of materials is facilitated.

- Impairment of maternal blood flow to or through the placenta is associated with fetal maldevelopment.

Campbell EA *et al.* (2006) Temporal expression profiling of the uterine luminal epithelium of the pseudo-pregnant mouse suggests receptivity to the fertilised egg is associated with complex transcriptional changes. *Human Reproduction* **21**, 2495–2513.

Das SK *et al.* (1994) Heparin-binding EGF-like growth factor gene is induced in the mouse uterus temporally by the blastocyst solely at the site of its apposition: a possible ligand for interaction with blastocyst EGF-receptor in implantation. *Development* **120**, 1071–1083.

Hamatani T *et al.* (2004) Dynamics of global gene expression changes during mouse preimplantation development. *Developmental Cell* **6**, 117–131.

Hempstock J *et al.* (2004) Endometrial glands as a source of nutrients, growth factors and cytokines during the first trimester of human pregnancy: a morphological and immunohistochemical study. *Reproductive Biology and Endocrinology* **2**, 58 <*http://www.rbej.com/content/2/1/58*>.

Kalinka J *et al.* (2005) Impact of prenatal tobacco smoke exposure, as measured by midgestation serum cotinine levels, on fetal biometry and umbilical flow velocity waveforms. *American Journal of Perinatology* **22**, 41–7.

Lee KY, DeMayo FJ (2004) Animal models of implantation. *Reproduction* **128**, 679–695.

Malik NM *et al.* (2001) Leptin requirement for conception, implantation, and gestation in the mouse. *Endocrinology* **142**, 5198–5202.

Sherwin R *et al.* (2006) Large-scale gene expression studies of the endometrium: what have we learnt? *Reproduction* **132**, 1–10.

Spencer TE *et al.* (2004) Implantation mechanisms: insights from the sheep. *Reproduction* **128**, 657–668.

Strumpf D *et al.* (2005) Cdx2 is required for correct cell fate specification and differentiation of trophectoderm in the mouse blastocyst. *Development* **132**, 2093–2102.

11 Maternal Recognition and Support of Pregnancy

If the implanting conceptus is to survive, it must signal its presence to the mother and prevent the withdrawal of progestagenic support that would normally occur with luteolysis. Moreover, in many species, that support must be not just briefly prolonged, but sustained over weeks or months. The mechanisms by which the endocrine support of pregnancy is first established and then sustained are the subjects of this chapter.

Maternal recognition of pregnancy requires that luteal life be prolonged

We saw in Chapter 5 that luteal survival depends on the balance between a positive luteotrophic complex and negative luteolytic factors, which, in species other than primates, seem to be uterine prostaglandins. If luteal life is to be prolonged, then clearly either normal luteolytic factors must be neutralized or normally dwindling luteotrophic factors must be stimulated or supplemented. In practice, both mechanisms are probably at work.

Chorionic gonadotrophin prolongs luteal life in primates

The primate blastocyst prolongs the life of the corpus luteum by production of a luteotrophic factor of its own, which takes over from the inadequate support provided by the pituitary luteinizing hormone (LH) present during the luteal phase (see Chapter 5). If blood samples from pregnant women 8–12 days after fertilization are compared with those taken from women in the comparable period of a non-pregnant cycle, they are found to contain rising levels of the glycoprotein *human chorionic gonadotrophin* (hCG; see Table 3.4). hCG is synthesized in the syncytiotrophoblast of the implanting blastocyst from as early as 6–7 days after fertilization and is released to pass into the maternal circulation (Fig. 11.1b). It is carried to the ovary where it binds to LH receptors on the luteal cells to exert a luteotrophic action, one part of which is sustained *progesterone output that itself actively promotes luteal survival by autocrine stimulation of luteal cells*—yet another example of positive feedback. In addition, production of *luteal relaxin* (Table 3.6) also rises and supports the transition to pregnancy. This combined luteotrophic stimulus overcomes any tendency to luteolysis. The evidence for this effect of hCG comes from two types of experiment.

If non-pregnant women are given daily injections of hCG, starting in the midluteal phase, regression of their corpora lutea is prevented or delayed and progestagen levels remain elevated. Conversely, antibodies specific to the terminal amino acid sequence unique to the hCG β-chain (or indeed to CG derived from baboons, rhesus monkeys and marmosets, which make bCG, rhCG and mCG, respectively) will bind to CG but not to LH. Injection of this antiserum throughout the luteal phase of a pregnant human or monkey cycle neutralizes CG production and luteal regression occurs on time (Fig. 11.1c). Female monkeys *actively* immunized to their own CG have normal LH levels and menstrual cycles, and fertile matings, but no pregnancies. These lines of evidence clearly implicate CG as necessary and sufficient for the prevention of luteal

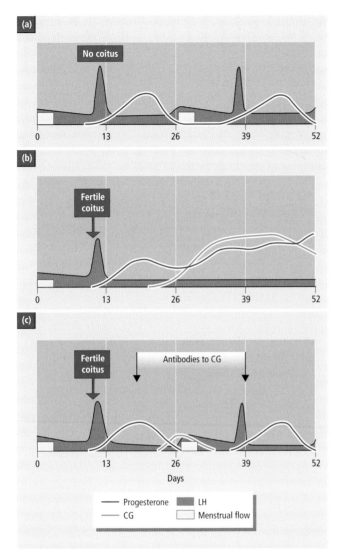

Fig. 11.1 Levels of hormones in the blood during two menstrual cycles of a higher primate. (a) Non-pregnant cycles. (b) Cycles in which fertile mating occurs (arrow). (c) Similar to (b) but passive administration of a highly specific antichorionic gonadotrophin (CG) antibody is given (arrowheads); depression of CG and loss of pregnancy occurs but there is no effect on LH levels or cyclicity.

regression during early pregnancy in the primate. So, detection of hCG in luteal phase blood or urine is taken as evidence of a *biochemical pregnancy*, later confirmed by ultrasound as a *clinical pregnancy* (Chapter 10).

Suppression of luteolytic activity prolongs luteal life in large domestic animals

In the large farm animals, luteolysis is normally induced by secretion of uterine prostaglandins (see Chapter 5). We saw that in the absence of these prostaglandins, for example

after hysterectomy, luteal life is prolonged or lasts indefinitely. So in these species, the luteotrophic support by the pituitary is presumably quite adequate. Not surprisingly, therefore, CGs have not been detected in the blood of pigs, cows and sheep bearing preimplantation conceptuses. The pig conceptus produces oestrogens from about day 12 onwards, and oestrogens are a major luteotrophic agent in this species (see Table 5.4). However, in the large farm animals the primary role of the conceptuses is to *suppress luteolytic activity* by neutralizing the action of prostaglandin $F_{2\alpha}$ ($PGF_{2\alpha}$).

In pregnant sheep and cattle, the levels of $PGF_{2\alpha}$ and its metabolites in the blood draining the uterus are reduced compared with those in non-pregnant animals. As we saw in Chapter 5, luteal oxytocin provides the stimulus for $PGF_{2\alpha}$ release, but the oxytocin receptors only appear in the epithelial and glandular cells of the uterus towards the end of the luteal phase. In the presence of a conceptus, however, oxytocin receptor expression is blocked, thereby preventing oxytocin stimulation of $PGF_{2\alpha}$ release (but not its synthesis, which persists). The oxytocin receptor depression is caused by the paracrine action of *trophoblast interferon* (IFN-τ; also called *trophoblastin* and *trophoblast protein 1* or *TP-1*), a peptide belonging to the type-1 interferon family of cytokines (Table 3.6). IFN-τ secretion from mononuclear trophoblast cells is restricted to the conceptus over precisely the period during which suppression of $PGF_{2\alpha}$ activity is required. Infusion of IFN-τ into non-pregnant uteri has antiluteolytic effects resembling the presence of a conceptus. IFN-τ acts via its receptors IFNAR1 and 2 to promote expression of the gene *IFN regulatory factor 2* (*IRF-2*), which is a powerful repressor of gene transcription. However, in parallel with its *repressor* role in the uterine epithelia, IFN-τ acts as a *promoter* in the endometrial stroma to activate expression of several genes, which seem to be important for sustaining pregnancy.

The detailed situation in the pig differs from that in ruminants, although the general principles are similar. Thus, in the non-pregnant cycle, oxytocin is involved in the exocrine release of $PGF_{2\alpha}$. However, the conceptus switches $PGF_{2\alpha}$ release from an endocrine to an exocrine route, so most of it no longer passes in the blood to the corpus luteum but is secreted into the uterine lumen, where it is metabolized. This diversionary secretion is mediated by two periods of oestrogen secretion from the pig conceptuses at around days 11–13 and 15–30 of pregnancy. In addition, the oestrogen promotes PGE production (which antagonizes the luteolytic action of $PGF_{2\alpha}$), and also promotes LH and prolactin receptors in the corpus luteum, thereby boosting the effective luteotrophic support. Its actions can be mimicked in non-pregnant pigs by oestrogen injections. Interestingly, the pig conceptus does not produce IFN-τ, but does secrete IFN-γ and δ. Neither is antiluteolytic, but they do, like IFN-τ in ruminants, seem to have a key role in sustaining early pregnancy.

Pregnancy hormones are required for the support of pregnancy

The successful establishment of pregnancy creates a new and extraordinary parabiotic liaison between mother and conceptus, which may last for a period of months in some species. In the human, in whom pregnancy approximates to 9 months, its course is often described as lasting three *trimesters* (a trimester being 3 months). Conventionally, human pregnancy is timed from the last menstrual period. Given that this event marks the beginning of a menstrual cycle rather than ovulation, a 12-week pregnancy is in fact only 10 weeks after ovulation and fertilization, and 8 weeks after corpus luteum salvage.

For the period of pregnancy, the conceptus is totally dependent on the mother for its protection and nutrition. It subverts many of her metabolic and physiological activities to its own ends, so that there is adequate mobilization of oxygen, salts and organic precursors to supply its needs. One way in which it achieves this is by inducing and taking part in the formation of the vascularized placenta where the bulk of these substances is exchanged for its own metabolic waste. During pregnancy, the mother is also prepared for the future requirements of the fetus and neonate. Thus, hypertrophy of the uterine musculature, which participates in fetal expulsion at parturition, and the development and maintenance of mammary glands for postpartum lactational nutrition, are both stimulated during pregnancy. This takeover of the mother's metabolism is controlled by the *pregnancy hormones*. These hormones were introduced in Chapter 3, where we noticed that pregnancy-specific variants of several existed, either through differential splicing of a single gene or through expression of gene duplication variants (LH and CG, GH-N and GH-V, prolactin and placental lactogens). The elaboration of these variants may reflect the fact that the needs of the mother and the fetus sometimes conflict, and so some competition for control of resources may be occurring. In the remainder of this chapter, we consider the nature and origin of these pregnancy hormones. It will become clear that the placenta can be thought of as a major and versatile endocrine gland. In Chapters 12–14, we will look at how, where and when the hormonal products of this gland achieve their effects.

The central role of progesterone

The extended secretion of progesterone is critical for the initiation of pregnancy. This absolute requirement for progesterone persists throughout pregnancy. Indeed, in some species, progesterone levels in maternal blood rise continuously as pregnancy proceeds (Fig. 11.2). Moreover, as pregnancy advances, the level of oestrogens in the maternal blood also rises (Fig. 11.2). These steroid hormones may reach plasma levels many times greater than those seen in a normal luteal phase. In many species, the ovarian corpora lutea under the control of the maternal pituitary continue to secrete an essential proportion of these steroids throughout pregnancy. Removal of either the ovary or pituitary at any time therefore results in pregnancy loss (Table 11.1, group C). In other species (Table 11.1, groups A and B), the whole of pregnancy clearly does not depend totally on steroids secreted by pituitary–ovarian interactions, because, at varying periods during pregnancy, one or both glands may be removed without inducing pregnancy loss. Where does the endocrine support come from in these species? Some of the clearest answers to this question have come from studies on human pregnancy, which shows the least dependence on the maternal ovarian–pituitary axis of any species. We will therefore examine the endocrinology of human pregnancy in some detail and discuss the evidence from other species in relation to the human pattern.

The human conceptus synthesizes steroid hormones

We saw in the first section of this chapter that within 2 weeks of fertilization the human conceptus synthesizes and releases the hormone hCG. This hormone then maintains the progestagenic activity of the corpus luteum. Within a further 2–3 weeks, the conceptus is also synthesizing all the steroidal hormones required for pregnancy, and although the maternal corpus luteum remains active for the whole of pregnancy, it can be dispensed with after only 4–5 weeks and plays only a trivial role in total progesterone output at later stages. *The human conceptus thus shows a remarkable endocrine emancipation.* It asserts its complete endocrine independence of the mother.

Our understanding of the role of the conceptus in steroidogenesis has come from several sources. For example, much has been learnt from observations on steroid output and interconversions in abnormal pregnancies, and from isolation of tissues from different parts of the normal conceptus and assessment of their steroid biosynthetic capacity *in vitro*. However, by far the most informative and important data have come from *in vivo* studies using the fetuses of induced pregnancy terminations. Direct sampling of umbilical and maternal blood, and the infusions of minute quantities of radiolabelled steroid precursors into the maternal, fetal or placental circulations, with subsequent analysis of their interconversions, has provided information of great clinical value about the sites of steroid synthesis and interconversion in the conceptus (Fig. 11.3).

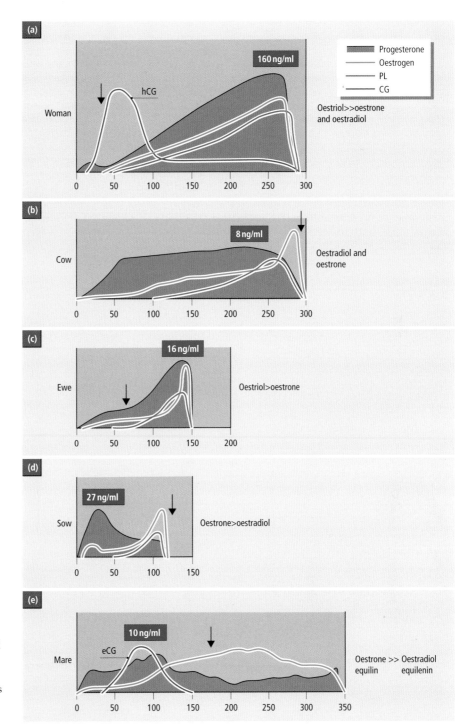

Fig. 11.2 Patterns of plasma hormones during pregnancy (in days) in various species. The maximal progesterone level is indicated in the blue box and the principal oestrogens are recorded to the right of each panel. PL, placental lactogen; hCG and eCG are human and equine chorionic gonadotrophins. The arrow indicates the time at which ovariectomy no longer terminates pregnancy.

Progesterone is secreted by the placental trophoblast

By late human pregnancy, the output of progesterone exceeds 200 mg/day. Blood absolute levels are high, partly due also to a threefold increase in transcortin, which increases the proportion of bound progesterone (see Table 3.9). From where in the conceptus does the progesterone come?

A clue comes from observations on pathological pregnancies, in which an embryo fails to develop but progesterone output is only marginally reduced. Thus, *chorio-carcinomas* or *hydatidiform moles* (malignant and benign tumours of the chorion, respectively) secrete progesterone in the absence of any embryonic tissue, suggesting that the placental trophoblast itself is the principal progesterone

Table 11.1 Dependence of pregnancy on maternal ovarian and pituitary function in various species.

Species	Duration of pregnancy (days)	Duration of non-pregnant luteal phase (days)	Day of pregnancy when hypophysectomy is without effect	Day of pregnancy when ovariectomy is without effect
Group A				
Human	260–270	12–14	?	40
Monkey (*M. mulatta*)	168	12–14	29	21
Sheep	147–150	16–18	50	55
Guinea-pig	60	16	3	28
Group B				
Rat	22	10–12	12	Term
Mouse	20–21	10–12	11	Term
Cat	63	30–60	Term?	50
Horse	330–340	20–21	?	150–200
*Group C**				
Cow	280–290	18–20	?	Term
Dog	61	61	Term?	Term?
Pig	115	16–18	Term	Term
Rabbit	31	12	Term	Term
Goat	150	16–18	Term	Term

*NB: These results do not mean that these species are solely dependent on pituitary and ovarian function. It is established that some are partially dependent on support from placental sources which are inadequate when acting alone (see Table 11.3).

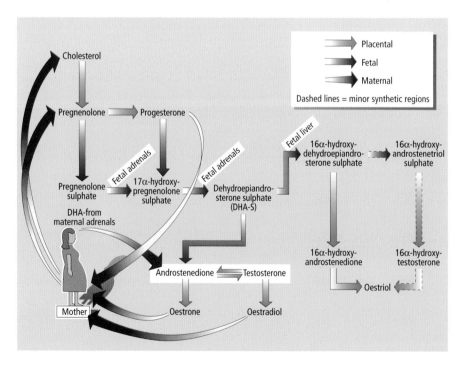

Fig. 11.3 Summary of the principal routes by which the human materno-feto-placental unit synthesizes oestrogens.

source. *In vitro* studies on the biosynthesis of progesterone by cultures of syncytiotrophoblast confirm this conclusion, and also indicate that the trophoblast can only use cholesterol (not acetate) as a substrate. The cholesterol is usually derived from the maternal rather than the fetal circulation. The rising output of progesterone through pregnancy appears to be completely autonomous; no external controlling mechanism has yet been discovered.

Clinical observations on patients whose ovaries have been removed at various times in early pregnancy indicate that the placenta is capable of synthesizing an adequate, supportive level of progesterone by 5–6 weeks. In the normal pregnant woman, there is a plateau, or even a slight fall, in the concentration of blood progesterone between 6 and 9 weeks. The plateau coincides with a marked fall in 17α-hydroxyprogesterone (an ovarian progestagen), indicating that over this period the placenta takes over progestagenic support. Both pregnenolone and progesterone pass from the placenta into both the fetal and maternal circulations, infused radiolabelled progestagens being distributed widely within the fetal and maternal tissues. The principal excreted metabolite of progesterone (15% of total) is *pregnanediol*, but its urinary level is not a useful indicator of fetal well-being and only a crude indicator of placental function. The failure to correlate progesterone output with fetal well-being is not surprising, as the fetus itself plays no part in progesterone synthesis. The poor correlation with placental function is mainly a result of the wide interindividual variation in the level of progesterone's urinary metabolites in normal pregnancies.

The human fetus and placenta cooperate to produce oestrogens

The conceptus is also the source of the high level of oestrogens in human pregnancy (Fig. 11.2). The principal oestrogen is not oestradiol 17β but the less potent oestriol (Table 11.2). Oestrogen output differs from that of progesterone, however, in that it is severely reduced in cases of choriocarcinoma and hydatidiform mole, in which a fetus is lacking. Moreover, although the incubation of placental tissue with radiolabelled cholesterol or pregnenolone yields labelled progesterone, no labelled oestrogens are produced. Clearly, the placenta alone is inadequate for synthesis of oestrogens. Could the fetus itself produce them?

When radiolabelled pregnenolone was infused into the circulation of isolated perfused human fetuses, little or no labelled oestrogen was produced. Therefore, the fetus alone cannot be the site of oestrogen synthesis. However, when labelled pregnenolone was injected into an intact fetoplacental unit, complete synthesis of oestrogens occurred. These observations show that the human fetus and placenta cooperate to produce oestrogens. A series of observations on the result of infusing various radiolabelled steroid substrates has shown that, while the placenta is capable of synthesizing oestrogens from C_{19} androgens, it is *not* capable of synthesizing its own androgens from progestagens. The *fetal adrenal*, in contrast, *can* synthesize the C_{19} androgens (DHA and some androstenedione) from progestagens but *cannot* aromatize them to oestrogens. These C_{19} steroids, which are made in a *special fetal zone* of the adrenal, must therefore pass to the placenta, which can then convert them to oestrogens. The principal pathways involved are summarized in Fig. 11.3. This cooperative organization is reminiscent of that observed between luteal and granulosa cells in the production of ovarian oestrogens (see Chapter 5).

Two important points should be noted about this cooperative event. First, the initial step in the *fetal handling* of *all steroids* arriving from the placenta or mother is *conjugation to sulfates*. This conjugation occurs mainly in the fetal liver but also in the adrenals. The conjugated steroid is then converted biosynthetically by the fetal adrenal to other steroid derivatives via sulfated intermediates. Conversely, the placenta takes conjugated steroids arriving from the fetus and deconjugates them, releasing free steroids into the maternal (and fetal) circulation. Thus, the *fetus sulfates* and the *placenta desulfates*. This apparently bizarre manoeuvre is in fact extremely important, as conjugated steroids are both water soluble and biologically inactive. The conjugation may protect the fetus against untoward steroidal penetration into, and activity within, fetal tissues (e.g. masculinization of females by weak androgens, see Chapter 1). Thus, this strategy permits the high ambient levels of steroid required by the *maternal organism* for the

Table 11.2 Plasma levels of various steroids in women during late pregnancy.

Steroid	Values in pregnancy (ng/ml)	Values in luteal phase of cycle (ng/ml)
Progesterone	125–200	11
Oestriol	7 ⎫ 113	—
Oestriol conjugates	106 ⎭	
Oestrone	7 ⎫ 53	0.2
Oestrone conjugates	46 ⎭	
Oestradiol 17β	10 ⎫ 15	0.2
Oestradiol conjugates	5 ⎭	

maintenance of pregnancy to coexist with the low level of active steroids essential for protection of the *fetal organism* from unwanted side effects. An X-linked placental sulfatase deficiency exists and is associated with deficiencies in the aromatization of C_{19} steroids to oestrogens, with a consequent maternal oestrogen deficiency.

Second, the placental synthesis of oestrone and oestradiol 17β can occur from DHA sulfate derived *either* from the fetal adrenal (40% but rising towards term) *or* from the maternal adrenal. Oestriol synthesis also occurs in the placenta but the 16α-hydroxylated substrate required comes *solely* from the *fetal* liver. It follows therefore that 16α-hydroxylated steroids, such as oestriol, should provide an indicator not only of *placental function* but also of *fetal well-being*. In pregnancies at risk, a consistent decline over a period of days of 16α-hydroxylated steroids correlates with fetal distress and may indicate that premature delivery should be induced. A parallel decline in oestradiol 17β is not seen because 50–60% of its synthesis by the placenta utilizes maternal not fetal DHA sulfate. In anencephalic fetuses, in which fetal adrenal function is impaired, the ratio of oestradiol+oestrone to oestriol is greatly increased, as would be expected. Thus, 16α-hydroxylated steroids can have a diagnostic value.

Corticosteroids rise during pregnancy under the influence of oestrogens

Blood levels of cortisol rise in pregnancy, and this rise can be mimicked by oestrogen injection into non-pregnant women. The elevated levels are partly due to a decrease in the metabolism of free cortisol, but predominantly due to an oestrogen-stimulated synthesis of transcortin from 3.5 mg/100 ml to 10 mg/100 ml. The transcortin binds both cortisol and progesterone.

The major placental protein hormones

Chorionic gonadotrophin is not required once placental steroid synthesis is established

We saw earlier in this chapter that hCG was critical for the initiation of pregnancy by extending luteal life from 2 to 6–7 weeks until placental steroids take over. The rising blood and urinary levels of hCG over this period can usefully be measured when testing for pregnancy, a positive test indicating a *biochemical pregnancy*. The action of hCG may be limited to this short-term luteal support, as its blood levels fall after 8 weeks (Fig. 11.2), correlating with the fall in 17α-hydroxyprogesterone (a luteal product) and the emancipation of the fetoplacental unit from ovarian dependence. Low levels of hCG remain detectable for the remainder of pregnancy (although in the rhesus monkey rhCG levels are trivial from 40 days onwards).

How the variation in CG output is controlled is uncertain. The placenta produces its own pulses of GnRH and the pulsatile output of CG is sensitive to exogenous GnRH pulses, suggesting a causal relationship. Moreover, inhibin A and progesterone depress, while activin A and oestrogen enhance, CG production. However, although the basic building blocks of an intraplacental control system are in place, just how they might be coordinated to give the observed temporal pattern of CG secretion remains to be elucidated.

The somatomammotrophins are synthesized by the placenta towards the end of the first trimester

As hCG levels decline, syncytiotrophoblastic expansion is associated from about 6–8 weeks with increased secretion of human placental lactogen (hPL) and the placental variants of human growth hormone (hGH-V and chorionic somatomammotrophin-like (CS) A, B and L; see Table 3.5). Blood levels then increase further during the last trimester. The nature of the physiological control of this switch in hormone production is unclear. As plasma levels of hGH-V rise, those of pituitary hGH fall, suggesting that the placental variant is exerting a negative feedback control systemically. Indeed, pregnancy survives in the face of maternal GH deficiency. Placental GH modulates maternal metabolism through stimulation of placental growth and the induction of placental IGF-1 to induce nutrient repartitioning to the fetus. A deficiency of placental GH is associated with fetal growth retardation. The placental GH does not itself enter the fetal circulation.

In addition, release of pituitary prolactin is stimulated by oestrogens (see Chapter 6), and maternal plasma concentrations reach over 200 ng/ml by the last trimester. Prolactin is also synthesized by the decidual tissue. Some synthesis is detectable by the spontaneous decidual cells that appear towards the end of each luteal phase (see Chapter 10), but much larger amounts are secreted between 10 and 30 weeks of pregnancy. Progesterone is implicated in the control of its secretion. Little decidual prolactin appears in either the fetal or maternal circulation. Most of it seems to pass into the amniotic fluid where it may have a role in maintaining the water and electrolyte balance of the fetus (see Chapter 12).

Different strategies achieve the endocrine support of pregnancy in other species

Dependence of steroid synthesis on the pituitary–ovarian axis varies among species. Elevated steroid levels are a feature of pregnancy in most mammals studied, although there is considerable variation in the patterns and absolute levels from species to species (Fig. 11.2). As we saw in Table 11.1, the degree of independence from the pituitary–ovarian axis also varies, but even in species such as the cow and the pig that require both pituitary and ovary to be present through-out pregnancy, there is a fetal steroid contribution (Table 11.3). Conceptuses of both the horse and the sheep become independent of the ovary by about one-third of the way through pregnancy. Both are comparable to the human, with a fetal source of DHA sulfate being deconjugated and aromatized by the placenta. In the horse, the principal oes-trogens formed are oestrone, together with two oestrogens found only in equids: *equilin* and *equilenin*. The fetal DHA sulfate used for aromatization in the horse is derived not from the fetal adrenal but from the hypertrophied intersti-tial tissues of the fetal gonads, which show a spectacular increase in weight between 100 and 300 days of gestation, regressing by birth. The sheep fetus, like the human, syn-thesizes sulfated DHA in the adrenal, and maternal sources of DHA may also be available. In addition, the sheep pla-centa, unlike the human placenta, can undertake conver-sion of progesterone to oestrogens, and this property is of great importance at parturition (see Chapter 13).

Protein hormones are actively synthesized by the placenta in many species. From the time of attachment (around 16–30 days; Table 10.1) biosynthesis of placental lactogens (PLs; Table 3.5) by the binucleate trophoblast cells of sheep, cow and goat conceptuses can be detected. This synthesis is reflected subsequently in their rising blood levels as pregnancy progresses (Fig. 11.2). However, these hormones are much more closely related to prolactin than hPL is to human prolactin, and so have less GH-like activity than does hPL. Placental GH-V synthesis occurs in sheep and goats (but not cows, which use fetal and maternal GH), roughly paralleling PL production and coming from the same binucleate cells. Together these two placental hor-mones act to stimulate the uterine glandular secretions, which remain so important throughout the pregnancy of large farm animals with their non-invasive, central implan-tations (Chapter 10). There is evidence that IFN-τ, directly or indirectly, may sensitize the glands to these hormones, independent of its actions in suppressing oxytocin receptor synthesis.

Between days 40 and 120 of pregnancy in the mare, a gonadotrophin with weak follicle-stimulating hormone and strong LH-like activity, called originally *pregnant mares' serum gonadotrophin* (PMSG) but now *equine chorionic gona-dotrophin* (eCG) on the basis of its structural similarity to other CGs, is secreted from the trophoblastic cells of the endometrial cups. How its secretion is controlled is not known, although the quantity of its secretion is determined by the genetic constitution of the mare. One effect of the eCG is to promote follicular growth and even secondary ovulation in the maternal ovaries between days 40 and 120 of pregnancy; as a result, secondary corpora lutea may develop. These remain an active source of progesterone until the decline of eCG and the take-over by placental progesterone at around 140–150 days.

In many species, but notably in the guinea-pig and pig, a cytokine called relaxin (a member of the insulin family; see Table 3.6) has been detected in blood at low levels during pregnancy, rising just before parturition. This hormone appears to be produced by the corpus luteum of pregnancy, and has also been detected in humans. Its actions will be discussed in the context of parturition (see Chapter 13). Finally, and also in the pig, placental oestro-gens continue to play a major role in the support of histio-trophic secretion, acting in part via induction of uterine IGF-1 and FGF7.

Table 11.3 Major sites of hormone synthesis during established pregnancy.

Species	Progestagens	Oestrogens	Gonadotrophins
Human	Placenta	Fetal adrenal and placenta	Placenta (hCG and hPL)
Horse			
early	Corpus luteum	Ovarian follicles	Placenta (eCG)
mid–late	Placenta	Fetal gonad and placenta	—
Sheep			
early	Ovary and placenta	Placenta (oestradiol and oestrone sulfate)	—
mid–late	Placenta	Ovary (oestrone), placenta (oestrone sulfate)	Placenta (oPL)
Cow	Ovary (and placenta)	Placenta (and ovary)	Pituitary and placenta later (for bPL)
Pig			
early	Ovary	Placenta	Pituitary
late	Ovary (and placenta)	Placenta	Pituitary

The richness of the endocrine placenta

The foregoing account captures the complexity of the placental endocrine gland. Nonetheless, it is a relatively impoverished account. The placenta resembles a 'mini-organism': it synthesizes hypothalamic releasing hormones (GnRH, CRF) and pituitary-like hormones (ACTH, oxytocin, vasopressin) together with a large range of cytokines (including TGFβ, activin A, inhibins A and B, IGF1 and 2, FGFs, EGF), vasoactive peptides (VEGF, endothelin), neurohormones (monoamines, neuropeptide Y) and metabolic hormones (leptin, grhelin). This list is far from exhaustive. Many of these hormones spill over into maternal and/or fetal blood. Others act locally within the placenta itself. It is not yet clear exactly what all these hormones do, as the complexity of their production is matched by the even greater complexity of their interactions. Some of these individual players we will pick up in later chapters, but for the moment grasp the extraordinary biosynthetic richness of this transient organ.

Summary

Three comments of general relevance need to be made when comparing the available data on pregnancy hormones. First, the tendency for the fetoplacental unit to take over endocrine control from the mother in whole or in part is seen in most species. Second, while the levels of plasma oestrogens and progesterone rise, there is great species variation in the absolute level achieved (compare 160 ng progesterone/ml in the human with 8 ng/ml in the cow). Third, the temporal patterns of plasma steroids recorded through pregnancy differ among various species. The large variation, both qualitative and quantitative, in plasma hormone levels is difficult to explain. This difficulty is compounded by the fact that we do not yet have a complete understanding of the functions of many of these hormones during pregnancy. These issues are addressed in Chapters 12–14.

FURTHER READING

Barnea ER *et al.* (eds) (1992) *The First Twelve Weeks of Gestation.* Springer-Verlag, Berlin.

Duncan WC (2000) The human corpus luteum: remodelling during luteolysis and maternal recognition of pregnancy. *Reviews of Reproduction* **5**, 12–17.

Spencer TE, Bazer FW (2004) Conceptus signals for establishment and maintenance of pregnancy. *Reproductive Biology and Endocrinology* **2**, 49 doi:10.1186/1477–7827–2–49.

KEY LEARNING POINTS

- The implanting conceptus must signal its presence to the mother and prevent the withdrawal of progestagenic support by luteolysis.

- The primate blastocyst prolongs the life of the corpus luteum by production of the luteotrophic factor: chorionic gonadotrophin (CG).

- CG is synthesized in the syncytiotrophoblast of the implanting primate blastocyst from as early as 6–7 days after fertilization and is carried to the ovary where it binds to LH receptors on the luteal cells to exert a luteotrophic action.

- Progesterone itself is luteotrophic, an example of positive feedback.

- CG falls after the first trimester and is no longer needed.

- In the large farm ruminants the conceptus suppresses luteolytic activity by neutralizing the oxytocin-dependent release of $PGF_{2\alpha}$ from uterine epithelial cells.

- It does so by producing trophoblast interferon which suppresses the development of oxytocin receptors in the uterine epithelial cells.

- In pigs, the conceptus produces oestrogen which has both antiluteolytic actions (diverting $PGF_{2\alpha}$ from endocrine to exocrine secretion) and luteotophic ones (promoting LH and prolactin receptors).

- In humans, the conceptus synthesizes all the steroidal hormones required for pregnancy from about 5–6 weeks of pregnancy.

- The placental trophoblast is the principal source of progesterone in human pregnancy.

- Human trophoblast also synthesizes oestrogens from C19 androgens, notably DHA.

- Human trophoblast cannot synthesize its own androgens from progestagens.

- The human fetal adrenal synthesizes the C19 androgens in the fetal zone of the adrenal but cannot aromatize them. These C19 steroids pass to the placenta, which converts them to oestrogens.

- The fetus conjugates steroids and the placenta deconjugates them.

- Corticosteroids rise during pregnancy under the influence of oestrogens.

- Somatomammotrophins (e.g. hPL, hGH-V) are synthesized by the placental trophoblast or decidua (prolactin) from 6–8 weeks of pregnancy.

- Dependence of steroid synthesis on the pituitary–ovarian axis varies among species, as does the pattern of hormones during pregnancy.

Steven DH (ed.) (1977) *Comparative Placentation*. Academic Press, New York.

Stouffer RL (2003) Progesterone as a mediator of gonadotrophin action in the corpus luteum: beyond steroidogenesis. *Human Reproduction Update* **9**, 99–117.

More advanced reading

Ashworth CJ *et al.* (2000) Placental leptin. *Reviews of Reproduction* **5**, 18–24.

Gootwine E (2004) Placental hormones and fetal–placental development. *Animal Reproduction Science* **82–83**, 551–566.

12 The Fetus and its Preparations for Birth

The fetus is not a quiescent, passively growing product of conception tucked neatly away in its protected uterine environment. Although undoubtedly dependent on the mother's nutrient supplies for its growth and survival, it nonetheless enjoys considerable independence in the regulation of its own development. Indeed, the fetus exerts profound effects on maternal physiology via hormones secreted by the fetal part of the placenta into the maternal circulation. These in part determine the mother's ability to meet the metabolic requirements of pregnancy. In addition, the fetus and mother must develop physiological mechanisms that anticipate the transition from a uterine to an external, independent existence at parturition. This extraordinary change of circumstance must be achieved while maintaining the internal environment of the neonate.

Placental, fetal and maternal factors determine fetal growth and well-being during pregnancy

The rate of fetal growth is relatively slow up to the 20th week of pregnancy but accelerates to reach a maximum around weeks 30–36, declining thereafter until birth (Fig. 12.1a). A postnatal peak in growth velocity occurs during week 8. Growth initially is through an increase in cell number, but from week 32 increase in cell size dominates. Protein accumulation occurs early in fetal development to reach its maximum, about 300 g, by week 35, and precedes fat deposition, most of which is subcutaneous, and which only comes to exceed the weight of protein by week 38. By term, some three times as much energy is stored as fat as is stored as protein. The relative amount of water (95% in

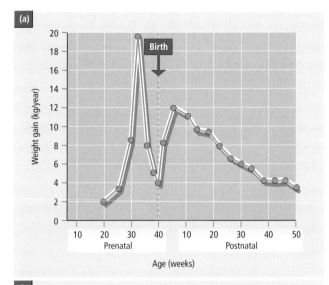

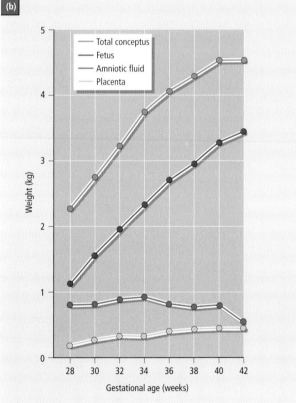

Fig. 12.1 (a) Change in velocity of growth in weight of singleton fetuses and children. (b) Weight changes of conceptus, fetus, placenta and amniotic fluid during pregnancy.

the young fetus) also decreases. Amniotic fluid also increases in volume until week 34 of pregnancy, after which time it declines. It is reasonable to assume that growth is one indicator of fetal well-being, and fetuses that develop poorly are said to suffer from *intrauterine growth retardation*

(*IUGR*). Babies may be of *low birthweight* (less than 2500 g) because they are born prematurely, because they arise from a multiple pregnancy (twins, triplets etc., usually also born prematurely) or, if born at full term, because of IUGR. As many as one-third of low-birthweight singleton babies come into the latter category and are said to be *small for gestational age* (SGA or sometime *small for dates*; defined as being of a weight that is two standard deviations below the weight expected of a baby of a particular gestational age).

It is important that the fetal growth trajectory balances the demands of the fetus with the capabilities of the mother. Too large a fetus brings a difficult delivery, risky for the mother. Too small a fetus brings both short-term and long-term problems for the fetus. Indeed, as we will see, the impact of an adverse maternal growth environment is not limited to the fetus, but can also 'programme' development in ways that influence postnatal function, and even health patterns later in life (see end of this chapter). An understanding of how growth is regulated is thus important for pregnancy management, the clinical care of small neonates, and the general health of the population. Mother, placenta and fetus are each implicated in the endocrine regulation of fetal growth.

In this chapter, we will see that the mother's needs are often placed secondary to those of fetal survival, the pregnancy hormones directing metabolic resources towards the placenta. However, we will also see that simple fetal survival can sometimes impose high costs, both short- and longer-term, for the surviving child.

Maternal contributions to growth control

The mother adapts to the demands of the conceptus by increasing her caloric intake and modifying her metabolic activity. The size and nature of these adaptations seem to occur largely in response to signals from the fetoplacental unit, although it is not completely clear how. However, the mother also seems to *constrain fetal growth*. Thus, maternal height, which is linked to uterine capacity and thus potential for growth, exerts a powerful influence on full-term birthweight. However, again it is not clear how this constraint is exercised. There is little evidence that fetal growth is increased by dietary supplements to well-nourished healthy women, suggesting that availability of nutrients is not limiting. Supplements, especially when given early in pregnancy, are only found to be of clear value in preventing SGA babies in poorer, undernourished women. Maternal uterine blood flow and/or placental size may be limiting, because although the placenta increases in size slowly and steadily until birth, the relatively rapid growth of the fetus before birth means that the ratio of placental weight to fetal weight falls significantly during the later stages of pregnancy (Fig. 12.1b). Perhaps the placenta limits the transport of nutrients to the fetus late in pregnancy and thereby underlies part of the fall in growth velocity after week 36 and the protection against fetal overgrowth? Certainly placental deficiencies seem to underlie IUGR, when both the placental surface area and specific uptake mechanisms are reduced significantly. For the non-pathological situation then, the question becomes: why does placental growth slow, and how is this regulated maternally?

Additional maternal factors that may affect birthweight include parity (primiparous mothers have smaller babies than multiparous mothers), maternal size, multiple pregnancy (more than one fetus carried simultaneously) and self-inflicted damage, for example smoking and drug and alcohol abuse (see Chapter 10 for discussion on blood flow and reactive oxygen species).

Fetal contributions to growth control

Fetal sex affects fetal growth, male fetuses being on average larger than females. The pattern of fetal growth is determined primarily through the *genome of the fetus*, but additional fetal and maternal factors modulate the effects of its expression. *Insulin-like growth factors 1 and 2* (IGFs or *somatomedins*; see Table 3.6) are produced by a range of fetal cell types, the mix of which varies with stage of development in species-specific ways. Synthesis of both IGFs rises with progress through pregnancy, IGF2 being present in fetal blood at 2–3-fold higher levels than IGF1. IGF1 provides a major direct endocrine stimulus to fetal growth through its anabolic effects; IGF2 may do so mainly indirectly by stimulating placental growth and transport mechanisms. Genetic knockout of either or both IGFs results in fetal growth retardation. Fetal IGF1 production is responsive to nutrient levels, declining when nutrients fall, and also to nutrient-sensitive hormones such as insulin, thyroxine and glucocorticoids, and thus matches fetal growth to nutrient supply. IGF1 production is not stimulated by fetal GH, probably because of a deficit in its receptors. Fetal thyroid hormones also stimulate growth in the latter part of pregnancy. Leptin levels, produced not only by adipocytes but also the syncytiotrophoblast and possibly other fetal tissues, rise during pregnancy and correlate strongly with fetal and placental growth rates, suggesting but not proving a functional link with growth.

Fetal metabolism depends critically on placental transport of essential nutrients

The main ingredient of the fetal diet is carbohydrate, and about half the calories needed for growth and metabolism come from glucose, the remainder coming equally from amino acids and from lactate formed from glucose in the placenta. If normal growth and development are to occur, the fetus must also be provided with the basic building materials: essential amino acids, fatty acids, vitamins and minerals. These must come from the mother, most via the placenta, but some across the amniotic membranes.

The discrete nature of the maternal and fetal circulations, separated by cellular and acellular layers, confers an important barrier property on the placenta. Simple diffusional exchange between the circulations will only therefore be significant in the case of low-molecular-weight molecules, such as blood gases, sodium ions, water and urea, or in the case of non-polar molecules, such as fatty acids and non-conjugated steroids. In contrast, hexose sugars, conjugated steroids, amino acids, nucleotides, water-soluble vitamins, plasma proteins, maternal cells, potentially infective agents such as viruses and bacteria, and molecules such as cholesterol (which are complexed and transferred in large lipoprotein particles) will not gain access to the fetal circulation unless either special transport mechanisms exist or the integrity of the barrier is breached. 'Bleeds' across the placenta are rare (except at parturition) and probably occur mainly in a fetomaternal direction. However, recent evidence suggests that less traumatic erosions of the integrity of the trophoblastic layer at the maternal–fetal interface may not be uncommon.

The identification of transfer routes between mother and fetus is difficult. The system is highly complex: both maternal and fetal components are dynamic and their physiology changes with the duration of pregnancy; the fetal, placental and maternal components may each utilize (or produce) the substance under study and so complicate quantitative measurements; there are several potential routes of transfer (amnion, chorioallantoic placenta, yolk sac placenta), each of which may also have some heterogeneity in its transport systems. Studies have used radiolabelled markers and serial sampling in intact materno-feto-placental units, perfused fetoplacental units, isolated placentae, cultured placental fragments or trophoblastic cells *in vitro*.

The factors that will influence exchange between mother and fetus include the thickness and organization of the tissues interposed between them; the maternal and fetal blood flows (already considered in Chapter 10); the fetal and maternal concentrations, and thereby the gradient, of the substances to be transported; and the types of transport mechanism available.

We saw in Chapter 10 that there is considerable interspecies variability in the microstructure of the layers separating maternal and fetal circulations (see Table 10.3 & Fig. 10.6). In addition, within a species, the facility with which diffusional exchange occurs varies during pregnancy. For example, in early pregnancy, terminal villi in the human placenta are large (150–200 μm in diameter) and the fetal vessel is located centrally beneath 10 μm of syncytiotrophoblast, so metabolites must diffuse a considerable distance. Furthermore, the syncytiotrophoblast is itself metabolically active and intercepts and utilizes maternal metabolites. As *pregnancy progresses*, the *villi thin* to 40 μm in diameter and the *fetal vessel occupies a more eccentric position*, indenting the overlying syncytiotrophoblast to leave only a 1–2 μm layer separating it from the maternal blood. This altered anatomical relationship increases the capacity for diffusional exchange and reduces consumption by the trophoblast of oxygen. A similar thinning of diffusional barriers also occurs in the synepitheliochorial placenta of sheep.

Although the interspecies differences in placental microstructure do influence the relative efficiency of diffusional exchange (e.g. diffusion of Na^+ is faster across the haemochorial than synepitheliochorial placenta), the more freely diffusible molecules such as O_2 are much more affected by blood flow than placental barrier thickness. The important point to appreciate about the microstructure of the placental interface is that it either permits adequate diffusional exchange (i.e. has a large safety factor) or employs special transport systems to promote selective transport of less freely diffusible, but essential, substances, such as glucose, fructose, amino acids and various proteins. Both methods of placental transport will be affected critically by the circulatory factors that were discussed in Chapter 10. Here we will now consider the transport mechanisms themselves, and the changes in maternal and fetal metabolism and physiology that determine the relative blood levels of metabolites, and thereby the gradients across the placental interface.

Oxygen and carbon dioxide

During pregnancy, maternal O_2 consumption at rest and during exercise is increased compared with non-pregnant females proportionate to the growing tissue mass of the conceptus. Physical working capacity and the efficiency with which work is performed are not affected significantly by pregnancy. Cardiac output (both stroke volume and rate) increases by about 30% during the first trimester, but little more thereafter. It is accommodated by a reduction of peripheral resistance by as much as 30% owing to the demands of the conceptus, and only a slight blood pressure increase (see also Chapter 10, 'Blood flow in the placenta'). Blood volume rises by up to 40% near term in humans, due partly to a 20–30% increase in erythrocytes and partly to increasing plasma volume (up 30–60%).

Maternal *pulmonary ventilation increases by 40%* during pregnancy, possibly because of a direct effect of progesterone on respiratory mechanisms in the brainstem. A decrease of about 25% in maternal Pco_2 results, with a corresponding fall in bicarbonate concentration, a slight increase in pH and greater changes in pH with exercise. The fetus requires O_2 in relatively continuous supply because fetal stores of the gas are very small: a 3-kg fetus near term requires 18 ml O_2/min, but stores are only 36 ml or 2 minutes' worth. In addition, the placenta itself is very active metabolically and consumes a massive 40–60% of the total glucose and O_2 supplied by the mother! Because it is a non-polar molecule, O_2 diffuses readily across the placental interface, as does the carbon dioxide (CO_2) generated by fetal metabolism, with its diffusion constant 20 times higher than that of O_2.

The gradients of the gases at the transplacental interface may be estimated from the figures shown in Table 12.1. Clearly the tension of O_2 in the fetal blood is low and that of CO_2 is high relative to the tension of the gases in maternal blood. Gradients to drive diffusional exchange therefore exist. However, inspection of Table 12.1 reveals that although the Po_2 in the oxygenated fetal venous blood leaving the placenta in the umbilical vein is relatively low, the O_2 saturation and content are not much less than in maternal arterial blood. Thus, a much lower O_2 tension leads to a very similar O_2 content, indicating that the 'O_2 trapping' properties of fetal blood must be more effective than those of maternal blood. This higher affinity of fetal blood is shown graphically in Fig. 12.2. How is it achieved?

Table 12.1 O_2 and CO_2 composition of human maternal and fetal blood.

	Maternal blood (arterial)	Fetal blood (venous)	Umbilical artery	Umbilical vein
Oxygen tension (Po_2) (mmHg)	90	35	15	30
Oxygen saturation (%)	95	70	25	65
Oxygen content (vol. %)	14	10	5	13
CO_2 tension (Pco_2) (mmHg)	30	35	53	40
pH	7.43	7.40	7.26	7.35

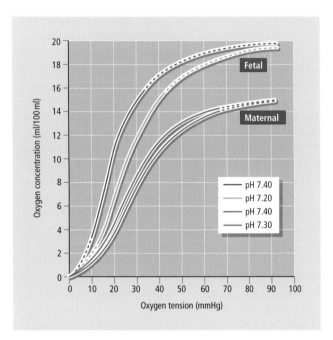

Fig. 12.2 The effect of varying oxygen tension on the oxygen content of human maternal and fetal blood under conditions likely to be encountered in the placenta. Note the greater oxygen concentration in fetal blood at any given Po_2. Note also that the pH shifts occurring in the placenta (falling pH in maternal blood and rising pH in fetal blood) will further facilitate unloading of oxygen from maternal blood and its uptake by fetal blood.

The earliest site of *erythropoiesis* in the implanting mammalian conceptus is the yolk sac mesoderm (see Fig. 10.8). The primitive *embryonic erythrocytes* formed are nucleated, and are replaced later by *fetal erythrocytes* (also nucleated) made in the liver. As parturition approaches, the spleen and bone marrow take over erythropoiesis. This latter transition is regulated by the rising levels of fetal cortisol occurring towards term (see later). Embryonic and fetal erythrocytes, like those of the adult, contain haemoglobin as the O_2-carrying molecule. The embryonic and fetal haemoglobins consist of four globin chains coupled to a haem group; however, they differ from the adult in that the constituent globin chains are not two α- and two β-chains. Rather, embryonic haemoglobin contains two ε- and two φ-chains, and fetal haemoglobin contains two α- and two γ-chains. Each globin chain is coded for by a different gene, and during development a programme of gene switching occurs to yield the embryonic, the fetal and the adult sequences. The switch from fetal to adult haemoglobins, like the site of erythropoiesis, is also regulated by fetal cortisol. It is this difference in globin chain composition that results in the different O_2-binding curves (Fig. 12.2).

In adults, the highly charged molecule 2,3-diphosphoglycerate (DPG) can bind to sites on the β-chain

that are exposed only on deoxygenation. This binding stabilizes the deoxyhaemoglobin, thereby reducing the opportunity for O_2 binding. Thus, a higher Po_2 is needed to load haemoglobin with O_2. The β-chain is lacking in embryonic and fetal haemoglobins, and its equivalents (the γ- and ε-chains) are relatively insensitive to DPG. Therefore, at any given Po_2, fetal and embryonic haemoglobins will bind more O_2 than will maternal haemoglobin. In some species, the fetal DPG levels may also be lower, which will further assist the O_2 loading process.

In addition, as Fig. 12.2 shows, a *double Bohr effect* occurs in the placenta to facilitate transfer of about 10% of the O_2 in a fetal direction. Thus, the fall in pH of maternal blood due to uptake of fetal CO_2 drives release of maternal O_2, and the rise in fetal pH due to the removal of its CO_2 facilitates uptake of O_2. Under non-pathological conditions the maternal Po_2 and placental perfusion are unlikely to be limiting, and thus the rate of transfer of O_2 across the placenta will vary simply with the Po_2 of the fetal blood in the umbilical circulation. Thus, *the level of fetal oxygenation will be regulated simply by the fetal requirement for O_2.*

Glucose and carbohydrate

The fetus has little capacity for gluconeogenesis largely because the necessary enzymes, although present, are inactive at low arterial Po_2. At birth, when arterial Po_2 rises, gluconeogenesis is initiated. The fetus must therefore obtain its glucose from maternal blood, whose glucose levels depend on maternal nutritional status and the integrated endocrine control mechanisms, which maintain free plasma glucose levels within narrow limits. Thus, the secretion of insulin from the maternal pancreas prevents glucose levels from rising too high by increasing glucose utilization for glycogen and fat synthesis and storage. Conversely, absorption of glucose from the gut and gluconeogenesis (by the utilization of glycogen stores under the action of catecholamines, corticosteroids, glucagon and growth hormone) help prevent maternal glucose levels from falling.

Early in gestation, progesterone increases maternal appetite and stimulates the deposition of glucose in fat stores. Later in pregnancy, placental lactogen uses its growth-hormone-like activity to mobilize fatty acids from these fat 'depots'. These fatty acids are important for maternal metabolism and essential for fetal growth, because later in pregnancy maternal tissues become progressively less sensitive to insulin. The consequences of this *insulin insensitivity* are twofold.

First, *latent diabetes mellitus* in women may appear for the first time from midpregnancy onwards. Second, the maternal blood glucose is taken up less by maternal tissues and more by placental transfer to the fetus. This transfer occurs by facilitated diffusion, in which specific carriers within both the maternal and the fetal surfaces of the trophoblast use concentration gradients to drive the transport of D-glucose, thereby enhancing diffusional rates to a maximum flux of 0.6 mmol/min/g placenta. The levels of fetal glucose are related simply and directly to those in the mother, as the carrier system saturates only at supraphysiological maternal serum concentrations (approx. 20 mmol/L). The placenta also utilizes metabolically a considerable amount of the 'in transit' glucose and generates lactate, some of which is distributed to the fetal circulation at about one-third the equivalent flux of glucose. Thus, it contributes significantly to fetal metabolism. Under normal conditions there is little *direct* flux of lactate from mother to fetus.

The rate at which glucose is utilized by growing fetal tissues is probably determined largely by the actions of fetal insulin secreted by its own pancreas in response to glucose load. If the load is high, as can occur in maternal diabetes mellitus, fetal growth and fat storage are promoted and overweight neonates result. The storage of glucose as glycogen, particularly in the fetal liver, is important if the metabolic needs of the neonate are to be provided until feeding begins. A progressive increase in the activity of the fetal adrenal cortex near term (see below) is especially important in promoting the deposition of liver glycogen (see Fig. 12.5). Indeed, fetal adrenal hypoactivity is associated with major reductions in liver glycogen stores, a situation reversed by corticosteroid replacement, while exogenous adrenocorticotrophic hormone (ACTH) or corticosteroids enhance liver glycogen content in normal fetuses.

The high concentration of glycogen in fetal cardiac muscle probably explains why the heart can maintain its contractile activity in the face of severe hypoxia. By contrast, the brain has no glycogen stores and therefore relies totally on a supply of circulating glucose. Thus, hypoglycaemia can have deleterious effects on the brain, especially if accompanied by hypoxia, and the risk is higher in a fetus with low cardiac glycogen reserves, as occurs through glucoprivation accompanying placental insufficiency. Postnatal hypoglycaemia may also be seen in babies born to a diabetic mother, as the reduction in the maternal supply of glucose at parturition is not immediately accompanied by a corresponding cut in the fetal hypersecretion of insulin. A sharp drop in neonatal blood glucose results. Fortunately, although neonatal hypoglycaemia is potentially a major cause of brain damage, it is highly treatable.

The storage of glucose as fat in the fetus is regulated primarily by insulin. Thus, when glucose levels are maintained optimally, such as occurs when maternal nutrition is good, the glucose available after the requirements for growth are fully met is diverted by fetal insulin into fat stores. In conditions where glucose supplies to the fetus are reduced, the needs of growth have priority over storage, glucose is released from fetal stores, and the newborn consequently has an emaciated appearance.

In addition to these storage depots of white fat, brown adipose tissue or *brown fat* is also found in the fetus, newborn and infant. It is deposited in five sites: (1) between the scapulae, in a thin diamond shape; (2) in small masses around blood vessels in the neck; (3) in the axillae; (4) in the mediastinum between the oesophagus and trachea, as well as around the internal mammary vessels; and (5) in a large mass around the kidneys and adrenal glands. It is different in structure to white fat, the lipid being distributed multilocularly and having large numbers of mitochondria-bearing prominent cristae. These deposits of brown fat are of immense importance in temperature regulation and can generate large quantities of heat, independent of increased muscular movement and shivering. Indeed, this form of heat production is termed *non-shivering thermogenesis*. As neonatal development proceeds, brown fat becomes less important thermogenically, and regresses.

Amino acids and urea

Amino acids in the adult are derived directly from digestion of both dietary and endogenous protein, and by interconversion from other amino acids. Deamination of amino acids during catabolism results in release of ammonia, levels of which are kept low by hepatic conversion to urea, which constitutes the major source of urinary nitrogen excretion. Traditionally, protein supplements have been considered an important and desirable feature of pregnancy diets, to cope with the increased protein synthetic demands of the growing conceptus. However, except in cases of extreme malnourishment, there is little or no evidence to support this view, and protein supplements appear largely to be used for conversion as energy sources.

As the fetus clearly does grow and thereby increases the total protein content of the pregnant mother, where do the required amino acids come from? There is no evidence for improved maternal digestion of dietary protein (which exceeds 95% normally). However, the efficiency of the intermediary metabolism of amino acids appears to increase. Thus, urea excretion falls markedly in pregnancy, suggesting that the same intake of dietary amino acids is being utilized more efficiently. A reduced capacity of the maternal liver to deaminate amino acids occurs during pregnancy as a result of progesterone action. Thus, the human conceptus, via its production of progesterone, regulates maternal metabolism of amino acids such that no extra dietary protein intake is required to support fetal growth. The 'extra' amino acids retained in the mother are transported actively to the fetal circulation, and fetal urea produced by the limited catabolism of fetal amino acids diffuses passively into maternal blood with its already lowered endogenous urea levels.

The fetal blood levels of most amino acids are higher than those in the mother, evidence of their active transport across the placenta. Moreover, experimental infusion studies indicate that transport is driven simply by the concentration of amino acids in maternal blood. Amino acid transporter proteins exist in the trophoblast membranes fronting both maternal and fetal circulations. So, amino acids are taken up actively from the maternal circulation, diffuse through the trophoblast and then are transported out into the fetal circulation. Numerous different classes of amino acid transporter, with differing amino acid specificities and transport kinetics and characteristics, have been identified in the two faces of the trophoblast, and their patterns of expression change during development in species-specific ways. Quite how this dynamic complexity is regulated is uncertain. There is evidence that at least part of the growth-promoting effects of the IGFs (especially IGF2) is mediated through stimulation of placental amino acid transport. Indeed, when the maternal amino acid supply is limited, the fetus signals this to the placenta by synthesizing more transporter in an attempt to make up for the deficit. Thus, the fetus seems to control the amino acid transporter levels.

Fatty acids

Maternal lipid metabolism changes during pregnancy, with major consequences for fetal growth and development. The largest requirement for essential fatty acids, and therefore for the supply of long-chain polyunsaturated fatty acids (LCPUFAs), occurs during the third trimester of pregnancy. The C20 and C22 LCPUFAs, arachidonic and docosahexanoic acids, are key components of all membranes and are incorporated into the structural lipids of the developing brain. They are synthesized by desaturation and elongation of linoleic and α-linoleic acids. If the normal development of maternal hyperlipidaemia and accumulation of lipids in maternal tissues is limited or prevented by hypothyroidism or diabetes early in pregnancy, fetal growth is reduced and brain development late in gestation can be irreversibly damaged.

Fetal demand for lipids is met by both placental transfer and endogenous synthesis. The placenta is almost impermeable to lipids except free fatty acids and ketone bodies. Studies on isolated, perfused human placentae have revealed the order of selectivity in the placental transfer of fatty acids to the fetal circulation to be: docosahexanoic > α-linoleic > linoleic > oleic > arachidonic.

This selectivity may explain why the total concentration of LCPUFAs is greater in the fetal than in the maternal circulation. Thus, the concentration of docosahexanoic acid in circulating fetal plasma is 14 times higher than that found in maternal plasma, but the concentration of essential fatty acids is similar or lower. The steady-state concentration of fatty acid in the fetal circulation is presumably a function of its delivery by the placenta, removal from the fetal circulation and, in the case of LCPUFAs, synthesis from their essential fatty acid precursors.

Water and electrolytes

During pregnancy, the elevated progesterone binds competitively to the maternal renal aldosterone receptor but does not activate it, leading to natriuresis. A compensatory 10-fold increase in aldosterone results, an exaggerated version of the luteal aldosterone rise observed in the menstrual cycle (see Chapter 8). In addition, oestrogens stimulate angiotensinogen output by the liver four- to sixfold, further stimulating aldosterone output. The net effect is an increase in maternal sodium and water retention.

Exchange of water between mother and fetus occurs at two main sites: the placenta and the remainder of the non-placental chorion where it abuts the amnion internally (Figs 10.8–10.10). The relative quantitative contributions of each route, particularly early in pregnancy, are unclear, although the placenta is suspected to be the main site of exchange. Most studies in humans and in animals indicate that both amnion and chorion are freely permeable to water molecules. There is no evidence for active transport or water secretion by the membranes themselves, so either diffusional or hydrostatic fluxes must account for water transfer. However, a *large* hydrostatic pressure difference between maternal and fetal circulations within the placenta cannot occur, because if it were large in the maternofetal direction, the fetal vessels would collapse and impair fetoplacental exchange, and if large in a fetomaternal direction, the fetus would dehydrate. Most likely, then, small or intermittent hydrostatic gradients are responsible for moving the large amounts of water necessary for the fetus.

There is a large measurable traffic of sodium and other electrolytes across the placenta in both directions. Much of this flux is in association with energy-dependent co-transport of other molecules via a transcellular route, but the evidence that this route is used primarily for ion accumulation, or even contributes significantly to net flux, is not secure, at least for humans. As ions can also diffuse, and so equilibrate, via a paracellular route, it is probable that the net flux is mainly driven by diffusion.

Significant quantities of water, sodium and other electrolytes may also cross the amniotic membranes. There is some evidence that the high concentration of decidual prolactin in the amniotic fluid of late pregnancy may assist this exchange.

Iron

Iron is present in fetal and maternal blood both in a free form and bound to the protein transferrin. However, fetal blood contains iron at 2–3 times the concentration of maternal blood. Since the iron-binding capacities are similar, the higher fetal concentration is due to more unbound iron, accumulated by active placental transport. Trophoblast contains intracellular iron in a ferritin complex as part of the transport process. In pregnancy, there is a 40–90% incidence of maternal serum iron deficiency, although anaemia is less frequent. Additional iron is required to provide an average 300 mg to the fetus, 50 mg to the placenta, 200 mg in blood loss after labour, and about 500 mg to increase the maternal haemoglobin mass. Iron absorption is enhanced from 10% in the first trimester to 30% or more in the third. A food intake of 12 mg/day and 10% absorption provides an estimated 335 mg, sufficient for the majority of pregnant women, but a supplement of 100–150 mg/day in the second half of pregnancy is recommended.

Calcium

Calcium (and phosphate) is transferred actively to the fetal circulation against a concentration gradient (differential 1 mg/dL) by a magnesium ATPase calcium pump. Ossification requires some 21 g of calcium, 80% of it accumulated in the last trimester at a daily rate of up to 150 mg/kg fetus, placing a considerable demand for calcium on the mother. However, the average daily maternal intake of calcium greatly exceeds adequacy and during pregnancy an increase of 30–35% maternal dietary calcium absorption occurs. The absorption efficiency increases further during lactation when higher levels of maternal parathormone (PTH) stimulate renal conversion of *vitamin D* to the active derivative 1,25-dihydroxyvitamin D. In addition, maternal mobilization of bone calcium increases. Overall, there is a positive calcium balance throughout pregnancy and lack of vitamin D is a more likely cause of *maternal osteomalacia* than is dietary deficiency of calcium. Maternal PTH, calcitonin and 1,25-dihydroxyvitamin D do not cross the placenta, but 25-hydroxyvitamin D does, where it is hydroxylated to its active form and is thought to stimulate osteoblastic activity—see below.

Vitamins

Folic acid and *vitamin B$_{12}$* are two essential dietary compounds with fundamental metabolic actions vital for normal fetal development. Folic acid and its coenzyme forms are involved in 1-carbon transfers, and thereby in nucleoprotein synthesis and amino acid metabolism. Vitamin B$_{12}$ is a cofactor in folate metabolism and in the metabolism of some fatty acids and branched amino acids. Both are provided at the expense of maternal stores, making fetal deficiency unlikely. However, vitamin deficiencies in the mother may affect the fetus indirectly via the resultant maternal metabolic disorders.

Red-cell folate activity accounts for 95% of the maternal blood folate, levels of which decrease progressively towards term. The incidence of folate deficiency is around 2% and that of megaloblastic anaemia is much lower. Folate blood levels in megaloblastic anaemias of pregnant women are generally less than in non-pregnant women. The precise consequence of folate deficiency for the fetus is uncertain, but appears to be associated with prematurity and abortion. Folic acid supplements are generally considered to be desirable in pregnancy as a means of preventing the development of maternal anaemia.

Vitamin B$_{12}$ is absorbed relatively slowly across the mucosa of the terminal ileum to be transported in blood mainly by transcobalamin II. Maternal serum levels of vitamin B$_{12}$ decrease during pregnancy, falling to a minimum at 16–20 weeks, but not low enough to be a true deficiency, which is rare in pregnancy. Indeed, vitamin B$_{12}$-deficient women are unlikely to become pregnant in the first place.

Bilirubin

Bilirubin is a lipid-soluble product of haemoglobin catabolism and is present in fetal, neonatal and adult plasma in both a free form and bound to serum albumin. In the mother, bilirubin passes in the blood to the liver where the enzyme *uridine diphosphate (UDP) glucuronyl-transferase* converts it to bilirubin *glucuronide*. This polar conjugate cannot cross the placenta but is excreted in the maternal bile (Fig. 12.3). The fetal liver lacks the conjugating enzyme until late in pregnancy in preparation for neonatal bilirubin excretion. So the non-conjugated bilirubin diffuses readily across the placenta down a concentration gradient, the mother's hepatic conjugation activity preventing its return to the fetus (Fig. 12.3).

Bilirubin transport and metabolism is important clinically. *Hyperbilirubinaemia* is common in the newborn and in its mild form (so-called 'physiological hyperbilirubinaemia') is known as *jaundice* because of the associated yellow colouration of the skin and mucous membranes. Its occurrence can be associated with accelerated red blood cell breakdown where an infant has a large blood volume, as can arise if the umbilical cord is clamped too late, when some 30% of babies may show jaundice. Or the effectiveness of bilirubin conjugation by the neonate may be

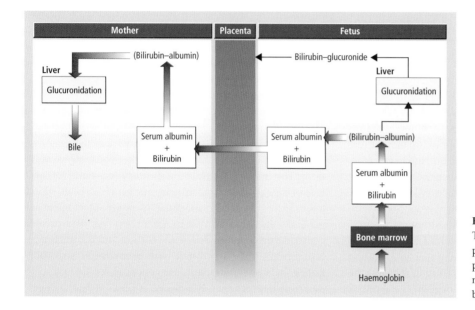

Fig. 12.3 The metabolism of bilirubin. The red arrows represent the principal route of metabolism during pregnancy. Fetal glucuronidation does not occur significantly until after birth.

depressed as a result of dehydration, low caloric intake or even the actions of steroid hormones, particularly progestagens, which actually inhibit conjugation.

Severe or pathological hyperbilirubinaemia may result in *encephalopathy*, also known as *kernicterus*. It may arise as a result of a much increased fetal red cell breakdown, such as occurs if the mother develops an immune response to fetal erythrocytes (see later in this chapter) or impairment of maternal bilirubin conjugation. Damage to the fetal liver as a result of injection of drugs, maternal diabetes, congenital defects and prematurity is also associated with poor conjugation of bilirubin. The hyperbilirubinaemia (or its consequences) may be prevented by a number of approaches: exposure to ultraviolet light (phototherapy) causes the breakdown of bilirubin to a non-toxic product; early feeding prevents hypoglycaemia and dehydration; early clamping of the umbilical cord decreases red cell volume and hence bilirubin plasma levels. If the above fail, or in severe cases, exchange transfusion is used.

Amniotic fluid is derived from maternal and fetal fluids

The composition and turnover of amniotic fluid have become a subject of renewed interest with the advent of the sampling procedure, *amniocentesis*, in the diagnosis of fetal abnormalities. The volume of amniotic fluid increases during pregnancy from about 15 ml at 8 weeks postconception to 450 ml at week 20, after which time net production declines to reach zero by week 34. The composition of amniotic fluid (Table 12.2) suggests that it is a dialysate of maternal and/or fetal fluids, save that the concentration of protein is only 5% that of serum. During the last trimes-

ter, total solute concentration in amniotic fluid falls, while the concentrations of urea, uric acid and creatinine increase. Amniotic fluid is in a dynamic state, complete exchange of its water component occurring every 3 h or so.

There are several routes by which water and solutes enter and leave the amniotic cavity. Exchange with the fetus occurs via its gastrointestinal, respiratory and urinary tracts, and until week 20 or so also with fetal extracellular fluid through the non-keratinized skin of the fetus. Thus, the fetus swallows from 7 ml of amniotic fluid per hour at week 16 to around 120 ml per hour at week 28. Radio-opaque dye injected into amniotic fluid becomes concentrated in the fetal stomach, presumably because after swallowing, most of the water is absorbed by the fetus. The fetal lungs produce a fluid that fills the alveoli and also contributes to amniotic fluid. Some 3–5 ml/h of hypotonic urine passes into the amniotic cavity at 25 weeks, rising to 26 ml/h (500–600 ml/day) by week 40, after which time it drops rapidly. The relative importance of these pathways for exchange at various times of gestation has not been determined, although the fetal kidney seems to be a principal source of amniotic fluid later in pregnancy. Renal agenesis causes *oligohydramnios* (insufficient amniotic fluid, *Potter's syndrome*), while excessive accumulation of amniotic fluid, *polyhydramnios*, is associated with impaired or no swallowing, for example in anencephaly or oesophageal atresia. In addition, the amniotic epithelium, which during the later stages of pregnancy fills the extraembryonic coelom and apposes both chorion and umbilical cord (see Fig. 10.9), is also a route of exchange. Indeed, the finding in rhesus monkeys that removal of the fetus does not prevent formation of amniotic fluid emphasizes this capability of the amnion.

Table 12.2 Compositions of amniotic fluid in early and late pregnancy and the full-term maternal and fetal serum.

Fluid	Total osmotic pressure (mosmols)	Na (mM)	Cl (mM)	K (mM)	Non-protein nitrogen (mg/100 ml)	Urea (mg/100 ml)	Uric acid (mg/100 ml)	Creatinine (mg/100 ml)	Protein (mg/100 ml)	Water (%)
Amniotic fluid (first and second trimester)	283	134	110	4.2	24	25	3.2	1.23	0.28	98.7
Amniotic fluid (third trimester)	262	126	105	4.0	27	34	5.6	2.17	0.26	98.8
Maternal serum (full term)	289	137	105	3.6	22	21	—	1.55	6.5	91.6
Fetal serum (full term)	290	140	106	4.5	23	25	3.6	1.02	5.5	—

The diagnostic value of amniotic fluid can be considerable. For example, the glycoprotein α-fetoprotein is normally present in very low concentrations, but is elevated markedly if the fetus has a defect in neural tube formation, as in spina bifida or anencephaly. The recovery of fetal cells in amniotic fluid allows fetal karyotyping for gross chromosomal abnormalities (e.g. Down's syndrome) and assessment of fetal genetic sex, or for diagnosis of various genetic disorders (e.g. those associated with Duchenne muscular dystrophy, phenylketonuria or haemophilia) using gene amplification techniques and DNA sequence analysis of candidate mutant genes. The recovery of amniotic fluid for these diagnostic tests is discussed further in Chapter 15 (Box 15.2).

Fetal systems develop and mature in preparation for postnatal life

The fetus must exist both for the present and for the future. The physiological basis of life within the maternal environment is very different from that experienced after parturition. The fetus must therefore develop mechanisms that anticipate this change and gear its own metabolism to adapt more or less instantaneously. A rising fetal output of corticosteroids towards term plays an important part in orchestrating the maturation of fetal physiology as well as its timing. Other critical anatomical and functional changes also occur. In this section, these various adaptations to uterine and then extrauterine life are considered.

The cardiovascular system

The fetal circulation differs from that in the adult because the placenta, not the lung, is the organ of gaseous exchange. Two fetal adaptations achieve this difference: (1) the two fetal ventricles pump not in series but in parallel; and (2) three vascular shunts divert the fetal circulation away from the lungs and towards the placenta. The design of these adaptations is such that conversion to the adult form of circulation is initiated instantaneously at the first breath taken by the newborn. The fetal circulation is shown in Fig. 12.4a. Oxygenated blood returns from the placenta and is carried into two channels. The larger of these is the ductus venosus, a fetal shunt that bypasses the hepatic circulation and delivers blood directly into the inferior vena cava. The smaller channel perfuses the liver and enters the inferior vena cava through the hepatic veins. The inferior vena cava carries blood to the right atrium where it is split into two streams by the crista dividens, the free edge of the interatrial septum, which projects from the foramen ovale. The larger stream passes through the foramen ovale, another fetal shunt, into the left atrium, thereby avoiding the pulmonary circulation. The smaller stream continues through the right atrium, as does coronary blood and blood returning from the head region via the superior vena cava. This blood flows into the right ventricle and out through the pulmonary artery. Thereafter, it also is split into two channels: the largest passing through yet a third fetal shunt, the ductus arteriosus, which carries blood to the aorta; while the smaller channel conveys blood to the fetal lungs. The small amount

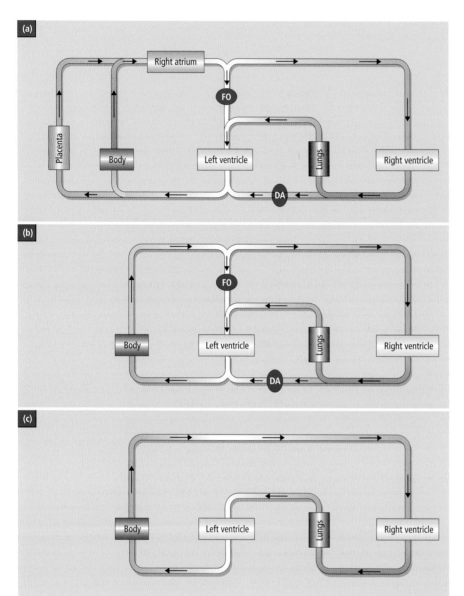

Fig. 12.4 Highly schematic representation of the circulations of: (a) the fetus; (b) the neonate; and (c) the adult. The transitory form in (b) occurs through the occasional opening of fetal shunts prior to their complete, anatomical closure. DA, ductus arteriosus; FO, foramen ovale.

of poorly oxygenated blood passing through the pulmonary circulation returns to the left side of the heart.

The combined cardiac output consists of about one-third from the left and two-thirds from the right ventricle. The three fetal vascular shunts combine in function to ensure the optimal distribution of oxygenated blood to the head and body. Thus, blood leaving the placenta in the umbilical vein is 90% saturated with O_2. Most of it is shunted past the liver to join with poorly oxygenated (20%) blood in the inferior vena cava, the resultant mix reaching the heart being 67% saturated. The blood shunted through the foramen ovale to the left atrium is joined by O_2-poor blood returning from the lungs. The resulting 62% saturated blood leaves the heart via the brachiocephalic artery to supply mainly the head region. The remainder of the O_2-

rich blood from the inferior vena cava enters the right atrium to mix with poorly oxygenated blood (31% saturated) returning from the head region via the superior vena cava. The blood thereby entering the pulmonary artery via the right ventricle is 52% saturated with O_2, and the largest proportion of it is shunted through the ductus arteriosus to join O_2-rich blood in the aorta to yield an O_2 saturation of 58% in the descending aorta. The effectiveness of the ductus arteriosus shunt results largely from the high pulmonary vascular resistance due to constriction of pulmonary arterioles in response to the low fetal O_2 tension (20–25 mmHg, compared with 80–100 mmHg in the adult).

The changes in the fetal circulation at birth involve closure of the three fetal shunts to replace the placental circulation with a pulmonary circulation (Fig. 12.4b,c). With the obliteration of the umbilical circulation, the ductus venosus ceases to carry blood to the heart. At the same time, a dramatic fall in pulmonary vascular resistance occurs as a result of inflation of the lungs with the first breath and the rise in pulmonary Po_2. Thus, overall, there is a net drop in pressure on the right side of the heart (with a loss of umbilical input and rise in pulmonary outflow) and a rise in pressure on the left side (with a return of pulmonary venous blood). This pressure imbalance leads to a brief reversal of blood flow through the ductus arteriosus, the muscular wall of which responds to the elevated Po_2 of neonatal blood by contracting. Prostaglandin E_2 (PGE_2) prevents this contraction and a drop in its levels at birth is involved in closure, which fails in about 6/10000 term neonates but more frequently with prematurity. Indomethacin can be used to treat a patent ductus arteriosus by inhibiting PGE_2. The foramen ovale has a flap valve over it in the left atrial chamber. In the fetus, this is maintained open by the stream of blood from the right atrium, but with the reversal of interatrial pressure, the flap is pressed against the interatrial wall, thereby separating the two sides of the heart to yield two pumps working in series. There is a recognizable, transitory form of circulation in the newborn that is the result of functional, rather than anatomical, closure of the foramen ovale and ductus arteriosus, and these shunts are able to reopen from time to time. The ductus venosus is closed permanently in most individuals within 3 months of birth and the ductus arteriosus by 1 year; the foramen ovale obliterates very slowly, and fails to close in about 10% of adults, in whom a probe may be passed through it. The rising cortisol levels observed as parturition approaches (see later) seem to underlie increases in fetal cardiac output, peripheral resistance and blood pressure towards term.

The respiratory system

The fetus spends at least 1–4 h each day making rapid respiratory movements which are irregular in amplitude and frequency and generate negative pressures of 25 mmHg or more in the chest. These occur in episodes of up to 30 min during rapid eye movement (REM) sleep (see 'The nervous system' below) but not during wakefulness or slow-wave sleep. They are purely diaphragmatic, moving amniotic fluid in and out of the lungs. Their functions may include an element of 'practice' of the reflex neuromuscular activities to be initiated in breathing at birth, and also promotion of the growth that follows lung distension. Prevention of fetal breathing, as occurs in congenital disorders of the nervous system or diaphragm, retards lung development to an extent that precludes support of extrauterine life.

The fetal lungs undergo major structural changes during pregnancy, and especially near parturition. Primitive air sacs are apparent in the lung mesenchyme from about week 20 and blood vessels appear around week 28. The pressure required to expand the fetal lung decreases as the time of birth approaches, largely due to the appearance of *surfactant*, which reduces the surface tension of pulmonary fluid. The surfactant is a phospholipid (a disaturated lecithin, mainly dipalmitoyl lecithin) attached to an apoprotein. It is synthesized by enzymes in the human fetal lung from weeks 18–20, but especially in the 2 months before birth. Its synthesis is promoted by fetal corticosteroids, which rise preterm (Fig. 12.5). They stimulate conversion of noradrenaline to adrenaline by activation of *phenylethanolamine N-methyl transferase* (PNMT) in both the adrenal medulla and, locally, in the lungs. Catecholamine receptor numbers in the lungs are also increased. Within the lungs, both water resorption and surfactant production rise. Failure to produce sufficient surfactant has serious consequences for lung expansion, as is seen in so-called *idiopathic respiratory distress syndrome* (or hyaline membrane disease). Lung maturation can be accelerated by injecting ACTH to stimulate fetal adrenal activity, or by administering potent corticosteroids to the mother. Such treatment is highly effective for infants about to be born prematurely.

To initiate normal, continuous breathing at birth, the first breath must overcome the viscosity and surface tension of fluid in the airways and also the resistance of lung tissues. Removal of fluids in respiratory pathways occurs through the mouth during vaginal delivery as a result of the rise in intrathoracic pressure, but this does not occur during Caesarean delivery. Remaining fluid is resorbed through the agency of pulmonary lymphatics and capillaries, helped by the cortisol/adrenaline stimulation. Prenatal episodic breathing is replaced rapidly with normal, continuous postnatal breathing, and the gaseous exchange function of the lungs is established within 15 min or so of birth.

The mechanisms bringing about the pronounced inspiratory effort at birth are varied. Cold exposure and tactile, gravitational, auditory and noxious stimuli may all enhance respiration at birth, but are not absolutely necessary for the initiation of continuous postnatal breathing. Whichever factors are important, they operate on a newborn in whom the neuromuscular activities of respiration and swallowing (see below), including the ejection of foreign bodies from the pharynx and trachea, have been rehearsed, and brainstem medullary respiratory rhythmicity has been established. Pulmonary stretch receptors and arterial and central chemoreceptor mechanisms are also functional by this time. Again, corticosteroids seem to be involved in their activation.

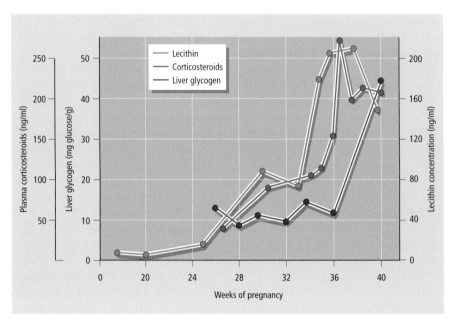

Fig. 12.5 Time course of concentrations of corticosteroids in plasma of umbilical cord, of lecithin in amniotic fluid, and of glycogen in fetal liver. Lecithin may be used as an indicator of surfactant production in the fetal lung. The rise in lecithin content of human amniotic fluid just before birth is reflected in the lecithin/sphingomyelin ratio test for monitoring fetal development and well-being. (Sphingomyelin is a phospholipid, the concentration of which does not change near term and serves therefore as a baseline against which to measure lecithin.) A ratio >2 indicates surfactant production is normal, and <2 indicates the fetus may have hyaline membrane disease (see text). The close temporal relationship between corticosteroid concentration in blood and amniotic lecithin levels indicates the causal relationship between the two. The increase in liver glycogen near term is also the result of the rise in corticosteroids, which induces the late cluster of fetal liver enzymes, including those required for glycogen synthesis.

The gastrointestinal system

The human fetus swallows large volumes of amniotic fluid daily (see earlier), which passes through the stomach to the large bowel. Water is absorbed readily through the small bowel as are electrolytes and other small molecules, such as glucose. Debris from fetal skin and larger molecules in amniotic fluid accumulate in the large bowel, together with sloughed cells from the small intestine and bile pigments, to form a green faecal mass, *meconium*. Defecation *in utero* does not normally occur. Maternofetal metabolism and the placental transport of metabolites was considered earlier.

The renal system

Although the placenta is the main organ of excretion, the fetal kidneys are functional during pregnancy and produce substantial quantities of hypotonic urine, the tubules being inefficient at sodium reabsorption. Fetal urine contributes to total amniotic fluid volume to the extent of about half a litre per day. Renal agenesis (Potter's syndrome) is associated with a marked reduction of amniotic fluid volume; however, affected fetuses survive to term and are born alive despite various growth and developmental defects.

At parturition, renal function must undergo a quite radical alteration, as the constant supply of water, sodium and other electrolytes through the placenta will be lost. Soon after birth, urine flow occurs at a high rate while sodium reabsorption is rather low, but urine flow is reduced over the following hours, rising again after a week. The neonatal glomerular filtration rate is only about one-third that expected for body size, and does not achieve maturity until 1.5–2 years of age. The newborn is in danger of hyponatraemia, as the ability to retain sodium ions (Na^+) is poor. Prematurity represents an important risk in this context, as the kidney leaks up to three times more Na^+ than that seen in babies born at term. The improvement seen in term babies reflects the action of rising fetal cortisol on Na^+,K^+-ATPase activity in cortical tubules. The embryonic changes in the genital tract and external genitalia during sex differentiation were discussed in Chapter 1.

The nervous system

Fetal hormones, particularly sex steroids and thyroxine (see Chapter 2 and below), have major effects on neural development but, in general, rather little is known about the development of function in the fetal brain. The fetus is clearly capable of responding to extraneous stimuli. Loud noises and intense light, noxious stimulation of the skin and rapid decreases in the temperature of its fluid environment will result not only in movement but also in autonomic responses, such as acceleration of heart rate. Presumably the level of stimulation in these sensory modalities is normally rather low and unvarying in the fluid-cushioned, constant temperature, light- and sound-attenuated chamber in which the fetus grows.

However, an important scientific, clinical and ethical issue concerning the development of sensory systems in the fetal brain is associated with the question 'When does a fetus feel pain?' Medical procedures during pregnancy (including amniocentesis), surgical procedures on the fetus itself and also the termination of pregnancy all may involve exposing the fetus to noxious stimuli and so an answer to the question is important. Clearly, an unambiguous definition of pain is required and this is obviously problematic in individuals who cannot speak and therefore cannot express what they are feeling. The International Association for the Study of Pain defines pain as 'an unpleasant sensory and emotional experience associated with actual or potential tissue damage' and also emphasizes the importance of experience related to past injury (i.e. cognitive factors). It has long been appreciated that, unlike simple touch or pressure, the response to noxious stimuli that we experience as pain critically involves an unpleasant affective experience. Thus, an important aspect of pain is its emotional component; take that away and a noxious stimulus, which can still damage tissue, is not necessarily 'painful'.

Given the obvious complexity of the neural processes subserving pain, focusing on neural maturation of a specific part of the brain's nociceptive system will not necessarily help the determination of when a fetus feels pain. But there is an emerging consensus among developmental neurobiologists that the establishment of thalamocortical connections (the pathway by which peripheral sensory information arrives at the cortex, where conscious sensation and feelings are processed) must be a critical event. The penetration of thalamic fibres into the developing cortex occurs between weeks 22 and 34 of gestation and evoked potential recordings have suggested that sensory impulses cannot reliably be detected in the cortex before week 29 of gestation. Such data have led to the suggestion that a fetus cannot 'feel' pain before the cerebral cortex is able to process incoming sensory, including noxious, information and that this is therefore most unlikely to be the case before about week 26 of gestation. Of course, even then it is impossible to know whether the fetus is consciously feeling pain since we have few data on the development or neural basis of consciousness. The multidimensionality of pain perception, involving sensory, emotional and cognitive factors, may in itself be the basis of conscious, painful experience, but it will remain difficult to attribute this to a fetus at any particular developmental age. Much importance is often ascribed to the fact that fetuses show clear nociceptive withdrawal reflexes at a much earlier stage, say by 15 weeks. But these generally reflect the fact that the spinal mechanisms mediating these simple reflexes are established at that time, occurring as they do in anencephalic fetuses. They cannot be taken to indicate the feeling of pain by the fetus. However, there is increasing evidence that noxious events early in development can have adverse effects on later neurodevelopmental events, indicating that noxious stimulation need not necessarily be consciously experienced in order to affect adversely the course of sensory development. It has therefore been suggested that some form of pain control be considered for medical procedures occurring particularly during the third trimester, in order to minimize any possible effects on later sensory development. More research and many more data are needed to clarify these important issues, especially if rational approaches to pain control in neonatal medicine are to be developed.

Fetal movements occur early in pregnancy, and these can be felt readily by mothers by week 14. The function of the movements is uncertain, but 'exercise', which will contribute to both muscle growth and limb development, is likely to be among them. During the long human gestation period, the innervation of muscles by motor nerves and partial maturation of both ascending sensory and descending motor systems in the central nervous system (CNS) means that some well-coordinated movements become possible late in pregnancy. A number of simple postural and other stereotyped reflexes is also apparent in the fetus from a relatively young gestational age. However, *complete myelination* of the long motor pathways, for example the corticospinal tract, does not occur until after birth, which is why fine movements of the fingers, for example apposition of fingers and thumb, are not possible until then.

The fetus shows periods of slow-wave and REM sleep between periods of wakefulness. The neonate sleeps for about 16 h each day, and spends a much greater proportion of this time in REM sleep than an adult does. This sleeping time progressively decreases over the first 2 years of life to about 12 h each day, and the proportion of REM sleep decreases to about one-quarter compared with slow-wave sleep.

Of tremendous clinical and sociological significance is the impact of drugs from the maternal circulation on the developing brain of the fetus. Many are lipid soluble and have no barrier to their free diffusion across the placenta and therefore into the brain as well. The immature status of the blood–brain barrier also ensures that other chemical agents may gain access to the fetal brain in a way not seen in the adult. Drugs such as opiates (heroin, morphine) and nicotine which may be taken and abused by pregnant women can produce dependence in their babies, including the appearance of withdrawal symptoms after birth. Painkilling drugs, which are sometimes given during labour, may depress the behavioural repertoire of the newborn; for example, sucking reflexes may be impaired. This may have adverse consequences for both lactation and mother–infant interaction (see Chapter 14).

Summary

In this section, we have examined how selected fetal systems operate during intrauterine life and prepare for the time of parturition and extrauterine survival. The mechanisms involved vary from the instantaneous (cardiovascular system) to the gradual (urinary system), with some occurring late in pregnancy (gastrointestinal and respiratory systems) and many regulated, like parturition itself (see Chapter 13), by endocrine events involving the fetal adrenal cortex. In the next section, we now examine aspects of fetal endocrine regulation more closely.

Fetal and neonatal neuroendocrine systems coordinate many aspects of fetal development and preparations for birth

It has already been emphasized that the fetoplacental endocrine system exerts important influences on maternal physiology (see Chapter 11 and this chapter). In contrast, the maternal endocrine system does not influence the fetus directly, except in pathological circumstances, and few maternal hormones other than unconjugated steroids and releasing hormones cross the placenta. In general, the fetal endocrine organs function by the end of the first trimester, from which time the fetus is autonomous in its endocrine requirements. Most of its hormones do not cross the placenta to the mother. The fetal endocrine system has a number of unique functions not apparent in the adult, for example in the differentiation of the reproductive tract, lungs, gastrointestinal system and even the brain itself.

The anterior pituitary

The anterior pituitary functions through most of fetal life. Growth hormone is produced by the fetal pituitary, but any role in the fetus is unclear as GH receptors are deficient and its role is probably taken by the IGFs (see earlier). Prolactin is present in amniotic fluid in concentrations 100-fold greater than those in either maternal or fetal circulations, but most of this prolactin is of decidual origin. After week 30 or so, the low levels of prolactin in fetal plasma rise markedly until term, presumably as a result of fetal pitui-

tary activity, but then decline neonatally after a brief postpartum rise. Its functions are unknown, although decidual prolactin may have a role in regulating the permeability of the chorion and amnion to water. It may also be an important cohormone in facilitating the effects of corticosteroids on the production of lung surfactant. The thyroid and adrenal regulating activities are discussed below and the gonadal regulating activity in Chapter 1.

The thyroid gland

During early pregnancy, hCG directly stimulates the maternal thyroid. Furthermore, oestrogen stimulates increased production of the thyroxine-binding globulin (TBG) and elevated albumin, which temporarily reduces free thyroxine. The negative feedback provokes an increase in thyroid stimulating hormone (TSH) secretion and hyperstimulation of the thyroid. In some women, these changes can lead to a transient thyrotoxicosis, commonly seen, for example, with trophoblastic tumours or in multiple pregnancy. Later in pregnancy, increased iodine clearance and thus relative iodine deficiency can occur, and lead to TSH rise and compensatory goitre. These changes may mask underlying thyroid pathologies.

Thyroxine (T_4) is essential for the normal development of the fetus. Maternal T_4 supports the needs of the conceptus through the first trimester, but only has limited transplacental access to the fetal circulation later and in amounts insufficient to meet fetal needs. Maternal iodine is required for the secretion of T_4 by the fetal thyroid under the influence of fetal TSH later in gestation to yield circulating T_4 levels exceeding those in the mother by term. Some of this iodine comes from placental deiodinase activity. Fetal hypothyroidism is associated with a bone age far behind chronological age, deficiency in body hair and, most important, behavioural retardation, since T_4 is essential for the normal differentiation of the CNS. Some maternal antithyroid antibodies can cross the placenta to affect the fetal thyroid.

Infusing TSH into fetal lambs early in gestation increases circulating levels of tri-iodothyronine (T_3) and prolactin, and these hormones are able to facilitate the effects of the relatively low circulating levels of corticosteroids which alone are insufficient to affect lung maturation. As TSH readily crosses the placenta, maternal treatment with glucosteroids and TSH has the potential to accelerate fetal lung maturation at a gestational age when the response to corticosteroids alone is attenuated.

The calcium-regulating hormones

The fetal parathyroid glands secrete two calcium-regulatory hormones: *parathormone* (PTH) and *parathormone related protein* (*PTHrP*). The latter is also secreted by the placenta and by fetal liver, skeletal growth plate and amnion. PTH's main function is to respond to lowered fetal blood levels of calcium, sensed via the parathyroidal *calcium sensing receptor* (*CaSR*). It acts on target cells via the PTH receptor (PPR) to mobilize calcium. In contrast, although PTHrP similarly regulates fetal blood calcium, its major novel function is the paracrine regulation of transplacental calcium transport. Although secretion of both is responsive to hypocalcaemia, the identity of the placental calcium sensitive receptor regulating PTHrP is unknown, as is the PPR-equivalent receptor by which it stimulates transport. Through their joint action, calcium inflow to the fetus maintains fetal blood calcium even at the expense of hypocalcaemic mothers. PTH levels peak in fetal blood in mid-gestation, falling towards term, probably because of increasing influx of maternal calcium, which thus becomes the main determinant of ossification rates. In mice genetically lacking parathryoids, the absence of PTH is compensated by increased secretion of PTHrP. In contrast, mice genetically null for PRHrP die at birth as a result of defective calcium transport and attendant mineralization problems. Calcitonin from thyroid parafollicular cells is at relatively high concentrations in fetal plasma in response to the relative fetal hypercalcaemia, and helps maintain ossification.

Glucagon and insulin

The endocrine pancreas is active early in pregnancy, glucagon (α-cells) and somatostatin (δ-cells) predominating at first, followed by insulin (β-cells), which is clearly present by 10 weeks in humans. Development of β-cell function appears to depend on anterior pituitary growth hormone and ACTH activity. Initially, each type of cell is clustered separately, and only later do β-cells become surrounded by α- and δ-cells. Abnormalities in early pancreatic development tend to affect α- and δ-cells preferentially, leading to relatively uncontrolled β-cell activity, hyperinsulinaemia and hypoglycaemia (*nesidioblastosis syndrome*). Insulin secretion from mid-pregnancy onwards responds positively to amino acids, glucose and short-chain fatty acids, and negatively to catecholamines. Details of how insulin acts in the fetus are given above under 'Glucose and carbohydrate'.

The adrenal gland

Fetal aldosterone levels rise late in pregnancy, but appear not to become responsive to a reduction in blood volume or nephrectomy until after birth. Atrial natriuretic factor (ANF) is also produced prenatally, perhaps under corticosteroid control, and is able to regulate Na$^+$ excretion. We have already encountered the importance of adrenal cortical activity for the fetus (in this chapter) and for the endocrine function of the placenta (see Chapter 11), and will do so again in Chapter 13 in the context of parturition. Fetal pituitary ACTH secretion is under the control of fetal hypothalamic corticotrophin-releasing factor (CRF) and changes in the content of CRF mRNA precede alterations in the circulating levels of ACTH and cortisol. There is evidence that fetal ACTH from the anterior pituitary has an inductive role in the growth and development of the adrenal cortex. Fetal serum ACTH concentrations are quite high during weeks 12–19 of gestation and gradually decline by around week 40. Very high levels are found again in the term fetus, probably as a stress response to parturition.

Cortisol is found in fetal blood by week 10 and levels increase as gestation proceeds, to be especially high during labour. After birth, the adrenal gland shows major structural changes. The fetal zone, which is responsible for the synthesis of dehydroepiandrosterone (DHEA—substrate for placental aromatization to oestrogen; Chapter 11), regresses during the first neonatal month, while the cortex proper differentiates into the distinctive three zones characteristic of the adult gland. Table 12.3 summarizes the actions of fetal corticosteroids, especially as parturition approaches and emphasizes its coordinating role during the transition from fetal to neonatal life.

Awareness of the importance of the rise in corticosteroid levels as term approaches for the final maturation of fetal systems has led to the use of synthetic analogues in premature babies or in women at risk of premature delivery (some 7% of pregnant women in Europe and North America). This use is not, however, without its dangers. Thus, acute exposure of the developing brain to high doses of corticosteroids can modify brain biochemistry in ways that may lead to enduring changes in the function of the hypothalamo–pituitary–adrenal axis and adverse impacts on mental health.

How does the fetus survive maternal immune rejection?

On the first page of this book, we discussed the particular value of sexual reproduction in generating genetic diversity. The whole edifice of sexual differentiation, reproductive cyclicity and pregnancy, with their social ramifications, is constructed on the basis of the biological advantages conferred by producing a genetically distinct individual. Yet we have now come full circle. For the genetically distinct individual will also be phenotypically unique. A component of this unique phenotype is the array of cell-surface glycoproteins that constitute the system of histocompatibility antigens. Thus, the biological advantages of genetic variation appear to confront and conflict with those of viviparity. The problem may be illustrated dramatically. If the skin of

Table 12.3 Functions of glucocorticosteroids secreted by the fetal adrenal cortex.

Function	Mechanism and/or relevant section
Lung maturation	Induction of enzymes necessary for surfactant synthesis, stimulation of alveolar water resorption and central respiratory mechanisms (see 'The respiratory system')
Parturition	Induction of placental oestrogen-synthesizing enzymes. Increase in oestradiol precursor (DHEA) concentrations (function of fetal zone) (Chapter 13)
Glucose storage and gluconeogenesis	Induction of enzyme systems in liver and myocardium (see 'Glucose and carbohydrate' and 'The gastrointestinal system')
Insulin secretion	Regulates maturation of fetal islets (see 'Glucose and carbohydrate')
Lactogenesis	Ductular–lobular–alveolar growth in pregnancy (Chapter 14)
Synthesis of adrenaline	Induction of phenylethanolamine-N-methyl transferase in adrenal medulla
Production of thyroxine	May promote conversion of T3 to T4
Haemoglobin formation	May promote 'switch' in production of fetal to adult haemoglobin and shift of haematopoiesis to bone marrow
Maturation of salt:water ratio	Activation of ANF? Stimulation of GFR regulation and reabsorption of Na

DHEA, dihydroepiandrosterone; GFR, glomerular filtration rate.

a newborn child is grafted to its mother, she rejects it. Why then did she not reject the whole fetus, grafted as it was onto the maternal uterus? Indeed, the pregnant mother is competent to respond immunologically to the fetus and examination of maternal blood in late pregnancy indicates that a regular feature of pregnancy is an immunological reaction against the conceptus. Even more striking, the active presensitization of the mother, by injecting or grafting paternal tissues, does not prejudice the establishment and maintenance of subsequent pregnancies by the same father. Thus, neither a generalized nor a specific depression of maternal immune responsiveness can adequately explain fetal survival. Several mechanisms have been proposed to explain the survival of the fetus *in utero*.

Does the fetus possess antigens?

This question is easily answered. The developing fetus does not lack target antigens. The major histocompatibility antigens (MHCs) appear on embryonic cells shortly after implantation and, although present in smaller amounts than in the adult, are detectable throughout pregnancy. Thus, grafting of fetal tissues to another individual (or to the mother) results in their rejection. They can elicit immune responses and be destroyed by them. However, the fetus is not normally in direct contact with the mother but is separated from her by the placenta—admittedly part of which originates from the conceptus. How effective is this separation, and could that explain the fetal survival?

Does the placenta intervene?

The fetus and its circulating blood are separated from the

mother by the investments of fetal membranes (see Fig. 10.9). The discrete nature of the fetal and maternal circulations prevents appreciable passage of maternal cells to the fetus. In many species, including the pig, sheep, cow and horse, antibody is also excluded. However, in humans and monkeys, immunoglobulin G (IgG) antibodies normally pass across the chorioallantoic placenta into the fetal circulation via a special transport mechanism. The maternal antibodies will include some directed against prevalent bacteria and viruses and will thus confer passive immunity on the fetus and afford the neonate temporary protection for a few weeks postnatally. (In rats, mice and rabbits, the yolk sac placenta performs this function, while in farm animals, a similar protection is afforded by antibodies transmitted postnatally in the milk; see Chapter 14.) However, in addition to antibodies reactive to bacteria, IgG antibodies directed against fetal antigens presumably could also be transferred. That such transfer does indeed occur is seen in cases of sensitization to the major blood group antigen called rhesus. A woman may lack the rhesus antigen (rhesus negative) and if she carries a fetus possessing it (rhesus positive), she may mount an IgG immune response to the antigen, particularly at parturition when extensive fetal bleeding into the mother may occur. In subsequent pregnancies, the IgG antibody is transferred across the placenta and destroys the fetal erythrocytes in a rhesus-positive fetus. Here, then, is a clear example of the mother rejecting her fetus immunologically. But the rhesus antigen is only one of many antigens by which mother and fetus may differ. Can we gain any clues from the rhesus example as to why fetuses are not normally rejected?

The rhesus antigen differs in two ways from most of the other cellular antigens expressed on fetal cells. First, the rhesus antigen is present only on red blood cells. Most of the other important histocompatibility and blood group antigens are also present on several other types of fetal cell and are thus widely distributed among the tissues of the fetus. Second, the rhesus antigen exists only as a structural component of the cell membrane. Other antigens, such as ABO blood group and major HLAs, seem to be present not only as structural membrane components but also in solution in the fluids of the fetus, such as the blood and amniotic fluid. Thus, if an antibody, or indeed the odd lymphocyte, directed against these other antigens should enter the fetal circulation, it could first be 'mopped up' harmlessly by free soluble antigen. Any remaining antibody will be distributed among a wide range of cell types and so would effectively be 'diluted out'. Any given single cell will be unlikely to bind a large number of antibody molecules and, as only the binding of a large number of antibodies will debilitate the cell, gross tissue damage is avoided. In the case of the rhesus antigen, 'mopping up' and 'diluting out' cannot occur and so the chance of tissue damage increases considerably with obvious pathological consequences.

So the placenta seems to provide at least a filter function, if not a barrier function, between maternal immune responsiveness and fetal antigenicity. However, the membranes separating the two organisms are themselves part of the conceptus, and therefore genetically alien to the mother, so why is it not rejected?

Does trophoblast antigenicity influence maternal immune responsiveness locally?

The outermost layer of the placenta is usually chorionic trophoblast, which is in intimate contact with the mother, in haemochorial placentae remarkably so as it is bathed in maternal blood. Moreover, extravillous trophoblast breaks away to invade maternal spiral arteries during the first trimester, and some of this invading tissue can become detached and be carried into the maternal circulation where it can be detected for several months. So, why does it not elicit a strong immune rejection response from the mother that might even endanger the fetus? After all, within the uterus and among the decidual cells there is even a conspicuous invasion of uterine natural killer cells (uNK cells) at implantation ready and waiting to do battle. Is the chorionic trophoblast able to resist maternal rejection and, together with its filter function, thereby protect the fetus? Studies on the antigenicity of the trophoblast have revealed convincing evidence that its surface lacks conventional class I and class II MHCs, the main ligands for immune receptors on the uNK cells. The syncytiotrophoblast that is in direct contact with maternal blood seems to lack any MHCs at all. However, the extravillous trophoblast cells

that invade the uterus and especially the termini of the spiral arteries express an array of unique HLA class I antigens: HLA-C, -G and -E. Of these, HLA-G is not apparently expressed by any other fetal or maternal cells. The precise ways in which these HLAs might function during an immune encounter with uNK cells is unclear.

There is some evidence that during pregnancy the quality of the local maternal immune response is different, perhaps modified by the high levels of pregnancy hormones. Helper T cells decline relative to suppressor cells, and the classes of immunoglobulin produced change their balance. It is possible that these qualitative changes contribute to the survival of the fetal 'graft', but they alone cannot easily provide a complete explanation.

A further possibility is that a more dramatic *local immune regulation* occurs in the close vicinity of the conceptus. Among the population of leucocytes in the uterus, *natural killer* (NK) cells predominate. Their number varies during the menstrual cycle, being sparse in the proliferative phase and high in the decidua during the early stages of gestation, particularly in the decidua basalis at the site where trophoblast cells invade the uterus. By contrast, T cells are sparse in the decidua and it is uncertain whether these decidual T cells recognize the antigens expressed by invading trophoblast. Even if they do, they appear to be relatively anergic either because of specific tolerance or because of some unique property of the local environment. There is circumstantial evidence that high local levels of progesterone, corticosteroids and/or chorionic gonadotrophin might modulate local responsiveness, and that a high local metabolism of tryptophan might do so, but in neither case is there decisive evidence as to *how* they might do so.

The relative scarcity of T cells and their apparent lack of immune reactivity to trophoblast suggest that NK cells may modulate the local allogeneic recognition by uterine dendritic cells of placental tissue. These NK cells express a variety of receptors that are capable of recognizing HLA class 1 molecules, including: (1) killer inhibitory receptors (KIRs), whose interaction with class 1 HLA molecules (specifically HLA-C and HLA-G) leads to signals that inhibit cytolysis or cytokine production; (2) killer activatory receptors (KARs) which transmit positive signals in the triggering of cytolysis or cytokine production; and (3) receptors encoded by NK-associated genes, known as CD94 and NKG2, both being membrane glycoproteins with an external lectin-like domain. It seems possible that decidual NK cells can recognize HLA-C or HLA-G expressed by the invading trophoblast via populations of KIRs, KARs and CD94, thereby leading to a combination of positive and negative signals that regulate cytokine production and cytolysis (Fig. 12.6). These decidual NK cells have been shown to produce a variety of cytokines and hence to have the potential to influence the growth, differentiation or

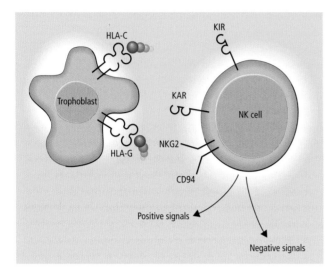

Fig. 12.6 Class I HLA molecules expressed by an invading human trophoblast and their potential receptors on decidual natural killer (NK) cells. The effector function of NK cells after target cell recognition may depend upon triggering positive or negative signals that alter their ability to kill invading cells or to produce cytokines.

migration of the invading trophoblast via a paracrine network that locally determines a balance between placental invasion and maternal resistance.

Summary

The protection of the fetus from the immune response of the mother appears to depend on: (1) an antigenically unique trophoblast forming the front-line defences, possibly via locally mediated depression of immune reactivity; (2) special populations of NK cells in the decidua that are able to recognize specific HLAs on invading trophoblast cells and via paracrine mechanisms regulate invasion and maternal immune resistance; (3) a complete (or, in humans, highly selective) barrier to the transmission of immune cells or antibodies from mother to fetus; and (4) properties of fetal antigens such that any aggressive immune cells or antibodies that get across the placenta are mopped up and diluted out before they can cause extensive tissue damage.

The mother 'programmes' the fetus to affect its postnatal physiological function

Epidemiological studies of human populations have shown that adverse pregnancy conditions can influence physiological function and disease patterns in adult life. Thus, poor maternal diet (low calorie, low protein and/or high saturated fats), maternal stress, hypoxia and placental insuffi-

Table 12.4 Adult diseases that have been associated with suboptimal intrauterine conditions.

Cardiovascular disease	Hypertension, coronary heart disease, stroke, atherosclerosis, coagulation disorders, pre-eclampsia
Metabolic disease	Impaired glucose tolerance, insulin resistance, dyslipidemia, obesity, type 2 diabetes
Reproductive problems	Polycystic ovary, early adrenarche/menarche, early menopause
Respiratory disease	Chronic obstructive pulmonary disease, asthma
Endocrine disease	Hypercortisolism, hypothyroidism
Nervous disease	Schizophrenia, dementia

ciency are associated with a constellation of overlapping adult pathologies, which together are often given the name *metabolic syndrome* (Table 12.4). This syndrome is experienced regardless of the contemporary exercise and obesity pattern of the adult concerned. Examination of the babies born to mothers experiencing these adverse conditions shows that frequently they are both disproportionate and smaller (*intrauterine growth retardation* or *IUGR*), although not necessarily so. Moreover, if postnatally they experience an early growth spurt, often called *catch-up growth*, then the chance of them having metabolic syndrome later in life is very high indeed. In addition, they are much more likely to be obese as children, often with poor appetite control and irritable behaviour patterns. It will not escape notice that these features characterize one of the major contemporary health problems internationally, an epidemic of child and adult obesity and associated pathologies sweeping through the more affluent modern world in all continents. Is it possible that there are *fetal origins for much of this adult disease*? And if so, what exactly is happening?

Experimental studies: cause, effect, mechanism

Controlled experimental studies in pregnant animals, in which a single variable such as diet can be altered and its impact on both size of offspring and adult health patterns assessed, clearly suggest a causal link. This observation has led to the concept of *developmental programming* of the fetus by the mother. Moreover, although the exact pattern of diseases generated may depend on the variable under study, it is more the balance among different pathologies that is influenced than the range of pathologies, which thus come as a constellation. Given the variety of precipitating conditions, it is tempting to think that their effects must be funnelled through a limited pathway to produce such a similar spectrum of pathologies. What might that pathway be? Again, controlled animal studies are most informative but have not yet provided an unambiguous answer.

It seems clear that maternal hormonal profiles are affected by many of the maternal stresses and that secondarily this affects both the endocrine exposure of and the endocrine activity in the fetus. Hormones are intimately involved in growth control and metabolic regulation and are thus plausible mediators of programming. Glucocorticoids are particularly implicated, since they are sensitive barometers of maternal stress and have widespread growth inhibitory effects on the fetus. Moreover, experimental overexposure to glucocorticoids mimics the effects of maternal stressors, the negative programming effects of which are also ameliorated by depression of maternal glucocorticoid responses. Consistent abnormalities in the glucocorticoid feedback loop involving hypothalamus, pituitary and adrenal have been described in the programmed offspring of stressed mothers.

However, programming can occur when maternal stresses are experienced for limited periods during pregnancy, including periovulatory, embryogenic and embryonic periods as well as fetal periods. This observation places some constraints on the underlying mechanism(s) that might affect adult physiology. For example, it is unlikely that the effects are exerted directly on the physiological systems regulating fetal metabolism, because these are not yet matured at these early stages. These sorts of observation make us wonder whether changes induced early in development leave some sort of memory trace, the impact of which is seen later in disturbed endocrine patterns?

One hypothetical memory trace might result from the impact of stressors on cell proliferation in the conceptus to affect the relative and/or absolute numbers of cells allocated to and within the different parts of the placenta and embryo. This might easily lead to disproportionality, small babies, and different organs (including the placenta) being affected differently depending on whether exposure to the stressor occurred during a rapid growth period in that organ.

Another memory trace for which some direct evidence exists is the epigenetic modification of gene promoters that affect the level of gene expressibility and thus activity in adults. We introduced the concept of epigenesis in Chapters 4 and 9, from which you will recall that two sorts of epigenetic modification can leave an imprint: the post-translational modification of chromatin histones, and the direct methylation of cytosines within the DNA sequence itself (Figure 9.9). This latter methylation of selected cytosines is a postreplicative event mediated by a methyl

transferase, and once initiated is then copied at each round of DNA replication as long as the maintenance methylase remains present. So it is this type of epigenetic modification that is most clearly heritable and a possible candidate for the maternally programmed memory trace. Indeed, in animal studies, experimental manipulation of nutritional factors and glucocorticoids or induction of placental insufficiency have all been shown to alter patterns of cytosine methylation in individual gene promoters at all stages of development. Moreover, these changed patterns then seem to persist into adulthood, and in some cases, have been associated with altered expression patterns at the level of functional proteins. So a programming route via epigenetic modification seems highly likely. Further analysis of individual genes and gene families is ongoing. Potentially interesting genes are the adipokines such as leptin, because of their association with obesity and their elevation during pregnancy in both maternal and fetal circulations. Resetting of the fetal leptin regulatory system, directly through epigenetic changes or indirectly down stream of such changes, to promote fat deposition might provide an explanation for child and adult obesity.

Finally, it is known that certain polymorphic variants of some genes involved in growth and metabolism predispose to metabolic syndrome, and environmental factors seem to interact with these to produce pathology. Analysis of the epigenetic modifications to these polymorphic variants under different maternal stressor conditions will be interesting. (There is further discussion of gene–environment interactions and epigensis in Chapter 14.)

For the moment, however, it is the case that we do not yet have a definitive answer to the question: by what mechanism(s) do maternal stressors influence adult health?

Why programming?

There is now convincing evidence that maternal programming of development occurs, even if we do not understand fully the mechanism(s) mediating it. What possible evolutionary reason could there be for programming adult ill health in this way? This is of course the wrong question. The process of evolution selects adaptively for those genotypes that result in phenotypes most able to survive and reproduce. There may well have been survival value in selecting for genes that reduced fetal growth in response to maternal nutritional stress as a way of preparing the offspring for optimized survival in a resource-poor world—a *predictive adaptive response*. Where the postnatal environment turns out to be nutritionally rich, the predictive adaptive response is inappropriate and catch-up growth predicates poorer middle-aged health despite survival to reproductive age. So perhaps the question we should really ask is: what do these studies mean for optimized maternal and neonatal nutrition during pregnancy, and by optimization can we avoid disruptive programming? We hope so. However, the worrying scenario is that the mother's metabolism has already, through her own lifetime experiences including that *in utero*, been set in ways that prevent useful manipulations to her diet from being effective in ameliorating adverse impacts on her offspring. Indeed, there is already some evidence for transgenerational effects of the maternal environment on patterns of offspring morbidity. Exactly how these effects are mediated is also uncertain, but is clearly of concern if the wave of obesity is to be addressed not simply symptomatically but also preventively. The health focus may have to be on regulating the postnatal diet to prevent the worst negative impact of maternal programming.

Summary

Viviparity provides the developing embryos with the optimal environment for growth. The uterus may be viewed as the ultimate 'nest': temperature controlled, a continuous supply of food and protection from predators. This environment is created at the mother's expense and her metabolism is brought, to varying degrees, under the control of the fetus, which to a large extent functions autonomously within its protected environment. It should, however, be clear from this account that we still have much to learn about fetal and maternal function in pregnancy and its control. Central to the maintenance of pregnancy is the trophoblast of the placenta. This remarkable tissue elaborates and secretes the steroid and protein hormones; it is involved in the transplacental passage of a variety of essential substances and also the products of metabolism, both by diffusion and by active transport; it acts as a selective barrier between the two circulations and presents an antigenically effectively inert tissue to the mother's immune system. The role of the trophoblast ends with delivery of the new infant but the mother still has a major and crucial role to play postnatally. This subject is discussed in the following two chapters.

KEY LEARNING POINTS

- The rate of fetal growth is relatively slow up to week 20 of gestation, but peaks in weeks 30–36 to decline thereafter until birth.

- Fetal growth and fetal and postnatal well-being are affected by fetal genetic make-up, insulin-like growth factors, maternal nutrition and maternal health and well-being.

- The transfer of nutrients, blood gases and other essential chemicals across the placenta from mother to fetus is influenced by the thickness of the placental interface, maternal and fetal blood flows, fetal and maternal concentrations of substances to be transported, and the types of transport mechanisms available.

- Maternal Po_2 and placental perfusion are not normally the rate-limiting factors affecting transfer of O_2 across the placenta; instead, the rate of transfer of O_2 across the placenta varies simply with the Po_2 of fetal blood.

- The fetus has little capacity for gluconeogenesis and must obtain glucose from maternal blood, the glucose levels of which depend on maternal nutritional status and endocrine control mechanisms.

- The rate at which glucose is utilized by fetal tissues is determined mainly by the actions of fetal insulin secreted by the pancreas in response to fetal glucose load.

- Storage of glucose as glycogen in the fetal liver is important to meet the metabolic needs of the neonate until feeding begins.

- Brown fat is critically important for thermogenesis in the newborn. It regresses during childhood.

- Fetal amino acids and urea are derived directly from digestion of dietary and endogenous protein; non-essential amino acids are derived by interconversion from other amino acids.

- The largest fetal requirement for essential fatty acids, and therefore for the supply of long-chain polyunsaturated fatty acids, occurs during the third trimester of pregnancy, and is met by both placental transfer and endogenous synthesis.

- Fetal deposition of long-chain polyunsaturated fatty acids is rapid during this period of maximum brain growth, and a failure to accomplish a specific component of neural growth owing to inadequacy of critical membrane lipids may result in irreversible brain damage.

- Exchange of water between mother and fetus occurs at two main sites: the placenta and the remaining non-placental chorion where it abuts the amnion internally.

- There is a large traffic of Na^+ and other electrolytes across the placenta in both directions.

- Significant quantities of water, Na^+ and other electrolytes may also cross the amniotic membranes.

- Fetal blood contains iron at two to three times the concentration of maternal blood, as a result of an increased concentration of unbound iron, which accumulates through active transport across the placenta.

- There is a high incidence of maternal iron deficiency and so additional iron intake in pregnancy is required.

- The fetus places a considerable demand for calcium on the mother, largely during ossification in the last trimester; calcium is transferred to the fetal circulation against a concentration gradient by a saturable active transport mechanism.

- Folic acid and vitamin B_{12} are vital for normal fetal development, and are provided for the fetus at the expense of maternal stores.

- Diffusion of bilirubin from fetus to mother, and maternal hepatic conjugation activities preventing its return to the fetus, ensure adequate elimination of fetal bilirubin. Hyperbilirubinaemia is common in the newborn and in its mild form is known as jaundice.

- The volume of amniotic fluid increases during pregnancy from about 15 ml at 8 weeks after conception to 450 ml at week 20, after which time net production declines to reach zero by week 34.

- Amniotic fluid is in a dynamic state, complete exchange of its water component occurring about every 3 h.

- The fetal circulation differs in two ways from that in the adult because the placenta, not the lung, is the organ of gaseous exchange: (1) the two fetal ventricles pump in parallel, not in series as in the adult; and (2) three vascular shunts divert the fetal circulation away from the lungs and towards the placenta.

- The changes in the fetal circulation at birth involve closure of the three fetal shunts, thereby replacing the placental circulation with a pulmonary circulation.

- The fetal lungs undergo major structural changes during pregnancy. The pressure required to expand the fetal lung decreases as the time of birth approaches, because surfactant reduces the surface tension of pulmonary fluid. Synthesis of surfactant is promoted by fetal corticosteroids.

- Fetal and neonatal neuroendocrine systems coordinate many aspects of fetal development and preparations for birth.

- Thyroxine is essential for the normal development of the fetus, including the brain. Fetal hypothyroidism is associated with a bone age far behind chronological age, deficiency in body hair and behavioural retardation.

- Fetal adrenal cortical activity is critical for inducing enzyme clusters, the production of lung surfactant, the endocrine function of the placenta and the timing of parturition.

- The endocrine pancreas is active early in pregnancy, glucagon and somatostatin predominating initially followed by insulin, which is clearly present by week 10 in humans.

- Maternal programming of fetal development adjusts fetal metabolic and growth responses to perceived ambient nutritional conditions. Should the actual conditions differ, the physiology of the neonate may be set inappropriately with consequences for the later development of cardiovascular and metabolic diseases.

- The protection of the fetus from the immune response of the mother appears to depend on: (1) an antigenically relatively inert trophoblast forming the front-line defences, possibly in association with local, endocrinologically mediated depression of immune reactivity; (2) special populations of natural killer cells in the decidua that are able to recognize specific HLA antigens on invading trophoblast cells and, via paracrine mechanisms, regulate invasion and maternal resistance; (3) a barrier to the transmission of immune cells or antibodies from mother to fetus; and (4) properties of fetal antigens such that aggressive immune cells or antibodies that do get across the placenta are mopped up and diluted out before they can cause extensive tissue damage.

FURTHER READING

General reading

Allegrucci C et al. (2005) Epigenetics and the germline. Reproduction 129, 137–149.

Fowden AL (2003) The insulin-like growth factors and fetoplacental growth. Placenta 24, 803–812.

Fowden AL, Forhead AJ (2004) Endocrine mechanisms of intrauterine programming. Reproduction 127, 515–526.

Fowden AL et al. (2006) Intrauterine programming of physiological systems: causes and consequences. Physiology 21, 29–37.

Gluckman PD, Hanson MA (2004) Living with the past: evolution, development, and patterns of disease. Science 305, 1733–1736.

Hay WW Jr (2006) Recent observations on the regulation of fetal metabolism by glucose. Journal of Physiology 572.1, 17–24.

Jansson T (2001) Amino acid transporters in the human placenta. Pediatric Research 49, 141–147.

Kudo Y, Boyd CA (2002) Human placental amino acid transporter genes: expression and function. Reproduction 124, 593–600.

Moffett A, Loke C (2006) Immunology of placentation in eutherian mammals. Nature Reviews in Immunology 6, 584–594.

Murphy VE et al. (2006) Endocrine regulation of human fetal growth: the role of the mother, placenta, and fetus. Endocrine Reviews 27, 141–169.

Owen D et al. (2005) Maternal adversity, glucocorticoids and programming of neuroendocrine function and behaviour. Neuroscience and Biobehavioral Reviews 29, 209–226.

Regnault TRH et al. (2005) Fetoplacental transport and utilization of amino acids in IUGR—a review. Placenta 26 (Suppl. A) doi:10.1016/j.placenta.2005.01.003

Sack J (2003) Thyroid function in pregnancy—maternal–fetal relationship in health and disease. Pediatric Endocrinological Reviews 1 (Suppl. 2), 170–176.

Vickaryous N, Whitelaw E (2005) The role of the early embryonic environment on epigenotype and phenotype. Reproduction, Fertility and Development 17, 335–340.

Waterland RA, Carza C (1999) Potential mechanisms of metabolic imprinting that lead to chronic disease. American Journal of Clinical Nutrition 69, 179–197.

Waterland RA, Jirtle RL (2004) Early nutrition, epigenetic changes at transposons and imprinted genes and enhanced susceptibility to adult chronic disease. Nutrition 20, 63–68.

Weinstock M (2005) The potential influence of maternal stress hormones on development and mental health of the offspring. *Brain, Behavior and Immunity* **19**, 296–308.

More advanced reading

Barker DJP (1997) The fetal origins of coronary heart disease. *Acta Paediatrica* **422** (Suppl.), 78–82.

Bass JK, Chan GM (2006) Calcium nutrition and metabolism during infancy. *Nutrition* **22**, 1057–1066.

Battaglia FC (ed.) (1997) *Placental Function and Fetal Nutrition*, Nestlé Nutrition Workshop Series, Vol. 39. Nestlé Ltd, Vevy/ Lippincott-Raven, Philadelphia.

Bloomfield FH *et al.* (2003) A periconceptional nutritional origin for noninfectious preterm birth. *Science* **300**, 606.

British Medical Journal (1996) Do fetuses feel pain: for debate. *British Medical Journal* **313**, 795–798: 'Fetal pain' is a misnomer. Derbyshire SWG, Furedi A p. 795. We don't know; better to err on the safe side from mid-gestation. Glover V, Fisk N p. 796; Reflex responses do not necessarily signify pain. Lloyd-Thomas AR, Fitzgerald M pp. 797–798.

Ciba Foundation Symposium 86 (1981) *The Fetus and Independent Life.* Excerpta Medica, Amsterdam.

Coceani E, Olley PM (1973) The response of the ductus arteriosus to prostaglandins. *Canadian Journal of Physiology and Pharmacology* **51**, 220–225.

Fitzgerald M (1994) Neurobiology of fetal and neonatal pain. In: *Textbook of Pain* (ed. P. Wall and R. Melzak), pp. 153–163. Churchill Livingstone, Edinburgh.

Gluckman PD (1986) The role of the pituitary hormones, growth factors and insulin in the regulation of fetal growth. *Oxford Reviews of Reproductive Biology* **8**, 1–60.

Gootwine E (2004) Placental hormones and fetal–placental development. *Animal Reproduction Science* **82–83**, 551–566.

Haggerty P *et al.* (1997) Long-chain polyunsaturated fatty acid transport across the perfused human placenta. *Placenta*, **18**, 635–642.

Henson MC, Castracane VD (2006) Leptin in pregnancy: an update. *Biology of Reproduction* **74**, 218–229.

Herrera E, Munilla MA (1997) Maternal lipid metabolism and its implications for fetal growth. In: *Placental Function and Fetal Nutrition*, Nestlé Nutrition Workshop Series, Vol. 39 (ed. F.C. Battaglia), pp. 169–182. Nestlé Ltd, Vevy/Lippincott-Raven, Philadelphia.

Jones CT (ed.) (1988) *Research in Perinatal Medicine* (VII): *Fetal and Neonatal Development*. Perinatology Press, Ithaca, NY.

Jumpsen J *et al.* (1997) Fetal lipid requirements: implications in fetal growth retardation. In: *Placental Function and Fetal Nutrition*, Nestlé Nutrition Workshop Series, Vol. 39 (ed. F.C. Battaglia), pp. 157–167. Nestlé Ltd, Vevy/Lippincott-Raven, Philadelphia.

Kapoor D, Jones TH (2005) Smoking and hormones in health and endocrine disorders. *European Journal of Endocrinology* **152**, 491–499.

McMillen IC *et al.* (2006) Regulation of leptin synthesis and secretion before birth: implications for the early programming of adult obesity. *Reproduction* **131**, 415–427.

Rodien P *et al.* (2004) Abnormal stimulation of the thyrotrophin receptor during gestation. *Human Reproduction Update* **10**, 95–105.

Sandman CA *et al.* (1994) Psychobiological influences of stress and HPA regulation on the human fetus and infant birth outcomes. *Annals of the New York Academy of Sciences* **739**, 198–210.

Tobias JH, Cooper C. (2004) PTH/PTHrP activity and the programming of skeletal development in utero. *Journal of Bone and Mineral Research* **19**, 177–182.

Weinstock M (1997) Does prenatal stress impair coping and regulation of hypothalamic–pituitary–adrenal axis? *Neuroscience and Biobehavioural Reviews* **21**, 1–10.

13 Parturition

In the previous chapters, we have described the events leading to the development of a mature fetus. In this chapter, we consider *parturition*. Factors affecting the onset and mechanism of parturition in women are poorly understood, despite intensive study. It is understandable that such an important event is difficult to study scientifically, and a lot of our knowledge has come from pharmacological interventions to facilitate overdue or difficult births or to delay or prevent premature ones. Whether these interventions help us to understand endogenous controls or mislead us wildly is unclear. More rigorous scientific data have been obtained from studies on other species, especially sheep. However, these species differ from the human in both the source and profile of their pregnancy hormones (see Chapter 11) and in many aspects of parturition, so at best they give us clues as to what questions to ask of the human situation—and then it is often unclear whether they are the appropriate questions!

The myometrium and cervix are the tissues most critically involved at parturition

Before the onset of parturition, the fetus lies within its fetal membranes in the uterus and is retained there by the cervix (Fig. 13.1). The successful maintenance of the pregnancy requires that spontaneous phasic myometrial contractions are suppressed and the cervical canal is firmly closed so as to provide physical support for the growing fetus. Thus, at term, two major physiological changes are necessary for the expulsion of the fetus to proceed smoothly. First, the cervix must undergo a structural change called *softening* or *ripening*, such that it becomes sufficiently compliant to allow the expulsion of the neonate: a change in role from support to birth canal. Second, but no less important, myometrial tone must change to allow coordinated *contractions of the body of the myometrium* (assisted later in labour by contractions of striated muscle in the abdominal wall and elsewhere) to increase intrauterine pressure. These contractions must be *periodic* not continuous in order to prevent pressure occlusion of the blood supply to the conceptus. In addition, they must be spatially organized so that contractions in the lower uterus adjacent to the cervix do not prevent entry into the birth canal. Before examining how each of these changes is physiologically regulated, we first consider the nature of changes that occur in each tissue and what influences them.

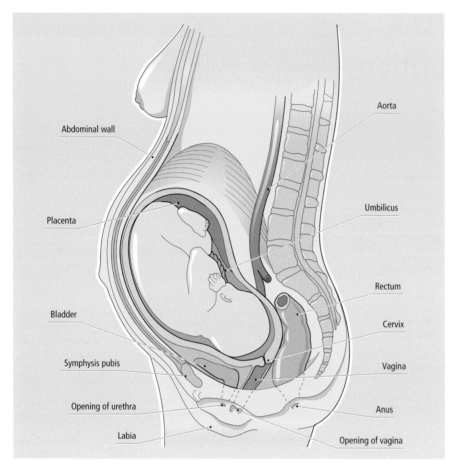

Fig. 13.1 Diagram of a sagittal section through the body of a pregnant woman. Notice particularly the size and position of the uterus, and how much of the abdomen it occupies.

The cervix

Softening of the uterine cervix is achieved by structural tissue changes

The cervix is of major importance in retaining the fetus in the uterus during pregnancy. This function is reflected in its high connective tissue content, which helps resist stretch. The connective tissue is derived from collagen fibre bundles embedded in a proteoglycan matrix. The cervical softening required in order for the fetus to move from the uterus to the outside world is achieved by two changes in the intercellular matrix: a reduction in collagen fibres and a marked increase in glycosaminoglycans (GAGs), which decreases the aggregation of those collagen fibres remaining. In the human cervix, keratan sulfate, which does not bind to collagen, increases peripartum, at the expense of dermatan sulfate, which binds collagen tightly. In consequence, collagen bundles 'loosen'. The activity of metalloproteinases in the cervix increases as parturition approaches and has been implicated in bringing about the cervical softening. There is also an influx of inflammatory cells following a rise in the levels of certain proinflammatory cytokines (interleukins 2 and 8).

Prostaglandins influence cervical softening

Prostaglandins can be shown to effect cervical ripening. Clinical trials have demonstrated that both prostaglandin E_2 (PGE_2) and prostaglandin $F_{2\alpha}$ ($PGF_{2\alpha}$) increase the compliance of the cervix when given intravaginally or intracervically. Moreover, they have been shown to affect collagen bundle content and associations in cervical biopsies. PGE_2 also induces a leucocytic migration into the cervix by inducing the release of interleukin 8 (IL8). The use of PGs clinically facilitates delivery during the induction of birth or the evacuation of a late abortus. However, their role in cervical softening during normal delivery is less certain, since no increase in their endogenous levels within the cervix is seen during spontaneous ripening. Moreover, it is unclear whether prostaglandin inhibitors block the process. Recently, NO has been proposed as a possible physiological ripener of the cervix. Indeed, in animal studies, the pharmacological inhibition of iNOS prevents ripening and, moreover, NO has been shown to stimulate local release of PGs. It is possible therefore that both NO and PGs are involved.

The myometrium

Myometrial contractility depends on its excitability and on calcium release

The myometrium consists of bundles of non-striated muscle fibres, intermixed with areolar tissue, nerves, blood and lymph vessels. During pregnancy, oestrogens stimulate an increase in myometrial bulk, primarily by increasing muscle cell size from about 50 to 500 µm (hypertrophy) and by increasing glycogen deposition. Functionally, this system of muscle cells behaves as a syncytium, cells being coupled electrically via specialized gap junctions or nexuses. These allow coordination of the spread of current and contraction through the myometrium. However, the extent to which this nexus functions to achieve contraction is under tight endocrine control. In order to understand this process, we first consider briefly the physiology of myometrial contractility.

The contraction of myometrial cells depends on a rise in intracellular calcium concentration, both by liberation from intracellular stores and by entry into the muscle cells from the extracellular fluid. The calcium then binds to regulatory sites on the contractile proteins, actin and myosin, to allow expression of ATPase activity, and hence contraction. This release of calcium is stimulated by the presence of action potentials within the muscle cell. In the myometrium, spontaneous depolarizing pacemaker potentials occur. If the magnitude of such potentials exceeds a critical threshold, a burst of action potentials is superimposed on the pacemaker, a sharp increase in intracellular calcium occurs and a contraction follows. Calcium is then pumped back into intracellular stores and out of the cell, and the muscle relaxes. Contractility can therefore be modulated by changing the pacemaker potentials, the relationship between these potentials and the threshold for spiking, and/or the effect of spiking on calcium release.

Myometrial contractility is influenced by progesterone, prostaglandins and oxytocin

Three types of hormone have been implicated in contractility regulation: progesterone stabilizes the membrane potential, prostaglandins E_2 and $F_{2\alpha}$ (PGE_2 and $PGF_{2\alpha}$) enhance calcium entry into cells, and oxytocin acts mainly by enhancing the liberation of calcium from intracellular stores. In contrast, another prostaglandin, PGI_2, operating through a different receptor subtype, relaxes smooth muscle including the myometrium. It is possible that the PGI_2 ensures that waves of myometrial relaxation are inter-spersed with contractility to maintain the blood supply to the fetus. In addition, PGI_2 may also play a role in relaxing the lower uterus.

Steroid hormones modulate the uterine actions of prostaglandin and oxytocin

Before considering the mechanisms underlying the control of parturition, we will briefly review the physiology of prostaglandin and oxytocin production and release, and in particular the impact of steroid hormones.

Prostaglandin activity is regulated by the changing oestradiol:progesterone ratio

As discussed in Chapter 3, PGs are biologically active lipids synthesized in most body tissues. They are essentially local hormones acting at or near their site of synthesis and are inactivated in the lung during one circulation in the bloodstream. The main prostaglandins produced by utero-placental tissues are PGE_2, $PGF_{2\alpha}$ and PGI_2. Factors that increase PG synthesis are believed to act primarily by altering the stability of membranes binding phospholipase A_2, thereby liberating the active enzyme (see Fig. 3.4). Those factors decreasing PG synthesis probably do the converse and stabilize membranes. It is interesting to note therefore that steroid hormones exert opposing effects on phospholipase A_2: oestrogens activate it, while progesterone stabilizes it. Thus, the high progesterone dominance during pregnancy provides a relatively quiescent uterine environment, and a rise in the *oestrogen:progesterone ratio* would result in increased production of arachidonic acid, and hence PG synthesis (see Fig. 3.4).

The oestrogen:progesterone ratio also affects the *release* of PGs. It does so indirectly via effects on oxytocin receptors. Thus, in the sheep, oestradiol has been shown to increase the number of endometrial oxytocin receptors, while progesterone has the reverse effect. Oxytocin then stimulates the release of PGs directly. Thus, a rising oestradiol:progesterone ratio can affect PG release via an oxytocin-dependent mechanism, independently of any alteration in circulating oxytocin levels. This *receptor regulation* may play an important role in parturition; indeed, in women, myometrial oxytocin receptor numbers double at this time. Thus, two routes to increased PG availability at parturition exist, and both can be induced by an increase in the oestrogen:progesterone ratio. In addition, there is evidence that uterine stretching also stimulates the appearance of receptors for PGs and oxytocin, but again only under low progesterone conditions. This stretch-induced response will thus further promote the transition to parturition.

Oxytocin is released from the posterior pituitary by stimulation of the uterine cervix and by myometrial contractions at parturition and is also influenced by the changing oestradiol:progesterone ratio

Oxytocin is a nonapeptide synthesized by magnocellular neurons in the supraoptic and paraventricular nuclei of the hypothalamus and transported axonally to the posterior lobe of the pituitary (see Fig. 3.7). Its release occurs in response to tactile stimulation of the reproductive tract, particularly the uterine cervix and myometrium. This neuroendocrine reflex has, as its afferent limb: (1) the sensory nerves from the vagina and cervix; (2) the ascending somatosensory pathways in the spinal cord (the anterolateral columns); and (3) an incompletely described projection through the brainstem and medial forebrain bundle that ultimately reaches the hypothalamic magnocellular nuclei. The efferent limb of the reflex is the blood-borne carriage of oxytocin to the uterus, where the hormone exerts its actions on myometrial contractility and cervical softening in interactions with both steroid hormones, PGs and perhaps NO. This reflex, called the *Ferguson reflex* (Fig. 13.2), is itself greatly *facilitated by a high plasma oestrogen: progesterone ratio*. This oestrogen-mediated reflex release of oxytocin resembles the coitus-induced release of prolactin seen in rats, which was discussed in Chapter 6. In the next chapter, we will see that stimulation of the nipple during suckling also causes the release of both oxytocin and prolactin via a similar reflex pathway and that these events are vital for lactation.

Summary

A rising oestrogen:progesterone ratio appears to be critical in promoting the action of PGs and oxytocin. In order to understand how the timing of parturition is controlled, we

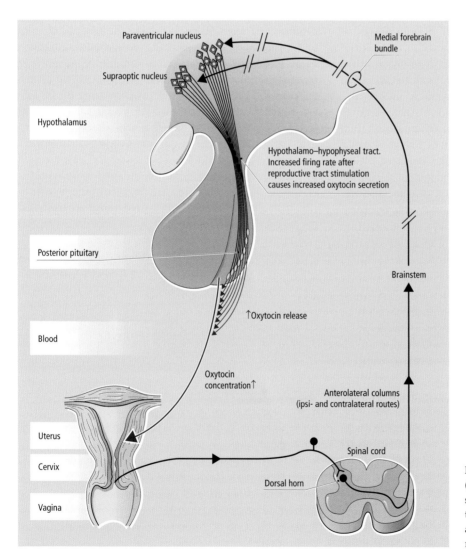

Fig. 13.2 The neuroendocrine reflex (Ferguson reflex) underlying oxytocin synthesis and secretion. Stretching of the uterus and cervix (black line) activates the reflex leading to oxytocin release (red lines)

need therefore to understand whether and how such a rise occurs.

Adrenal glucocorticoids exert major controls on the timing of onset of parturition

We look first at the best-studied model of parturition: the sheep. In this species, we now have a good idea of the main sequence of changes that occur leading up to parturition. Moreover, this species seems to provide a reasonable model for most other species. We will see that, in these species, the *fetus* itself determines the timing of parturition through maturational changes in the fetal hypothalamic–pituitary–adrenal axis. We will then try to apply that understanding to the human—but with only limited success.

The sheep fetus controls the timing of parturition via the hypothalamo–pituitary–adrenal placental axis

The fetal pituitary–adrenal axis plays the dominant role in timing the onset of parturition in the sheep. Thus, fetal hypophysectomy, stalk section or bilateral adrenalectomy all prolong pregnancy indefinitely. In contrast, administration to the fetus of sufficient ACTH or dexamethasone (a synthetic glucocorticoid) induces parturition prematurely. Fetal lambs show a marked increase in plasma concentrations of ACTH during the last 15–20 days of pregnancy, associated with a doubling in weight of the fetal adrenal. This increased ACTH output is driven by the hypothalamus via the parvocellular neurons of the paraventricular nucleus (see Fig. 6.2), which show a corresponding increase in synthesis of corticotrophin-releasing hormone (CRH). Accordingly, neurosurgical lesions of the fetal paraventricular nucleus carried out *in utero* delay the onset of parturition. Together, these data indicate firmly the importance of fetal hypothalamic–pituitary–adrenal interactions in timing the onset of parturition via cortisol secretion. It is assumed that the fetal growth and/or maturation trajectory in some way times the activation of the CRH increase. Quite how it does this is unclear. In contrast, the mechanism of cortisol action is established.

Sheep depend on the placenta for steroid hormone production in the later stages of pregnancy (see Table 11.1), and it is in the placenta that the fetal cortisol acts. The rise in cortisol is closely followed by a rise in fetal prostaglandin PGE$_2$ (see Fig. 3.3), which is synthesized in trophoblast cells. The PGE$_2$ then in turn activates placental enzymes 17α-hydroxylase, steroid C-17/C-20 lyase and probably also aromatases (see Figs 3.3 & 13.3). The effect of this activation is to divert placental progesterone synthesis into the synthesis of oestrogens. Progesterone then falls precipitously and the maternal oestrogen:progesterone ratio rises. This increase leads to a relaxation of the progesterone

depression of myometrial excitability and so the now large fetus can stretch the myometrium and increase contractions, which in turn induce oxytocin release from the maternal neurohypophysis, thereby reinforcing both PG release and myometrial contractility. Moreover, stretching also induces activation of a cluster of myometrial genes including those encoding receptors for oxytocin and PGs, thereby sensitising the myometrium to both. That PGs provide the final link in this chain of events resulting in myometrial contractions is emphasized by the finding that in sheep PG inhibitors block naturally occurring myometrial contractions as well as those induced by ACTH, cortisol or dexamethasone.

Other domestic and experimental animals studied seem to correspond broadly to the sheep model. Thus, the fetal adrenal times the onset of parturition and the rising cortisol leads to parturition by increasing the oestrogen:progesterone ratio. There are, however, some differences in the physiological processes linking these two events, and these differences simply reflect the different interspecific patterns of endocrine support of pregnancy described in Chapter 11. For example, the goat depends throughout pregnancy on progesterone from the corpus luteum, not the placenta (see Table 11.1). In the goat, fetal corticosteroids are observed to rise, as in the sheep. However, the caprine corticosteroids induce *placental aromatizing enzymes* that convert DHEA and DHEA sulfate (also derived from the fetal adrenal) to oestrogens, which in turn enhance the

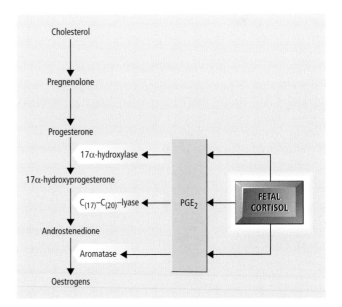

Fig. 13.3 Pattern of oestrogen synthesis in the placenta of the sheep. Cortisol secreted from the fetal adrenal activates PGE$_2$, which enhances conversion of progesterone to oestrogens by activating the enzymes 17α-hydroxylase, C-17/C-20-lyase and, possibly, aromatases.

local synthesis and release of PGs in the placenta. The PGs cause corpus luteum regression and plasma concentrations of progesterone to plummet. Rising fetal corticosteroid levels may also close down production of *caprine placental lactogen* (cPL) during the last 15 days of pregnancy, thereby removing an important luteotrophic stimulus. However, it is not clear exactly how the corticosteroids shut off cPL synthesis or how important this shut-off is for parturition, given the pituitary luteotrophic support in the goat. Overall, a higher oestrogen:progesterone ratio is the end result, as in the sheep.

We have a reasonable understanding of the control of parturition in animals. What is the situation in women?

The endocrine mechanisms causing parturition in women are not understood

Despite the background of animal research summarized above, for women there remains little consensus as to the timing mechanism for parturition. CRH levels rise exponentially towards term. However, the placenta also produces CRH, and in pregnancies with anencephalic fetuses, with their attendant absence of fetal CRH, gestation is not reliably prolonged, so a fetal hypothalamic–pituitary timing mechanism seems unlikely to be obligatory. Plasma cortisol concentrations in the fetus and in the amniotic fluid rise during the last few weeks of normal pregnancy. For example, corticosteroid sulfate concentrations in the amniotic fluid rise after week 30 of gestation, and this is paralleled by alterations in the palmitate/stearate ratio that provides an index of lung maturation (see Chapter 12). Fetal adrenal hypoplasia may be associated with postmaturity, but not necessarily so, and gestation and parturition within the normal range of variation have been seen in fetuses with congenital absence of adrenal glands. Infusions of ACTH or synthetic glucocorticoids do not apparently induce parturition in women. Thus, the evidence for cortisol triggering human parturition is also very weak.

Moreover, unlike in the sheep, maternal plasma progesterone concentrations do not generally fall at human parturition, and the oestrogen:progesterone ratio does not show a reliable increase. It is possible that local changes in the oestrogen:progesterone ratio, without detectable changes in their circulating plasma levels, are more important. Thus, changes in the local metabolic stability or interconversion of steroids have been proposed. Perhaps more significant, there is a suggestion that an increase in the ratio of progesterone A:B receptors, coupled with a decline in a progesterone receptor coactivator, may increasingly blind the uterus to some of the actions of progesterone. One consequence of progesterone action is the suppression of oestrogen α-receptor synthesis, and indeed this receptor is observed to rise in the uterus as parturition approaches.

Such a change locally might amount to the uterus 'seeing' a shifting steroid ratio away from progesterone and towards oestrogen. However, what the stimulus for these tissue changes might be is unclear.

An increase of $PGF_{2\alpha}$ in amniotic fluid has been demonstrated before the onset of human labour, and levels do progressively increase as parturition proceeds and cervical dilatation increases. The cause of the early increase in PG levels, as will be clear from the above account, is not immediately apparent. However, the observation that the number of myometrial oxytocin receptors can be up to five times higher around the time of parturition compared to the non-pregnant myometrium, even in the absence of obvious changes in the oestrogen:progesterone ratio, is consistent with an oxytocin-mediated increase in PG secretion. Surprisingly, experiments in non-human primates, notably the rhesus monkey, have not particularly clarified the mechanisms of parturition occurring in women: the situation is just as complex and difficult to unravel in that species.

Summary

In most mammals, the onset of parturition is timed primarily by the fetus via secretions of the adrenal cortex. Although the exact consequences of this increased secretion of fetal cortisol may vary slightly in different species, the general result is an increasing ratio of oestrogen to progesterone, which stimulates the synthesis and release of PGs in the uterus. PGs are important players in the mechanical events of parturition, myometrial contractions and cervical ripening. Oxytocin further enhances the synthesis and release of PGs as parturition proceeds. In women, some of these changes are observed but not the rising oestrogen:progesterone ratio, which may effectively vary locally in the uterine tissues by mechanisms not understood.

Relaxin is a pregnancy hormone that may influence parturition

The existence of relaxin was first postulated in the 1920s to explain the phenomenon in some species of prenatal separation of the *maternal pubic symphysis* caused by relaxation of the interpubic ligament; hence the name relaxin and its implied role as an aid to parturition. Relaxin has now been identified as a cytokine related to insulin (see Table 3.6). There is considerable interspecies variation (>50%) in its amino acid composition and peptide chain lengths.

The corpus luteum is a major source of relaxin

There are substantial species differences in the source of relaxin; for example, in guinea-pigs it is produced mainly in the uterus, whereas in rabbits and horses it is produced in the placenta. The major source of relaxin in the human, pig, cow, sheep, rat and mouse is apparently the corpus luteum, where it is stored in cytoplasmic granules of the granulosa-derived large lutein cells. Removal of the corpus luteum causes systemic levels of relaxin to fall. It is secreted in relatively small amounts during most of pregnancy, and released in large amounts immediately before parturition, accompanied by degranulation of luteal cells. In pregnant women, relaxin is detectable in the blood as early as weeks 7–10, but maximum plasma concentrations are seen during weeks 38–42. The acute release of relaxin antepartum is probably a consequence of luteolysis. Plasma relaxin levels are apparently not elevated in women during labour induced with either $PGF_{2\alpha}$ or oxytocin.

Relaxin influences cervical softening and mammary development in non-primate species

The marked species differences in relaxin structure make it unwise to extrapolate its actions in rats and pigs, which have been most studied, to humans and other animals. Two clear and unequivocal actions have been established in rats and pigs. First, relaxin promotes growth and softening of the uterine cervix, thereby facilitating delivery. Second, relaxin promotes growth and development of the mammary apparatus: in rats by stimulating nipple development, and in sows by developing the glandular parenchyma (see Chapter 14). Many other actions have been proposed for relaxin, including separation of the innominate bones in several species, but they are less clearly proven.

Labour has three stages

In the above account, we have discussed those factors that determine the onset of labour, which is the process by which the mother expels the fetus. *Premature or preterm labour* in women is said to occur after legal viability (24 weeks) but before 37 weeks of gestation. Labour *at term* occurs between 37 and 42 weeks. After this time, labour is called *post-term*. The process of labour is divided into three stages. The *first stage* begins with its onset (regular painful contractions, and dilation and shortening of the cervix) and ends when the *uterine cervix is fully dilated*. It may further be divided into a *latent* phase, when the cervix slowly dilates to about 3 cm, and an *active* phase thereafter when the dilatation of the cervix occurs more rapidly. The *second stage* of labour begins at full dilation of the cervix and ends with complete *delivery* of the fetus. The *third stage* begins with completion of fetal expulsion and ends with delivery of the placenta.

With the onset of labour, large contractions of the uterine musculature occur. These are regular, occur at shorter and

shorter intervals and result in intrauterine pressures of 50–100 mmHg, compared with about 10 mmHg between contractions. One of the functions of these contractions is to retract the lower uterine segment and cervix upwards to allow the vagina and uterus to become one continuous *birth canal*, through which fetal expulsion occurs. This phenomenon of *brachystasis* reflects the properties of myometrial cells. Thus, shortening of each muscle cell during contraction is followed during relaxation by a failure to regain its initial length. With each subsequent contraction, further shortening of the cell occurs and so, eventually, each myometrial cell becomes shorter and broader, the fundal musculature becomes thicker, and uterine volume decreases. The lower uterine segment does not take part in these contractions and remains quite passive during labour. As a result of this muscular phenomenon the lower segment moves upwards, and is therefore retracted. This event may be palpated abdominally because the junction between the two uterine segments (the physiological *retraction ring*, marked because of the contrast between thick myometrium above and thin lower uterine segment below) gradually moves upwards. During this time the cervix softens and, when fully dilated, can no longer be pulled upwards because of its attachment to uterine and uterosacral ligaments and pubocervical fascia.

Moving into the second stage of labour, the fully dilated cervix is drawn up to just below the level of the pelvic inlet. Subsequent uterine contractions, and the resultant decrease in uterine volume, push the fetus downwards and through the pelvis (see Fig. 13.4 for summary). This whole process of labour varies in duration between individuals but usually takes less than 8 h in multipari and 14 h in primipari. The first stage occupies much of this time and the second stage should generally last less than 1 h. A few minutes after delivery of the fetus and clamping of the umbilical cord, the placenta becomes detached from the uterine wall as the result of a myometrial contraction. Within a short time, the placenta will be completely expelled by uterine contractions, a process often aided by the midwife or obstetrician by use of pharmacological doses of oxytocic agents or ergometrine and by steadily pulling on the umbilical cord (active management of the third stage of labour).

Fetal monitoring can reveal fetal distress during labour and indicate the need for Caesarean section

Parturition is a time of vulnerability for the fetus as it undergoes the transition to neonatality. The necessary adjustments that it must make to its own cardiovascular and respiratory systems (see Chapter 12) are preceded by a period of dwindling maternal support as labour

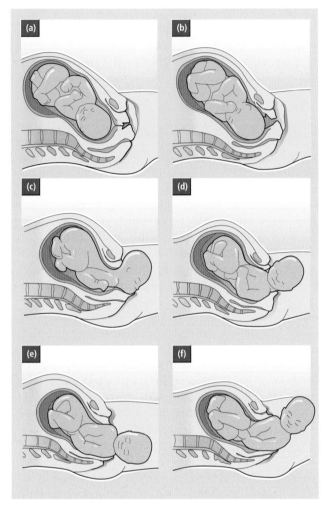

Fig. 13.4 Normal labour showing: (a) engagement and flexion of the head; (b) internal rotation; (c) delivery by extension of the head after dilation of the cervix; (d–f) sequential delivery of the shoulders.

progresses. If this period is unduly protracted, the effectiveness of metabolic exchange can decline such as to cause fetal distress and asphyxia. The traditional obstetric approach has been to monitor the fetal heart rate by intermittent auscultation with a Pinard obstetric stethoscope, and to resort to Caesarean section if necessary. Continuous electronic monitoring of fetal heart rate and/or sampling of fetal scalp blood pH is now more widely used in making the decision as to whether the fetus is genuinely hypoxic. However, although introduction of this technique has improved survival rates in difficult cases, its effectiveness in routine cases is debatable. Some studies report a tendency to resort to Caesarean section more readily, thus increasing the use of this delivery procedure disproportionately. However, the likely increase in the use of monitoring procedures in the future, together with advances in understanding the fetal events underlying the resultant traces, should continue to benefit obstetric practice.

HIV can be transmitted during pregnancy, at parturition and in breast milk

In Chapter 12, we considered the placenta as a fetal–maternal barrier or, more properly, a filter, as it shows selectivity in its transmission properties. It has become important to assess the extent to which human immunodeficiency virus (HIV) can cross the placental filter from an infected mother to infect her fetus. Numerous studies show clearly and unambiguously that HIV is transmitted from mother to baby (*vertical transmission*). If neonates born to mothers who are HIV antibody positive are tested for the presence of anti-HIV antibodies, 100% of them test positive. This result is not surprising, as we saw in Chapter 12 that maternal antibodies can cross the human placenta and provide a source of *passive* immune protection against infection. These antibodies decline over a 6-month period, and if after this time babies are retested for the presence of antibodies to HIV only a proportion of them remain positive. These antibodies are not of maternal origin, but reflect the baby's own *active* immune response to HIV. Sensitive tests for the direct detection of virus confirm that in these babies, but only in these babies, virus is present in addition to antibody. The proportion of babies that carry virus in this way varies in different populations, being highest in East African populations (c.25–35%), intermediate in the USA (c.15–25%), and lowest in Western Europe (c.15–20%). The reasons for this variation are uncertain, but may include the effects of cofactors such as maternal diet, vitamin A deficiency, other infections and inflammations, intravenous drug abuse, general health and socioeconomic status, as well as the virulence of the viral subtype, maternal immune status and viral load during pregnancy and parturition. The question is: how has the virus arrived in the baby?

In principle, three routes are available: transplacental, parturitional and lactational. It is clear from direct analysis of fetal and placental tissues for virus, that infection can occur *in utero*, and that, in principle, both free virus and cells infected with virus can cross the placenta. However, this is likely to be a *low-frequency route* of transmission. There is little doubt from the results of controlled studies, in which HIV-positive mothers using exclusively either breast- or bottle-feeding are compared, that HIV transmission can be halved with bottle-feeding, clearly implicating milk during lactation as a route of infective transmission. However, it is important to note that abandonment of breast-feeding can, in poorer communities, have its own severe health costs, affecting the dietary intake and level of infection in infants, which can erode any clear advantage of reduced HIV transmission.

What about parturition? There is evidence that the birth canal can be a major repository of infectious agents and that maternal bleeding at parturition can also expose neonates to HIV. Among twins delivered to infected mothers, the first-born has a higher infection rate than the second. To test the idea that birth canal infections might occur, trials are being undertaken in which disinfectant viricidal swabbing of the birth canal occurs in advance of delivery. Studies comparing Caesarean and natural deliveries have produced conflicting, and as yet unresolved, outcomes. Overall, there is a clear impression that delivery is a time of high risk for infectious transmission to the baby. That risk is also shared, albeit at a much reduced level, by the midwife and obstetrician. However, unlike the baby, the medical staff can protect themselves with gloves, masks, visors and protective gowns. There are as yet no reported cases of health-care workers being infected with HIV during delivery.

For the babies yet to be born to HIV antibody-positive mothers, there is some good news. A multicentre controlled trial, using matched asymptomatic HIV antibody-positive pregnant women, compared maternoneonatal HIV transmission rates from women who had been treated with either AZT (zidovudine) or placebo. Treatment consisted of oral AZT for up to two trimesters and intravenous AZT infusions during parturition, and their delivered neonates were treated for 6 weeks postnatally (all babies were bottle-fed). The trial was terminated when a reduction in HIV transmission from 25% to 8% was found with use of AZT. Further analysis of the data from this trial suggests that limiting the dosage of AZT over the period of parturition gives maximum protection to the neonate. With the development of a wider range of drugs to suppress HIV viral load, in particular the protease inhibitors, the prospects for preventing vertical transmission look good for those who can afford the drugs. For the poor, where most vertical transmission occurs, this is not the case. It also remains to prove that different drugs and drug combinations do not cause developmental anomalies. If they do, an HIV-positive mother who is undergoing drug therapy to protect herself from the consequences of HIV infection, might have to cease taking medication for at least the first trimester, which might compromise her own future health by allowing drug-resistant variants of HIV to emerge.

Summary

Once born, inspected, and sexed, the fruit of the past 13 chapters enters into a period of prolonged parental care during which, early on, its nutritional requirements are usually provided by the lactating mother. These topics are the subject of the next chapter.

KEY LEARNING POINTS

- Contractility of the uterine myometrium is regulated by progesterone via effects on excitability, and by prostaglandins (PGs) and oxytocin via changes in myometrial intracellular calcium.

- The relatively firm non-pregnant uterine cervix must soften or 'ripen' at parturition to allow passage of the fetus; these changes are thought to be mediated by PGs and nitric oxide.

- Changes in the oestrogen/progesterone ratio late in pregnancy cause changes in PG synthesis, release and action in many species.

- Part of this effect is mediated by increasing the levels of oxytocin receptors, as oxytocin induces PG release.

- Mechanical stimulation of the cervix and contractions of the myometrium cause the secretion of oxytocin from the posterior pituitary and a high oestrogen:progesterone ratio facilitates this release.

- Timing of the onset of parturition in animals is determined largely by the fetus via increased secretion of CRH, ACTH and glucocorticoids.

- Fetal glucocorticoids bring about changes in the oestrogen: progesterone ratio via different mechanisms in different species.

- In sheep, increased fetal glucocorticoid secretion causes a rise in placental PGE_2 output which in turn activates enzymes that convert placental progesterone to oestrogen, thereby increasing the oestrogen:progesterone ratio.

- In goats, increased fetal glucocorticoid secretion causes an increased output of $PGF_{2\alpha}$ by the placenta, which induces luteal regression and thereby parturition by removing the progesterone 'block' on uterine contractions.

- In women, predictable changes in fetal adrenal glucocorticoid secretion and oestrogen/progesterone ratios at the onset of parturition have not been reliably established.

- In women there may be changes in the ratio of tissue receptors for progesterone and oestrogen such that the tissue 'sees' less progesterone and more oestrogen, but what causes this receptor change is not clear.

- In women, PGs and oxytocin are implicated in the cervicouterine changes at parturition.

- The cytokine, relaxin, is secreted by the corpus luteum and has effects on cervical softening and mammary development in some non-primate species, but not in humans.

Continued

- Term labour occurs between 37 and 42 weeks of gestation.

- Premature labour occurs between 24 and 37 weeks of gestation.

- Post-term labour occurs after 42 weeks of gestation.

- There are three stages of labour.

- Fetal monitoring can reveal fetal distress during parturition.

- HIV may be transmitted vertically between mother and fetus *in utero*; this is a low-frequency route of viral transmission.

- HIV may be transmitted vertically between mother and fetus at parturition; this route is important.

- HIV may also be transmitted via breast-feeding; bottle-feeding can reduce vertical transmission.

- Treatment of pregnant and parturient women with anti-HIV drugs can reduce vertical transmission.

FURTHER READING

General reading

Brown AG *et al.* (2004) Mechanisms underlying 'functional' progesterone withdrawal at parturition. *Annals of the New York Academy of Sciences* **1034**, 36–49.

Bulletti C *et al.* (1997) The uterus: endometrium and myometrium. *Annals of the New York Academy of Sciences* **828** (especially Part VIII, pp. 230–284).

Challis JRG (2002) Prostaglandins and mechanisms of preterm birth. *Reproduction* **124**, 1–17.

Hertelendy F, Zakar T (2004) Prostaglandins and the myometrium and cervix. *Prostaglandins, Leukotrienes and Essential Fatty Acids* **70**, 207–222.

Mesiano S (2004) Myometrial progesterone responsiveness and the control of human parturition. *Journal of the Society for Gynecological Investigation* **11**, 193–202.

Thijssen JHH (2005) Progesterone receptors in the human uterus and their possible role in parturition. *Journal of Steroid Biochemistry and Molecular Biology* **97**, 397–400.

More advanced reading

Challis JR *et al.* (2005) Fetal signals and parturition. *Journal of Obstetrical and Gynaecological Research* **31**, 492–499.

Hertelendy F, Zakar T (2004) Regulation of myometrial smooth muscle functions. *Current Pharmaceutical Design* **10**, 2499–2517.

Jayaraman P, Haigwood NL (2006) Animal models for perinatal transmission of HIV-1. *Frontiers in Bioscience* **11**, 2828–2844.

Rezapour M *et al.* (1997) Sex steroid receptors and human parturition. *Obstetrics and Gynaecology* **89**, 918–924.

Sherwood OD (2004) Relaxin's physiological roles and other diverse actions. *Endocrine Reviews* **25**, 205–234.

Weems CW *et al.* (2006) Prostaglandins and reproduction in female farm animals. *Veterinary Journal* **171**, 206–228.

Wood CE (2005) Estrogen/hypothalamus–pituitary–adrenal axis interactions in the fetus: the interplay between placenta and fetal brain. *Journal of Obstetrical and Gynaecological Research* **12**, 67–76.

14 Lactation and Maternal Behaviour

Mammals are characterized by lactation. In this chapter, we consider the early postnatal events ensuring the survival of the newborn, including the provision of food via the process of lactation and associated nursing, and the relatively extended period of parental care that most mammals provide—a protective environment in which the young can grow and gradually attain independence.

Lactation provides a primary source of nutrition and protection for the newborn

Among the many changes occurring in the mother during pregnancy are those that involve the breast. In most species, this process is as vital to the success of reproduction as gamete production and fertilization, since a failure to lactate will result in early postnatal death of the young. We describe the factors that induce, control and regulate breast development, lactation and milk removal by the young, primarily in the human female. We refer to other species only when data in the human are lacking, or when important differences between species are apparent.

Breast development from birth through puberty to pregnancy occurs under endocrine influences

The human mammary gland comprises 15–20 lobulated masses of glandular (or parenchymatous) tissue, fibrous tissue connecting the *lobes* and adipose tissue between them. Each lobe is made up of *lobules of alveoli*, blood vessels and *lactiferous ducts*. The basic pattern of breast structure shown in Fig. 14.1 is common to all species, even though the number of mammary glands, their size, location and shape vary greatly. The sow, for example, has up to 18 mammary glands (9 pairs), while in the cow and goat their pairs of glands (2 and 1, respectively) are closely apposed within an abdominal udder. In addition, there is some variation in the pattern of the duct system (Fig. 14.2). The alveolar walls are formed by a single layer of cuboidal to columnar epithelial cells, their shape depending on the

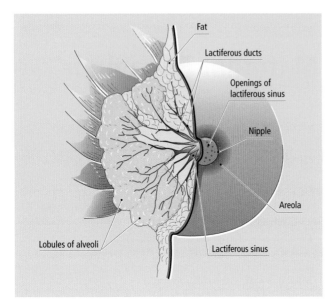

Fig. 14.1 Dissection of the lateral half of the right breast of a pregnant woman. When fully developed, the lobules consist of clusters of rounded alveoli, which open into the smallest branches of milk-collecting ducts. These, in turn, unite to form larger, lactiferous ducts, each draining a lobe of the gland. The lactiferous ducts converge towards the areola beneath which they form dilations, or lactiferous sinuses, that serve as small reservoirs for milk. After narrowing in diameter, each lactiferous sinus runs separately through the nipple (or papilla) to open directly upon its surface. The skin of the areola and nipple is pigmented brown and wrinkled. Also opening onto the peripheral area of the areola are small ducts from the Montgomery glands, which are large sebaceous glands whose secretions probably have a lubricative function during suckling.

fullness or emptiness of the alveolar lumen (Fig. 14.3). It is these cells that are responsible for milk synthesis and secretion during lactation. The *myoepithelial* cells situated between the epithelial cells and the basement membrane have a contractile function, and are important for moving milk from the alveoli into the ducts before it is ejected (see the section on the milk ejection reflex below).

At birth, the mammary gland consists almost entirely of lactiferous ducts with few, if any, alveoli. Apart from a little branching, the breast remains in this state until puberty (see Chapter 7). At this time, and under the action primarily of *oestrogens*, the lactiferous ducts sprout and branch, and their ends form small, solid, spheroidal masses of granular polyhedral cells, which later develop into true alveoli. As menstrual cycles establish themselves, successive exposure of mammary tissue to oestrogen and progesterone induces additional, if limited, ductal–lobular–alveolar growth, and the breasts increase in size as a result of the deposition of fat and growth of connective tissue. Adrenal corticoster-

oids may also contribute to duct development at this time.

Cyclic changes to the breast occur in non-pregnant women and are especially evident premenstrually, when there may be an appreciable increase in breast volume and tenderness (see Chapter 8). In addition, some secretory activity may occur in the alveoli and small amounts of secretory material can be expressed from the non-pregnant breast during the premenstrual period. Mammary development in non-pregnant women is extensive compared with other mammals, including non-human primates, in which appreciable mammary growth is not achieved until the middle or end of pregnancy. In light of this difference, it is not surprising that the hormonal requirements for human breast development during pregnancy also differ from those in other animals. Thus, in other species, notably rodents, a complex of sex steroids, adrenal steroids, growth hormone, prolactin and placental lactogen combine to induce mammary growth, reflecting the relatively poor mammary development before pregnancy. In women, neither placental lactogen nor growth hormone is essential. Rather, during early pregnancy, and under the influence of oestradiol, progesterone and possibly insulin and prolactin, the previously developed ductular–lobular–alveolar system undergoes considerable hypertrophy. Growth factors may play a significant role in regulating mammary growth. Epidermal growth factor and transforming growth factor α, in particular, are able to stimulate the growth of normal mammary cells *in vivo* and *in vitro*, and have been localized to, or are synthesized in, mammary tissues. Their activities seem to be under the regulatory control of mammogenic hormones.

Under these hormonal influences, prominent lobules form in the breast, and the lumina of the alveoli become dilated. Differentiation of the alveolar cells to the form shown in Fig. 14.4 occurs during midpregnancy at a time when duct and lobule proliferation has largely ended. The epithelial cells contain substantial amounts of secretory material from the end of the fourth month of human pregnancy, and the mammary gland is fully developed for lactation, awaiting only the endocrine changes described below for full activation.

Breast milk is a rich source of nutrients, energy and immune protection

Milk *fat* is synthesized in the smooth endoplasmic reticulum of the alveolar epithelial cells and passes in membrane-bound droplets of increasing size towards the luminal surface of the cell (Fig. 14.4). The droplet then pushes against the cell membrane, causing it to bulge and lose its microvilli. Gradually the cell membrane behind the lipid droplet constricts to form a 'neck' of cytoplasm, which

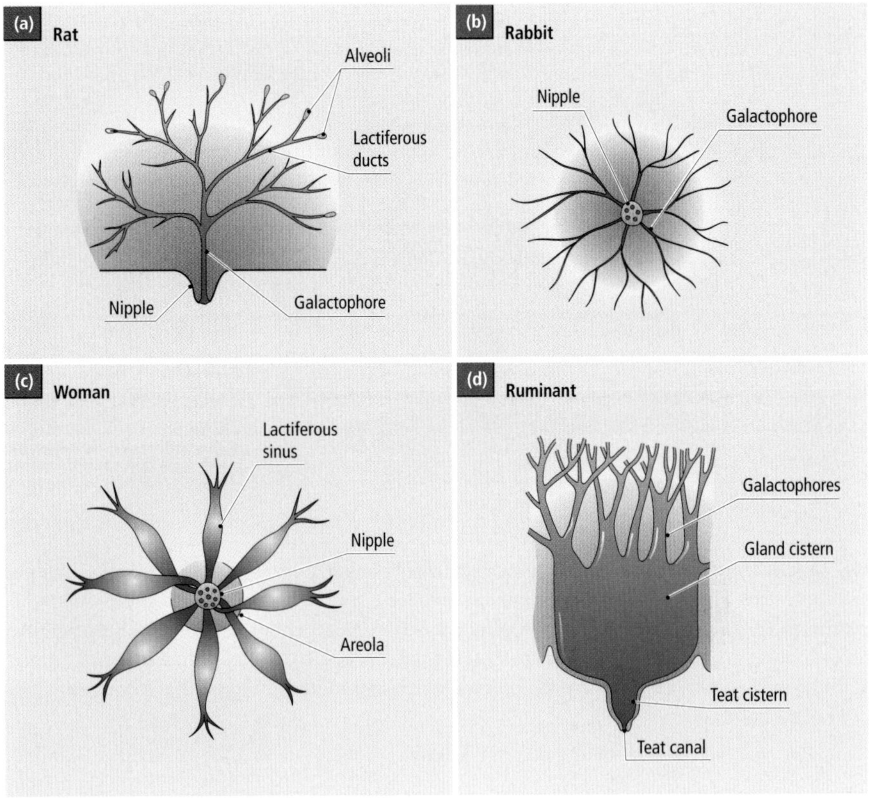

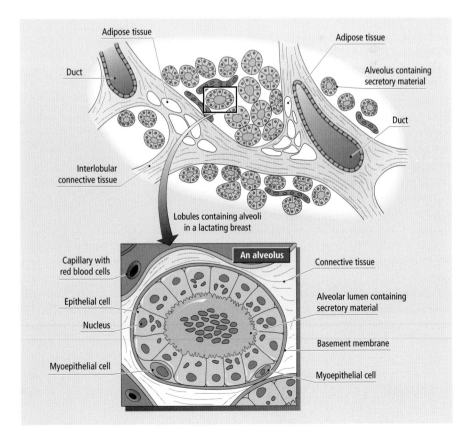

Fig. 14.2 Different patterns of the ductular system in the mammary glands of four mammals. (a) The rat, in which the lactiferous ducts unite to form a single galactophore, which opens at the nipple. (b) The rabbit, in which a number of lactiferous ducts unite to form several galactophores. (c) The human female, in which one lactiferous duct drains each of 15–20 mammary lobes, dilating as a lactiferous sinus before emerging at the nipple. (d) The ruminant, in which, in the udder, the galactophores open into a large reservoir or gland cistern, which opens into a smaller teat cistern and thence to the surface via a teat canal.

Fig. 14.3 Microscopic structure of (above) lobules in a lactating mammary gland and (below) a high-power view of an alveolus. Note the rich vascular supply from which the single layer of secretory epithelial cells draws precursors used in the synthesis of milk. The myoepithelial cells situated between the basement membrane and epithelial cells form a contractile basket around each alveolus.

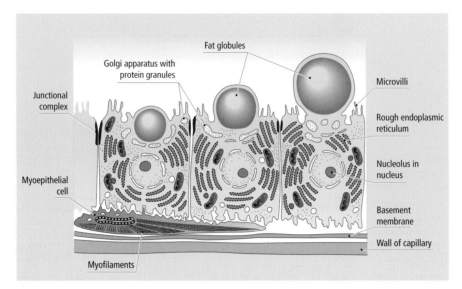

Fig. 14.4 Schematic drawing of the ultrastructure of secretory alveolar epithelial cells. The position of the myoepithelial cell can be seen (compare with Fig. 14.3). Adjoining alveolar cells are connected by junctional complexes near their luminal surfaces, which themselves bear numerous microvilli. The cell cytoplasm is rich in rough endoplasmic reticulum, particularly in the basal part of the cell. Many mitochondria are present and the large Golgi apparatus is situated nearer the luminal surface and close to the cell nucleus. The fat globules and protein granules are the cellular secretory products destined for the alveolar lumen. Their manner of extrusion from the cell is also indicated.

ultimately is pinched off, releasing membrane-enclosed lipid into the alveolar lumen (Fig. 14.4). In contrast, milk *protein* passes through the Golgi apparatus into vacuoles, and is released by exocytosis (Fig. 14.4). Both release processes depend on activation of the *prolactin* receptors present on the alveolar cells (see later).

The composition of milk varies with time *postpartum*. Up to 40 ml/day of a yellowish, sticky secretion called *colostrum* is secreted during the first week postpartum. It contains less water-soluble vitamins (B complex, C), fat and lactose than mature milk, but greater amounts of proteins, some minerals and fat-soluble vitamins (A, D, E, K), and immunoglobulins (IgGs). During a transitional phase of 2–3 weeks, the concentrations of IgGs and total proteins decline, while lactose, fat and the total calorific value of the breast milk increase to yield mature milk, the contents of which are summarized in Table 14.1 (see also discussion on transmission of human immunodeficiency virus in Chapter 13).

One or two features of human milk will be emphasized here. The main energy source in this milk is fat, which is almost completely digestible, partly because it is present as small, well-emulsified fat globules. Milk fat is also an important carrier for vitamins A and D. *Lactose* (milk sugar) is the predominant carbohydrate in milk. It is less sweet than common sugars and is important for promoting intestinal growth of *Lactobacillus bifidus* flora (lactic acid-producing), as well as providing an essential component (*galactose*)

Table 14.1 Some contents of human mature milk.

Water	Approximately 90 gm%
Lactose	Approximately 7 gm%
Fat	Including essential fatty acids, saturated fatty acids, unsaturated fatty acids
Amino acids	Including essential amino acids
Protein	Including lactalbumin and lactoglobulin
Minerals	Including calcium, iron, magnesium, potassium, sodium, phosphorus, sulfur
Vitamins	Including A, B1, B2, B12, C, D, E, K
pH	7.0
Energy value	650 kcal/100 ml

for myelin formation in nervous tissue. Lactose is formed within the Golgi apparatus of alveolar cells and is dependent on a combination of α-*lactalbumin* (the whey protein) and the enzyme *galactosyltransferase*, which together form *lactose synthetase*. The sugar passes to the alveolar lumen with the protein granules. Galactosyltransferase activity is stimulated by prolactin (see later).

The newborn gut is a sterile environment and thus the first influx of breast milk provides an acute dose of richly varied antigenic stimulation including bacterial and viral antigens. The gut epithelium and its underlying and intraepithelial immunocompetent cells provide the major line of first defence via local innate and adaptive proinflammatory responses. These responses must be balanced to ensure that potential infections can be neutralized but excessive inflammation, with its potential for tissue-damaging consequences, prevented. Breast-feeding is associated with a lower incidence of gastrointestinal infection and allergic disease. Breast milk contains a number of agents that modulate the inflammatory response of the gut. Some such as immunoglobulins, lysozyme and lactoferrin may help to process or neutralize antigens, and others may act to influence the innate immune response itself by selective activation of receptors (such as the Toll-like receptor or TLR family) that lead to controlled proinflammatory responses.

A changing oestrogen : progesterone ratio and prolactin initiate and maintain milk secretion

Although the human breasts are sufficiently developed and the alveoli adequately differentiated to begin milk secretion by month 4 of pregnancy, copious milk secretion characterizing full lactation does not occur until after parturition. Why? The disappearance of oestrogen and progesterone, and perhaps also of human placental lactogen (hPL), from the maternal circulation occurring at or soon after parturition holds the key to the initiation of lactation (*lactogenesis*). Although prolactin increases in plasma concentration throughout pregnancy and reaches a maximum at term (Fig. 14.5), the breast is simply *not responsive* to it until *after* steroid levels, particularly progesterone, fall. The steroids, helped perhaps by hPL, appear to inhibit milk secretion by acting directly on mammary tissue, probably on the alveolar cells.

After parturition, prolactin levels also fall but more slowly. In the absence of suckling, the newly initiated milk secretion will last, if scantily, for 3 or 4 weeks, during which period blood prolactin concentrations remain well above normal. However, if prolactin levels are to remain elevated and full lactation is to continue with copious milk secretion (*lactopoiesis*), *nipple stimulation by suckling is essential*. Suckling achieves this release of prolactin from the anterior lobe of the pituitary via a neuroendocrine reflex. Denervation of the nipple prevents prolactin release in response to nipple stimulation (see also discussion of suckling-induced delay of implantation, Chapter 10). The afferent limb of this reflex consists of neural pathways conveying sensory information from the nipples via the anterolateral columns in the spinal cord through the brainstem to the hypothalamus (Fig. 14.6). In the hypothalamus, this leads to a reduction in secretion of dopamine (prolactin inhibitory factor, PIF) into the portal vessels during nipple stimulation (see Chapter 6). In addition, experiments in suckling rats have revealed a marked increase in the secretion of vasoactive intestinal polypep-

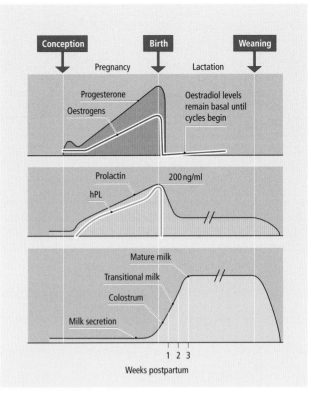

Fig. 14.5 The sequence of hormone changes in the maternal circulation which underlie the onset of lactation in women. Withdrawal of oestrogen and progesterone is critical and removes a block to prolactin-induced milk secretion in the gland. Withdrawal of human placental lactogen (hPL) may have a similar function but this is less certain.

tide (VIP) into the portal vessels, which may facilitate prolactin secretion in the absence of dopamine, which sensitizes the lactotrophs to VIP, indicating that the two mechanisms may interact positively. The amount of prolactin released is determined by the strength and duration of nipple stimulation during suckling. Suckling at both breasts simultaneously, when feeding twins for example, induces a greater release of prolactin than occurs during stimulation of one breast.

The circulating plasma concentration of prolactin during lactation appears, more than any other factor, to determine the amount of milk secreted in women. Thus, declining milk secretion in women can be boosted, with consequent breast engorgement, by treatments that release prolactin (see Chapter 6). Clearly, nipple stimulation during suckling fulfils a most important function in lactopoiesis. In other species, additional hormones (growth hormone, insulin and adrenal steroids among them) may be essential for the successful maintenance of lactation.

The fact that nipple stimulation during a feed induces prolactin release, which subsequently induces further milk

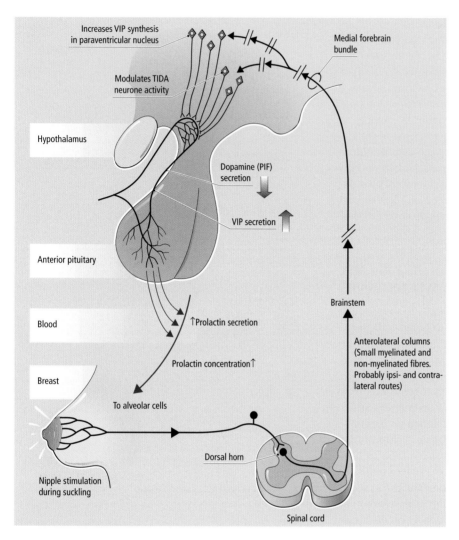

Fig. 14.6 Somatosensory pathways in the suckling-induced reflex release of prolactin. The exact route taken by sensory information between the brainstem and hypothalamus is not certain. Tuberoinfundibular dopamine (TIDA) neurone activity is modulated as a result of the arrival of this somatosensory-derived input to reduce PIF output, which increases prolactin output and also sensitizes the lactotrophs to VIP, the output of which from VIP-containing neurones in the paraventricular nucleus is increased during suckling.

secretion, suggests that *the baby actually orders its next meal during its current one.*

Summary

We have seen that development of the ductular–alveolar system and milk-secreting capacity of the mammary glands during pregnancy is under the influence of adrenal, ovarian and placental steroids. The initiation of milk secretion depends on the presence of high levels of prolactin and withdrawal of oestrogen and progesterone. The maintenance of milk secretion then depends, in women, solely on the continued secretion of prolactin, maintained by nipple stimulation during suckling. These events are summarized in Table 14.2. Having produced milk, the mother must deliver it to the neonate. In the next section, we describe how the suckling infant removes milk from the breast, and the *milk ejection reflex* (MER) which subserves this task.

The milk ejection reflex enables a suckling infant to remove milk from the breast

Milk removal involves transport of milk from the alveolar lumina to the nipple (or teat) where it becomes available to, and is removed by, the suckling infant. The MER, which underlies this function, has much in common with the reflexly induced release of prolactin described above.

The MER is a neurosecretory mechanism engaged by suckling

Stimulation of the nipple during suckling probably represents the most potent stimulus to milk ejection. The sensory information so generated travels via the spinal cord and brainstem to activate *oxytocin neurons* in the paraventricular and supraoptic nuclei in the hypothalamus (Fig. 14.7). This input boosts not only the synthesis of oxytocin but also its release from the posterior pituitary into the bloodstream.

Table 14.2 Summary of events leading to full lactation in the human.

Hormone or activity	Effect
Early to mid-pregnancy	
Oestrogen, progesterone and corticosteroids	Ductular–lobular–alveolar growth. Considerable branching of the duct systems until mid-pregnancy. Followed by considerable differentiation of epithelial stem cells into a true alveolar secretory epithelium
Oestrogen and progesterone (hPL?)	Little or no milk secretion occurs due to the inhibitory effects of these hormones on prolactin stimulation of alveolar cells. *Continues until . . .*
Late pregnancy and term	
Oestrogen and progesterone	Pronounced alveolar epithelial cell differentiation
Steroid and prolactin levels high	Colostrum secretion. *Steroids begin to fall at . . .*
Parturition	
Oestrogen and progesterone fall precipitously. Prolactin levels decline but basal concentrations remain high	Stimulation of active secretion of colostrum and, over 20 days or so, secretion of mature milk. Full lactation initiated
Suckling	Induces episodic prolactin release at each feed. Maintains milk secretion by promoting synthesis of lipids, milk (particularly α-lactalbumin) and lactose

On reaching the mammary gland, oxytocin causes contraction of the myoepithelial cells surrounding the alveoli to induce the expulsion of milk into the ducts and a build-up of intramammary pressure (*milk let-down* or 'draught'), which may cause milk to spurt from the nipple or teat.

Although touch and pressure at the nipple are very potent stimuli to oxytocin release and milk let-down, the MER can be *conditioned* to occur in response to other stimuli, such as a baby's hungry cry or, in cows, the rattling of a milk bucket. Such *conditioned* hormone secretion does not seem to occur in the case of prolactin, where nipple stimulation seems to be the only effective inducer. The fact that the cow's udder contains, in the gland cistern (see Fig. 14.2), all the milk obtainable during milking emphasizes that let-down is due to the increase in mammary pressure resulting from the expulsion of milk from alveoli to fine ducts, rather than any sudden increase in milk secretion as was once thought. The same situation applies to women.

In Chapter 13, we described how stimulation of the female's reproductive tract, particularly the vagina and cervix, also induces the release of oxytocin. The oxytocin release so induced explains the phenomenon of milk ejection during coitus in lactating women and the rather ancient, but otherwise puzzling practice of blowing air into a cow's vagina to induce milk draught! The MER is particularly susceptible to inhibition by physical and psychological stresses; discomfort immediately after parturition or worry and uncertainty about breast-feeding are potentially

important inhibitors of the successful initiation and early maintenance of lactation. The way in which 'stress' inhibits the MER is not clear, but may involve inhibition of oxytocin release, and/or the release of catecholamines, such as adrenaline, and activation of the sympathetic nervous system. Constriction of mammary blood vessels induced by adrenergic stimulation might limit access of oxytocin to the myoepithelial cells.

The afferent route taken by sensory information arising at the nipple (or reproductive tract) is quite well established from research on rodents. It involves the peripheral sensory nerves, which enter the spinal cord via the dorsal roots, and a number of synaptic relays in the dorsal horn before transmission via the anterolateral columns. These pathways contain fibres destined for various sites in the thalamus and spinal cord and, in particular, the brainstem reticular formation. From this point, the route to the hypothalamic, magnocellular paraventricular and supraoptic nuclei (see Fig. 6.2) is not entirely clear, but the *midbrain peripeduncular nucleus* appears to be an important relay. Fibres then run via the *medial forebrain bundle*, which courses through the lateral hypothalamus, to reach the magnocellular nuclei.

Babies express milk from the nipple or teat during suckling

The mechanics of suckling have been the subject of considerable debate. Many workers hold that infants obtain milk

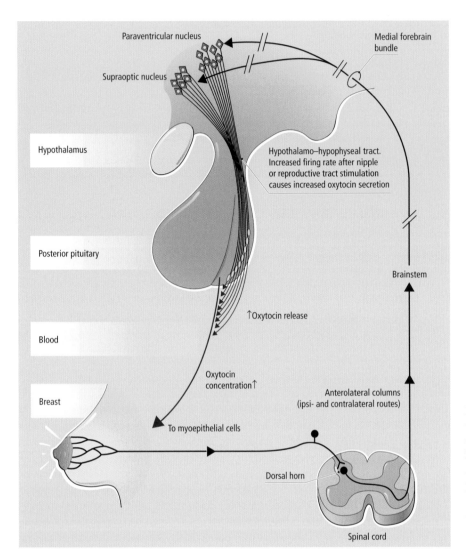

Fig. 14.7 Somatosensory pathways in the suckling-induced reflex release of oxytocin. The brainstem–hypothalamic route taken by the sensory information is uncertain, but probably involves an important relay in the midbrain peripeduncular nucleus before travelling in the medial forebrain bundle to reach the magnocellular nuclei.

from the breast by actively sucking, and that an airtight seal between lips and breast is essential for the negative pressure-dependent transfer of milk. However, X-ray cinematographic evidence suggests that this may not be the case and that milk is obtained by *expressing* it from the nipple or teat, sucking merely aiding the process. Thus, in the human, the nipple and areola are drawn out to form a teat, which is compressed between the infant's tongue and hard palate. The milk is then *stripped* out of this 'teat' by the tongue compressing the nipple from base to apex against the hard palate. Pressure on the base of the teat is then released, allowing its rapid refill with milk due to the oxytocin-induced increase in intramammary pressure that subserves let-down. There are undoubtedly species differences in this process, and young also readily adapt to alternative means of obtaining milk. Bottle-feeding using stiff teats, for

example, requires more sucking than stripping, and calves or human infants learn this skill rapidly.

Summary

Removal of milk from the breast is dependent on the suckling-induced MER. By this means, stimulation of the nipple and other cues associated with nursing induce the release of oxytocin from the neurohypophysis. This hormone stimulates contraction of the myoepithelial cells, which surround each alveolus, forcing milk out of the alveoli into the smaller lactiferous ducts. The resulting increase in intramammary pressure results in milk let-down, causing milk to spurt from the nipple and to be removed from the breast by the suckling infant. The neural pathways mediating the MER are not completely understood, but are likely to be complicated, particularly when mediating psychological factors associated with the induction or inhibition of the MER.

Fertility is reduced during lactation

Lactation can continue for months. During this period, menstruation and ovulation return more slowly than in non-lactating women. Rarely will either occur before 6 weeks postpartum, normal reproductive function usually re-establishing itself by 3–6 months. However, menstruation itself is a poor indicator of fertility during this period, and conception often occurs in lactating women without an intervening menstruation. Approximately half of all contraceptively unprotected nursing mothers become pregnant during 9 months of lactation. This period of postpartum lactational amenorrhoea and anovulation is probably mediated primarily by prolactin, which can suppress the initiation of cyclic release of gonadotrophins, as discussed more fully in the contexts of hyperprolactinaemia (which characterizes lactation) in Chapter 6 and of facultative delayed implantation (see Chapter 10).

Cessation of lactation may be achieved pharmacologically or naturally

Lactation can be suppressed by dopamine receptor agonists

It may be necessary to suppress lactation in women for a variety of reasons. Nursing may be contra-indicated for clinical reasons, for example the mother may be HIV antibody positive (see Chapter 13) or may simply prefer not to breast-feed her baby. Stillbirth or abortion after 4 months of pregnancy will be followed by unnecessary lactation. A number of traditional methods for suppressing lactation may still be employed today, including breast-binding, application of ice packs or treatment with sex steroids to antagonize the effects of prolactin. However, the most widely used lactation suppressants used today are dopamine D_2 receptor agonists, such as bromocriptine or cabergoline, which markedly depress prolactin and hence milk secretion (see Chapter 6).

The breast involutes when lactation ceases

When the suckling stimulus is discontinued, milk accumulates in the alveoli and small lactiferous ducts, causing distension and mechanical atrophy of the epithelial structures, rupture of the alveolar walls and the attendant formation of large hollow spaces in the mammary tissue. The alveolar distension also compresses capillaries, resulting in alveolar hypoxia and reduction in nutrient supply. Milk

secretion is therefore suppressed not so much by the fall in plasma prolactin (as suckling frequency diminishes), but as a consequence of the effects of local mechanical factors. As desquamated alveolar cells and glandular debris become phagocytosed, the lobular–acinar structures become smaller and fewer, and the ductular system in the breast again begins to predominate. The alveolar lumina decrease in size and may eventually disappear, and their lining changes from the secretory single-layered to a non-secretory, two-layered type of epithelium, previously seen before pregnancy. This whole involutional process takes about 3 months, but is more intense if nursing is stopped suddenly rather than reduced in frequency as during gradual weaning.

Although these changes in the mammary gland are pronounced, they differ markedly from those in postmenopausal women. In the latter, there is clear structural atrophy of the breast rather than a transition to a period of inactivity. The breasts invariably remain larger after lactation than they were before pregnancy because of the increased deposition of fat and connective tissue that occurs between these two time points.

Breast- or bottle-feeding?

In addition to its higher nutritional value than artificial or cow's milk, breast-feeding has many clearly documented benefits (Box 14.1). Moreover, newborn infants seem to prefer breast to artificial milk if given the choice. Increasingly, for premature babies, which are at particular risk of infection and malnutrition, it is recommended that colostrums or breast milk be included as part of their diet, with beneficial outcomes. Contra-indications to breast-feeding may include the risk of serious infection transmission (see Chapter 13 for HIV discussion). Currently, a 6-month exclusive breast-feeding period is recommended as optimal for an infant's lifetime health (Box 14.1). However, observed rates of initiation and especially of maintenance of breast-feeding in Americo-European societies fall far short of this ideal. For example, in the UK only around 70% of mothers initiated and only 30% had maintained any breast-feeding by 6 months, most of these non-exclusively. Among factors reported by women to reduce breast-feeding are nipple soreness and difficulties in milk production, lack of good cultural and/or family support for breast-feeding, midwife behaviour (especially undue pressure to breast-feed), inconvenience (especially in working mothers) and lack of maternal self-confidence. Most mothers are well aware of the benefits of breast-feeding, and not surprisingly therefore health campaigns based simply on provision of information have not prevented premature termination of breast-feeding. Indeed, public health campaigns have generally not been very successful, although antenatal and

BOX 14.1 Benefits claimed for exclusive breast-feeding

For the infant

- Reduced incidence and duration of diarrhoeal illnesses, respiratory infection, and occurrence of otitis media and recurrent otitis media.
- Reduced risk of developing an allergy to cow's milk.
- Improved visual acuity and psychomotor development, which may be caused by polyunsaturated fatty acids in the milk, particularly docosahexaenoic acid.
- Higher IQ scores, which may be the result of factors present in milk or to greater maternal stimulation of infant during contact.
- Reduced malocclusion due to better jaw shape and development.
- Possible protection against neonatal necrotizing enterocolitis, bacteraemia, meningitis, botulism and urinary tract infection.
- Possible reduced risk of autoimmune disease, such as diabetes mellitus type I and inflammatory bowel disease.
- Possible reduced risk of sudden infant death syndrome and of adiposity later in childhood.

For the mother

- Early initiation of breast-feeding after birth promotes maternal recovery from childbirth; accelerates uterine involution and reduces the risk of haemorrhaging, thereby reducing maternal mortality; and preserves

maternal haemoglobin stores through reduced blood loss, leading to improved iron status.
- Prolonged period of postpartum infertility, leading to increased spacing between successive pregnancies if no contraceptives are used.
- Possible accelerated weight loss and return to prepregnancy body weight.
- Reduced risk of premenopausal breast cancer.
- Possible reduced risk of ovarian cancer.
- Possible improved bone mineralization and thereby decreased risk of postmenopausal hip fracture.

Duration?

Research has shown that there is no risk from exclusive breast-feeding for at least 6 months. WHO, the UK Department of Health and UNICEF all recommend 6 months exclusive breast-feeding as optimal for health. However, the individual circumstances of the mother and infant need to be taken into account when assessing whether this period of breast-feeding can be achieved.

Further reading

Michaelsen KF *et al.* (2003) *Feeding and Nutrition of Infants and Young Children: Guidelines for WHO European Region with Emphasis on Former Soviet Countries.* WHO Regional Publications, European Series, No. 87. World Health Organization, Geneva.

Kramer MS, Kakuma R. (2002) Optimal duration of exclusive breastfeeding. *Cochrane Database of Systematic Reviews, Issue 1.* Art. No.:CD003517. doi: 10.1002/14651858.CD0037517

---

postnatal support that boosts maternal confidence and assertiveness and builds peer support networks has helped increase the duration of breast-feeding.

Maternal behaviour appears promptly around parturition and is critical for survival of the newborn

In Chapter 2, we described how important the influence of behavioural interactions between a growing infant and its parents could be in forming a sexual and gender identity. This example illustrates the vital role that parents play in ensuring not only the very survival of their offspring but also their social development. Early on, the mother is of special importance and she displays a range of interrelated patterns of maternal behaviour so that her offspring is given protection, warmth, food and affection. The infant, however, is not merely the passive receiver of all this attention, but an active participant in a two-way interaction, eliciting by its own actions appropriate responses from its mother. Our understanding of how parental care operates effectively, particularly in humans, is far from complete.

Here, we examine some of the important features in a comparative setting in order to reveal some of the general principles involved.

Patterns of maternal behaviour change with time and vary with the state of maturity of the newborn

Maternal behaviour may be considered to occur in three sequential stages: (1) behaviour preparatory to arrival of the young displayed during gestation, for example nest building; (2) behaviour concerned with the care and protection of the young early after parturition and associated with lactation; and (3) behaviour associated with the progressive independence of the young and associated with weaning.

Gestational behaviour

During gestation many mammals enter a phase of nest-building activity that is highly characteristic for each species. Very often at this time, the female may show a marked increase in aggression and defend the area in which the nest has been made. Females of few species, human females among them, will accept the sexual advances of males as gestation proceeds.

Postparturient behaviour

After birth, the females of all mammalian species are critical for the survival of their young, because of their lactational role. The other roles of the mother during the early postnatal period vary from species to species depending on how developmentally advanced the young are at birth. Those species in which the young are very immature, notably the marsupials, show little change in their behaviour at parturition. The young crawls into the mother's pouch and attaches to a teat, and the mother, apart from cleaning her pouch more often, shows little additional maternal behaviour, apparently not recognizing her own as distinct from other young at this time. Young who are born naked and blind (e.g. mice, rats, rabbits, ferrets and bears), so-called *altricial* young, have food and warmth provided by their suckling mothers in nests. Maternal retrieval forms an important element of behaviour in these species, often elicited and directed by ultrasonic calls from misplaced young. *Semi-altricial* young are those born with hair and sight (e.g. carnivores, non-human primates), but have poorly developed motor skills and may need to be carried by their parents. The parents may have nests or dens in which the female stays with the young most of the time (e.g. the canids), the males returning periodically to the nest to regurgitate food, initially for the non-excursive mothers, but later for the young as well. Primates do not normally leave their young in nests, but carry them around, the infants having well-developed clinging reflexes. Males often help in this task. Ungulates, guinea-pigs and aquatic mammals give birth to *precocious* young, which can move about well and, to some extent, fend for themselves. The mother–infant bond in these species seems to reflect more a need for contact rather than nourishment; mothers appear to recognize their own young quickly, and thereafter will feed only them.

Weaning behaviour

As infants grow, there is a gradual change in the behaviours of both them and their mother, which ultimately results in independence. During this time, infants tend to move away from the mother more often and to greater distances. Mothers, on the other hand, retrieve them less and encourage this exploration by rejecting them more often. Suckling occurs less frequently, lactation ceases and the infant is weaned and, in the human, enters childhood (see Chapter 7). In solitary species, the young move away from their mother quite rapidly, the females stop maintaining the nest and the temporary family aggregation disintegrates. In more social, group-living species, the young become independent of, and are rejected by, their mothers, but are progressively integrated within the group. In humans, childhood is an extended phase in which parental support remains essential for survival.

Maternal behaviour therefore comprises a complex and variable pattern of interaction between mother and young, adapted to the social and environmental context in which it occurs. Despite or perhaps because of this variety, little is known in detail of the mechanisms underlying the onset and maintenance of the mother–infant bond in many species.

In non-primates both exposure to young and sex hormones influence maternal behaviour

A prevailing belief in studies of maternal behaviour has been that the distinctive profile of pregnancy hormones (progesterone, oestradiol and prolactin/placental lactogen) must be involved in nest building before birth, and in the prompt appearance of maternal behaviour directed so selectively towards the mother's own young after birth. However, the evidence challenges this belief. Thus, ovariectomized, hypophysectomized female rats and even castrated or intact male rats, will all develop elements of the 'maternal' behaviour pattern when exposed to pups for a period of about 4–7 days. This *pup stimulation*, in which attributes of the pups evoke behavioural changes in the adults, is often called *sensitization* and can occur independently of any hormonal factor. It is also generally accepted that continuing maternal behaviour in the normal, postpartum lactating female is not dependent on hormones, as postpartum ovariectomy and hypophysectomy are not followed by any *decline* in behaviour (other than via endocrine effects on lactation, which must be taken into account). Thus, hormones do not seem to be *required* for either the *initiation* or the *maintenance* of maternal behaviour. Neither do they seem to influence the naturally occurring *withdrawal* of maternal behaviour, as both sensitized and lactating 'mothers' show a similar decline in their maternal care over a period of 10–20 days postpartum, avoiding nursing and increasing their rejection of pups.

Hormones facilitate but are not essential for the initiation and maintenance of maternal behaviour

It would be quite wrong, however, to suppose that hormones have *no* influence on elements of maternal behaviour. Non-postpartum females (or males) require several days of exposure to pups before they display such behaviour, whereas *postpartum* females display all elements of maternal behaviour *immediately* after delivery. Perhaps the hormones of gestation, and particularly the changes occurring before parturition, are important determinants of the *prompt onset* of maternal behaviour. Sequences of injections of oestradiol, progesterone and prolactin, to mimic the changes seen during pregnancy, induce a more rapid onset of maternal behaviour in virgin females presented with pups. Oestradiol appears to be the most important hormone in this regard. However, although eliciting a more rapid response, this treatment has never adequately mimicked the *immediacy* of maternal care following normal delivery. Clearly, there is something special about parturition itself that renders the mother uniquely sensitive to the newborn. Experiments on sheep have shown that this is indeed the case.

Parturition itself influences the onset of maternal behaviour

Non-parturient ewes, or parturient ewes 2h or more after having given birth, will not accept or nurse an orphaned lamb even if they are oestrogen primed. They can be induced to do so with 50% or so success by being made temporarily anosmic by use of a nasal spray, or alternatively by draping the pelt of the ewe's own dead lamb over an orphaned lamb that requires fostering. Olfactory cues from the lamb apparently, then, prevent it from being nursed by any mother, other than its own. The parturient ewe *will* accept an alien lamb and nurse it along with her own, *provided it is presented within 2h or so of the ewe having herself given birth*. The reason for this seems to be that the ewe has an altered olfactory responsiveness to the lamb during the immediate postpartum period. There are two possible mechanisms. Perhaps the ewe can selectively recognize the odour of her own lamb and respond only to it (or to an alien lamb presented in that period). Alternatively, the ewe may be functionally anosmic in the immediate postpartum period and therefore does not respond negatively to an alien lamb by rejecting it. The latter explanation seems more likely, but in either case, how is this olfactory mechanism brought into play? In an ingenious experiment, stimulation of the cervix and distension of the vagina (using a vibrator or the bladder of a rugby football, respectively) in oestrogen-primed non-parturient ewes caused the immediate (within minutes) display of maternal behaviour towards alien lambs (Fig. 14.8). The same immediate response has now been seen to occur in rats: cervical stimulation of virgin, oestrogen-treated females caused maternal behaviour within minutes of exposure to pups. Thus, mechanical stimulation of the reproductive tract, especially the cervix, during parturition may be a critical trigger for the neural mechanisms underlying the rapid induction of maternal behaviour.

Specific neural mechanisms underlie maternal behaviour

The neural basis of maternal behaviour has been studied mainly in rats and sheep. Given the impact of sex steroids on the rapid induction of maternal behaviour, it is not sur-

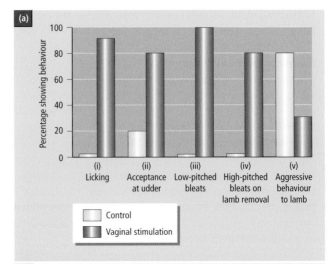

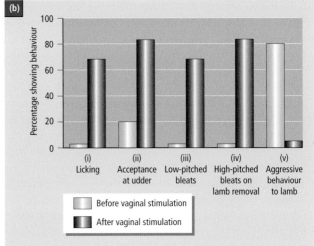

Fig. 14.8 (a) The effects of vaginal stimulation on the maternal behaviour of non-pregnant ewes. After stimulation, ewes: (i) lick the alien lambs; (ii) allow them to suckle at the udder; (iii) emit low-pitched bleats characteristic of a maternal ewe; or (iv) emit high-pitched bleats, indicating distress, if the lamb is removed; and (v) exhibit a marked decrease in aggression towards the lamb. (b) Here, the controls in (a), who showed little or no maternal behaviour, were subjected to vaginal stimulation at the end of the observation period. As can be seen, their change in behaviour towards the alien lamb immediately afterwards is dramatic.

prising that the *medial preoptic area* appears to be of major importance, bilateral lesioning of it severely impairing pup retrieval, nest building and nursing responses in postpartum female rats. Moreover, implantation of oestradiol in this area facilitated maternal behaviour in hypophysectomized or ovariectomized female rats. Recently a direct correlation has been shown between high-quality maternal care and higher expression levels in the medial preoptic area of the oestrogen α-receptor.

In addition, the medial preoptic area receives projections from the *medial amygdala*, either directly or via the *bed nucleus* of the *stria terminalis*. The amygdala is an important structure in mediating the effects of olfactory cues from the *accessory olfactory bulb*, which is the principal recipient of the special kind of olfactory information processed by the *vomeronasal organ* in non-primate species. Thus, this route is potentially important for maternal olfactory recognition of offspring. Lesions of the medial amygdala *facilitate* maternal behaviour by reducing its latency of onset in female rats exposed to pups. Thus, removal of either the receipt of olfactory information by peripheral anosmia or its central transfer by amygdalectomy reduces the time required for pup stimulation to sensitize maternal responses.

The extremely rapid onset of maternal behaviour at parturition, when the steroid hormone environment of the brain is optimal for pups to elicit maternal responses, suggests that a hormone-primed neural mechanism might operate. Experimental data suggest involvement of a *central oxytocinergic* neural system, activated in parallel with the peripheral oxytocin hormonal system at parturition. Oxytocin synthesis is not restricted to the magnocellular neurons of the paraventricular and supraoptic nuclei, but also occurs in the parvocellular neurons of the medial paraventricular nucleus which project to diverse areas of the brain, including the olfactory bulb, septal nuclei, amygdala and autonomic regions of the brainstem and spinal cord. This central oxytocin system functions independently of the neurohypophyseal oxytocin system, even though it may be activated by common stimuli, such as cervical stimulation during parturition. Oxytocin gene expression in these neurons is regulated by sex steroids, as is the expression of oxytocin receptors in some target neurons; indeed oxytocin mRNA is elevated in the parvocellular paraventricular nucleus at parturition—a time when oxytocin receptors are also increased in the ventromedial hypothalamus and bed nucleus of the stria terminalis.

Central, but not peripheral, administration of oxytocin to virgin female rats induces full maternal behaviour within a very few minutes, provided there has been prior 'priming' with gonadal steroids. The change in behaviour is dramatic, treated females switching from having no interest in pups to a relentless pursuit of nest building, retrieval, licking and other pup-orientated maternal responses. Moreover, maternal behaviour at parturition can be prevented by prior treatment with oxytocin receptor antagonists, but these antagonists do not have any effect once maternal behaviour is established. Thus, in rats at least, oxytocin released centrally at parturition induces maternal behaviour in a way that is coordinated with its peripheral effects in the uterus during labour and on mammary tissue for milk ejection. It has also been demonstrated that the cervicovaginal stimulation that so effectively induces maternal behaviour in nulliparous ewes (see above) is also associated with large increases in the central release of oxytocin. Indeed, at parturition, cerebrospinal fluid concentrations of oxytocin may reach those found in the plasma. These data suggest that central oxytocin may be a common mediator of the induction of maternal behaviour in many species, as summarized in Fig. 14.9. It is not known whether such neuroendocrine mechanisms, especially those involving central oxytocin, are also important for the onset of maternal behaviour in primate species, including women.

Summary

The sequence of events influencing the display of maternal behaviour in non-primates appears to be: (1) exposure to hormones, particularly oestradiol, during late pregnancy; (2) parturition or cervical stimulation itself; (3) the release of oxytocin within key areas of the forebrain; and (4) continuing exposure to the newborn and growing infant(s). Maternal behaviour will be displayed in the absence of either (1) or (2), but with reduced success. The realization that cervical stimulation has such dramatic effects has already had an impact on sheep farming. It has also provided a stimulus to studies of maternal behaviour in women, where implications for the success of mother–infant bonding following non-vaginal deliveries are obvious. Indeed, mother–infant bonding after Caesarean delivery may differ from that seen after vaginal delivery, but it is unclear whether this is related to differences in cervicovaginal stimulation. We will now examine in more detail how our understanding of non-primate maternal behaviour helps studies in humans and other primates.

In primates, mother–infant interaction changes dynamically

Baby monkeys spend most of their first few months (or years in apes) of life clinging tenaciously to their mothers, and occasionally fathers, aunts and juveniles, in characteristic ventro-ventral, back-riding or arm-cradled positions. This *clinging reflex* requires a well-developed motor capability. Similarly, a well-developed *rooting reflex*, also seen in human babies, by which the head turns towards a tactile stimulus around the mouth, particularly the cheeks, ensures that the infant gains the nipple for suckling. Clinging and rooting reflexes are present immediately after birth, and are elicited by cues from the mother. *Contact comfort* is also an important determinant of an infant monkey's early goal-directed movements, as experiments using surrogate mothers have shown. Thus, a 'cuddly' towelling-covered wire model is much preferred to a bare wire surrogate, even if the latter can provide milk. Similarly, a warm,

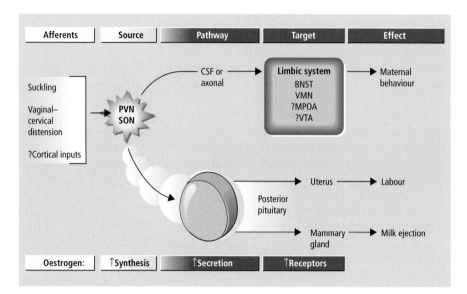

Fig. 14.9 Schematic summary of parallel central and peripheral oxytocin pathways activated at parturition. Oxytocin synthesized in magnocellular paraventricular nuclei (PVN) and supraoptic nuclei (SON) is transported to and released from the neurohypophysis into the peripheral circulation to affect the contractility of the uterus during parturition and the mammary alveoli to influence milk let-down. Oxytocin released either into the cerebrospinal fluid (CSF) or from the terminals of parvocellular oxytocin neurons in various structures such as the bed nucleus of the stria terminalis (BNST), ventromedial nucleus (VMN) of the hypothalamus, medial preoptic area (MPOA), olfactory bulb and midbrain ventral tegmental area (VTA) (in the region of the dopamine neurones there) may be involved with the initiation of maternal behaviour. Oestrogen increases the synthesis, release and binding of oxytocin to its receptors, but not necessarily by direct actions.

moving, milk-providing surrogate is preferred to one lacking these attributes. It is inferred that babies prefer such cues from the feelings of security and comfort generated. Human infant behaviour towards a warm, rocking mother or soft blanket is comparable.

Clinging, contact comfort and rooting behaviours emphasize the baby's contribution to the interactions at the earliest moments after birth, and help establish the bond with the mother, as well as securing warmth, contact and food with only minimal help from her. The mother must also keep her infant clean and protect it. Such behaviour is elicited quite specifically by the infant, which emphasizes that the close contact at suckling forms the focal point around which subsequent patterns of maternal behaviour develop. Although the baby initiates contact by clinging, the mother clearly derives considerable rewards too, as evidenced by the fact that a mother will carry her dead baby around for some days and show distress when it is removed.

Initially, an infant does not respond to its mother as an individual. Its filial responses can be elicited by a wide range of stimuli (fur, nipples, etc.), usually, but not necessarily, associated with its own mother's body. Eventually the range of stimuli eliciting responses in a baby becomes narrowed to those from its mother alone. Similar processes occur in human babies. Olfactory cues seem to be of par-

ticular importance in the mechanisms by which babies recognize their mothers and vice versa. Communication between mother and infant takes several forms, and these reinforce both mutual recognition and the mother–infant bond. Thus, baby monkeys make characteristic vocalizations, for example 'whoos' when separated from their mothers and 'geckers' when frightened or denied access to the nipple. The mother usually responds rapidly to such vocalizations with physical contact, giving an immediate soothing effect. There are obvious parallels with human babies who have characteristic cry patterns when in pain, frightened, hungry or in a temper, and who are soothed by close contact with their mothers. Mothers can distinguish the different types of crying and learn to respond appropriately. Undoubtedly, there are many more subtle and, as yet, poorly understood means of communication between mother and infant, for example facial expressions such as 'grins' in monkeys, and smiles in human babies which contribute to the mother–infant bond.

As an infant grows and begins to move away from its mother, it is essential that it understands and complies with its mother's signals concerning potential hazards, for example proximity of a predator. Thus, communication between mother and infant changes in parallel with, and often as a consequence of, an infant's cognitive and motor development. However, the gradual process of gaining independence from the mother and exploring the environment, including play with other infants, in turn influences cognitive development. Extreme fear of strangers and novel surroundings could easily result in an infant never leaving its mother and thus failing to gain experience of the wider world in which it must live. Indeed, monkeys reared in isolation show great fear of novel stimuli, probably because their cognitive development has been restricted and impaired. It is in this context, then, that the delicate balance between a mother's rejection of her infant and the latter's curiosity and exploratory tendencies assume importance. The mother's proximity and availability allow the infant to resolve the conflict between explore–retreat tendencies and so increase its familiarity with strange objects while assessing their safety or hostility (Fig. 14.10). If, during this time, a more prolonged separation of the infant from its mother is imposed by taking her away, devastating effects can follow. The baby shows considerable distress, withdraws into a hunched, depressed posture and decreases its motor activity. Reuniting the pair is followed by a period of intense contact, but with eventual and gradual rejection of the infant by the mother to re-establish preseparation patterns and levels of interaction. The longer the separation the more severe and potentially enduring the effects, and the mother's behaviour is then critical in restoring the infant's security. It is important to emphasize, however, that because mother–infant separation *can* have long-term behavioural effects, it *need not necessarily* have them and many factors may influence the final outcome.

In social primates, females have plenty of opportunity to learn and 'rehearse' skills they will subsequently need as mothers. They will watch other monkeys, particularly their mothers, holding infants and may even 'practise' by holding siblings themselves. Experiments demonstrate that females reared in a socially deprived environment make poor, aggressive and rejecting mothers. There may be important parallels in disturbances of parental care in humans.

In humans, attachment behaviour secures a bond between mother and infant

It is beyond the scope of this book to do credit to the wealth of data on mother–infant interaction in humans. However, one or two aspects are presented as they amplify some of the comparative data described above.

Maternal attitudes, psychophysiology and behaviour change during pregnancy so that even mothers with initially negative attitudes towards being pregnant generally become more positive by about 5 months. Whether the increasing concentrations of oestrogens, progesterone and opioids are involved is unclear. In addition, the abrupt changes in hormones occurring around parturition may influence parental behaviour. Cortisol is particularly impli-

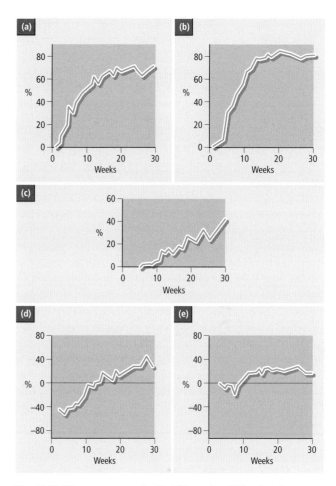

Fig. 14.10 The course over the first 30 weeks of life of mother–infant interaction in small captive groups of rhesus monkeys. (a) Total time infant spent off mother as a percentage of total time watched. (b) Time spent out of arm's reach (>60 cm) of mother. (c) Relative frequency of rejections (ratio of numbers of occasions on which infant attempted to gain ventro-ventral contact and was rejected, to number of occasions on which it made contact on mother's initiative, on its own initiative or attempted unsuccessfully to gain contact). (d) Infant's role in ventro-ventral contacts (number of contacts made on infant's initiative, as a percentage of total number made, minus number of contacts broken by infant, as a percentage of total number broken). (e) Infant's role in the maintenance of proximity. Note that, initially, the infant stays on the mother all the time, clasping her ventro-ventrally, but gradually it spends more time off her, both at hand and also out of arm's reach. Early on, the mother is primarily responsible for the close contact, restricting the infant's sorties by hanging on to a tail or foot. During this time, therefore, the infant is responsible for breaking, and the mother for making, contact. Later, however, the infant becomes primarily responsible for making contact, as the mother rejects its approaches more often and initiates contact less often.

cated, being high in pregnancy, peaking at parturition and then declining over the first week postpartum. Cortisol release is associated with high affect, and postpartum cortisol levels correlate positively with maternal responsiveness. Evidence for the role of oxytocin in the initiation of human parental bonding remains circumstantial. During the postpartum period and the fall in hormone levels, 40–80% of women experience mood changes, the intensity of which is thought to arise from the endocrine change and the type of which (depression, elation) to depend on circumstances.

Despite the almost folklorish assertion that newborn babies cannot see, they clearly can, and direct their attentive responses selectively to specific visual stimuli. Stimuli associated with the human face seem especially important and there is good evidence for facial mimicry in babies just a few hours old. Observations of early maternal behaviour after home deliveries show that immediately postpartum mothers pick up their infant, stroke its face and start breastfeeding while gazing intently into its face. In hospital deliveries, the pattern differs only slightly, mothers particularly exploring their baby's extremities, but still with considerable emphasis on eye-to-eye contact. This early period of intense eye-to-eye contact and physical exploration may be very important. But the interaction is not one way; the baby emits signals to the mother that evoke her maternal responses and willingness to nurse. Thus, there is a reciprocity in mother–infant interaction important in establishing their bond and leading subsequently to mutual recognition.

In addition to the stimuli associated with the mother's face being important for eventual maternal recognition by her infant, olfaction is used by human neonates to differentiate between their own and another mother. In experiments in which a 6-day-old infant was presented with breast pads (which had absorbed milk) from its own mother or from an 'alien' lactating female, significantly more time was spent turning towards its own mother's pad. Babies, particularly when several weeks old, attune to their mother's facial expressions when they talk and coo. In one study, a 4-week-old infant, with a blind mother who had never been sighted and displayed a mask-like face during speech, tended to avert his eyes and face from his mother when she leaned over to talk to him. When interacting with other, sighted, individuals, however, this was not the case. The normal interaction had therefore been distorted, but not completely so, as other modes of communication (verbal–auditory, in particular) were used successfully to overcome this interaction deficit.

The essential contribution of the baby to the bond between it and its mother is highlighted when babies display behaviour that disrupts the relationship. A baby who cries and shows avoidance responses when picked up may very easily induce feelings of frustration, confusion and anxiety in the parents. They may, in fact, feel rejected by the infant, quite the opposite to what is usually encountered when examining the occurrence of rejection in a mother–infant dyad. The behaviour displayed subsequently by the 'rejected' parents will affect their infant's developing behaviour and so the path is potentially set for an unsatisfactory and enduring pattern of interaction between them.

The effects of early separation on subsequent mother–infant interaction in rhesus monkeys may be paralleled in humans. Enforced early separation of women from their newborn babies for periods of up to 3 weeks, as might occur after premature delivery, can be associated with differences in *attachment behaviour* (bonding) when compared with mothers similarly separated from their babies, but allowed additional contact during the first few days after birth. Modern paediatric practice takes account of such findings, and where possible ensures as much contact as is practicable between mothers and their babies. Again, it must be emphasized that although postnatal separation of mother and baby can have delayed and long-lasting effects, it need not necessarily do so.

Summary

There is still much to learn about the mechanisms regulating the onset, course and maintenance of human parental care. The brief account above is not intended to represent the 'way' a mother or father should behave towards their baby, or to say that adverse consequences will necessarily result if they do not behave in this way. However, by studying the behaviour of both human and non-human primate mother–infant pairs, we may begin to understand what factors contribute to the success and richness of the mother–infant bond. Equally, we may discover what contributes to its breakdown, and how failure to establish an adequate bond at an appropriate time leads to disturbed behaviour in the parents or the infant, or both, later on. Given the pervasive effects of good or bad parental care on subsequent social and, indeed, parental behaviour, the importance of such research is obvious. Recent research in genetics is beginning to shed some light on this subject.

Genetics and maternal care

We have seen how aspects of parental care can influence the long-term behaviour of the offspring. However, one reliable but puzzling feature of this work is the variability in the response among different offspring exposed to an apparently similar level and quality of parental care. In addition, we do not yet have a clear understanding of exactly how these early events produce such lasting responses—the underlying causal mechanism(s). Might there be useful genetic explanations? The sequencing of the genomes of various species provides a powerful first step along a path that should lead to explanations as to just how environmental signals interact with genes to produce distinctive phenotypes. Here we give just two sorts of examples relevant to maternal care of how this work is progressing.

The impact of maternal care can depend on the genetic make-up of the offspring

An explanation for at least part of the variability in offspring responses to specific patterns of maternal care may lie in the subtle influences exerted by different genetic polymorphisms. A polymorphism is a sequence variation within the gene or its regulatory regions that does not prevent the expression of a functional protein (thus the allele is still considered to be a 'wild type' allele) but may affect the properties of the mRNA and/or the protein in subtle ways that become revealed only in particular circumstances—such as, for example, exposure to certain infectious agents. In the context of maternal behaviour, two recent prospective studies on children from birth to adulthood have been informative, both studies having now been independently confirmed.

In the first study, it was found that patterns of antisocial behaviour were higher in young men who were maltreated as children. However, not all maltreated young men showed this response to the same extent (Fig. 14.11a). The highest levels of antisocial behaviour were associated with the presence of a genetic polymorphism in the promoter of the gene monoamine oxidase A (MAOA)—but this relationship only emerged as significant when the boys had been maltreated. This polymorphism resulted in lower levels of gene and enzyme activity in the brain. Now, MAOA is an enzyme that controls the destruction of monaminergic neurotransmitters, such as noradrenaline, serotonin (5-HT), and dopamine, reducing their level. Both MAOA deficit and elevated levels of these neurotransmitters are associated with increased aggression. So, one interpretation of these results is that childhood abuse interacts with MAOA activity to influence the susceptibility of the maltreated child to expression of antisocial behaviour.

A second example from the same prospective study examined how childhood abuse might interact with genetic polymorphisms to influence patterns of depression later in life. This time the gene examined encoded the serotonin transporter, a gene pertinent for depression because current pharmacotherapies target selective serotonin reuptake. The polymorphism studied was in the gene promoter region and was characterized as being long or short, the latter

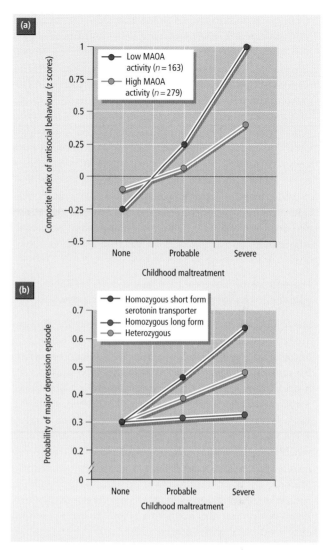

Fig. 14.11 (a) Summary plot of the relationship between antisocial behaviour as adults and the maltreatment of boys in childhood (3 and 11 years) who either had high or low monoamine oxidase A (MAOA) activity. Note that severe maltreatment is strongly associated with high levels of antisocial behaviour in boys with low MAOA activity, but much less so for boys with high MAOA activity. (b) A similar plot for adult depressive episodes (18–26 years) in adults homozygous or heterozygous for the 5-HT transporter. (Redrawn and adapted from Caspi A et al. (2002) *Science* **297**, 851–854 and Caspi A et al. (2003) *Science* **301**, 386–389.)

polymorphism showing lower transcriptional efficiency. When childhood maltreatment had occurred, children with one or two short alleles had a significantly elevated probability of a major depressive episode compared with children having two long alleles (Fig. 14.11b). Again, this significant difference in depression only emerged with childhood maltreatment.

These studies focused on genes with a strong probability of involvement in the psychiatric behaviour under study. It is not claimed that these polymorphic variations can provide the sole explanation for population variations in responses to behaviours experienced in childhood. The value of these studies is that they offer us paradigms for studying how parental behaviours might interact with genetic susceptibilities to produce different behaviour patterns later in life. Of course the outstanding question then becomes: just how might their interaction function to create this enduring change in behaviour? One answer to that question may lie in another remarkable recent study that again involves genetic expression. In this case, however, we are not dealing with polymorphisms but with epigenetics.

The pattern of maternal care may induce heritable epigenetic changes in the chromatin of the newborn

Studies in rats have shown that one consequence of high-quality postpartum maternal care is a lowered sensitivity of the offspring to stressors later in life—greater resilience. In contrast, offspring that experience low-quality care become more sensitive to stressors and show higher acute corticosteroid responses—they stress easily. Indeed, stable lines of rats have been bred in which the mothers consistently show low-quality or high-quality mothering with reliable effects on their offspring. However, if the offspring of low-quality-care mothers are cross-fostered at birth to high-quality mothers, then they grow up with relatively robust reactions to stressors, and vice versa. This experiment shows that the mothering seems to have a causal effect on the subsequent stress behaviour.

A recent study asked where and how the memory of maternal care quality was laid down. It found that the offspring experiencing high-quality care showed increased sensitivity of the hypothalamic–pituitary–adrenal (HPA) axis to negative feedback by glucocorticoids and a damped anxiety/stress response compared to offspring that had experienced low-quality care. The increased glucocorticoid feedback sensitivity was associated with a greater expression of glucocorticoid receptors in the hippocampus. These findings appeared to locate at least one site of enduring maternal effect, but what caused this difference in expression? The answer found was surprising, and involved epigenetic changes to chromatin.

You will recall that there are several mechanisms by which epigenetic imprinting can be achieved. It can involve variation in the histone subtypes making up the chromatin, various post-translational modifications to histones, and also direct methylation of certain cytosine residues in the DNA itself (see Fig. 9.9). It is the latter sort of epigenetic imprint that was described here. Thus, when the promoter

region of the hippocampal glucocorticoid receptor was analysed for its cytosine methylation pattern, it was found that those offspring that had experienced high-quality care had much lower levels of cytosine methylation at certain key bases in the promoter sequence. Moreover, this lower level of methylation was found regardless of whether the neonates had been born of high-care mothers or had been cross-fostered to them from low-care mothers immediately after birth. This latter control is very important, because had they been left with their birth mothers, they would have had high methylation levels as adults. This result implies that the lower methylation levels were determined by high-quality maternal care and were in turn (at least in part) responsible for offspring anxiety behaviour—a chain of causality. This conclusion was further strengthened by the experimentally induced reduction in the methylation levels of the glucocorticoid receptor promoter in the adult hippocampus, which converted easily stressed animals to more stressor-resilient ones. Conversely, increasing the methylation levels in the adult offspring of good mothers rendered them less resilient to stressors.

This study leaves many questions of mechanism unanswered. There are also questions about the specificity of the responses. However, the study offers an example of how a complex environmental input (maternal care) can operate epigenetically to influence chromatin organization and thereby patterns or levels of gene expression in ways that are heritable across cell generations and have a subtle effect on a complex behavioural phenotype. If these sorts of epigenetically induced change were applied to genes with polymorphic variations, then it might enhance further an underlying difference in expressivity that could also explain the results with MAOA and 5-HTT.

One question that hangs in the air from these findings is why such a system might have evolved. It is interesting to speculate that we might we be seeing a behavioural version of the maternal metabolic programming described in Chapter 12. Thus, in a high-stressor environment, mothers may become more stressed and so give less good care to their offspring. Their offspring then pick up this signal through epigenetic modifications so that in adulthood their own responsiveness to stressors is heightened. In consequence, their chances of survival to sexual maturity, and thus reproduction, might increase, but this survival may be at the expense of their longer-term health and welfare.

FURTHER READING

General reading

Bainham A *et al.* (1999) *What is a Parent*? Hart Publishing, Oxford.

KEY LEARNING POINTS

- Lactation provides the primary source of nutrition for the newborn and is also the focus around which mother–infant bonding occurs.

- The breast develops during pregnancy under the influence of several hormones, especially sex steroids, prolactin and insulin in women.

- Alveoli are grouped together in lobules and these are responsible for secreting milk which is conveyed to the nipple via lactiferous ducts.

- Milk contains water, lactose, fats, amino acids, proteins, minerals and vitamins with an energy value of 650 kcal/100 ml.

- Milk, and especially colostrums, contains a range of immunoprotective agents that assists the sterile gut of the newborn to give a controlled innate immune response to the antigenic load experienced with the first milk intake.

- Falling levels of progesterone late in pregnancy and high circulating levels of prolactin are key events in lactogenesis—the initiation of lactation.

- Maintenance of milk secretion, lactopoiesis, depends on elevated levels of prolactin secretion which are achieved through nipple stimulation by the suckling infant.

- Stimulation of the nipple by suckling is the primary stimulus to the milk ejection reflex which is mediated by the release of oxytocin from the posterior pituitary and causes contractions of alveolar smooth muscle cells.

- Fertility is suppressed by lactation and is mediated by the high levels of prolactin which suppress cyclic gonadotrophin secretion.

- Lactation can be suppressed by treatment with dopamine D_2 receptor agonists, which prevent prolactin secretion and hence lactopoiesis.

- When lactation ceases the breast gradually involutes.

- There are clear medical advantages to breast-feeding, including bonding and secure attachment, immune protection and healthier nutrition. These may outweigh risks of maternal infection transmission.

- The rapid induction of maternal behaviour at parturition is critical for survival of the young.

- Stimuli from the newborn of many species are critical in inducing maternal responses; they are able to do so even in nulliparous females, but with a long latency.

- Exposure to sex steroids during pregnancy greatly hastens the onset of maternal behaviour in response to cues from the newborn.

- Parturition itself and the associated stimulation of the cervix is also a potent stimulus to the onset of maternal behaviour.

- The release of oxytocin from neurons within the brain appears to be a common neural mechanism underlying maternal behaviour. Oxytocin levels in the cerebrospinal fluid are high at parturition and can be elevated by cervical stimulation. Infusions of oxytocin can induce maternal behaviour within seconds in females who have been exposed previously to oestrogens. Oxytocin receptor antagonists prevent the induction of maternal behaviour at parturition.

- Very little is known of the neuroendocrine mechanisms underlying maternal behaviour in non-human primates and in women.

- Mother–infant interaction soon after parturition supports the formation of a close bond between mother and infant that forms the focal point for maternal behaviour.

- In monkeys, infants gradually gain independence from their mothers through a dynamic interaction which involves the infant leaving the mother progressively more often to explore its environment and the gradual rejection of the infant's approaches to the mother for contact.

- In humans the period of maternal care is prolonged and complex. The mechanisms that induce maternal responses and maintain this long period of maternal (and paternal) care are not clearly understood. They undoubtedly also depend increasingly on cognitive processes, in addition to any neuroendocrine influences around the time of parturition.

- The quality of parental care can impact differently on offspring depending on their genetic make-up, such that some offspring may be genetically more susceptible to enduring effects of parental care quality.

- Parental care may also impose epigenetic imprints on genes in the neonate that heritably affect the gene expressivity later in life with consequences for subsequent behaviour.

Carter CS, Altemus M (1997) Integrative functions of lactational hormones in social behaviour and stress management. *Annals of the New York Academy of Sciences* **807**, 164–174.

Carter CS *et al.* (1997) *The Integrative Neurobiology of Affiliation.* Annals of the New York Academy of Sciences, Vol. 807. New York Academy of Sciences, New York.

Howie PW *et al.* (1990) Protective effect of breast-feeding against infection. *British Medical Journal* **300**, 11–16.

Insell TR *et al.* (1997) Central oxytocin and reproductive behaviours. *Reviews of Reproduction* **2**, 28–37.

Nowak R *et al.* (2000) Role of mother–young interactions in the survival of offspring in domestic mammals. *Reviews of Reproduction* **5**, 153–163.

Owen D *et al.* (2005) Maternal adversity, glucocorticoids and programming of neuroendocrine function and behaviour. *Neuroscience and Biobehavioral Reviews* **29**, 209–226.

Rutter M (2006) *Genes and Behviour Nature–Nurture Interplay Explained.* Blackwell Publishing, Oxford.

Weaver ICG *et al.* (2006) Maternal care effects on the hippocampal transcriptome and anxiety-mediated behaviors in the offspring that are reversible in adulthood. *Proceedings of the National Academy of Sciences of the USA* **103**, 3480–3485.

Zhang T-Z *et al.* (2006) Maternal programming of defensive responses through sustained effects on gene expression. *Biological Psychology* **73**, 72–89.

More advanced reading (see also Box)

Bowlby J (1973) *Attachment and Loss*, Vol. 2. Hogarth, London.

Bowlby J (1980) *Attachment and Loss*, Vol. 3. Hogarth, London.

Bowlby J (1982) *Attachment and Loss,* Vol. 1, 2nd edn. Hogarth, London.

Caspi A *et al.* (2002) Role of genotype in the cycle of violence in maltreated children. *Science* **297**, 851–854.

Caspi A *et al.* (2003) Influence of life stress on depression: moderation by a polymorphism in the 5-HTT gene. *Science* **301**, 386–389.

Champagne FA *et al.* (2006) Maternal care associated with methylation of the estrogen receptor-1β promoter and estrogen receptor-expression in the medial preoptic area of female offspring. *Endocrinology* **147**, 2909–2915.

Ciba Foundation Symposium 33 (1975) (New Series) *Parent–Infant Interaction.* Elsevier, Amsterdam.

Corter CM, Fleming AS (1995) Psychobiology of maternal behaviour in human beings. In: *Handbook of Parenting*, Vol. 2 (ed. M.H. Bornstein), pp. 87–115. Lawrence Erlbaum Associates, Mahwah, NJ.

Harlow HF, Suomi SJ (1970) Nature of love—simplified. *American Journal of Psychology* **25**, 161–168.

Harlow HF, Zimmerman RR (1959) Affectional responses in the infant monkey. *Science* **130**, 421–432.

Hinde RA (1974) *Biological Bases of Human Social Behaviour.* McGraw-Hill, New York.

Keverne EB *et al.* (1983) Vaginal stimulation: an important determinant of maternal bonding in sheep. *Science* **219**, 81–83.

Kools EJ *et al.* (2005) A breast-feeding promotion and support programme: a randomised trial in the Netherlands. *Preventive Medicine* **40**, 60–70.

LeBouder E *et al.* (2006) Modulation of neonatal microbial recognition: TLR-mediated innate immune responses are specifically and differentially modulated by human milk. *Journal of Immunology* **176**, 3742–3752.

Marlier L, Schaal B (2005) Human newborns prefer human milk: conspecific milk odor is attractive without postnatal exposure. *Child Development* **76**, 155–168.

Reeve, JR *et al.* (2004) A preliminary study on the use of experiential learning to support women's choices about infant feeding. *European Journal of Obstetrics and Gynaecology and Reproductive Biology* **113**, 199–203.

Weaver IC *et al.* (2004) Epigenetic programming by maternal behavior. *Nature Neuroscience* **7**, 847–854.

Weaver ICG *et al.* (2005) Reversal of maternal programming of stress responses in adult offspring through methyl supplementation: altering epigenetic marking later in life. *Journal of Neuroscience* **25**, 11045–11054.

CHAPTER 15

15 Fertility

In the preceding chapters, we have attempted to describe the important mechanisms that underlie the establishment of sex, the attainment of sexual maturity, the production and successful interaction of male and female gametes, the initiation and maintenance of pregnancy and the production and care of the newborn. These processes absorb much of our physical, physiological and behavioural energies. Reproduction and its associated activities permeate all aspects of our lives. This ramification of sex, in turn, makes it highly susceptible to social and environmental influences, and these influences can be of adaptive value, as we have seen at several points in the book. However, although the adaptive value of sensitivity to environmental and social signals seems undeniable for the reproductive efficiency of the species as a whole, it is not necessarily so for the individual. In contemporary human society, the increasing emphasis on individual rights and welfare has prompted a more sympathetic attitude towards the fertility of the individual, both its limitation and its encouragement. Moreover, sexual interaction among humans is not related directly and exclusively to fertility, but rather has evolved a wider social role. Sexuality and its expression has, in its own right and independent of any reproductive considerations, become an important element within human society

(see Chapter 2). In this final chapter, therefore, we stand back from a detailed consideration of the mechanisms of reproduction and look instead at human fertility patterns, and at the factors, both natural and artificial, that may influence them. We draw heavily on examples of the reproductive mechanisms described earlier to illustrate our points, and so the chapter cross-refers extensively.

Fertility, fecundibility and fecundity

To begin with, some definitions are necessary. The *fertility* of an individual, a couple or a population refers to the number of children born, and the *fertility rate* of a population is the number of births in a defined period of time divided by the number of women of reproductive age. Women rather than men are used in this calculation because their reproductive potential is limiting. Thus, fertility is a measure of *actual outcome* of the reproductive process. In contrast, *fecundibility* is defined as the probability of conceiving in a menstrual cycle in a woman who has regular periods and engages in regular unprotected sex, whether or not conception goes to term. Conception is indicated by either a biochemical pregnancy (positive human chorionic gonadotrophin test) and/or a clinical pregnancy (from an

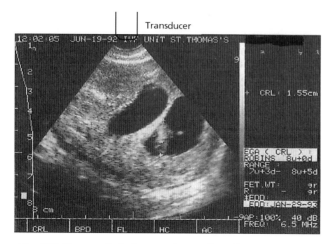
Transducer

Fig. 15.1 Transvaginal ultrasound scan of a twin gestation in a woman 8 weeks pregnant. Both sacs can be seen on this longitudinal section, although only one embryo (in the lower right-hand sac) is visible in this plane. The gestational age of the embryos can be determined from measurement of the crown/ rump length (between the white crosses).

ultrasound scan: Fig. 15.1). Finally, *fecundity* is a measure of the capacity to both conceive *and* produce a live birth under the same circumstances. Both fecundibility and fecundity are therefore measures of the *reproductive potential* of women.

Reliable estimates of human fecundibility have come recently from prospective population-based Chinese and European studies. These recruited couples, mostly with women under 35, using no contraception and trained to detect the most fertile 6 days around ovulation and to try for pregnancy every cycle during this period. Cumulative conception rates of around 50% after 2 cycles and 85% by 6 months were observed. Approximately half the remaining couples conceived within a year, leaving a residual 5% or so couples as clinically subfertile. Comparable data from prospective studies of fecundity are limited, but, together with reliable retrospective studies, suggest that 10–15% of all clinically diagnosed pregnancies end in spontaneous miscarriage. Thus, human fecundibility and fecundity rates of around 25% and 22% per cycle seem reasonable estimates for women of reproductive age. In reality, the fertility of a population or individual will rarely reach its theoretical maximum (fecundity), because of constraints placed on reproductive efficiency. It is the nature of these constraints that concerns us in this chapter.

The effects of natural constraints such as age and senescence on fertility and fecundity will be considered first. We will see that, for women, puberty and menopause mark the limits of the period of fertility. However, within this period, most women are not continuously reproducing. Traditionally three factors have limited their fertility: (1) social or religious practices and traditions, (2) the use of contraception and induced pregnancy termination, and (3) pathology (infertility or subfertility).

Age, senescence and reproductive capacity

Ageing should be distinguished from senescence. Ageing begins at conception and is a description of what happens with the passage of time. *Senescence* describes deterioration related to dysfunction and disease. Typically, reproductive senescence begins during middle age, but its onset and time course vary widely among individuals of the same age. Both men and women experience a number of senescent changes to the central nervous system (CNS), which, as we have seen, has an important regulatory role in reproductive and sexual function. Recent evidence suggests that the weak androgenic hormone dihydroepiandrosterone (DHEA), produced in large amounts by the adrenal, may have neuroprotective effects which might be reduced in some elderly people and thus might account for a reduced capacity to repair and sustain neurons, thereby contributing to the senescence of CNS function. In women, a major change occurs at the *menopause*, defined as the last menstrual cycle, and this results from the exhaustion of functional ovarian follicles and is thus primarily part of the ageing process. However, senescent changes in the reproductive potential of women may precede this landmark. Most men, in contrast, do not experience gametic exhaustion or a sudden fall-off in fertility as part of the ageing process, there being no evidence for a male equivalent of the menopause, despite popular claims to the contrary. They do, however, experience senescent changes, which, as for women, show a great variation among individuals.

Women

Menarche

The fertility of a woman varies with her age. Menstrual cycles begin during puberty, and menarche marks the earliest expression of the potential fertility of the female with its implication that a full ovarian and uterine cycle has been achieved. Failure of menarche indicates a diagnosis of primary amenorrhoea. This may result from a failure of normal maturation of the underlying neuroendocrine mechanisms (see Chapter 7); from primary defects in the gonad, such as dysgenesis or agenesis due to chromosomal abnormality (e.g. Turner's syndrome and true hermaphroditism, Chapter 1); or from primary defects in the genital tract, such as lack of patency between the uterus and vagina (cryptomenorrhoea or hidden menses) or, indeed, the absence of internal genitalia as seen in androgen insensitivity syndrome (see Chapters 1 & 3). However, even in most women, early menstrual cycles are rarely regular. Some

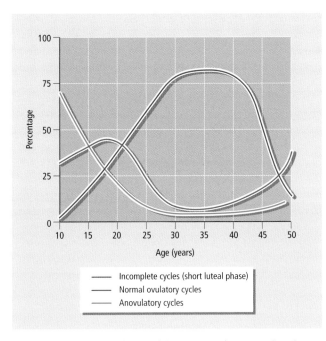

Fig. 15.2 Relative incidence of three types of menstrual cycle with age of woman.

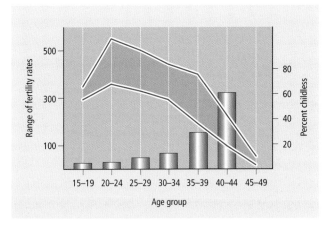

Fig. 15.3 Rates of fertility (red range) and childlessness (blue bars) by age of woman. The fertility rate data were collected from populations of married women in which, it is alleged, no efforts were made to limit reproduction. The range reflects the different circumstances of the populations, drawn from different parts of the world. These data approach a measure of fecundity by age in humans. The histograms show the proportions of women remaining childless after first marriage at the ages indicated despite continuing attempts to deliver a child. Note the sharp rise above 35 years, implying a fall in fecundity from this time onwards.

cycles are anovulatory and may lack, or have abbreviated, luteal phases (Fig. 15.2). In general, the follicular phase tends to become shorter with age and the luteal phase tends to lengthen, for reasons that are unclear.

The cause of the climacteric and menopause

Fertility is highest in women in their twenties and declines thereafter (Fig. 15.3). This decline could, in principle, be due to a reduction in fecundity or to changes in sexual behaviour resulting in older women having a reduced chance of, or inclination for, unprotected sex. Measures of the risk of childlessness in women of different ages at marriage, who then try actively to have offspring, are also shown in Fig. 15.3, and suggest a real decrease in fecundity. It is clear that the ability to sustain a pregnancy through to successful parturition declines slowly to the age of 35 years, but rapidly thereafter when increasing frequencies of failed ovulation, early pregnancy loss, perinatal or neonatal mortality, low birthweights, maternal hypertension and congenital malformations especially, but not exclusively, due to fetal chromosomal imbalance are encountered. Maternal oocytes, stored in second meiotic metaphase since fetal life, show evidence of increased meiotic spindle instability and chromosomal dispersal, and are the major contributor to this decline in fecundity. Accordingly, it is not surprising that irregular menstrual cycles may begin to reappear in some women in their early forties and mark the onset of the climacteric, a period of reproductive change that may last for up to 10 years before the last menstrual cycle (the

menopause). This secondary amenorrhoea occurs at a mean age of 52 years in the USA. Symptoms associated with the climacteric can include mood changes, irritability, loss of libido and hot flushes. The climacteric reflects declining numbers of ovarian follicles and their reduced responsiveness to gonadotrophins, and is a direct consequence of the fixed number of oocytes a woman has arising from the early termination of mitotic proliferation in female germ cells (Chapter 1, but see also Box 5.1).

The final cessation of reproductive life is, thus, a function of ovarian failure, although senescent changes to hypothalamic and pituitary cells may also make a contribution to the climacteric dsymenorrhoea. Premature loss of oocytes, and thus premature menopause, occurs in about 2% of women, in some as early as their late teens and early twenties. The causes of premature menopause are unclear, although in some women a familial element exists. With the decreasing numbers of small preantral/early antral follicles, the secretion of follicular inhibin B declines early in the climacteric, elevating FSH levels because of the reduced negative feedback. These elevated FSH levels can then temporarily salvage a greater proportion of the small follicles and can shorten the follicular phase. During this period, enough antral follicles still survive for adequate levels of inhibin A and oestrogen to rise. Only in latter part of the climacteric, as menopause approaches, do inhibin A and oestrogen also fall, and then LH rises too. Paradoxically,

Table 15.1 Steroidogenesis in the postmenopausal woman. Change from resting plasma concentrations (%).

Hormone	Dexamethasone suppression (% decrease)	hCG stimulation (% increase)
Oestradiol	>50	0
Oestrone	>75	10
Progesterone	>75	10
17α-OH progesterone	53	42*
Dehydroepiandrosterone	65	60*
Androstenedione	70	10
Testosterone	40	60*
Dihydrotestosterone	>30	—

Dexamethasone inhibits adrenal cortical steroidogenesis by depressing output of ACTH, so the degree of reduction in plasma steroid levels shown suggests the degree of adrenal contribution which is high. hCG provides a gonadotrophic stimulus to the ovaries, so the degree of increase in plasma steroid levels shown suggests the degree to which the ovaries are able normally to secrete the hormones. In the second column, there are only three significant changes from baseline (asterisked).

androgen levels may rise after the menopause, as a result of adrenal synthesis combined with increasing LH-responsive ovarian interstitial cell synthesis, and this may lead to hirsutism and further exacerbate the adverse effects of lowered oestrogen on the cardiovascular system. Postmenopausal hormone levels and responsiveness are shown in Fig. 6.8 and Table 15.1.

The consequences of the menopause

The physical, functional and emotional changes of the climacteric and menopause are driven directly or indirectly by these ovarian changes. Oestrogen withdrawal is responsible for: vasomotor changes, such as 'hot flushes' and 'night sweats'; changes in ratios of blood lipids, associated with an increased risk of coronary thrombosis; reduction in size of the uterus and breasts; and a reduction in vaginal lubrication and a rise in the pH of vaginal fluids, in consequence of which discomfort during intercourse (dyspareunia) and atrophic vaginitis may occur. The antiparathormone activity of oestrogen is also lost at this time, resulting in increased bone catabolism, osteoporosis and more brittle bones. These symptoms of the menopause may be prevented or reduced by oestrogen treatment (hormone replacement therapy, HRT). However, the results of recent trials have contra-indicated HRT as a routine treatment, as it can be associated with increased risks of breast cancer, cardiac disease and cerebrovascular accident

that more than offset the advantages of reduced osteoporotic fractures. Whether or not to receive HRT and for how long is a matter for consultation between patient and doctor, when individual variables and circumstances can be discussed.

A number of behavioural changes may occur during the climacteric, for example depression, tension, anxiety and mental confusion. However, these changes may not be related directly to effects of steroid withdrawal on the brain, but rather may result secondarily from difficulties in psychological adjustment to a changing role and status, and in part from insomnia due to night sweats. Loss of libido is common and may be related to dyspareunia due to vaginal dryness. In Chapter 8, we discussed the relationship between androgens and libido: given the rising postmenopausal androgens, libido might be expected to rise in at least some women, but findings are not consistent.

Oocyte donation and the postmenopausal woman

Regardless of the time of the menopause, women can nonetheless, if provided with an oocyte (or conceptus) from a donor woman (or couple), carry a pregnancy to term successfully. The early part of this pregnancy requires administration of exogenous hormones: first, to build up the regressed reproductive tract (see Chapter 8); and, second, to mimic luteal support until the fetoplacental unit takes over endocrine control (see Chapter 11). The capacity of women in their forties to sixties to give birth after oocyte donation therapy emphasizes that the primary reproductive ageing process is oocyte and follicle loss. Senescent changes in other tissues, such as the uterus, may reduce the likelihood of a successful pregnancy outcome in some women, although the effects are statistically marginal and suggest a case-by-case approach to patients be adopted.

Men

There is a reproductive deterioration with age, although much of it may be due to senescence. Thus, fertile spermatozoa can be produced well beyond the age of 40, and in most men throughout life. Nonetheless, semen volume and the motility, quantity and quality of spermatozoa decline steadily throughout adult male life from the early twenties, but with no obvious sudden change equivalent to the menopause in women (Fig. 15.4a). Studies of sperm fertilizing capacity in IVF procedures, in which the oocyte providers were under 30, show little evidence of age-related functional decline in spermatozoa until after the age of 40. However, we must be cautious when extrapolating this to the general population who are not experiencing problems conceiving. There is some evidence to suggest that the incidence of certain congenital malformations

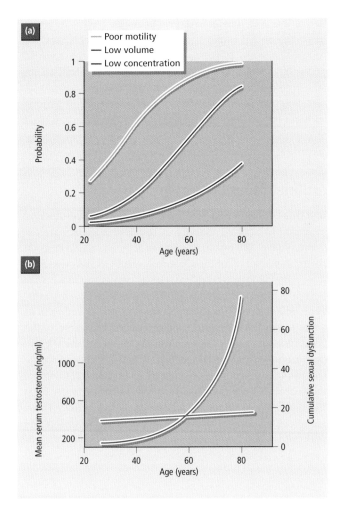

Fig. 15.4 Reproduction and ageing in males. (a) Probability of having various semen parameters by age (sperm motility < 50%; semen volume < 2 ml; concentration < 20 × 10⁶); (b) Note that although there is no obvious fall in testosterone with age, the cumulative incidence of sexual problems in men rises steadily and becomes marked after 40 years. (Redrawn and adapted from Eskenazi B *et al.* (2003) The association of age and semen quality in healthy men. *Human Reproduction* **18**, 447–454.)

increases with paternal age, although the effect seems to be less than with maternal age. This increase may be due to the much higher levels of spontaneous mutation observed in spermatogenic cells from ageing men. In addition, loss of libido, erectile dysfunction and failure to achieve orgasm occur with higher frequency from 30–40 years onwards (Fig. 15.4b), mostly resulting from senescent or iatrogenic factors, such as diabetes, pharmacological control of high blood pressure and neurodegeneration (see Chapter 9 for the biology of erectile dysfunction and its treatment).

There is little evidence for a fall with age in testosterone to below the threshold levels required for behavioural effects (see Fig. 8.16; Fig. 15.4b). However, as men age

beyond 60, atypical patterns of LH and testosterone pulses and a changed responsivity of LH to GnRH occur with higher frequency, and feedback control by testosterone seems more erratic. Some (disputed) evidence for a fall in the proportion of free/bound testosterone has been proposed to lead to a decline in *available* androgens, and a reduced responsivity of androgen receptors has been proposed to contribute to impaired androgen efficacy. All of these changes are thought primarily to be senescent. The muscle wasting and increased adiposity seen with age are plausibly related to a reduced anabolic effectiveness of androgens. Given the uncertainty about the exact underlying causes of male reproductive dysfunction with age, there is currently little evidence to support androgen therapy, the effectiveness of which remains unproven.

Social constraints on fertility

There is a rich literature on the sociology, anthropology and history of reproduction, which is too large for this book to cover comprehensively. It is an important body of knowledge for public health management, as all studies show that the simple availability of educational information about scientific and medical technology is not in itself sufficient to change sexual and reproductive behaviours. A further element, namely the *motivation* required for a change in behaviour to occur, is critically dependent on an individual's social network, values, beliefs and self-esteem, and the peer pressures that reinforce these. Among the important social variables that may influence fertility in either direction are:

1 the accepted social roles of men and women, the perceived and legal balance of power between them and, in particular, the extent to which women are educated and have economic independence

2 the age of women at marriage and at birth of the first child, and the maternal mortality rate

3 the accepted size of the family, availability of child care, and the preferred sex ratio, which may also be influenced by inheritance patterns

4 the desirability of spacing children and the anticipated child mortality pattern

5 the perceived economic advantages of a given family size

6 the permitted or expected frequency of intercourse in relation to the point in the menstrual cycle, the time of year or religious calendar, age of partners, social conditions and opportunities, and the delivery or suckling of children

7 the extent to which maternal lactation (with its consequent hyperprolactinaemia and depression of fertility, see Chapters 6 & 14) is replaced by use of milk substitutes or wet nurses

8 the acceptability of sexual interactions outside (or to the exclusion of) the usual framework in which successful pregnancy might result, emphasizing the sexual rather than the reproductive function of coition (e.g. prostitution, extra-partner sexual affairs, atypical patterns of sexual expression) (Chapter 2)

9 the social role and status of celibacy

10 the social, ethical and legal acceptability of reproduction outside of a tightly controlled social structure such as the nuclear or extended family (single or unmarried mothers, lesbian and gay couples)

11 the incidence of divorce and the attendant delay before remarriage

12 the strength with which religious beliefs are held by, or imposed on, the individual, which may also affect access to education, information, contraception, pregnancy termination and assisted reproductive technologies (see next sections).

Each of these factors will affect, to varying degrees, the overall fertility of the individual woman, couple or population, and the various factors will interact with each other. For example, high economic expectations coupled with low infant mortality and gender equality tend to reduce fertility by both delaying birth of the first child and reducing overall family size. Perhaps the single largest change that has occurred in most societies over the past century is the fall in expected infant mortality arising from improved diet and hygiene and the introduction of antibiotics and prophylactic immunization. However, this fall has led to a corresponding rise in the numbers of women surviving beyond puberty and, thus, to an increased fecundity of the popula-tion as a whole. The time lag between the decline in infant mortality and the reproductive adjustment to it, via the compensatory social factors listed above, has led to a world population explosion. Indeed, it is not clear that social adjustment alone is adequate to correct this imbalance. The increased use of artificial constraints on fertility in various societies has become an essential part of the social response to population growth, so as to regulate individual fertility according to desired or imposed social patterns.

Artificial control of fertility

The three socially accepted artificial controls over fertility available to varying extents in different societies are (1) *contraception*, (2) induced *pregnancy termination*, and (3) *sterilization*. Not all of these controls are 100% effective and, thus, some of them should be seen as regulating fertility by delaying births or increasing the interval between births. Their relative cost-effectiveness for both the population as a whole and the individual in particular is, of course, of the greatest importance. The main methods of fertility regulation used worldwide are shown in Table 15.2, and in the UK in 2004–05 by age of woman in Fig. 15.5. However, these global figures mask the wide variation with local traditions, some of which will be captured below. These variations emphasize that fertility control methods interact with cultural and economic factors to determine usage patterns. Special issues arise when considering fertility control for young people (Box 15.1).

Table 15.2 Range of pregnancy rates and patterns of usage for various forms of contraception.

	Pregnancy rate*	Use in less developed countries†	Use in more developed countries†
Oral contraception	<1–3	6	17
Progesterone-only pill	1–4		
Injectable	<1	3	0.1
IUCD (copper)	<1–2	16	8
Progesterone-releasing copper IUCD	<<1		
Male condom	2–15	3	15
Female condom	5–15		
Cap/diaphragm + spermicide	4–8		
Sterilization (female)	<<<1	22	10
Sterilization (male)	<<<1	4	7
None		40	30

*Expressed as number per 100 woman years of exposure (i.e. 100 women for 1 fertile year).
†Expressed as percentage of couples, but only where data are available (taken from United Nations data, 2001).

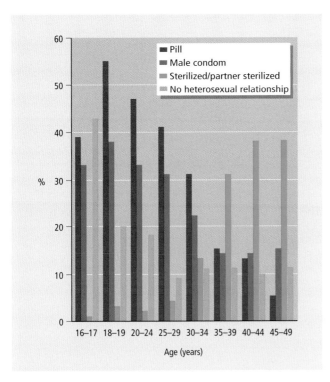

Fig. 15.5 The major fertility control methods used by UK women aged 16–49 in 2004–2005 (based on the Office of National Statistics Report).

Sterilization

Sterilization should be entered into as an irreversible procedure. It is therefore the method of fertility limitation selected by individuals or couples who have achieved their desired family size or who, for eugenic or health reasons, want to avoid reproduction. If there is any question of the person requesting sterilization not having the mental capacity to consent, the case should be referred to the courts for judgment to establish whether the procedure is in the best interests of the person concerned and not for the convenience of others.

Vasectomy

In men, sterilization involves *vasoligation* (ligation with a clip: not recommended) or *vasectomy* (preferred: removal of part of the vas deferens, see Chapters 8 & 9, with the ends overlapped and tied together or in conjunction with diathermy, both additional procedures to minimize spontaneous vas deferens reanastomosis). The vas is accessed through a small incision in the scrotum under local anaesthesia as an outpatient procedure. Aspermic ejaculates result within 2–3 months. Only 1/2000 men father a child after vasectomy, usually because they cease contraceptive

use too early. Sperm production is unaffected, and so the spermatozoa and small volume of fluid that continues to pass out of the epididymides can build up and lead to a local granuloma. Certain consequences follow: first, there is about twice the incidence of chronic or intermittent tenderness in the scrotal region, sufficient to cause distress in about 6% of cases; second, in 50% of men the leakage of spermatozoal debris into the systemic circulation from the site of inflammation induces an immune response to their own spermatozoa, but there is no evidence that this has ill-effects; third, in several species of experimental animal (but not in men), a progressive decline in spermatogenic output occurs. Some success with the surgical reversal of vasectomy has been achieved, but recent developments in the technology of assisted conception now make the infertility resulting from vasectomy potentially fully reversible (see 'Oligospermia' below). Psychological factors, particularly arising from the erroneous equation of *fertility* with *potency*, may result in anxiety that leads to erectile dysfunction after vasectomy in some men. This fear also prevents many men from accepting the procedure. Sexual arousal and ejaculation are, of course, independent of sperm release.

Tubal occlusion

In women, sterilization involves ligation (preferably by clipping with a Filshie clip or ring, or less desirably by *diathermy*—electrocoagulation). A general anaesthetic is usually required. The surgical approach is generally made with the use of a *laparoscope* on day patients through two small incisions in the lower abdominal wall, but larger incisions may be needed in women who are obese or have had previous abdominal surgery or infections (*mini-laparotomy*). *Hysteroscopic sterilization* involves the paravaginal insertion of a small titanium coil into the oviduct, around which tissue grows to block the tubes, a new procedure still undergoing evaluation. The operation has a low failure rate, but around 1/200 women (1 in 300–500 with a Filshie clip) will become pregnant, with increased risk of tubal pregnancy, especially after diathermy. Although it also cannot be easily reversed surgically, the new techniques of assisted reproduction (see later) allow the infertility to be circumvented. Sterilization may also be accomplished by hysterectomy, especially in premenopausal women troubled by irregular, painful or heavy menses or pathology of the uterus, such as fibroids or premalignant disease. Unwanted effects of sterilization can include: incidental surgical trauma at the time of the procedure; persistent pain at the site of the ligation; the very slight risk (1/12000) of mortality attendant on use of general anaesthesia; and psychological disturbance associated with loss of fecundity and the perception that femininity or womanhood may also have been damaged.

BOX 15.1 Fertility control for young people

- *The legal definition of 'young person'* varies with different jurisdictions, as do the legal requirements for doctors when dealing with them. In the UK for example, a child is a person who has not reached the age of 18 in England, Wales and Northern Ireland, but a person below the age of 16 in Scotland. The age at which young people can legally consent to sexual intercourse also varies from 12 to 18 across Europe, sometimes depending on whether partners of the same sex or the opposite sex are involved. It is essential that medical practitioners understand the local legal situation, but are also aware that people from overseas may not know of possible conflicts with the legal situation in their own country of residence.
- *Unwanted teenage pregnancy and genitourinary disease* (especially HIV and hepatitis infection, but also chlamydial infection with its attendant infertility consequences—see later) provide major stimuli to sexual health and relationship education for young people. For example, in England in 2001, a conception rate of 4.25% for 15–17 year old women was accompanied by a 56% induced termination rate. There is clear evidence that effective education works to delay first sexual experience, reduce unwanted pregnancy rates, and enhance self-esteem and relationship skills. The political will to implement national effective educational schemes is very variable across different countries, with corresponding differences in the effectiveness of programmes and the prevalence of unwanted pregnancies.
- *Professional clinical practice* requires that everyone, regardless of age, should be viewed as potentially autonomous and competent to give informed consent, and all decisions taken within local laws must be taken for the young person's benefit, and not for the convenience of other parties. Clinicians must therefore assess competence. However, children should not be encouraged to have intercourse below the legal age of consent, should have all pertinent health and legal issues of doing so explained to them, and should be encouraged to include their parents or carers in any decision about contraception or pregnancy termination, and be supported in doing so. The confidentiality of the consultation, and its limits (where coercion, maltreatment or exploitation is suspected) should be made clear.

Further reading

Baldo M et al. (1994) *Does Sex Education Lead to Earlier or Increased Sexual Activity in Youth?* WHO Global Programme on AIDS.

Bastable R, Sheather J (2005) Mandatory reporting to the police of all sexually active under-13s: new protocols may undermine confidential sexual health services for young people. *British Medical Journal* **331**, 918–919.

Faculty of Family Planning and Reproductive Health Care Clinical Effectiveness Unit (2004) Contraceptive choices for young people. *Journal of Family Planning and Reproductive Health Care* **30**, 237–251.

Herring J (2006) pp. 208–210 in *Medical Law and Ethics*. Oxford University Press, Oxford.

Ingham R (2004) Sexual health and young people: the contribution and role of psychology. In: *Sexuality Repositioned: Diversity and the Law* (ed. B. Brooks-Gordon et al.), pp. 235–260. Hart Publishing, Oxford.

Kirby D (1999) Sexuality and sex education at home and school. *Adolescent Medicine* **10**, 195–209.

O'Sullivan I et al. (2005) *Contraception and Sexual Health, 2004/05.* Office for National Statistics, London.

Contraception

Contraception differs formally from sterilization only in its potential or actual ease of reversibility and thereby in the control that the individual exerts over its use. It is, thus, the artificial control of choice for those who wish to delay the expression of fertility or to exercise it with discrimination. The methods currently available are listed in Table 15.2, together with estimates of their efficiency, expressed in terms of their failure rates. The reported rates vary widely, depending on the education, motivation and experience of the users, and their differential access to technology, good hygiene, education and medical follow-up. A breakdown of the main methods used to regulate fertility in the UK by women aged 16–49 is given in Fig. 15.5. Note the dominance of oral contraception, condom use and sterilization and that the balance of each varies with female age, a marked shift to sterilization occurring from 34 years, reflecting the differing objectives of fertility limitation.

Even the most cursory glance through these data makes evident the complexity of contraceptive use, reflecting in turn the variety of needs, resources and beliefs available to those exercising usage.

Natural methods

Contraceptive approaches that rely on coital technique, rather than the use of technical or pharmaceutical aids, straddle the boundary between social and artificial approaches to fertility control. In consequence, such approaches seem to pose particular problems for theologians and lawyers when prescribing or proscribing sexual behaviours. For example, of the techniques listed below, only the rhythm method is sanctioned by the Roman Catholic church on the grounds that the other approaches are 'unnatural'. All the methods described below occur naturally in the biological sense, if not in the theological sense.

The rhythm method. For many centuries common belief wrongly equated menstruation with the period of maximum fertility. In fact, of course, ovulation occurs approximately midcycle. However, given the potential life of spermatozoa in the cervix of several days and a 24-h fertilizable life of the oocyte (see Chapter 9), coition should be avoided through much of the first part of the cycle (Fig. 15.6). Moreover, the timing for this method is counted *back* from the small postovulatory rise in temperature of 0.2–0.6 °C (Fig. 15.6). Thus, the approach is retrospective and will only be safe if the woman's cycle is sufficiently constant, which it often is not, especially given its susceptibility to emotional or stressful disturbances (see Chapter 6). These factors, and the high motivation required by the sexual partners, make for a high failure rate, being some 20-fold less effective than oral contraceptives at their worst. Additionally, there are (disputed) claims of a significantly increased frequency of pregnancy loss and genetic abnormalities in conceptuses derived by fertilization of aged eggs occurring in couples using this method of fertility control (see Chapter 9 and 'Spontaneous pregnancy loss' below). Only around 1% of women now use this method in the UK, but as many as 15% in some parts of eastern Europe.

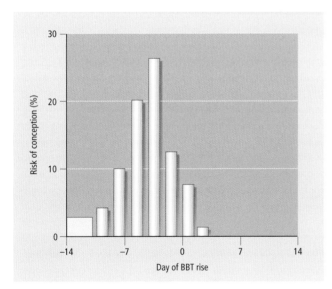

Fig. 15.6 The percentage risk of conception at different times during the unprotected cycle of women using the rhythm method, plotted as days before or after the day of rise in basal body temperature (BBT) (day 0). Coital interactions during much of the first part of the cycle carry a substantial risk of pregnancy. Only the period after the BBT rise until the end of the period of menstrual flow is truly safe. This extended period of risk is due to the potential longevity of spermatozoa in the female tract and variability in the length of the follicular phase in some women. Pink area represents menstrual flow.

Coitus interruptus. The withdrawal of the penis from the vagina during copulation but before ejaculation has been, and remains, one of the most frequently used forms of contraception, and the technique is credited (together with abortion) as being responsible for much of the decline in birth rate at the time of the industrial revolution in Europe. Failures occur, due both to lack of adequate control by men at the moment of ejaculation and to insemination with spermatozoa that leak from the urethra before ejaculation or persist from a prior ejaculation. It is difficult to estimate the true usage prevalence, but figures of 30% for southern and 1% for northern Europe are claimed.

Masturbation and other forms of sexual interaction. Mutual masturbation is one commonly employed means of reducing the incidence of pregnancy, and is highly effective as such. It is also free of risks of transmission of human immunodeficiency virus (HIV) as long as fresh semen or vaginal fluids are not subsequently rubbed manually into the vagina, anus or skin lesions. Oral and anal sex are commonly used in many societies to gain sexual pleasure without risking fertility. Although the evidence linking oral sex to HIV transmission is weak and disputed, other genital infections, such as herpes, hepatitis and gonorrhoea are readily spread by this sexual practice. Oral sex (unprotected by use of a condom) is, however, clearly low risk for HIV transmission in either direction when compared with unprotected vaginal or anal sex. In the latter case, the epithelia lining the anus and rectum are more easily damaged than the vaginal epithelium, making bleeding more frequent and infection transmission to both the penetrated and penetrating partners more common. High-strength condoms (see below) substantially reduce the risk of transmission of infection anally. There is some evidence that circumcision may reduce the transmission of HIV to men.

Caps, diaphragms and spermicidal foams, jellies, creams and sponges

The combination of both a physical seal at the cervix between the vagina and the uterus, and a spermicide at the site of seminal deposition, has been used for over a century. The method became popular initially as, for the first time, it gave women some control over the use of contraception. However, the method has decreased in popularity with the development of more effective and convenient methods of contraception, and is now used by only 1% of women in the UK.

The diaphragm (Fig. 15.7), via its sprung margin, occludes the top of the vagina including the cervix. The smaller 'Dutch' or cervical cap fits directly over and around the cervical os, where it is held by suction. These devices can be fitted well in advance of intercourse, and should be left in place for at least 6 hours after coitus. As neither of them

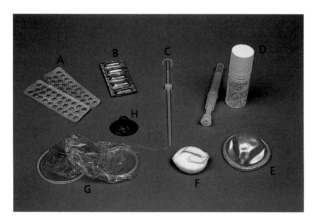

Fig. 15.7 Contraceptives. A, Two packs of oral contraceptives. B, Pack of vaginal spermicidal suppositories. C, Intrauterine contraceptive device (IUCD) (Copper T) emerging from its insertion catheter. Note that the IUCD is not entirely within the catheter; the two serrated arms remain exposed as the cannula is inserted through the cervix into the uterine lumen until the arms reach the fundus. When so located there, the insertion catheter is withdrawn leaving the IUCD in place with the thread tail on its end passing through the cervix. D, Spermicidal contraceptive foam with its applicator for insertion into the vagina. E, A diaphragm. F, Vaginal contraceptive sponge impregnated with spermicide. G, Female condom (Femidom). H, Male condom.

gives a perfect barrier, but will reduce the chances of spermatozoal passage deeper into the genital tract, they should only be used together with spermicides, which must be delivered into the vagina and/or placed in the device just before its insertion. Spermicides are available as foams or pessaries. It is not advised to use spermicides and spermicidally impregnated sponges *alone* for contraception. All spermicides contain nonoxinol-9, which can cause some epithelial disruption when used frequently, and so spermicides are not advised for use by women at risk of HIV transmission.

These contraceptive approaches give more control to the female partner and their use is relatively independent of intercourse compared with the condom (see below). They also offer protection from pelvic inflammatory disease. Their disadvantages are the requirements for careful fitting and training in use, high motivation, good hygiene and a willingness of women to touch their own internal genitalia. When used by motivated women they can be very effective, but otherwise can be of relatively low efficiency, clinical trials suggesting six-cycle pregnancy rates of around 7–10% (Table 15.2).

Condoms

Condoms (Fig. 15.7) are the commonest form of mechanical contraceptive in use (Fig. 15.5), particularly since their pro-

motion with the appearance of HIV (see Chapter 8). The improved strength, lubrication and design of modern condoms has considerably enhanced their efficiency and durability. Condoms are cheap, readily available and relatively easy to use, and also give protection against venereal diseases. Good use is crucial to their success (see Table 15.3).

The *female condom* has been marketed (under the brand name Femidom). It resembles an extra-large lubricated condom with a rimmed structure at the closed end, akin to the rim of a diaphragm, which fits into the vagina, thus protecting the cervical os in the vaginal vault (Fig. 15.7). It combines the protective advantages of the penile condom with many of the advantages of the diaphragm. Unlike the diaphragm, it does not require fitting or complex training in its use. Its user-friendliness and effectiveness remain the subject of research, but in general it is less effective than a properly used male condom, and is not popular.

Steroidal contraceptives for women

Since the initial development of the female 'pill' in the 1960s, a range of steroid-based contraceptives has been developed (Table 15.4), the oral pill being most popular in the UK (Fig. 15.5). Synthetic steroids, as described in Chapter 3 (Table 3.7), are used in these preparations as their half-lives in the body are longer and their effects therefore sustained. The general underlying principle is the suppression of ovulation by the negative and antipositive feedback effects of progesterone (with or without oestrogen) on the pituitary and hypothalamus (see Chapter 6). Additionally, progesterone can exert direct antifertility effects on the female genital tract to suppress sperm penetration through cervical mucus (Chapter 8) and endometrial receptivity (Chapter 10).

When considering these methods, it is important to remember that, 'naturally', female mammals living with males will not experience a series of oestrous cycles but will be pregnant or nursing for much of their fertile lives, and so will experience extended exposure to higher levels of oestrogens and progestagens. Humans, in contrast, are *atypical in being reproductively cyclic*, especially in modern developed societies. The steroidal contraceptives, in essence, mimic the continuous exposure to steroids experienced during pregnancy, during which of course the hypothalamic–pituitary axis is suppressed (see Chapters 6 & 11), and so, paradoxically, may take the endocrine status of women closer to that of most other female mammals.

The variables to consider in any steroidal contraceptive are: the *nature* of the steroidal components (oestrogens + progestagens, or progestagens only?); the *potency* and *dose* of the synthetic steroid(s) used; and the *duration of exposure* to steroids of different types or doses. A maximal contra-

Table 15.3 Condom use.

Do	Don't
Use kite-marked only	Don't use after 5 years old or exposed to excessive heat or UV light
Use water-based lubricants (KY jelly, glycerol, spermicides such as nonoxynol-9*)	Don't use oil-based lubricants (vaseline, baby oil, suntan lotions)
Use only once	Don't allow penis to become flaccid inside partner
Take care not to tear or snag condom	Don't have genital/anal contact after condom removal, unless penis washed
Put on penis before any genital/anal contact	Don't use ordinary strength condoms if having anal intercourse
Use spermicides/bacteriocides/viricides (foams, pessaries, sponges)	
Use condoms if risk of HIV, hepatitis, herpes, gonorrhoea, chlamydia or cervical dysplasia	

*Note: frequent use of nonoxynol can result in a mild inflammatory response of vaginal epithelium, which can increase risk of viral transmission.

ceptive effect and complete continuous amenorrhoea is provided by *high* doses of *both* types of steroid *continuously* present. However, against this optimal contraceptive regimen must be balanced: the side effects of the steroids (as also observed during pregnancy: Chapters 8 & 11); a woman's perception and concern about what is happening to her reproductive system when it is closed down completely such that menstruation ceases; and the requirement that reproductive capacity be recovered reasonably rapidly when contraceptive practice ceases. How can each of the potential variables be adjusted to maintain effective contraception while minimizing or eliminating the influence of these non-contraceptive concerns?

Combined oestrogen/progestagen contraception. Progesterone alone can suppress ovulation, but it does so with variable efficiency unless present constantly (see later). Oestrogen addition exerts an additional negative feedback effect of its own and also promotes the development of progesterone receptors (see Chapter 8), which renders the progestagens in the contraceptive more effective. Thus, the *combined oral contraceptive* (COC) uses, as its name implies, both types of steroid (Table 15.4). This contraceptive is usually taken for 21 days, during which time the output of endogenous gonadotrophins, follicular growth and thus ovarian oestrogen are completely suppressed (Fig. 15.8). The exogenous hormones develop and maintain the endometrial lining. This period of suppression is then followed by a 7-day break, with either no pills or placebo pills. During this period, the endometrium breaks down, which leads to a *withdrawal bleeding* that *simulates* menstruation. This withdrawal bleeding is important to many women psychologically, as it 'confirms' their cyclicity and lack of pregnancy (although, of course, it does not reflect a true ovarian cycle).

Without it, some women will discontinue contraceptive use, and so it is of importance for *compliance*, an essential element of a contraceptive's effectiveness. However, the absence of exogenous steroids for 7 days results in a reawakening of the woman's own hypothalamic–pituitary axis, a rising output of gonadotrophins and follicular development (Fig. 15.8). Indeed, towards the end of the 7-day pill-free period, some women can come dangerously close to ovulating. A failure to take the first active pill of the new series, or interference with its effectiveness (e.g. vomiting it up), can lead to contraceptive failure. This 21 days on, 7 days off regimen is called *monocyclic*. For more assured contraceptive efficiency, and for women who experience severe withdrawal symptoms (quasimenstrual tension) or for whom a regular bleed is socially or medically difficult, a recommended alternative is the use of the pill on a *bi-* or *tricyclic* regimen, in which the relative durations of active pill : placebo are 42 : 7 or 63 : 7 days, respectively. Such regimens, of course, lose the 'regular cycle' appearance, important for some pill users. (*Note:* these regimens should not be confused with bi- and triphasic pills, see below.)

It will be clear from this discussion that the regimen to be used is best tailored to the psychological, physical and social condition and needs of each woman. This personal tailoring also extends to the potency and dose of the constituent steroids used. Individual women react differently to the same preparation, some being more sensitive than others and so requiring lower doses or less potent preparations. The level and balance of oestrogens (now 20–35 μg ethinyl oestradiol) and progestagens (norethisterone and levonorgestrel; desogestrel and gestodene; norgestimate; and drospirenone) varies in different preparations, thereby offering a range of contraceptives to suit women with

Table 15.4 Steroid-based contraceptives for women.

	Oral COC*	Oral POP†	Injectables	Implants	LNG IUS‡
Administration					
Frequency	Daily	Daily	2- to 3-monthly	5-yearly	3 months
Relative progestagen dose	Low	Ultra-low	High	Ultra-low	Ultra-low
Blood levels	Rapidly fluctuating	Rapidly fluctuating	Initial peak then decline	Constant	Constant
How does it work?					
Ovary: ovulation suppressed§	+++	+	++	++	–
Cervical mucus: sperm penetrability down	Yes	Yes	Yes	Yes	Yes
Endometrium: receptivity to blastocyst down	Yes	Yes	Yes	Yes	Yes
User failure rates (%)	0.2–3	3–5	0.5–1	0.1	0.1
Menstrual pattern	Regular	Often irregular	Irregular	Irregular	Irregular
Amenorrhoea during use	Rare	Occasional	Common	Common	Usual
Reversibility					
Immediate termination possible?	Yes	Yes	No	Yes	Yes
By woman herself at any time?	Yes	Yes	No	No	No
Time to first likely conception from first omitted dose/removal	3 months	c.1 month	3–6 months	c.1 month	c.1 month
Usage rates in the UK (%)	18	5	3		1

*COC, combined (oestrogen and progestagen) oral contraceptive.
†POP, progesterone only pill.
‡LNG IUS, levonorgestrel-releasing intrauterine system.
§By two mechanisms—no preovulatory follicles formed and/or no LH surges occur.
Data adapted from Guillebaud J (1993) *Contraception: Your Questions Answered*. Churchill Livingstone, Edinburgh.

different clinical histories and physiologies. As a rule of thumb, it is best to go for the lowest dose of steroids possible, and this may be estimated as being just above the dose that gives *breakthrough bleeding*, an endometrial blood loss occurring *while the woman is taking an active preparation*. Breakthrough bleeding reflects inadequate support for the endometrium by the exogenous contraceptive steroids, and provides an indication of the woman's sensitivity to their action.

Other variants of the oral contraceptive include changing the ratio of oestrogen to progesterone in different pills during the 21-day cycle. The intention here is to mimic the natural cycle more closely. The now discontinued *sequential oral contraceptives* used oestrogens only for 7–14 days and a combined oestrogen–progestagen mix for 14 or 7 days, followed by 7 pill-free days. However, these pills required

higher doses of oestrogen and were less efficient contraceptively. In contrast, *biphasic and triphasic oral contraceptives* combine the mimicry of a normal cycle attempted in sequential preparations with the contraceptive efficiency of monocyclic COCs. Thus, in biphasic preparations, both oestrogen and progestagen are given for the first half of the cycle, but the progestagen dose is stepped up at midcycle. The contraceptive efficiency is as good as in the conventional combined tablets, but the doses of steroid used are lower. In triphasic preparations, 5 or 6 days have low oestrogen and low progestagen, a further 5 or 6 days have both oestrogen and progestagen slightly elevated, and the remaining 10 days have low oestrogen and doubled progestagen. These preparations place increasing emphasis on the capacity of progestagens to block the positive feedback effect of oestrogen and less on direct negative feedback

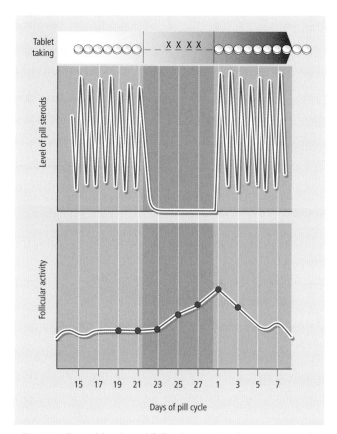

Fig. 15.8 Steroid levels and follicular activity during monocyclic use of the combined oral contraceptive. The days of pill-taking are indicated at the top by small pill symbols, while the pill-free days are dashed. 'X' indicates the days of withdrawal bleeding. The profile of synthetic steroids in the blood (upper panel) reflects the episodic (daily) taking of the pill. Levels fall rapidly when pill-taking ceases. The lower panel shows follicular activity measurable by ultrasound scan (see Fig. 15.11) and reflected in the output of endogenous steroids. Activity is low while the pill is taken, but note how rapidly follicles develop when pill-taking ceases, so reducing negative feedback and leading to rising gonadotrophin output. Resumption of pill-taking leads to immediate suppression. Note that a failure to resume pill-taking on time leaves a woman potentially vulnerable to ovulation and pregnancy.

effects (see Chapter 6). In consequence, oestrogen levels are lower and a more normal 'cycle' is achieved.

A *transdermal patch contraceptive* combining norgelstromin and ethinyl oestradiol (Evra) has been licensed. Each patch is applied for 7 days and then replaced by a new patch. After three patches, a 7-day patch-free period allows breakthrough bleeding. The contraceptive effectiveness is similar to that of triphasics, and self-reported compliance was higher. Side effects were more marked than for oral contraceptives for the first two to three cycles of use, but not thereafter.

Progestagen-only contraception. These contraceptives may be taken daily by an oral route or given by injection subcutaneously for continuous release over a period of 8 weeks, or as implants for up to 5 years. In addition, progesterone-impregnated IUCDs are available (see below and Table 15.4). Some 8% of women in the UK use one of these approaches. Progesterone-only pills (POPs) are taken continuously, contain low doses of progestagen, and work primarily by effects on cervical mucus and perhaps the endometrium (see Chapters 8 & 10). However, in a significant proportion of users (around 20%), ovulation is suppressed, and, in around 40%, follicular–luteal activity is abnormal. In all users, irregular bleeding may occur. Because the dose of progesterone used is small and the pill is taken daily, side effects are relatively few compared with COCs, although weight gain can be problematic because of progesterone's anabolic effects (see Chapter 8). However, the effect of the progesterone on cervical mucus lasts for only 22–26 h. Therefore, if the woman is significantly delayed in taking her daily pill, fertility returns. This requirement for a highly organized lifestyle and level of commitment is reflected in the much more variable contraceptive effectiveness.

Implanted depot progestagens, in contrast, are extremely effective contraceptives and used by millions of women worldwide, although less so in more developed countries (8% in UK). Implants lasting 5 years (levonorgestrel), 3 years (etonogestrel), or 2 years (nestorone) are available commercially in silicon capsules or rods (crystalline steroid). Follicular growth and ovulation are disrupted (Chapter 5), and any luteal phase function is inadequate, and this is the primary mechanism of contraceptive action, any effect on mucus and the endometrium being secondary. No major adverse effects have been reported, the method is fully reversible, and, despite some irregular bleeding, there appears to be high user satisfaction.

Injectable progestagens lie between orals and implants, and include depot medroxyprogesterone acetate (DMPA; renew every 12 weeks) and norethisterone enantate (NETEN; renew every 8 weeks). Injectables provide faster release systems that generate relatively high, ovulation-suppressing levels of steroid initially, which fall to mucus-affecting levels as the time for the next injection approaches. Their use is often associated with irregular bleeding and weight gain, with the positive side effect of reduced iron loss and anaemia.

(See also levonorgestrel-releasing intrauterine system or LNG IUS under IUCD below.)

Side effects of steroidal contraceptives. We have stressed the balance between contraceptive efficiency and unwanted side effects. Some of the unwanted side effects are social or psychological, such as the need either for a regular bleed or for no bleed at all, or a requirement for highly organized self-administration or the availability of good medical care. Other minor side effects can include weight gain, headaches, libido changes and acne, each of which will be specific for an individual woman and will vary with different preparations. All of these factors are extremely important, as marrying the physiology, psychology and social condition of the woman to her contraceptive is the key element in providing effective and *acceptable* contraception for her.

However, beyond these elements, there has also been widespread concern and discussion about more severe life-threatening side effects of steroidal contraceptives. There are two general points that need to be made emphatically. First, the life-threatening risk associated with modern steroidal contraception is fourfold lower than that from pregnancy, childbirth and pregnancy termination, and much less than that associated with driving a car. Second, there is little evidence that steroidal contraceptives *cause* life-threatening conditions, but they may be co-associated with *other* causal agents to promote *their* effects. Because these co-associated factors are known, the risk can be quantified for each woman.

There is evidence that the oestrogen in COCs increases clotting factors and blood coagulability (see Chapter 8), although they also increase fibrinolytic activity but *only* in the absence of smoking. The current increased risk of venous thromboembolism in women taking low-dose oestrogen monophasic COCs is estimated as threefold relative risk, but the absolute risk is small, increasing from 5 to 15 per 100 000 woman-years of use, and there is no increase in mortality. The companion progestagen in the COC influences relative risk, desogestrel and gestodene counteracting the prothrombotic effects of ethinyl oestradiol less than do levonorgestrel or norethisterone. None of the progesterone-only contraceptives increases the risk of venous thromboembolism. Thus two main general factors contraindicate combined steroidal contraception: smoking and obesity (body mass index > 30), especially in older women; and a history of thromboembolic or cardiovascular disease. Additionally, migraine, breast and liver tumours, and severe cirrhosis make COCs unacceptable. Finally, women should discontinue COC usage at least 4 weeks before major surgery or immobilization. For all of these cases, progesterone-only contraception can be considered (see below).

The broad effects of modern steroidal contraceptives on cancers are neutral. Benign breast cancer and carcinomas of endometrium and ovary (both very serious conditions) are *reduced* in pill users. A slight increase in hepatic carcinoma occurs, as does breast cancer, among women who have taken the pill for several years before the age of 25, an outcome perhaps related to the effects of progestagens on cell division in the postpubertal, developing breast. Increased cervical dysplasia is also reported, but may be secondary to increased coital activity without condoms rather than a direct effect of steroids. These observations emphasize the value of regular cervical smear and breast examinations in women on steroidal contraceptives.

The latent diabetes revealed in some women during pregnancy (see Chapter 12) can also become evident in users of steroidal contraceptives, who should therefore only use low-dose oestrogen preparations under careful supervision.

A plus for most women on steroidal contraception is the reduced incidence of pelvic inflammatory disease, a potent cause of infertility (see later). It is not clear why this is so, as genitourinary infections of the vagina are, if anything, increased. One idea is that infectious agents hitch a ride on spermatozoa, but the hostility of cervical mucus prevents their passage further into the female genital tract.

Postcoital emergency contraception

Postcoital emergency contraception was discussed in Chapter 8 (see Box 8.2) and antiprogestagens below.

Antiprogestagens

Antiprogestagens such as mifepristone (also called RU486, see Table 3.7) act as a luteal phase contraceptive and early abortifacient. It functions by occupying and blocking progesterone receptors but does not block follicular growth and oestrogen output. A putative advantage of mifepristone is that it might only be needed once a month to target particular points in the cycle. Trials to test this possibility show that administration early in the luteal phase (as emergency contraception within 120 hours after coitus) prevented most pregnancies. When taken at the mid or late luteal phase when implantation has occurred, RU486 fails to induce menses in a significant portion of cases. It is thus not as useful as modern COCs and progesterone-only contraceptives.

Steroidal contraceptives for men

Just as in the female, the output of gonadotrophin-releasing hormone (GnRH) and/or gonadotrophins can be suppressed in the male via negative feedback using androgens, progesterone or the continuous administration of a GnRH analogue (Table 3.7). In the latter two cases, endogenous androgens are depressed, reducing masculinizing stimulation and libido, both unacceptable side effects. Thus, all contraceptive preparations for men include synthetic androgen itself. However, trials have been disappointing. Trials using weekly injections of testosterone enanthate produced azoospermia in 2/3 of men and oligospermia (as little as 3×10^6/ml of semen) in the rest. However, androgen levels were very high, and there were large individual and ethnic variations in response. Combination of implants of testosterone with oral, injected or implanted progestagen has proved more promising, with severe oligopsermia ($<1 \times 10^6$/ml) in most men. Side effects include acne, weight gain and oily skin, which may affect long-term compliance. There is also some concern that treatment with the high doses of testosterone required may exacerbate the risk of prostatic hyperplasia, which is quite common in older men. It seems unlikely that hormonal contraception for men will have a major impact on fertility control.

Intrauterine contraceptive devices (IUCD or IUD)

Modern IUCDs, used by around 5% of UK women (Table 15.2), are made of copper, the older purely plastic models being no longer in use. The T380A (T Safe 380A in UK) is the gold standard among those models available. IUCDs function as foreign bodies within the uterus to produce a low-grade, local, chronic inflammatory response, the composition of the uterine luminal fluid resembling a serum transudate containing large numbers of invading leucocytes. The use of copper enhances contraceptive effectiveness because, in addition to copper's inflammatory effects, it also has specific spermotoxic and embryotoxic effects. There is a broad correlation between the capacity of the IUCD to induce inflammation and its efficiency as a contraceptive. Such a uterine environment reduces transport of viable sperm to the oviduct and thereby fertilization, is toxic for oocytes and any fertilized eggs that do form, and impairs implantation and decidualization. In addition, luteal life may be abbreviated because of premature prostaglandin release in some species (see Chapter 6). Overall, most but not all the contraceptive effect is thought to be prefertilization. These multiple sites of action make the IUCD highly effective, the copper T380A being as effective as the combined oral contraceptive (Table 15.2).

For obvious reasons, contraindications to IUCD insertion include a history of pelvic inflammatory disease, heavy or painful periods, and anatomical abnormality of the uterus. Possible complications following IUCD insertion are: heavy menstrual or irregular uterine blood loss (*dysmenorrhoea*); uterine pain or muscular spasm; and rarely (<0.01%) uterine perforation. Earlier suggestions to avoid IUCD insertion in nulliparous women seem to be without foundation, probably because copper IUCDs are smaller than plastic ones and produce fewer side effects and spontaneous expulsions. Immediately after insertion, but not thereafter, there is an elevated risk of pelvic inflammatory disease. Unnoticed expulsion of the IUCD can also occur (up to 1/20 in the first year of use), as can rare pregnancies with the IUCD still in place. There is no evidence of any effect of IUCD use on subsequent fertility or increased risk of reproductive

tract cancer. The skills required for insertion, and the desirability of regular monitoring of patients, mean that trained and available medical or paramedical staff are needed. The IUCD is a widely used and very effective contraceptive device, and is also highly effective as a postcoital contraceptive (see Box 8.2).

An extra twist to the contraceptive action of the IUCD is to combine a plastic T-shaped IUCD with steroidal contraception by use of the progesterone-impregnated IUCD (*levonorgestrel-releasing intrauterine system or LNG IUS*). The IUS delivers progesterone directly to its major peripheral sites of action: cervical mucus and the endometrium, leading to amenorrhoea, and so it is also used to regulate severe bleeding (*menorrhagia*; see Table 15.4).

The future

A range of variably effective sexual techniques, devices and pharmaceutical preparations now exists to limit reproduction. The use of these, tailored to the needs of the individual or couple concerned, should be adequate for effective control of fertility, high acceptability and good compliance. The problem is not with the technology but with its use, issues of education, support and motivation being paramount. It is unlikely, given the restrictions on clinical trials imposed in recent years, that a totally new range of contraceptive approaches will be available in the near future. Most advances have come from modifying and refining existing methods in the light of evidence-based practice.

Considerable research into immunological contraceptive approaches is ongoing. For example, active immunity to the specific β-chain terminal sequence of human chorionic gonadotrophin (hCG) neutralizes the embryonic hormone but leaves LH unaffected, thereby giving normal (or slightly lengthened) cycles and protection against pregnancy (see Chapter 11). Results of advanced trials using this approach have been encouraging. No side effects have been noted, and the immunity declines after about 6 months in the absence of a booster injection, so the approach should be reversible. Alternatively, immunity to antigens on spermatozoa, in semen or on the zona pellucida is known, from clinical and experimental studies on primates, to be associated with infertility. Such an approach has been harnessed for contraceptive use, using immunization to recombinant proteins of the zona pellucida and an epididymidal protein called eppin. However, there is a reasonable reluctance to tinker with the body's immune system until more is understood about its natural regulation. Uncontrollable side effects, such as a wider autoimmune response, might develop after extended use of a 'contraceptive vaccine', particularly one that utilizes cellular or cell-associated antigens. Moreover, there is wide variation among individuals in immune responsiveness, which makes for a corresponding and unacceptable variation in contraceptive effectiveness.

More speculative are approaches to the control of implantation deriving from our increased understanding of the cytokines involved (Chapter 9). The potent antipregnancy effects of knocking out genes for some of these cytokines have encouraged speculation that anticytokines might provide a good route to contraception. However, this possibility seems to be some way off.

Pregnancy termination

Clinical termination of pregnancy (abortion) is appropriate for women whose mental or physical health would be put at risk by a continuing pregnancy. Pregnancy termination is also, whether performed legally or illegally, an approach to fertility control in many communities, especially where contraception is not readily available or is unreliable. In the UK, it is estimated that at least one-third of women will have had a pregnancy termination by the age of 45. The legal position concerning medical termination is complex and details vary widely in different jurisdictions. Where fetal abnormality is suspected (through age of mother, a parent with a balanced translocation, exposure of the mother to potential teratogens, prior evidence of familial risk or as a result of a suspicious ultrasound scan) confirmatory tests may be recommended clinically which may include chorionic villous sampling and/or amniotic fluid sampling (amniocentesis). See Box 15.2 for more details.

About 40% of UK terminations are carried out in the first trimester (or 3 months) of pregnancy. Up to 9 weeks of pregnancy, medical terminations are recommended using antiprogestagens (such as mifepristone/RU486: see below) plus a prostaglandin E1 analogue (misoprostol). From 7 to 12 weeks, surgical termination most usually by vacuum aspiration is used. Failure rates using these approaches are low (<1%), as are complications, such as major blood loss, incomplete aspiration or damage to the cervix or uterus. The side effects of postoperative infection and damage to the uterus or cervix may affect subsequent fertility. After 12 weeks, surgical termination by dilatation and physical evacuation is recommended.

Risks versus effectiveness

Individuals require control over their fertility to be 100% effective at each sexual encounter, with zero risk of side effects. In practice, this requirement is not always achieved using conventional coital techniques with existing methods of fertility control. Thus, resort to multiple, or hierarchical, levels of fertility control tends to occur. Social regulation of sexual encounters is followed by use of natural or barrier

---

BOX 15.2 Chorionic villous sampling (CVS) and amniocentesis

- *Some 5% of pregnant women* are offered one of these invasive prenatal diagnostic tests, usually for chromosomal analysis of the conceptus. There are small associated risks that are related strongly to operator experience, which should ideally exceed a minimum of 10 procedures per year and be audited.
- *Amniocentesis* is more commonly offered, and mostly undertaken after 15 weeks of pregnancy (advised only exceptionally at earlier times). An ultrasound-guided 0.9 mm (20 gauge) needle tip is inserted transabdominally. Ultrasound guidance reduces maternal blood contamination, and damage to maternal and fetal organs. The aspirated fluid sample is spun and divided into amniocyte cells, which are considered fetal in origin, and the overlying liquid. The cells are tested cytogenetically, and the fluid can be examined (especially in third trimester) for evidence of rhesus disease, lung maturity, infection, and insulin levels. Women who are HIV positive should avoid amniocentesis if possible as the chance of maternofetal transmission increases. There is an associated miscarriage rate of around 1% in amniocentesis carried out later than 15 weeks of pregancy.
- *Before 15 weeks of pregnancy, CVS is safer than amniocentesis.* It is usually undertaken between 10 and 13 weeks of gestation, and is considered unsafe earlier. Overall, CVS is usually regarded as less safe than amniocentesis, but the evidence is variable. CVS involves ultrasound-guided aspiration of placental tissue, usually transcervically but sometimes (especially if done later than 13 weeks) via a percutaneous transabdominal route. The placental/trophoblastic tissue sample may be taken by aspiration or microforceps.

---

techniques. Failure of these approaches leads to use of postcoital contraception or to menstrual regulation. There should be little need for unwanted pregnancy in more sophisticated societies, given the cumulative contraceptive efficiency of these various approaches.

With the use of some contraceptive approaches there may be attendant risks to health, well-being or even life. However, although these risks should not be minimized, their impact is often somewhat exaggerated. For example, many of the contraindications to the use of steroidal contraceptives, such as thromboembolic episodes, cardiovascular problems or latent diabetes, also apply to pregnancy or the surgical procedures required for sterilization. Among groups not at risk from steroidal contraceptives, pregnancy itself and abortion constitute much greater risks to health and life. Thus, the balance of risks must be evaluated for each individual. The optimal situation is a combination of well-educated general practitioners, a readily available range of contraceptives, and easy and rapid access to early clinical pregnancy termination. Sadly, this combination is rare anywhere, and in most of the world it is simply not available.

Subfertility

Couples or individuals are described as subfertile when they fail to conceive within the time scale expected from the fecundibility level for their age group (see earlier). Conventionally, couples having frequent, unprotected intercourse are not defined as being clinically subfertile until they have *failed to conceive within 1 year*. The recent prospective fecundibility studies reported earlier may lead to revision of this criterion for women under 35, since fecundity estimates were 20% per cycle. Subfertility may be contributed to by either or both partners, a relatively minor problem for each sometimes becoming a more serious problem for both. Conventionally, a clinical investigation attempts to *locate* the subfertility to the male, the female or the couple, and to *categorize* it as *primary* or *secondary subfertility*. If neither partner has conceived or fathered a pregnancy before, the subfertility of each and of the couple is said to be primary. If either or both have parented a pregnancy with another partner previously, then subfertility is primary for the couple only, and secondary for each individual. Where the couple has had a previous pregnancy (whether or not it went to term) but now are having problems conceiving, their subfertility is described as secondary.

Estimates of the prevalence of subfertility are rough and ready, as many factors, especially the age distribution of the population, impinge on it. Conventionally, 10–15% of couples are said to experience difficulty with conception and successful delivery of a healthy child, but the prospective studies on women mostly under 35 suggested only 5%. The higher conventional estimate may reflect the increased proportion of older women trying to conceive.

Causes of subfertility

The causes of subfertility vary greatly with socioeconomic and geographical factors. The male and female partners contribute more or less equally to the problem, but for many couples the diagnosis is 'unexplained subfertility', a catch-all diagnostic category that in part reveals our ignorance (Fig. 15.9). Psychological factors causing sexual dysfunction (such as erectile dysfunction, vaginal spasm, premature ejaculation and disorders of sexual identity) are not uncommon among infertile patients, but they may often be responses to, rather than the primary causes of, the infertile state.

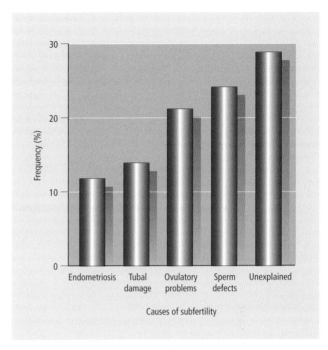

Fig. 15.9 Causes of subfertility in UK couples, expressed as a percentage frequency distribution.

Three major classes of disorder account for about 75–80% of all explicable cases of infertility (Fig. 15.9): disorders of the female tract (in particular blocked or damaged Fallopian tubes); disorders of ovulation; and poor quality or quantity of spermatozoa. In addition, there is evidence that human fertility patterns are influenced by the substantial (20–25%) loss of clinically diagnosed pregnancies in both fertile and subfertile couples.

Approaches to treatment

For a couple wishing to have a child, a diagnosis of subfertility can be protracted, stressful and socially isolating, as are many of the therapeutic options available. Moreover, for many couples, the biological clock is ticking and so pressure for early results builds. The increasing desperation of the couple combined with an eagerness of clinical staff to appear helpful and media hype about new developments can inflate expectations unrealistically. Although great strides have been made in treating subfertility, it is important for couples to realize at the outset that most treatment attempts end in failure, and that recourse to multiple lines of treatment, often through a hierarchy of different approaches, may be used, each treatment serving itself as a diagnostic tool to refine understanding of the couple's condition. Given that most couples fund their treatment, wholly or in part, the stresses of uncertainty and of the clock ticking are often compounded by financial stress.

The emphasis that clinics and the media place on 'success' rates in treating subfertility implies for many couples who leave treatment childless that they have failed. For this reason, it is useful to talk of outcome or live baby rates, and to build into the consultations from the outset both realism and serious discussion of options, including acceptance of the state of childlessness. The best clinics will view a successful treatment as one in which the total experience of the couple has been positive regardless of the precise outcome. Fortunately, more clinics are now adopting this approach, being attentive to the psychosocial support and honest informational needs of the couple and the attitudes underlying the actions and words of the whole subfertility team.

Certain general factors predispose to reduced fertility and need to be explored sensitively, with support and advice, early on. Key adverse factors to consider are poor communication or conflicting desires between the partners being treated, lack of knowledge about how and when best to conceive, obesity (especially in the woman), smoking, moderate to excessive alcoholic consumption, drug use, excessive caffeine intake, poor diet, and stress (occupational or social). Studies show that simply attending to adverse factors can result in spontaneous pregnancies without technical intervention, as well as enhancing the chance of pregnancy after more technological treatments.

A general outline of approaches to treatment is given below for different conditions, emphasizing the underlying biology explored in earlier chapters.

Disorders of the female tract

Tubal damage is often a consequence of pelvic infection, being associated with sexually transmitted disease such as untreated frank or asymptomatic gonorrhoea or chlamydial infection, tuberculosis, or sepsis following a termination or a completed pregnancy. Tubal infection leads to loss of cilia on the intraluminal cells, causing impaired oocyte and spermatozoal transport, and to extraoviducal scarring, leading to adhesions that restrict oviducal movement and oocyte pick-up, or may result in physical blockage of the fimbrial ends of the tubes (Chapter 9).

The diagnosis of *tubal obstruction* is preferably made by X-ray (*hysterosalpingogram*) using a radio-opaque dye or by instilling a small volume of fluid into the cavity of the uterus, observed using ultrasound (*sonohysterography*). Both are less invasive than visual assessment of the intra-abdominal pelvic organs with a laparoscope and by attempting to insufflate dye from the cervix through the tubes under direct vision, which may be advised if predisposing co-morbidities are present.

At present, microsurgical treatment for this large group of patients has limited success for mild disease only, and

requires a centre with high expertise for good outcomes. More effective therapy is provided by aspiration of oocytes from the ovary and *in vitro fertilization* (IVF) (Fig. 15.10), followed by placement of the conceptuses into the uterus, thereby bypassing the damaged tubes. When IVF technology is to be used, follicular growth is usually controlled exogenously by: (1) shutting down the woman's own hypothalamic activity via several days' administration of GnRH analogue (such as buserelin, see Table 3.7 & Chapter 6); (2) then administering a recombinant FSH preparation; and (3) monitoring follicular growth by ultrasound scanning of the ovary (Fig. 15.11). Intrafollicular oocytes are recovered when almost fully matured using a needle inserted through the vault of the vagina under continuous monitoring by transvaginal ultrasound scanning. The needle is inserted into each follicle which is then flushed with warm culture medium, and the oocyte collected by aspiration with its cumulus cells into a sterile receptacle. Spermatozoa are provided from the male partner by masturbation or, if obstructive azoospermia is present, by sampling the epididymis or extracting spermatozoa from a biopsy of the testis (see later).

Endometriosis, in which endometrial tissue grows inappropriately in ectopic sites such as the oviduct, ovary or peritoneal cavity, may cause a severe reaction in which the body responds by scarring and adhesion formation. It is often associated with dyspareunia and dysmenorrhoea, and its origins and pathogenesis remain unclear. Treatment is by laparoscopic ablation, and even when the endometriosis is minimal treatment almost halves the time to conception.

Uterine absence or malformation, or health problems in the female partner that make carrying a pregnancy unwise, can be circumvented by *surrogacy*. In *partial surrogacy*, the male partner provides sperm to inseminate the surrogate mother, who provides the oocyte. Partial surrogacy would be used where ovarian damage or absence has occurred, and does not *require* medical intervention, but is most safely undertaken with medical assistance. Full or complete surrogacy involves use of IVF with the gametes of the *commissioning couple* to produce a conceptus for transfer to the surrogate woman's uterus. Legal regulation of surrogacy arrangements varies among different jurisdictions, but in general (and in the UK) the birth mother rather than the commissioning couple/mother has the prior legal claim regardless of the source of the oocyte.

Disorders of ovulation

This general classification covers a range of disorders. Primary amenorrhoea was discussed earlier, as was premature menopause through early ovarian failure. Here we consider only disorders relating to malfunction of the matured reproductive system: namely, absent cycles (*sec-

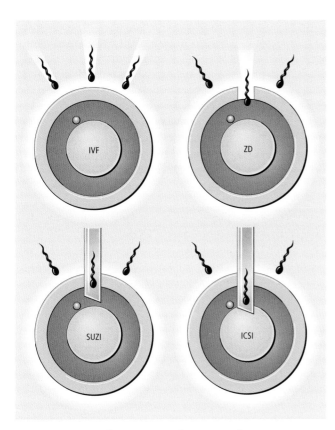

Fig. 15.10 Assisted conception techniques used to overcome infertility. In IVF, oocytes (shown as pink) are recovered from the female partner's ovary (or by donation from another female), usually after hormonally induced stimulation, and spermatozoa are recovered from the male partner (or by donation from another male). The two are then mixed *in vitro* for 24–48 h; the oocytes that have been fertilized are identified by the appearance of pronuclei and passage through cleavage to two to four cells, and up to two fertilized zygotes are placed in the uterus via a transcervical catheter. Any fertilized oocytes remaining may be frozen with reasonable success for later use, should this be necessary. After IVF, average pregnancy rates per treatment cycle initiated at established clinics in the UK are about 25%. Zona drilling (ZD) is identical to IVF except that prior to insemination a small hole is made in the zona pellucida (shown as grey) mechanically, by laser or by local application of a zona-dissolving chemical, to facilitate the access of spermatozoa to the oocyte. This approach is useful if the seminal quality is poor or if the oocytes are surrounded by particularly tough zonae, but can lead to polyspermy. The hole may also facilitate the escape of the blastocyst from the zona pellucida prior to attachment and implantation (see Chapter 10). Subzonal insemination (SUZI) involves the placement of one or more spermatozoa under the zona pellucida using a micropipette, while intracytoplasmic injection (ICSI) involves use of the micropipette to inject a single spermatozoon into the ooplasm. Both these techniques are useful for men with very low sperm numbers, ICSI being useful where there are no motile spermatozoa or even only epididymidal or testicular spermatozoa or spermatids (e.g. in obstructive azoospermia).

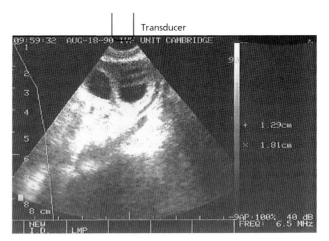

Transducer

Fig. 15.11 Transvaginal ultrasound scan of a human ovary showing two developing follicles, the largest of which has an average diameter of about 1.6 mm.

ondary amenorrhoea) and irregular cycles (*oligomenorrhoea*), both of which are indicative of *anovulatory cycles*. As the hypothalamus plays such a key role in regulating ovarian function via the pituitary, it is not surprising that these conditions are often associated with stress, obesity, strenuous exercise, anorexia nervosa or use of various drugs, such as neuroleptics or tranquillizers, and may resolve if the primary cause is removed or its effects alleviated. Indeed, in one study, merely taking women into clinical care and giving placebo treatments resulted in 30% of cases having successful pregnancies! Many other patients, although classified as oligomenorrhoeic or secondarily amenorrhoeic, have never had entirely normal cycles and could therefore represent failures of terminal maturation of the neuroendocrine system at puberty.

The endocrine features of a normal menstrual cycle were described in Chapter 6, and the associated cyclical changes in the woman's anatomy and physiology in Chapter 8. An ideal clinical investigation would examine all of these through at least one cycle, but such a procedure would be time-consuming, costly and inconvenient. In practice, therefore, a more limited range of preliminary tests is applied in an attempt to locate the endocrine defect. In the patient with cycles, a midluteal phase measurement of progesterone is the simplest screening test to give an indication as to whether or not she is ovulating. Several underlying causes of ovulation disorders can be identified.

Hyperprolactinaemia

Hyperprolactinaemia is a relatively common cause of menstrual irregularity and ovulation failure (discussed in Chapter 6 in some detail). Diagnosis is by two or more blood samples ideally taken at the same time of day under non-stressful conditions. Magnetic resonance imaging

(MRI) may also be performed to look for evidence of changes in the sella turcica caused by enlarging pituitary tumours, which may press on the optic chiasma. However, most cases of hyperprolactinaemia are due to microadenomas, which are unseen with routine imaging and are without effects on the visual system. Hyperprolactinaemia not requiring surgery is treated with bromocriptine or cabergoline, both dopamine D_2 receptor agonists.

Hypothalamic–pituitary insufficiency

Deficiency of GnRH in reaching the pituitary results in depressed gonadotrophin and oestrogen levels and failure of ovulation with oligo- or amenorrhoea (*hypogonadotrophic hypogonadism*). Ultrasonically, quiescent ovaries and a thin endometrium will be identified. Patients can be treated therapeutically with exogenous gonadotrophins, but the use of a pump to deliver pulsatile infusions of GnRH subcutaneously (as described experimentally in Chapters 6 & 7) is a more physiological approach and does not carry the same risk of multiple pregnancy.

Idiopathic anovulation

In other cases, gonadotrophin secretion seems to be occurring within the normal range, but is insufficient to support a normal cycle, probably as a result of ovarian insensitivity. In consequence, oestrogen levels fail to rise appropriately and ultrasonography of the ovary reveals antral follicles that fail to mature fully. Most cases will respond to therapy with exogenous gonadotrophins to recruit or maintain follicular growth and oestrogen output. The endogenous LH surge is usually attenuated and, hence, is supplemented or replaced by an injection of hCG (to mimic the ovulating effect of LH). However, the appropriate doses of gonadotrophins can be difficult to gauge and slight overdosing can lead to multiple ovulations and implantations or, in some cases, to *ovarian hyperstimulation*. Their use should be accompanied by ovarian ultrasound monitoring to measure follicle size and number and to adjust gonadotrophin doses accordingly.

Because of these difficulties and the cost of using gonadotrophins, a simpler regimen using antioestrogens, such as oral *clomiphene citrate* or *tamxifen*, tends to be used initially. Antioestrogens act on the hypothalamus to compete with endogenous oestrogen and thereby reduce its negative feedback, resulting in elevated gonadotrophins. Clomiphene also stimulates aromatase activity in the ovary, and the ovarian oestrogen produced then stimulates granulosa cell proliferation and development of LH receptors (see Chapter 5), and thereby ovarian responsiveness. Clomiphene tablets are administered early in the follicular phase, usually on days 2–6 or 5–9 of the cycle, and yield positive ovulatory responses in around 70% of anovulatory women (especially when they are not obese).

An assessment as to whether treatment with clomiphene or gonadotrophins is likely to be of greatest use is made with the *progesterone challenge test*, which estimates the circulating levels of oestrogen (as a marker of follicular maturation) and thus the likelihood of responsiveness to clomiphene. A synthetic progestagen is administered to the amenorrhoeic or oligomenorrhoeic woman for about 5 days and then stopped. If sufficient levels of natural oestrogen are present to prime the endometrium to respond to the progestagen, a withdrawal bleed will be precipitated. Absence of a bleed indicates low endogenous oestrogens and the likelihood that gonadotrophins may be more successful than clomiphene.

Polycystic ovarian syndrome (PCOS)

This distinct and common syndrome (found in 5–10% of women of reproductive age) is also associated with anovulatory cycles, but in addition with hyperandrogenism and secondary insulin resistance. PCOS is characterized by 2–3 times the normal number of preantral growing follicles that then arrest at the early antral stage, no dominant follicles being selected. Tonically elevated LH (but *not* FSH, which distinguishes this syndrome from secondary ovarian failure and (early) menopausal onset, see above) is also seen. The primary cause of ovarian failure of this kind is not known, but is thought to be a thecal cell defect in androgen biosynthesis. These ovaries are often exquisitely sensitive to clomiphene and gonadotrophins, and ovarian hyperstimulation is a real risk.

Treatment by surgical removal of part of the ovary (*wedge resection*) was recommended in the past. This procedure apparently produced an acute reduction in the prevailing high level of follicular circulating androgens, perhaps reinstating more normal feedback relationships and the possibility of an LH surge and ovulation. However, the precise sequence of events is far from clear, and the procedure has fallen out of favour because of the associated damage to the oviducts and postoperative adhesion formation. More recently, a variant procedure, involving the drilling of small holes in the ovary using diathermy or a laser, has achieved remarkably good results. Carefully monitored antioestroegn (clomiphene) therapy can achieve the same effect, possibly by stimulating aromatization of androgens within the granulosa cells.

'Anovulatory' cycles that are endocrinologically 'normal'

Luteinization can occur with the oocyte remaining *in situ*, the so-called *luteinized unruptured follicle syndrome* (LUF), and, in circumstances such as these, the cycle may appear normal but be infertile. There is some evidence that oocytes recovered from follicles laparascopically in women classified in this way are deficient when *in vitro* fertilization is attempted.

Abbreviated luteal phase

Some women with evidence of ovulation nonetheless show slow or reduced rises in progesterone, associated with infertility. This pattern is observed more frequently in women who have undergone gonadotrophin therapy. Whether it is due to a deficiency in the maturation of granulosa cells leading to poor luteinization, or is a primary defect, for example, in the development of LH or prolactin receptors, is unclear (see Chapter 5). However, as it is not yet clear whether, in women, either LH or prolactin are luteotrophic, a deficiency in these cannot be invoked by way of explanation. Treatment with progesterone during the luteal phase is, more often than not, unhelpful.

Absence of viable oocytes

Premature menopause, non-fertile attempts at reproduction during the climacteric or after the menopause, or female genetic abnormality can be treated by use of donor oocytes.

Oligospermia

Oligospermia (strictly meaning too few spermatozoa) is a term usually expanded to include a wide range of defects in semen quality, such as *asthenozoospermia* (reduced motility) and *teratozoospermia* (abnormal morphologies). Although each of these deficiencies may occur individually, they are usually associated (oligo-asthenoteratozoospermia), reflecting a general deficiency in spermatogenesis (Table 15.5). Total absence of spermatozoa in the ejaculate (*azoospermia*) may be due to deficient production (*aspermatogenesis*) or deficient transport (*obstructive azoospermia*). Deficiencies in the seminal plasma volume or composition usually reflect disease or malfunction of the accessory glands, such as the prostate or seminal vesicle.

A systematic and quantitative assessment of semen quality (either ejaculated or after recovery from the cervix postcoitally) is an essential part of an infertility examina-

tion and should be repeated at least once after 2–3 months. In addition, the availability of laparoscopically recovered human oocytes or of zona-free hamster oocytes on which to assay sperm function diagnostically can be exploited. It has been proposed recently that sperm counts in men from several developed countries may have declined during the last few decades, the suggestion being that environmental toxins, including some that appear to have oestrogenic metabolites, might have a causal role (see Chapter 3).

Causes

Characteristically, hypospermatogenesis is associated with smaller testes (<20 ml volume) of softer consistency and can result from dietary deficiency, X-irradiation, heating of the testis, exposure to a range of chemicals (notably cadmium, antimitotic drugs used in tumour therapy, insecticides and antiparasitic drugs), and excessive alcohol intake. Removal of the offending agent may restore spermatogenesis from the stem cell population of spermatogonia, if this is undamaged (see Box 4.1). Irreversible forms of hypospermatogenesis include: cryptorchid testes (see Chapter 1); genetic abnormalities such as XXY, XYY, some autosomal translocations and an increasing number of identified deletions on the Y-chromosome; and germ cell aplasia of unknown cause, often with hyalinization of tubules or as a sequel to severe orchitis or to prolonged and intense drug therapy for tumours. In all these patients (except those with Klinefelter's syndrome), testosterone and LH levels may well be in the normal range. FSH levels, however, tend to be elevated, probably because of the absence of inhibin production (see Chapter 6). In general, elevated FSH is associated with a poor prognosis. Hypospermatogenesis due to a primary neuroendocrine deficit is relatively rare in men and is easily recognized. Treatment may be attempted with exogenous GnRH or gonadotrophins or with bromocriptine, but success is not high.

Obstructive azoospermia is not associated with obvious endocrine disorder, and testes are of normal size and

Table 15.5 Characteristics associated with 'normal' and 'subfertile' semen.

Criterion	Normal	Subfertile
Volume (ml)	2–5	<2
Sperm concentration (no./ml)	$50–150 \times 10^6$	$<20 \times 10^6$
Total sperm no. per ejaculate	$100–700 \times 10^6$	$<40 \times 10^6$
Spermatozal vitality	>75% live	<75% live
Spermatozoa swimming forward vigorously	>50%	<50%
Abnormal spermatozoa	>30%	>70%
Viscosity after 60 min (liquefaction)	Low	High
White blood cells (no./ml sperm cells)	Low	$>10^6$

consistency. Obstruction to sperm transport usually occurs in the epididymides, as a congenital disorder (for example, heterozygosity for cystic fibrosis) or secondary to infection with, for example, gonorrhoea or tuberculosis.

Abnormal, slow-swimming or dead spermatozoa in the ejaculate, as distinct from low numbers, might also result from suboptimal spermatogenesis and is certainly increased, for example, in cases of *varicocoele* (varicosity of the spermatic vein), genetic abnormality, maintained elevated scrotal temperatures, deficiencies in spermatozoal maturation, genital tract infections, and cytotoxic factors or antisperm antibodies in the fluids of the accessory glands.

Treatments

Couples with mild male factor problems can be offered six cycles of *uterine insemination* (or fallopian sperm perfusion) at mid-cycle (with or without exogenous ovarian stimulation, depending on the female partner). *Donor sperm insemination* can be offered in the complete absence of spermatozoa, or where the male partner has an infectious disease (such as HIV) or genetic reasons for not reproducing, or in cases of hypospermia where use of IVF type procedures is not acceptable.

IVF and variants of it have provided useful routes for circumventing hypospermatogenesis by avoiding the dilution of spermatozoa that would occur during their passage through the female genital tract (see Chapter 9). In IVF small numbers of recovered viable spermatozoa are concentrated around the oocyte(s) to promote fertilization, which may be further enhanced by making a small hole in the zona pellucida (*zona drilling* or *ZD*) to encourage sperm entry. Alternatively, oocytes and spermatozoa are mixed and then transferred laparoscopically into the oviduct where fertilization occurs *in vivo* in a procedure called *gamete intrafallopian transfer* (*GIFT*).

Further variants of IVF have allowed successful pregnancies in cases where there are very few or no spermatozoa in the ejaculate, or where all or most of the spermatozoa in the ejaculate are immotile or clumped. A single spermatozoon, or even spermatid, is picked up in a micropipette and injected either under the zona (*subzonal injection* or *SUZI*) or directly into the ooplasm (*intracytoplasmic sperm injection* or *ICSI*). Sometimes sperm must be recovered from the epididymis (*percutaneous epididymidal sperm aspiration* or *PESA*) or testis (*testicular sperm extraction* or *TESE*). These approaches are summarized in Fig. 15.10. They are not without controversy. For those oligospermic conditions with a genetic component, transmission to any male offspring would occur unless selection of only female conceptuses for transfer was undertaken. In addition, about 50% of obstructive azoospermia cases are associated with heterozygosity for cystic fibrosis (CF), which raises the possibility of transmission of CF to offspring. Men with obstructive azoospermia can also be offered microsurgical correction to restore patency, although with variable outcome, reflecting the important role that the epididymis plays in spermatozoal maturation (see Chapter 9).

Miscarriage

The earliest sign that implantation is likely to have occurred comes from the detection in the blood, and later in the urine, of hCG during the period 18–30 days after the initiation of the last menstrual flow (see Chapter 11). This observation leads to the diagnosis of a *biochemical pregnancy*, although some tumours may also produce hCG. Definitive evidence of a *clinical pregnancy* is obtained by ultrasonographic investigation from as early as 5 weeks, at which time the presence and number of gestational sacs can be assessed (see Fig. 15.1). Using an ultrasound probe in the vagina, fetal heartbeat should be detected by 7 weeks after the last menstrual period. However, fertilization and the early development of the conceptus does not lead inevitably to a sustained pregnancy. Loss of the human conceptus is common and can occur at any stage, either because of its inherent deficiencies or as the result of environmental insult or inadequate maternal support.

The scale of the losses

We pointed out, at the beginning of this chapter that one out of every three cycles in which frequent, unprotected intercourse over the fertile period occurred nonetheless failed to yield a pregnancy. It seems likely that some of this failure can be accounted for by very early loss of the conceptus rather than failure of fertilization. Thus, in one study, human conceptuses were recovered by *uterine lavage* (flushing fluid through the uterus) 4.5 days after the detection of ovulation and the insemination of spermatozoa. Only 20% of the conceptuses recovered were blastocysts, the rest being retarded or abnormal. Moreover, of those conceptions surviving to the blastocyst stage and signalling their presence by the production of hCG, between 8 and 25% may fail, as this proportion of menstrual cycles is characterized by detectable but transient levels of hCG during the latter part of the (often slightly prolonged) luteal phase. This hCG is assumed to derive from lost periimplantation conceptuses. Such a loss could arise from (1) production of abnormal conceptuses that develop to the blastocyst but then fail, (2) from a failure of the uterine–conceptus interaction at implantation, or (3) failure of the corpus luteum to respond adequately to the hCG stimulation. There is some evidence to suggest that the hCG rise is delayed slightly in those cycles destined to fail, which suggests that an embryonic deficiency in its production may be responsible. Of pregnancies that survive further to be detected clinically, some 10–15% miscarry subsequently,

BOX 15.3 Recurrent miscarriage

Recurrent miscarriage is defined as the loss of three or more consecutive pregnancies. In *primary recurrent miscarriage*, the first three pregnancies are affected, whereas *secondary recurrent miscarriage* follows one or more live births. In the UK, about 1% of pregnant women experience the condition. The two main independent risk factors are maternal age and previous miscarriage.

Factors associated with recurrent miscarriage

- In 3–5% of couples, one partner carries a *balanced chromosomal reciprocal (called Robertsonian) translocation*, which gives a 40–50% chance of an unaffected pregnancy. Preimplantation genetic diagnosis is a high-tech, high-cost option.
- *Uterine anatomical anomalies* are associated with 2–38% of recurrent miscarriages, the range reflecting different study thresholds for inclusion of anomalies. The miscarriages tend to be late rather than early.
- *Antibodies to phospholipids (aPLs)*. Up to 20 antibodies can be detected directed against phospholipid-binding proteins of which two are associated with recurrent miscarriage: anticardiolipin and lupus anticoagulant. These are associated with early (pre-10 week) recurrent miscarriage, as well as later loss of normal fetuses and

severe pre-eclampsia. APLs inhibit trophoblast function and differentiation and are also associated with thrombosis of the uteroplacental vasculature later in pregnancy. Combined treatment with aspirin and low-dose heparin improves outcome to 70% live births, but also increases the risk of pregnancy complications and so needs careful monitoring.
- *Endocrine anomalies* do not seem to be a major cause of recurrent miscarriage, and there is no evidence that progesterone or hCG therapy improves outcomes.
- Where none of the above associated factors is present (unexplained recurrent miscarriage; c.50%) supportive care can result in live births, but the older the mother and the more miscarriages, the lower the likelihood of this outcome.

Further reading

Porter TF, Scott JR (2005) Evidence-based care of recurrent miscarriage. Best practice and research. *Clinical Obstetrics and Gynaecology* **19**, 85–101.
Regan L *et al.* (1989) Influence of past reproductive performance on risk of spontaneous abortion. *British Medical Journal* **299**, 541–545.
Stirrat GM (1990) Recurrent miscarriage. *Lancet* **336**, 673–675.
Royal College of Obstetricians and Gynaecologists Guideline 17 (2003) *The Investigation and Treatment of Couples with Recurrent Miscarriage*. RCOG Press, London.

---

the vast majority during the first trimester, some unfortunate couples experiencing recurrent miscarriage (Box 15.3). Overall, the cumulative outcome of such losses makes it possible that over 60% of human conceptions do not survive to birth. Why are they lost?

Abnormal conceptuses

After IVF, and culture of fertilized oocytes in the clinical laboratory during therapeutic IVF, only 20–40% result in blastocysts (a similar proportion to that found *in vivo* after lavage, as quoted above). This early developmental failure of the conceptus is associated with abnormalities of chromosomal distribution or number, many of the conceptuses examined having whole sets of chromosomes missing or duplicated, individual chromosomes gone astray, cells lacking nuclei or having multiple nuclei, or a mixture of cells of differing genetic constitution (*genetic mosaics*).

A high level of genetic abnormality is also detected in recognized clinical pregnancies (in 0.5% of all live births, 5% of still births and 40–60% of spontaneous miscarriages, especially those occurring in the first trimester). These figures mean that around 10% of *recognized* pregnancies are identified as being chromosomally abnormal. The type of each genetic abnormality observed, and its approximate incidence in spontaneous miscarriages, is recorded in Table 15.6. Three major classes of chromosomal abnormality are repre-

sented: *translocations* (i.e. structural rearrangements of chromosomes); *errors of ploidy* (i.e. deletions or duplications of a complete set of haploid chromosomes); and *errors of chromosome number or somy* (i.e. loss or gain of a single sex chromosome or autosome). It is clear from Table 15.6 that some types of abnormality are more common in miscarriage and others are compatible with survival to birth. It is also clear that some types of abnormality are missing altogether (e.g. haploids) or are underrepresented (e.g. autosomal and sex chromosomal monosomies, which might be expected to occur with the same frequency as trisomies, since when one nucleus gains a chromosome at division the other will lose one). It is likely that these types of abnormality are lethal very early in development (lack of genetic material being deleterious earlier than excess). Indeed, analysis of early mouse development confirms that most monosomic and haploid conceptuses die at preimplantation or early postimplantation stages, whereas trisomic, triploid and tetraploid conceptuses survive for longer. It has been calculated from clinical data, and by extrapolation from data derived from comparative studies, that 50% or more of all human conceptions may result in genetically abnormal embryos and fetuses.

Clearly this massive loss cannot be due entirely to constitutional genetic defects in all the germ cells of one or both parents, and many, if not most, genetic abnormalities in fetuses have indeed been shown to arise at, or shortly after,

Table 15.6 Incidence of chromosomal abnormalities in spontaneously aborted human conceptions.

	No. per 100 aborted conceptions	Surviving to birth (%)
Triploidy (three sets of chromosomes)	12–15	<0.01
Tetraploidy (four sets of chromosomes)	3–5	<0.01
Sex chromosome trisomies (three sex chromosomes)	<1	>99
Sex chromosome monosomies (one sex chromosome)	10	<1
Trisomy for one or two autosomes	20–40	3
Monosomy for one or two autosomes	1	None
Structural rearrangement of chromosomes	2–3	35

fertilization. For example, disorders of ploidy are likely to result from failure of polar body formation (10–20% of triploids), from polyspermy (80–90% of triploids) or from failure of one early cleavage division (tetraploidy, see Chapter 9). Many of the mono- and trisomic conceptuses also arise from abnormalities of oocyte meiotic divisions. As we saw in Chapter 9, these events are sensitive to a number of environmental perturbations, in particular, the age of the oocyte in hours postovulation, and exposure of the female to alcohol or anaesthesia around the time of ovulation. Other chromosomal abnormalities in the conceptus arise from events in the ovary or testis that affect gametes directly, well in advance of the acute events of fertilization and early cleavage. For example, abnormalities may be induced by exposure to X-irradiation or mutagenic chemicals, and such exposure correlates with a subsequently increased natural abortion rate. Moreover, an increased incidence of fetal abnormality is observed with increasing maternal age, which may reflect the fact that oocytes are maintained in a prolonged dictyate stage (see Chapter 5) during which they are susceptible to such damage. Oocytes seem to have much less effective surveillance systems than somatic cells for detecting chromosome distribution abnormalities, meaning that genetically flawed oocytes survive to be fertilized. Spermatogenic cells, in contrast, are highly sensitive to chromosomal anomalies, but lack the effective DNA repair systems of somatic cells, and consequently show three-fold higher mutation rates. At first sight, it seems curious that the germ line is less well genetically policed than somatic cells. Is it possible that we have evolved a system that encourages genetic diversity generation and relies on effective screening out of the failures during pregnancy—truly evolution in action with each throw of the fertilization dice?

In addition to genetic causes of embryonic and fetal loss, the conceptus may commence development normally but become deformed or incompetent as a result of environmental insult; for example, direct exposure of the fetus to X-irradiation, to certain viruses, such as rubella (German measles) or cytomegalovirus, and to certain *teratogenic drugs*, such as thalidomide, dilantin or 6-mercaptopurine. These agents are frequently active only at restricted periods of development, most during some point in the first or second trimester. Additionally, women who smoke or who drink heavily put fetal development at risk, especially in the third trimester, by impairing intercirculatory exchange within the placenta (see Chapter 10). Unfortunately, unlike most genetic disorders, these environmental insults to the fetus often result not in miscarriage but in the birth of deformed children. However, fortunately, as the insults are environmental, they are also, in principle, preventable.

Maternal problems

Of the 40–50% of miscarriages that are not clearly ascribable to genetic or induced defects of the conceptus itself, many are of uncertain origin. Clearly ascribable are miscarriages resulting from anatomical problems, such as cervical incompetence or implantation in eccentric uterine positions or ectopically. It is also being increasingly recognized that autoimmune disease in the mother such as systemic lupus erythematosus and antiphospholipid syndrome is associated with recurrent miscarriage and these negative effects can be ameliorated by use of low-dose aspirin or heparin. Haemolytic diseases of the fetus and neonate account for a diminishing proportion of fetal loss in Europe. Immunological incompatibility of mother and fetus at either the ABO or rhesus blood group loci poses the major problem (see Chapter 12). However, recognition of incompatibility during the first pregnancy, in which sensitization of the mother to these fetal antigens is most likely around parturition, allows prophylactic administration of antibody passively to the mother. The antibody mops up any antigen released by fetal bleeds late in pregnancy and prevents active immunization of the mother.

Paradoxically, incompatibility of mother and fetus at the major histocompatibility antigen (HLA) loci may favour a successful outcome of pregnancy. The reasons for this are obscure. However, compatibility at these loci predisposes the mother to the condition of *pre-eclampsia* (also called *toxaemia* or *gestosis*). Pre-eclampsia is characteristically a disease of first pregnancies and is more common in the last trimester in which maternal diastolic blood pressure is periodically or continuously elevated, and oedema and, in severe cases, albuminuria occur. Severe pre-eclampsia can lead to the convulsive state of *eclampsia*. Throughout, both mother and fetus are at risk, but with the improved survival and care of prematurely delivered neonates, fewer losses from eclampsia are occurring in developed countries.

Assisted reproductive technologies (ART)

Over the past 20 years, the plight of the infertile has been taken much more seriously by the medical profession. There is little doubt that this change of attitude has stemmed from the pioneering work of Bob Edwards and Patrick Steptoe in the development of IVF technology that led to the first IVF birth of Louise Brown in 1979 (she is now a mother herself!). Over 2 million people worldwide exist as a result of the reproductive technologies that have subsequently been refined or developed. Those ARTs mentioned in this book include ICSI, GIFT, SUZI, ZD, ICSI, TESE and PESA, DI, oocyte donation, and surrogacy. This capacity to help infertile people has also been a major stimulus to clinical research, as a result of which we now know much more about the basic science underlying human reproduction, and we are less reliant on animal models, essential though these remain. Now we can: freeze and thaw conceptuses and retain their viability; remove individual blastomeres from early 8-cell stages and test their DNA for the presence of faulty genes (*preimplantation genetic diagnosis* or *PGD*) or chromosome anomalies (*preimplantation genetic screening* or *PGS*), thereby offering the initiation of an unaffected pregnancy to affected couples; produce (in animals) at least some viable conceptuses by *somatic cell nuclear transfer* (*SCNT*), thereby potentially generating 'genetic clones'; and persuade the pluriblast cells from the blastocyst to proliferate *in vitro* as embryonal stem cells (ES cells). It is a tribute to the vision of Bob Edwards (the dedicatee of this book) that he predicted and even achieved most of these major advances himself some 30–40 years ago: one of the landmark contributions to human medicine and health in the twentieth century.

Despite the large numbers of healthy people born of ART, there nonetheless remain some lingering concerns about the longer-term safety of these novel technologies. These concerns have been fuelled by the increased understanding we now have of how the early developmental environment can influence patterns of health and behaviour later in life and even transgenerationally, and the role that epigenetics can play in mediating these influences (Chapters 12 & 14). These concerns emerge into the media

from time to time, often in alarmist terms and out of context. What is the evidence that actually bears on this concern?

There is one clearly established and highly significant adverse clinical outcome of ART, namely an increase in multiple births, which can constitute 25% or more of ART outcomes. Pregnancies carrying more than one conceptus show markedly increased maternal and child morbidity. This increase in multiple births in recent years comes from two sources: (1) induced ovulation for ovulatory disorders, and (2) placement of more than one conceptus into the uterus after IVF/ICSI to increase the chance of a pregnancy occurring. Multiple pregnancy is entirely avoidable and unnecessary, and only a single conceptus should be transferred in most cases.

IVF babies also have slightly lower birthweights and are slightly premature, although the differences are so small as to be statistically non-significant when only singleton babies are compared. (Multiple pregnancies always produce babies with highly significantly lowered birthweights simply as a result of there being more than one fetus for the mother to carry.) Birthweight deficit is thus not thought to be problematic.

Studies on the psychological adjustment and emotional well-being of children born of IVF reveal that if anything they score higher than control babies conceived naturally. Plausibly this may be related to the intense effort and commitment of their parents in producing them in the first place.

A significant increase in prevalence of congenital abnormalities in IVF babies has been reported in a meta-analysis of various retrospective comparative population studies. The data equate to one additional congenital abnormality over normal for every 60–250 ART babies born. This increased risk did not appear to be related to multiple births, and was similar for both minor and severe defects. Does the ART cause these defects, or are they a consequence of the parental genetic status that may underlie or predispose to the infertility? Since male genital tract defects are commonly reported in IVF babies, at least part of the increased incidence may relate to the parental infertility itself.

In retrospective analyses, the prevalence of defects in parental imprinting (Chapter 1) is higher among IVF babies than in the general population. However, the absolute prevalence is extremely low so numbers are very small. These studies are retrospective and thus not optimally controlled, and it is also unclear, should the difference turn out to be real, what the explanation might be. Did ART cause the imprinting errors? Or are certain types of infertility associated with a higher probability of imprinting error? Current clinical advice is that there is no proven reason for concern. Thus, overall, there appears to be a small but significant increased risk of problematic outcome amongst ART-produced babies, aside from the well-established substantial risk increase arising from multiple pregnancy. There are certainly features of ART procedures that give cause for concern that the procedures themselves might be responsible for at least some of this increased risk. Thus, the freezing and thawing of embryos, any delay in the fertilization of oocytes, the culture media composition and the risk of exposure to reactive oxygen species, variations in laboratory temperature and its effects on maternal meiotic spindle stability, and the medications used to induce ovulation could each impact adversely on outcome if not carefully and skillfully managed and monitored. It is also possible that some of the increased risk may arise from the underlying infertility of the couples seeking treatment, rather than the treatments themselves. Perhaps examining outcome data more carefully to discriminate between different types of infertility would be useful, since tubal damage secondary to infection is a very different sort of pathology from azoopsermia. Where does this leave us when talking with prospective patients for ART therapy?

What is reasonably clear is that doctors should properly discuss the increased risks from whatever source. However, it is a matter of concern that patients remain willing to accept the established risks arising from multiple pregnancy in order to increase their chances of conceiving at all. This suggests that among at least some patients, their desperation for a child is leading them to rash decisions, and so it seems unlikely that the other smaller and less well understood risks will deter them from undergoing ART at all. The second major conclusion from the evidence base is that much better quality analysis is needed, both from existing retrospective data and ideally from high-quality prospective matched cohort studies. The continuing and careful monitoring of children conceived after assisted reproductive therapies for any long-term health impacts is essential if we are to improve the quality of our evidence base from which to offer advice.

Reproduction, sexuality, ethics and the law

Humans, like many other primates and some cetaceans and insectivores, but unlike most other mammals, do not confine their sexual activity to one narrow phase of the cycle at or around the time of ovulation. Neither do humans confine their sexual activity to vaginal penetrative sex with a member of the 'opposite' gender. Thus, for humans, coition and the expression of sexuality have a biological function over and above that of reproduction. The nature of that function in evolutionary terms remains a matter for debate, but the clear biological separability of coital sex from procreation is undeniable. Moreover, through humankind's own talents and capabilities, whether viewed as evolved or God-given or both, this separability has been further enhanced. Thus, the development of methods for

reducing fertility or overcoming and circumventing infertility has further divorced reproduction from the sexual act. Reproduction may be commenced outside of the body, doctors and scientists becoming essential agents in the process. Oocytes, spermatozoa or embryos may be donated by individuals other than the partners being treated, leading to unusual patterns of 'parenting'; indeed, the very definition of a parent is being challenged. Thus, a woman may carry a fetus derived from gametes neither or only one of which came from her or her partner (*gamete* or *embryo donation*). A woman might carry a fetus derived from IVF with the purpose of giving it at delivery to two other parents, one or both of whom may be genetically related to the child (*surrogacy*). Parents may both be women or both men, only one of them being related genetically to the child. A woman may carry a pregnancy well after her menopause. Genetic parenthood after death by use of frozen gametes or embryos is real. Reproductive cloning has approached feasibility.

This blurring of boundaries between genetic and social parents, between the expression of sexuality and procreation, between conventional and novel patterns of parenting is confusing for many, and challenging for traditional religions and social values. This challenge derives from the fact that religious, social and legal control of sexual and reproductive activities has been a feature of all human societies, as these activities bear heavily on patterns of inheritance, power and individual freedom of expression, as well as on individual and social health. Thus, these new possibilities appear to threaten many established aspects of social structure. Clear ethical thinking about their impact is required, and not simply reactive assertion, if sensible legal controls on their use are to be enacted. Such legal responses are already occurring with variably sensible outcomes in many countries. What are the key ethical issues that have influenced these discussions and decisions? There is insufficient space here to do justice to the arguments, but some of the main points are summarized, not all of which are universally accepted, but all of which can form the basis for reflection and discussion.

• First, it is not legitimate to resort to ethical arguments that equate traditional with natural and novel with unnatural. What is possible biologically is natural and what is happening is therefore natural.

• Second, there is a presumption that individual liberty to choose how to act sexually and reproductively should be protected, as long as others are not affected adversely.

• Third, with this liberty goes the moral responsibility to protect the welfare of the parties practising sexual and reproductive interactions and also of any children that might be born as a result. This means that the adult parties should give adequate and informed consent to their mutual activity, and should not be placed under duress. The interests and welfare of any child born, and of the 'siblings' of any child born (or not born), must be taken into account. Such a process must consider the prevailing social values and how these will affect both society's perception of the child and the ability of the child to form a clear and positive identity. It will also take into account the genetic health of the child.

• Fourth, there is a general acceptance, based on biological and ethical arguments, that humans acquire an individual status of personhood progressively, not suddenly. There is no moment at which a human being exists where one did not before, just as there was no moment in evolution at which humankind existed where no humans had existed before.

• Fifth, and arising from this consideration, the status of the human gametes, preimplantation conceptus, embryo and early fetus differs from that of both existing humans and non-humans. Human material with the potential for development into an individual demands respect for that potential while not having the moral or legal rights accorded to an existing human; where conflict arises between the needs of a potential mother and those of her developing embryo/fetus, there is a presumption in favour of the mother's rights until such time that the fetus becomes capable of an independent existence.

• Sixth, there is a presumed right to parenthood, although not at any cost.

• Seventh, there is a presumption that individuals should be treated confidentially and should have control over the reproductive information held about them.

• Eighth, there is also a presumption that it is better not to withhold from individuals information about their origins, if, for example, they are conceived by techniques of assisted conception; and that genetic information should be stored securely and made available so that genetic incest can be avoided.

• Ninth, there should be a limit on the numbers of children produced from donated gametes and embryos from one individual, so as to limit the chances of genetic incest occurring subsequently.

• Finally, there is a presumption that it is better to exist than not to exist.

In the UK, in which much of the pioneering medical and scientific work that has led to this reproductive revolution has occurred, ethical debate and legal action also came early—indeed, it was initiated by Bob Edwards himself in the 1960s. There is currently in place, through the Human Fertilization and Embryology Act of 1990, a Human Fertilization and Embryology Authority (HFEA) set up to regulate the generation, use and storage of human embryos *in vitro*, the storage and use of human gametes *in vitro* for later therapeutic use, and the use of human embryos and of human fertilization *in vitro* in research. Many of the other issues raised above are also being brought to the HFEA. This body represents an attempt to protect the human individual, society and conceptus from exploitation and excess, by applying ethical principles to biological and medical problems through legal processes. It is being observed with interest by many other states as a possible model of enlightened regulation to copy or react against.

Conclusion

Our failure to control fertility adequately, concomitant with our success in decreasing neonatal and infant mortality, has, for much of humanity, replaced one tragedy by another. The spectre of deprivation, starvation, mass migration and war is still all too real for much of the world's population. One of the greatest indictments of medical science has been the relative neglect of, and belated initiation of, research in human reproduction, human sexuality and the associated clinical disciplines. The social and religious conservatism that has delayed or prevented analysis of these subjects means that much of our knowledge is recent or incomplete. Indeed, many of the pioneers in this area of scientific study are still alive. Echoes of this conservatism recur in debates on the ethics of the so-called 'test-tube babies', abortion, PGD, contraception, attitudes to sexual behaviour and the response to AIDS. More important, however, are the continuing effects of social and religious attitudes on the effective application of the knowledge that has accrued from such a relatively brief period of rigorous scientific and medical study. Deliberate policies to promote reproduction in some countries fearful of racial imbalance, and the frustration of family planning programmes in others, are sadly as much a feature of the so-called civilized world as of countries struggling to improve the economic circumstances of their inhabitants. Throughout this book I have refrained from imposing a personal view on the account of the science of reproduction. However, I do hope that study of this book will help students training to take a place in the medical and scientific professions to realize just how pervasive the reproductive process is, both for the individual and through society at large, and how an adequate understanding and control of it represents a crucial element in the survival and well-being of both.

FURTHER READING

General reading

Bancroft J (2005) The endocrinology of sexual arousal. *Journal of Endocrinology* **186**, 411–427.
Brinsden PR (2003) Gestational surrogacy. *Human Reproduction Update* **5**, 483–491.

KEY LEARNING POINTS

- Fertility, fecundibility and fecundity are measures of the actual and potential reproductive outputs of females.

- Reproductive fertility is time limited, especially in women, in whom optimum fecundity is restricted to 15–35 years.

- The menopause marks the end of fecundity in women and is preceded by the climacteric, a time of declining fecundity.

- Loss of female fecundity is due to abnormalities in and then exhaustion of oocytes.

- In men, the decline in reproductive function is progressive and more extended, and is largely the result of senescent changes, not loss of germ cells.

- Social and legal constraints on fertility and the expression of sexuality exist in most human communities.

- Sterilization involves vasectomy in men and tubal occlusion or section in women.

- Contraception can be achieved without mechanical or chemical intervention by behavioural approaches.

- Physical barriers to fertility (caps, diaphragms, condoms, spermicides) are more effective and provide better protection against genitourinary infection.

- Some steroidal contraceptives combine synthetic oestrogens and progestagens (COCs), and may be administered orally or transdermally.

- Other steroidal contraceptives use progestagens alone, and may be administered orally, by injection, by implant or by an impregnated IUCD.

- Most oral contraceptives are relatively safe and effective if taken responsibly and with medical advice.

- Oral contraceptives work by suppressing ovulation and/or sperm and embryo transport in the female tract.

- Steroidal contraceptives for men are still in clinical trials and use synthetic androgens with or without progestagens to suppress FSH output, but are not promising.

- Clinical termination of pregnancy may be used to control fertility where contraception is lacking or ineffective. Early (medical or surgical) termination is preferable to late (surgical) termination on maternal health grounds.

- A contraceptive strategy needs to be tailored to the needs and circumstances of each individual, which is reflected in the wide variation by age and geography in use of different contraceptive approaches.

- Approximately 10–15% of couples experience clinical subfertility.

- Clinical subfertility is defined as failure to conceive after 12 months of unprotected intercourse.

- Men and women contribute more or less equally to subfertility problems.

- Major causes of subfertility are blocked oviducts, ovulatory disorders and a- or hypozoospermia, but around 25% of cases are unexplained.

- Spontaneous miscarriage occurs in about 10–15% of clinically diagnosed pregnancies.

- At least 60% of all human conceptions are probably lost before term.

- Approximately 50% of these lost conceptuses are probably genetically abnormal.

- A range of techniques is now available to help the infertile including induced ovulation, IVF, ICSI, GIFT, SUZI, ZD, ICSI, TESE and PESA.

- There is evidence to indicate that the risk of maternal and paediatric morbidity is higher for ART-produced than for natural pregnancy and most of this increased risk arises from the higher prevalence of multiple pregnancy.

- Clear ethical reasoning is required to chart a moral path through the new assisted reproductive technologies and the new family patterns they are generating.

Brosens I et al. (2004) Investigation of the infertile couple: when is the appropriate time to explore female infertility? *Human Reproduction* **19**, 1689–1692.

Crosignani PG, Rubin B (1994) Male sterility and subfertility: guidelines for management. *Human Reproduction* **9**, 1260–1264.

Croxatto HB (2003) Mifepristone for luteal phase contraception. *Contraception* **68**, 483–488.

Dunson DB et al. (2002) Changes with age in the level and duration of fertility in the menstrual cycle. *Human Reproduction* **17**, 1399–1403.

Dunstan GR (1990) *The Human Embryo: Aristotle and the Arabic and European Traditions*. University of Exeter Press, Exeter.

Edwards RG (1980) *Conception in the Human Female*. Academic Press, New York.

Edwards RG (ed.) (1994) New concepts in fertility control. *Human Reproduction* **9** (Suppl. 2).

ESHRE Capri Workshop Group (2003) Hormonal contraception without estrogens. *Human Reproduction Update* **9**, 373–386.

Fertility Assessment and Treatment for People with Fertility Problems (2004) National Collaborating Centre for Women's and Children's Health, RCOG Press, London.

Frye CA (2006) An overview of oral contraceptives: mechanism of action and clinical use. *Neurology* **66** (6, Suppl. 3), S29–S36.

Guillebaud J (1993) *Contraception: Your Questions Answered*, 2nd edn. Churchill Livingstone, Edinburgh.

Guillebaud J (1997) *The Pill and Other Forms of Hormonal Contraception*. Oxford University Press, Oxford.

Herbert J (1997) Stress, the brain and mental illness. *British Medical Journal* **315**, 530–535.

Human Fertilization and Embryology Authority (1997) *Sixth Annual Report*. Paxton House, Artillery Lane, London E1 7LS <http://www.hfea.gov.uk>

Johnson MH (1998) Should the use of assisted reproduction techniques be deregulated? The UK experience: options for change. *Human Reproduction* **13**, 1769–1776.

Johnson MH (2001) The developmental basis of identity. *Studies in the History and Philosophy of Biology and Biomedical Sciences* **32**, 601–617.

Johnson MH (2005) The problematic in-vitro embryo in the age of epigenetics. *Reproductive BioMedicine* **10** (Suppl. 1), 88–96.

Johnson MH (2006) Escaping the tyranny of the embryo? A new approach to ART regulation based on UK and Australian experiences. *Human Reproduction* **21**, 2756–2765.

Kamischke A, Nieschlag E (2004) Progress towards hormonal male contraception. *Trends in Pharmacological Sciences* **25**, 49–57.

Klein J, Sauer MV (2002) Oocyte donation. Best practice and research. *Clinical Obstetrics and Gynaecology* **16**, 277–291.

Lenton EA, Woodward AJ (1988) The endocrinology of conception cycles and implantation in women. *Journal of Reproduction and Fertility* **36** (Suppl.), 1–15.

Long-acting Reversible Contraception (2005) National Institute for Health and Clinical Excellence, London.

Macklon NS *et al.* (2002) Conception to ongoing pregnancy: the 'black box' of early pregnancy loss. *Human Reproduction Update* **8**, 333–343.

Meirik O *et al.* (2003) Implantable contraceptives for women. *Human Reproduction Update* **9**, 49–59.

O'Sullivan I *et al.* (2005) *Contraception and Sexual Health, 2004/05.* Office for National Statistics, London.

Pitkin J *et al.* (2005) Managing the menopause: British Menopause Society Council consensus statement on hormone replacement therapy. *Journal of the British Menopause Society* **11**, 152–6.

RCOG (2004) *Male and Female Sterilisation.* Evidence-based Clinical Guideline Number 4. Royal College of Obstetricians and Gynaecologists, RCOG Press, London.

Santoro N (2005) The menopausal transition. *American Journal of Medicine* **118** (12B), 8S–13S.

Simon C (1996) Potential molecular mechanisms for the contraceptive control of implantation. *Molecular Human Reproduction* **2**, 475–480.

Taylor AS, Braude PR (1994) The role of the GP in the investigation and treatment of subfertility. In: *The Diplomate.* Royal College of Obstetrics and Gynaecology Press, London.

Swales AKE, Spears N (2005) Genomic imprinting and reproduction. *Reproduction* **130**, 389–399.

Thacker PD (2004) Biological clock ticks for men, too: genetic defects linked to sperm of older fathers. *Journal of the American Medical Association* **291**, 1683–1685.

The Care of Women Requesting Induced Abortion (2004) Evidence-based Clinical Guideline Number 7. Royal College of Obstetricians and Gynaecologists, RCOG Press, London.

Veldhuis JD *et al.* (2005) Mechanisms of ensemble failure of the male gonadal axis in aging. *Journal of Endocrinological Investigation* **28** (Suppl. 3), 8–13.

More advanced reading (see also Boxes)

Adashi EY *et al.* (2003) Infertility therapy-associated multiple pregnancies (birth): an ongoing epidemic. *Reproductive BioMedicine* **7**, 515–542.

Arce J-C *et al.* (2005) Resolving methodological and clinical issues in the design of efficacy trials in assisted reproductive technologies: a mini-review. *Human Reproduction* **20**, 1757–1771.

Bainham A *et al.* (eds) (1999) *What Is a Parent? A Socio-legal Analysis.* Hart Publishing, Oxford.

Battaglia DE *et al.* (1996) Influence of maternal age on spindle assembly in oocytes from naturally cycling women. *Human Reproduction* **11**, 2217–2222.

Bonduelle M *et al.* (2005) A multi-centre cohort study of the physical health of 5-year-old children conceived after intracytoplasmic sperm injection, in vitro fertilization and natural conception. *Human Reproduction* **20**, 413–419.

Cook R, Day Sclater S (eds) (2003) *Surrogate Motherhood.* Hart Publishing, Oxford.

de La Rochebrochard E, Thonneau P (2002) Paternal age and maternal age are risk factors for miscarriage; results of a multicentre European study. *Human Reproduction* **17**, 1649–1656.

De Rycke M *et al.* (2002) Epigenetic risks related to assisted reproductive technologies. Risk analysis and epigenetic inheritance. *Human Reproduction* **17**, 2487–2494.

Dennis J, Hampton N (2002) *IUDs: Which Device?* RCOG Press, London.

Devroey P, Van Steirteghem A (2004) A review of ten years experience of ICSI. *Human Reproduction Update* **10**, 19–28.

Edwards RG *et al.* (1969) Early stages of fertilization *in vitro* of human oocytes matured *in vitro*. *Nature* **221**, 632–635.

Eskenazi B *et al.* (2003) The association of age and semen quality in healthy men. *Human Reproduction* **18**, 447–454.

Faculty of Family Planning and Reproductive Health Care Clinical Effectiveness Unit (2003) *New Product Review Norelgestromin/Ethinyl Oestradiol Transdermal Contraceptive System (Evra).* RCOG, London.

Faculty of Family Planning and Reproductive Health Care Clinical Effectiveness Unit (2003) First prescription of combined oral contraception. *Journal of Family Planning and Reproductive Health Care* **29**, 209–223.

Faculty of Family Planning and Reproductive Health Care Clinical Effectiveness Unit (2004) The copper intrauterine device as long-term contraception. *Journal of Family Planning and Reproductive Health Care* **30**, 29–42.

Faculty of Family Planning and Reproductive Health Care Clinical Effectiveness Unit (2004) The levonorgestrel-releasing intrauterine system (LNG-IUS) in contraception and reproductive health. *Journal of Family Planning and Reproductive Health Care* **30**, 99–109.

Fretts RC (2006) Etiology and prevention of stillbirth. *American Journal of Obstetrics and Gynecology* **193**, 1923–1935.

Gnoth C *et al.* (2003) Time to pregnancy: results of the German prospective study and impact on the management of infertility. *Human Reproduction* **18**, 1959–1966.

Golombok S *et al.* (2002) The European study of assisted reproduction families: the transition to adolescence. *Human Reproduction* **17**, 830–840.

Hansen M *et al.* (2005) Assisted reproduction and the risk of birth defects—a systematic review. *Human Reproduction* **20**, 328–338.

Hunt PA, Hassold TJ (2002) Sex matters in meiosis. *Science* **296**, 2181–2183.

Liu PY, Handelsman DJ (2003) The present and future state of hormonal treatment for male infertility. *Human Reproduction Update* **9**, 9–23.

Liverman CT, Blazer DG (eds) (2004) *Testosterone and Aging: Clinical Research Directions.* IOM Committee on Assessing the Need for Clinical Trials of Testosterone Replacement Therapy, Institute of Medicine. The National Academies Press, Washington, DC.

McElreavey K *et al.* (2006) Y chromosome variants and male reproductive function. *International Journal of Andrology* **29**, 298–303.

Norman RJ *et al.* (2004) Improving reproductive performance in overweight/obese women with effective weight management. *Human Reproduction Update* **10**, 267–280.

O'Rand MG *et al.* (2004) Reversible immunocontraception in male monkeys immunized with Eppin. *Science* **306**, 1189–1190.

Sammartino A *et al.* (2005) Osteoporosis and cardiovascular disease: benefit–risk of hormone replacement therapy. *Journal of Endocrinological Investigation* **28** (Suppl. 10), 80–84.

Sauer MV, Kavic SM (2006) Oocyte and embryo donation 2006: reviewing two decades of innovation and controversy. *Reproductive BioMedicine* **12**, 153–162.

Schiavi RC *et al.* (1990) Healthy aging and male sexual function. *American Journal of Psychiatry* **147**, 766–771.

Stanford JB, Mikolajczyk RT (2002) Mechanisms of action of intrauterine devices: update and estimation of postfertilization effects. *American Journal of Obstetrics and Gynecology* **187**, 1699–1708.

Steptoe PC, Edwards RG (1978) Birth after the reimplantation of a human embryo. *Lancet* **2**, 366.

United Nations Department of Economic and Social Affairs Population Division (2001) *World Population Prospects: The 2000 Revision.* ST/ESA/SER.A/204. Sales No. E.01. XIII.12. United Nations, New York.

Venous Thromboembolism and Hormonal Contraception (2004) Guideline No. 40, Royal College of Obstetricians and Gynaecologists, London.

Wang X *et al.* (2003) Conception, early pregnancy loss, and time to clinical pregnancy: a population-based prospective study. *Fertility and Sterility* **79**, 577–584.

Yin W, Gore AC (2006) Neuroendocrine control of reproductive aging: roles of GnRH neurones. *Reproduction* **131**, 403–414.

Zhu JL *et al.* (2005) Paternal age and congenital malformations. *Human Reproduction* **20**, 3173–3177.

Index

delays 198–9
  messages mediating attachment 199–
    200, *200*
  messages mediating invasion 200–1,
    201
  overview of timing issues 193–7
  spatial organization 193–7
  timing window 198
nutrition mechanisms 202–6
  and blood flow 206–9
oxygen requirements 206–8
  haemotrophic vs. histiotrophic
    support 206–8
synthesis of steroid hormones 214–20
twin and chimaeric organizations
    192–3
see also implantation processes
    (conceptus)
condensation mechanisms 67
condoms 284, *285*
congenital adrenal hyperplasia (CAH) *see*
    androgen insensitivity syndrome
    (AIS)
contraception 282–90
  barrier creams 283–4
  caps and diaphragms 283–4
  condoms 284
  'morning-after' pill 150
  natural methods 282–3
  types and rates of use *280*
  for young people 282
'controller' gene *see* SRY gene
coprophiliac sexualities *31*
copying behaviours 28
corpora cavernosa *173*
corporeal crura 173, *173*
corpus albicans 91
corpus luteum *81*, 91–2, 250–1
  endocrine support 91
corticosteroids 39
  biosynthesis deficiencies 39
  concentrations in umbilical cord *234*
  functions in fetus *238*
  levels during pregnancy 218
  levels in fetus 237
corticotrophin *see* adrenocorticotrophic
    hormone (ACTH)
corticotrophin-releasing factor (CRF) 237
cortisol
  biosynthesis 39, *40*
  fetal 237
  roles
    onset of parturition 249, *249*
    parental behaviour patterns 269–70
cortisol-binding gobulins *57*
courtships 30–1
Cowper's gland *173*
Cox2 enzyme 200

CRE-binding transcription factors 69
CREB expression 69
CREM-controlled genes 69
CREs *see* cAMP responsive elements
    (CREs)
CRF *see* corticotrophin-releasing factor
    (CRF)
CRISP1 180
cross-dressing *31*
cryptorchidism 14
CSF *see* cytostatic factor (CSF)
cultural influences, on reproduction 30–1
cumulus oophorus 86
cyclin B 182
cycloxygenase *43*
cyproterone *52*, 157
cyritestins 180
cytokines 43–4
  classification *46–7*
  and follicular development *85*
  paracrine actions 77
  and parturition 250–1
  properties *46–7*
  and spermatogenesis 64
  see also Müllerian inhibiting hormone
    (MIH)
cytokinesis 63
cytostatic factor (CSF) 182
cytotrophoblasts *194*, 195

danazol *52*
Dax1 gene 6
daylight and fertility 123–5
  circadian rhythms 123–4
  circannual rhythms in seasonal breeders
    124–5
decidualization processes (conceptus) *194*,
    195–6
defeminization, sex hormone exposure
    studies 24
dehydroepiandrosterone (DHEA) *41*, 137,
    155, 276
  fetal 237
dehydrogenase *40*
Denver system classification 4
depot contraceptives 287
17, 20-desmolase 39
desogestrel *52*
11-desoxycortisol 39
detumescence 172, 174
dexamethasone *278*
DHEA *see* dehydroepiandrosterone
    (DHEA)
diabetes mellitus 226–7
diapause 198–9
diaphragma sellae 102
diaphragms 283–4
dieldrin 51

5α-dihydrotestosterone *41*, 148, 169
diploidy 181–2, 183
DNA, genetic determinants of sex 4–6
DNA bending 6
DNA synthesis, in spermatogenesis 65–6,
    66
dominance hierarchies 127–9
dopamine 49, *51*
  and control of prolactin 120, *120–1*
dromostanolone *52*
drug use, impact on fetus 235–6
dry orgasms 174
'Dutch' cap 283

ED *see* erectile dysfunction
Edwards, Bob 299
EGF receptors 199
EGFs *see* epidermal growth factors (EGFs)
eicosanoids 39–42
ejaculate, composition *171*
ejaculation mechanisms 174
electrolytes, fetal requirements 228–9
embryo development
  conceptus stages 189–209
    early differentiation *203–4*
embryogen *see* conceptus
emergency contraception 150
emotions, neurophysiology 27
endocrine effects *see* hormones
endocrine secretion 37
endometriosis 292
endometrium changes, oestrogen actions
    150–2, *151*
β-endorphin 45, 49, 116, 165
endosulfan 51
endothelins *47*, 93
environmental influences on reproduction
    122–9
Eomes genes 193
epiblasts *193*
epidermal growth factor (EGF) receptors
    199
epidermal growth factors (EGFs) 37–8, *46*,
    199–200
  and mammary growth 256
epididymis 168–70
  changes to spermatazoa *170*
epigenetic imprints 185–6, 241, 272
epiregulin 199
EPOR model (Masters and Johnson)
    171–2
equilin *215*, 219
erectile dysfunction (ED) 172–3
  treatments 172–3
erectile response 172–4
  hormonal control mechanisms 157–8,
    158
erotic arousal 31–2